ADVANCES IN PROSTATE CANCER

Edited by **Gerhard Hamilton**

Advances in Prostate Cancer
http://dx.doi.org/10.5772/45948
Edited by Gerhard Hamilton

Contributors

Glenn Tisman, Elba Vazquez, Geraldine Gueron, Javier Cotignola, Miguel Álvarez-Múgica, Ugo Rovigatti, Vildan Bozok Çetintaş, Burçin Tezcanlı Kaymaz, Buket Kosova, Soon Cheol Ahn, Hak-Jong Choi, Kwang-Youn Kim, Sun-Nyoung Yu, Sang-Hun Kim, Sung-Sik Chun, Yeong-Min Park, Yong-Lark Choi, Sun-Yi Lee, Prada, Peng Lee, Mandeep Singh, Yirong Li, Garrett Daniels, Sujata Persad, Jacqueline R Ha, YuHao D Huang, Amit Persad, Meyers, Jutta Engel, Martin Dörr, Anne Schlesinger-Raab, Guangchao Sui, Daniel Stovall, Mario Bernardo-Filho, Mauro Luis Barbosa Júnior, Adele Holloway, Suyin Paulynn Chin, Joanne L Dickinson, Luis Espinoza, Jorge Salvador, Vânia Moreira, Samuel Silvestre, Shinji Kariya, Tine Hajdinjak, Luke Robles, Cheryl Dawn Helgason, Francesco Crea, Pier-Luc Clermont, Zachary Klaassen, Ray S. King, Kelvin A. Moses, Rabii Madi, Martha Terris, Manuela Iezzi, Rossano Lattanzio, Alessia Lamolinara, Mauro Piantelli, James Norris, Faik Atroshi, Sarah Rudman, Christopher Sweeney, Gerhard Hamilton

Published by InTech

Janeza Trdine 9, 51000 Rijeka, Croatia

Publishing Process Manager Iva Simcic
Technical Editor InTech DTP team
Cover InTech Design team

Additional hard copies can be obtained from orders@intechopen.com

Advances in Prostate Cancer, Edited by Gerhard Hamilton
p. cm.
ISBN 978-953-51-0932-7

For EU product safety concerns:
IN TECH d.o.o., Prolaz Marije Krucifikse Kozulić 3, 51000 Rijeka, Croatia,
info@intechopen.com or visit our website at intechopen.com.

Meet the editor

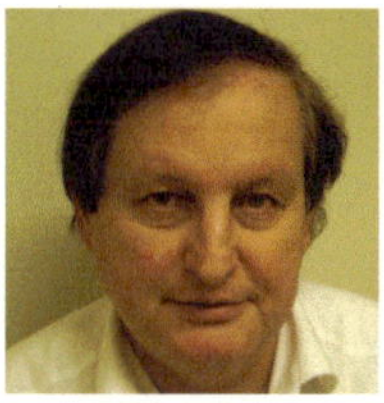

Dr. Gerhard Hamilton studied biochemistry at the University of Vienna, Austria. After finishing his doctoral thesis he got a position in the research laboratories of the Department of Surgery at the University Medical School of Vienna and obtained the degree of associate professor in 1996. His scientific publications comprise the fields of organ transplantation, burn care, sepsis and oncology. Recent research projects have focussed on preclinical characterization of anticancer compounds and mechanisms of drug resistance. Furthermore, special topics are assessment of diagnostic testing based on cytokeratin fragments in colorectal and prostate cancer and intermittent androgen suppression. In addition, Dr. Hamilton has been the scientific coordinator of the "Ludwig Boltzmann Cluster of Translational Oncology" Vienna, Austria since 2006.

Contents

Preface

"Advances in Prostate Cancer" is an addition to the InTech collection of three previous books about prostate cancer and aims at providing a comprehensive overview of specific aspects of the latest research and current knowledge relating to this tumor entity to scientists and clinicians. For this purpose a series of research articles, clinical investigations and reviews that deal with a wide range of relevant aspects pertinent to the epidemiology, diagnosis, patient care, treatment and basic biology of prostate cancer were included. Thereby this book aptly adds to the other InTech titles in the field of oncology, that describe advances in cancer therapy, diagnosis and treatment of various cancers with reference to the cancer stem cell concept.

The numerous participating authors of this book shared their expertise in epidemiology and etiology, as well as supportive care, which comprises the handling of psychological challenges and effects of physiotherapy in coping with the consequences of prostate cancer treatment. State-of-the-art radiation therapy is moreover discussed as well as the significance of testosterone and PSA measurements, the latter in form of a novel internet "App" that helps to interpret the time course of the marker determinations on the outcome. After many years of limited means to treat advanced prostate cancer several new agents such as CYP17 inhibitors and new cytotoxic drugs, as well as a cancer vaccine, became available, which poses new questions in regard to patient selection and appropriate choice of medical care. These topics comprehensively discussed in several chapters are supplemented by a review of the current state of intermittent androgen suppression versus continuous hormone ablation. These chapters are complemented by a number of discussions on the some characteristics of the cell biology of prostate cancer, including cancer stem cells, inflammatory processes, roles of androgen receptor and diverse non-androgen gene transcripts and, furthermore, cell adhesion proteins. This book is therefore destined to all cancer researchers and therapists who intend to understand the current status of cell biology and treatment of prostate cancer.

As editor of this book, I would like to acknowledge the significant efforts made by all of the contributing authors for their excellent work as well as the entire Intech editorial team in publishing of this volume. I would like to dedicate this book to the "Ludwig Boltzmann Society" and, in particular, to Prof. Dr. Gerhard Baumgartner whose long-standing support has allowed for the successful realization of many scientific projects. Last but not least, I would like to thank my wife for her personal support and great patience at all times.

Gerhard Hamilton, PhD
Ludwig Boltzmann Cluster of Translational Oncology

Section 1

Epidemiology and Etiology

Chapter 1

Epidemiology of Prostate Cancer

Martin Dörr, Anne Schlesinger-Raab and Jutta Engel

Additional information is available at the end of the chapter

http://dx.doi.org/10.5772/45948

1. Introduction

This chapter presents the current state of prostate cancer epidemiology and compares data from different regions. The data are taken from several sources:

Globocan 2008 [1] gives a glance on the worldwide situation in cancer epidemiology and permits the comparison of more and less developed regions in every continent.

The "Surveillance, Epidemiology and End Results" Program (SEER) [2] in the USA and the Robert Koch Institute (RKI) [3] in Germany present epidemiologic data of highly industrialized nations with maximally developed medical systems.

The Munich Cancer Registry (MCR) [4], a population-based clinical cancer registry of Upper Bavaria, an area of 4.5 million inhabitants in the South of Germany, presents detailed analyses of clinical data, distributions of prognostic factors and therapy, and survival analyses. Data of the MCR have also contributed to the publication "Cancer Incidence in Five Continents, Volume IX" [5].

2. Incidence and mortality

In Table 1 absolute numbers and age-standardized rates of incidence and mortality are presented for selected regions and countries [1]. In 2008 it was estimated that nearly every seventh case of male malignoma was prostate cancer (899 thousand new cases, 13.6% of the total). Therefore, in men prostate cancer was the second most diagnosed cancer after lung cancer. Approximately three quarters of these cases were diagnosed in more developed countries. The highest incidence rates were measured in Australia, New Zealand, Northern and Western Europe and Northern America. Moderate incidence rates were found in South

America and Eastern Europe. The lowest incidence rates were reported from South-Central Asia.

Region	Incidence absolute	Incidence ASR (W)	Mortality absolute	Mortality ASR (W)
World	899	27.9	258	7.4
More developed regions	644	61.7	136	10.5
Less developed regions	255	11.9	121	5.6
Asia	133.2	7.2	59.6	3.2
North America	213.7	85.7	32.6	9.9
Central America	20.5	34.8	8.1	12.6
South America	84.1	50.2	29.2	16.2
Australia and New Zealand	21.0	104.2	4.0	15.4
Central and Eastern Europe	58.4	29.1	23.1	10.9
Northern Europe	64.9	73.1	17.4	15.4
Southern Europe	79.5	50.0	20.4	10.4
Western Europe	167.9	93.1	28.7	12.4
Germany	70.8	82.7	12.2	11.7
Japan	38.7	22.7	10.0	5.0
USA	186.3	83.8	28.6	9.7
Brazil	41.6	50.3	14.4	16.3
China	33.8	4.3	14.3	1.8
India	14.6	3.7	10.4	2.5
Russian Federation	22.1	26.1	9.5	10.8
SouthAfricanRepublic	7.5	59.7	2.5	20.8

Absolute numbers in thousands; ASR (W): age standardised rate per 100,000 by world standard

Table 1. Absolute numbers and age-standardised rates of incidence and mortality for selected regions and countries [1]

Despite its high proportion of cancer diagnoses, prostate cancer is the cause of cancer specific death in only every 16th case (258 thousand deaths, 6.1% of the total). This places prostate cancer on the sixth position of cancer-specific causes of death, topped by lung, liver, stomach, colorectal and oesophageal cancer. These deaths occur almost equally in both, more developed and less developed regions, thus leading to a twofold higher mortality rate in the more developed regions.

2.1. Incidence and mortality trends

Table 2 shows the current incidence and mortality of the USA [2], Germany [7, 8] and the Munich Cancer Registry [4]. These rates have changed considerably over time. Time series of more developed countries show that the incidence rates experience a drastic rise from 1985 to 1995 and remain at this high level. In the USA incidence (by world standard per 100,000) increases slowly from 1975 until 1985 (from 50 to 65). Then it rises rapidly reaching a peak of 135 in 1992. Then it decreased, since 1995 more slowly, but it remains on a higher level than before the peak (around 110). In Germany incidence is rising continuously since 1988 (from 30 to 75). The main explanation for these trends is the broad use of prostate specific antigen (PSA) testing as a screening method and performing biopsies, which started in the mid-1980s in the USA and in the early 1990s in Germany.

	USA (SEER, NCHS) [2, 6]	Germany (RKI) [7, 8]	MCR [4]
Absolute incidence	241.7	70.8	2.9
Crude incidence		157.7	145.1
Incidence ASR (W)	106.1	82.7	76.4
Mortality ASR (W)	10.2	11.7	13.3*
Lifetime risk(%)	16.2	13.0	
Median age at diagnosis(years)	67.0	69.5	67.2
Median age at death(years)	80.0		76.7
5-year overall survival(%)		77.0	79.2
5-year relative survival(%)	99.2	92.0	93.4
10-year overall survival(%)			58.2
10-year relative survival(%)	98.3		87.8

Absolute numbers in thousands

ASR (W): age standardised rate per 100,000 by world standard

Incidence and mortality from cohorts of 2008 (all regions)

Absolute incidence numbers of the USA are estimates of SEER data from 2012

* Mortality ASR (W) for singular prostate cancers is 9.9

median ages from cohorts of 2005-2009 (all regions)

5-year survival from cohorts of 2002-2008 (SEER and MCR)

10-year survival from cohorts of 1998-2008 (SEER and MCR)

Table 2. Epidemiologic basic numbers

In the USA, mortality initially increases slightly from 1975 and since 1992 it is decreasing more rapidly (from 14 over 17 to 10). In Germany the mortality rate (by world standard per 100,000) stays stable at 13.

2.2. Age distribution and age-specific incidence and mortality rate

Nearly all patients (≈ 99%) who are diagnosed with prostate cancer have reached an age of fifty or higher. The age distribution at diagnosis describes a positively skewed unimodal distribution with its modus at the age group 65-69. This age group contributes to nearly 25% of all prostate cancer cases. The risk of getting prostate cancer increases nearly exponentially with increasing age. This makes prostate cancer one of the most distinctive cancers in aging populations (Figure 1) with a ASIR of 800-1000 per 100,000 in the elderly of 70 years and older.

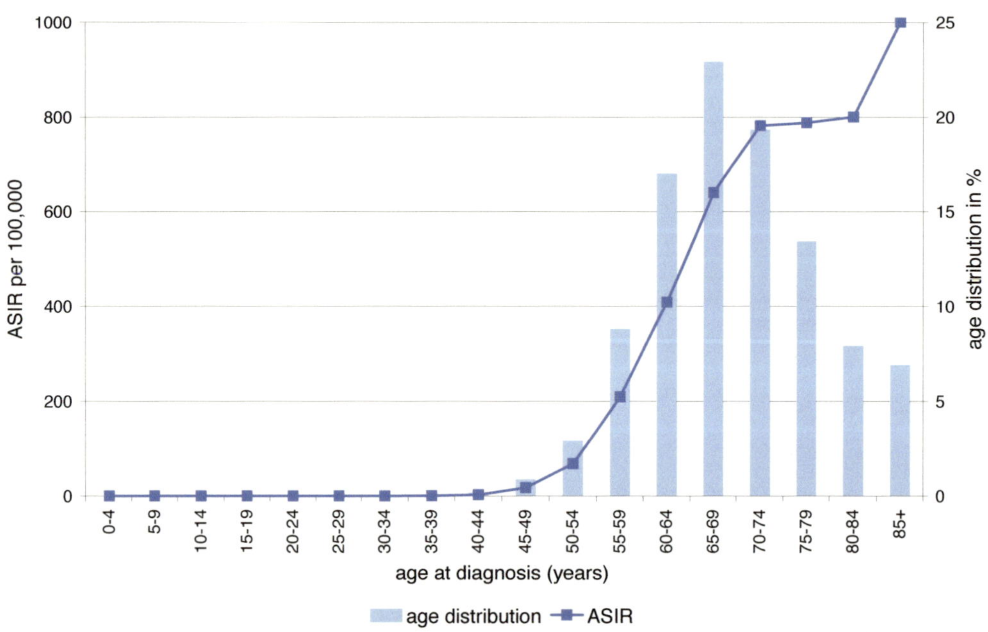

Figure 1. Age distribution at diagnosis and age-specific incidence rate (ASIR) of prostate cancer (1998-2008) [4]

Nearly all patients who died of prostate cancer (singular initial malignoma) have reached an age of fifty-five or higher. The distribution of age at death describes a negatively skewed unimodal distribution with its modus at the highest age group 85+. Here the age-specific mortality rates (ASMR) can perfectly be described by an exponential function. The risk of dying by prostate cancer increases accelerated with increasing age (Figure 2). The ASMR reaches 450 per 100,000 for men with an age of 80-84 and already 600 per 100,000 for men older than 84.

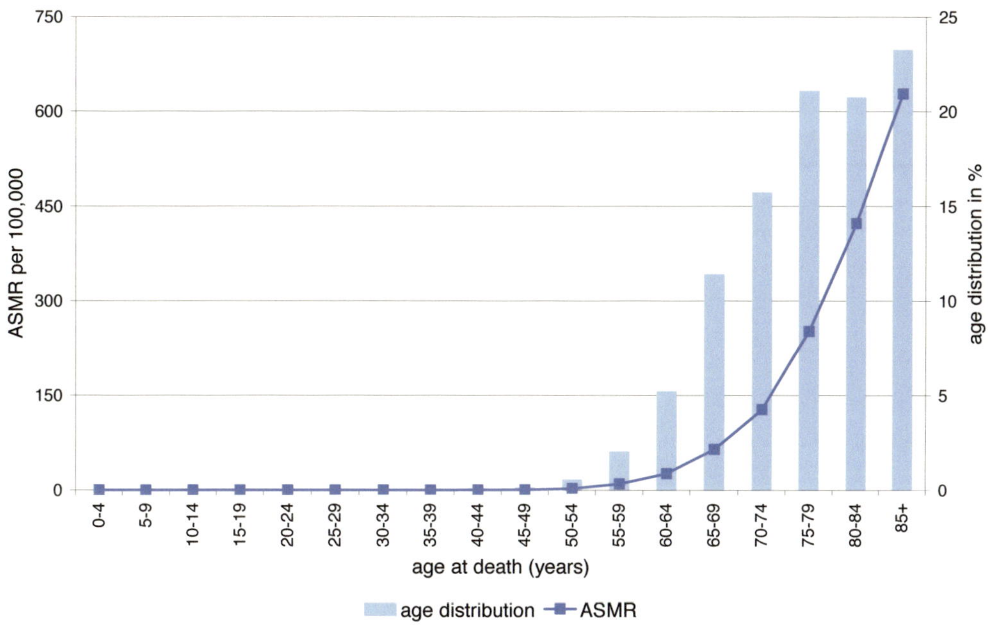

Figure 2. Age distribution at death and age-specific mortality rate (ASMR) of prostate cancer (1998-2009) [4]

3. Prognostic factors

According to Table 3 the conditional age distributions of the combined T categories 2 until 4 have the same shape and the modus at the age group of 65 until 69. These distributions are shifted slightly towards higher ages with the increasing T category. This simply reflects that it takes time to develop an advanced tumour. However, in those patients diagnosed with T1 category (clinically) the age distribution appears to be totally different. Here 80% of the men are older than 64 (about 60% within the other T categories) and every third man is older than 74.

Lymph node category (N), distant primary metastases (M), Gleason Score, initial PSA value and Gleason Score are positively correlated with the combined T category: the higher the T category, the higher the PSA value, the higher the Gleason Score and the higher the porportion of regional or distant metastases.

A positive lymph node status is mostly diagnosed when the tumour has spread through the prostatic capsule. Nearly 20% of those men with T3 and almost 50% with T4 tumours therefore are diagnosed with lymph node metastasis.

	T category				
	T1 % (n=1826 13.3%)	T2 % (n=8219 59.9%)	T3 % (n=3164 23.0%)	T4 % (n=503 3.7%)	All % (n=13712 100%)
Age (years)					
<50	0.5	2.3	1.4	1.8	1.8
50 - 54	1.5	4.5	3.5	3.0	3.8
55 - 59	3.0	11.0	10.2	11.1	9.8
60 - 64	9.7	20.2	18.2	15.1	18.2
65 - 69	20.9	31.4	32.8	26.4	30.1
70 - 74	26.1	20.2	23.1	19.7	21.7
≥75	38.3	10.4	10.8	22.9	14.7
Lymph node status					
N+	2.5	1.6	18.4	45.1	7.3
N0	40.6	85.2	73.5	33.6	76.2
NX	56.9	13.2	8.1	21.2	16.5
Metastasis status					
M0	97.4	98.8	95.4	72.6	96.9
M1	2.6	1.2	4.6	27.4	3.1
PSA value (ng/ml)					
< 4	25.8	13.2	7.8	3.7	13.2
4 - <10	42.0	60.7	41.5	18.9	52.4
10 - <20	17.5	18.3	24.9	15.7	19.7
≥20	14.7	7.8	25.7	61.8	14.8
Gleason Score					
2 - 4	14.3	1.6	0.2	0.2	2.9
5 - 6	54.8	48.1	12.3	4.2	39.1
7	19.1	40.5	49.4	26.6	39.3
8 - 10	11.8	9.8	38.2	68.9	18.7

Presented numbers are column-wise percentages.

T category is a combination of cT and pT.

The disease cohort is limited to 2005-2009 to provide best current estimators.

Table 3. Prognostic factors by T category [4]

Although, only 2.4% of all prostate cancer cases have primary distant metastases, already 25% of the T4 patients are diagnosed with metastases.

About 50% of the men with prostate cancer have a PSA value of 4 to 10 ng/ml at initial diagnosis.

According to Figure 3aa shift from capsule exceeding tumours to capsule limited tumours took place in the 1990s. In the late 1980s about 15% of the diagnosed tumours were staged T4, some 45% T3 and nearly 25% T2. In the 2000s only some 5% of the diagnosed tumours were staged T4, good 20% T3 and about 60% T2. The T1 category was unaffected and oscillated around 12% during the whole time period. It seems that PSA-Screening has considerably lowered the proportion of locally advanced tumours.

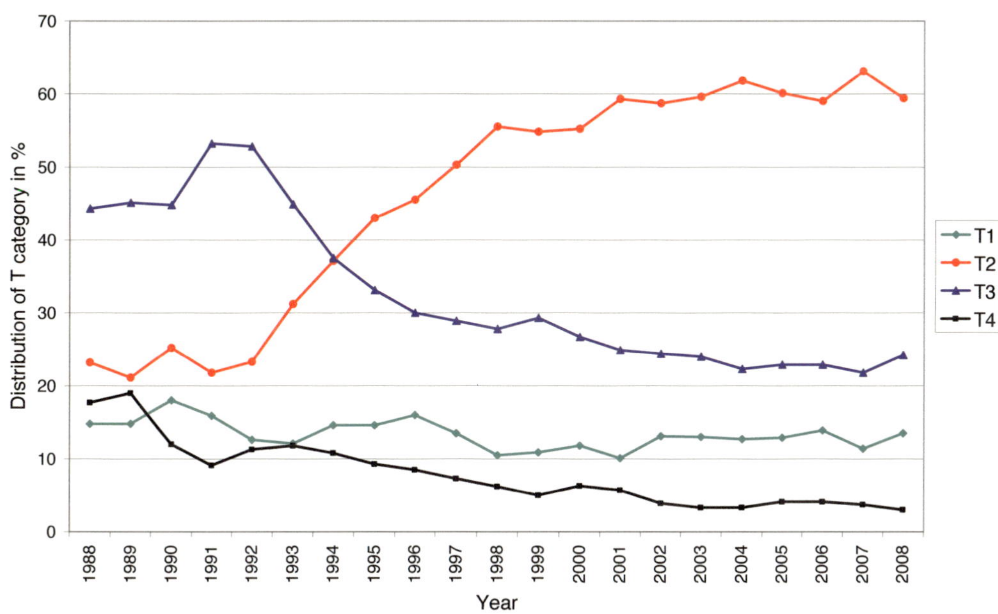

Figure 3. Distribution of T category over time (n = 35544) [4]. T category is a combination of cT and pT.

4. Therapy

Table 4 presents in detail the effects of combined T category on the choice of therapy. Guidelines [9] note that radical prostatectomy, radiation therapy and hormone therapy in combination with radiation therapy are the main primary treatment options when the tumour remains within the prostate capsule (T2) or does not invade nearby structures other than the seminal vesicles or the bladder neck (T3). A spreading prostate cancer should be treated with a hormone therapy. Active surveillance (AS) and watchful waiting (WW) are only noteworthy initial therapy strategies for tumours detected in an early stage. Although these are accepted treatment options in localised prostate cancer, they are seldom chosen compared to radical prostatectomy and hormone therapy. Transurethral resection of the prostate is not an appropriate surgical treatment option in prostate cancer but its proportion in T1 category (46.7%) indicates a greater proportion of incidentally found prostate cancers during a treatment of benign hyperplasia. Without further surgical or hormone therapy, one could classify these cases into the AS or WW groups.

	T category				
	T1 % (n=1826 13.3%)	T2 % (n=8219 59.9%)	T3 % (n=3164 23.0%)	T4 % (n=503 3.7%)	All % (n=13712 100%)
Initial therapy					
RPE		74.9	65.9	31.3	61.8
TUR	47.2	3.2	2.5	11.4	9.0
HIFU	4.5	3.4	0.8	0.2	2.8
XRT	16.6	6.1	9.8	12.7	8.5
Hormone	23.7	11.6	20.3	44.2	16.4
AS and WW	8.0	0.8	0.7	0.2	1.6

Presented numbers are column-wise percentages.

T category is a combination of cT and pT.

The disease cohort is limited to 2005-2009 to provide best current estimators.

RPE: radical prostatectomy, TUR: transurethral resection of the prostate, HIFU: high-intensity focused ultrasound, XRT: radiation therapy, Hormone: hormone therapy, AS: active surveillance, WW: watchful waiting

Table 4. Initial therapy by T category [4]

As Figure 4 shows impressively, initial therapy strategies have changed noticeably over the last 20 years. In the late 1980's radical prostatectomy was the initial therapy in about 25% of all treatments. Its rate increased continuously and finally reaches almost 60%, making this the most selected initial therapy per year since 1995. The curve of hormone therapy developed oppositely. To be more precise: hormone therapy was the most selected treatment till 1994. From 65% in 1989 it continuously decreased to now 20%. Radiation therapy (XRT) slightly increased to 10% as initial therapy. Finally, within the whole time span transurethral resection of the prostate (TUR) remains stable at a proportion of nearly 10%.

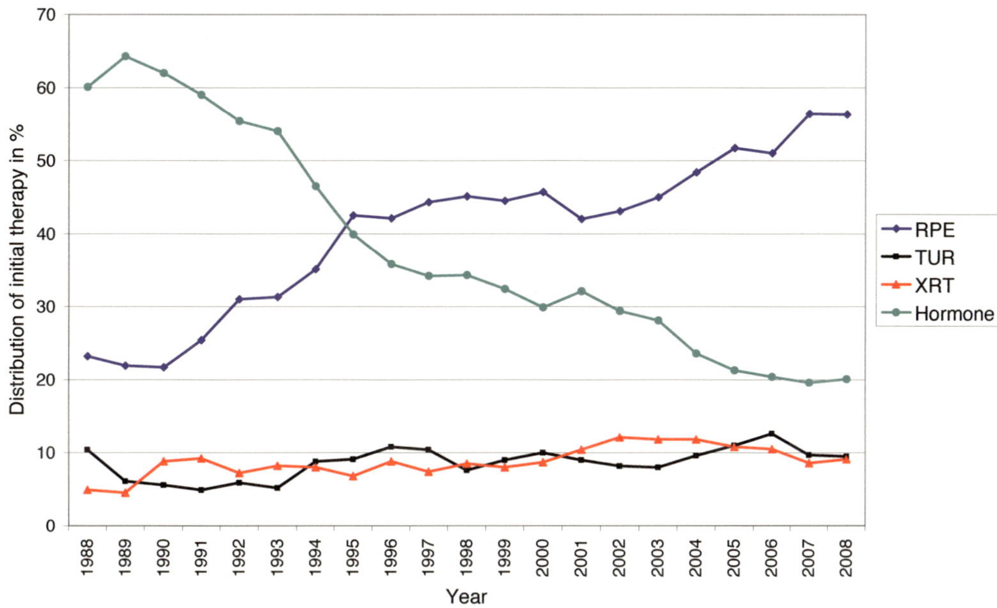

Figure 4. Distribution of initial therapy strategies over time (n = 35544) [4]. RPE: radical prostatectomy, XRT: radiation therapy, Hormone: hormone therapy, TUR: transurethral resection of the prostate

5. Survival

The following figures mainly present the relative survival (RS) curves, an estimator for the cancer specific survival. This is calculated by dividing the overall survival (OS) of the observed cohort by the expected survival of a normal population with the same distribution regarding birth-date and sex.

When looking at the influence of the year of diagnosis on the overall survival (Figure 5) or relative survival (Figure 6) only the curve of patients with a diagnosis in the years 1998 until 1992 noticeably differs from the other ones. Here the 5- and 10-year relative survival was 85.0% and 74.3%, respectively. In the group of patients diagnosed between 1993 and 1997 the 5- and 10-year relative survival was 94.9% and 88.6% in the group of 1998-2002 the 5- and 10-year relative survival was 94.0% and 84.1% and in the recent group of 2003-2008 the 5-year relative survival was 92.1%. Therefore, the following survival analyses are presented for patients with a diagnosis between 1998 - 2008.

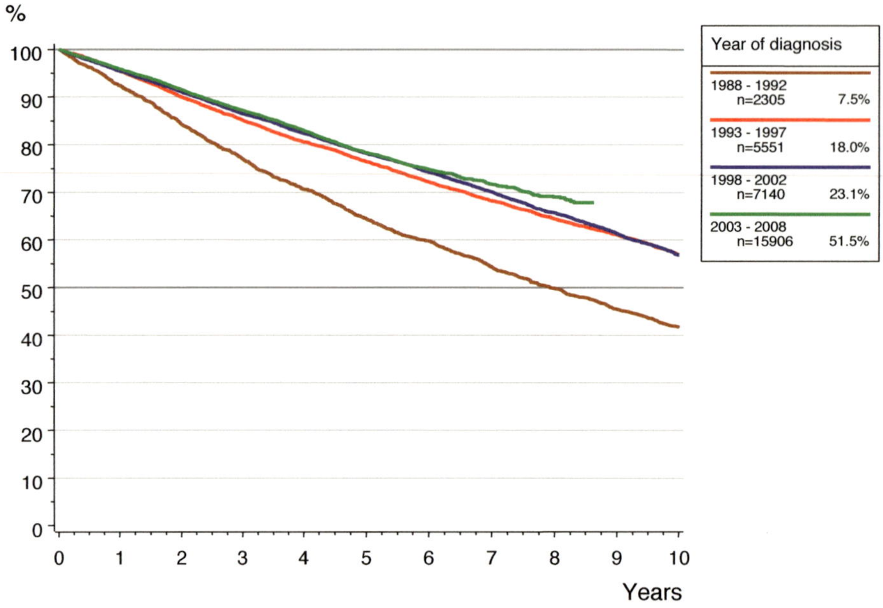

Figure 5. Overall survival by year of diagnosis (n=30902) [4]

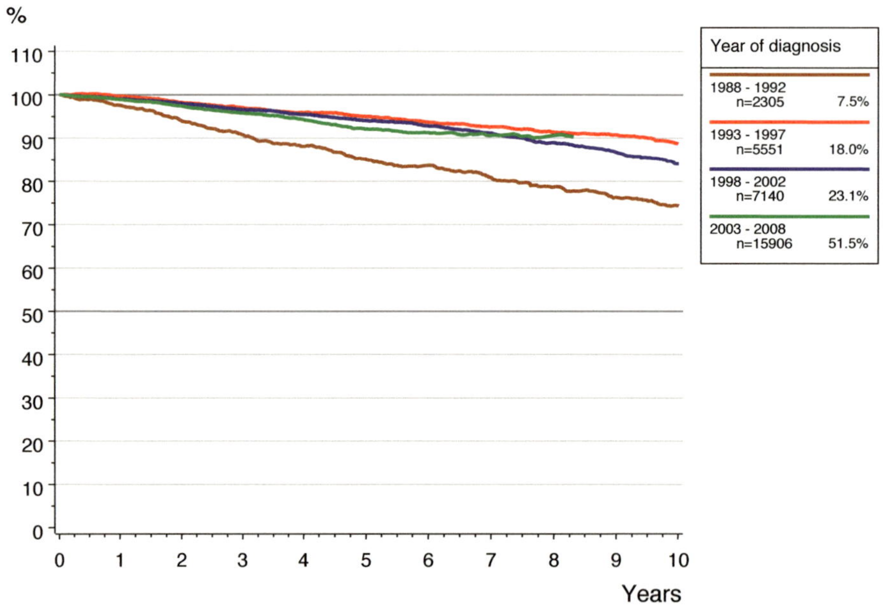

Figure 6. Relative survival by year of diagnosis (n=30902) [4]. Relative survival is the quotient of overall survival and expected survival and thus an estimator for the cancer specific survival.

The complete cohort of prostate cancer patients with a diagnosis between 1998 and 2008 (Figure 7) shows a 5-year overall survival of 78.8% and a 10-year overall survival of 57.7%. The relative survival is 93.6% and 84.1%, respectively. For comparison: SEER data show a 5-year relative survival of 99.2% for patients diagnosed between 2002 and 2008 and a 10-year relative survival of 98.3% for the cohort of 1998 – 2008.

Figure 8 presents the relative survival by the combined T category. As expected, patients with a T2-staging perform better than patients with a T1-Staging. The 5- and 10-year relative survival is 102.0% and 94.0% in T1, 104.9% and 108.8% in T2, 97.6% and 89.5% in T3 and 61.4% and 43.8% in T4, respectively. Relative survival can exceed 100%, because prostate cancer patients benefit from the better treatment of comorbidities during aftercare.

Lymph node status (N category) is an important prognostic factor. As Figure 9 shows, a positive lymph node status (N+) reduces the relative survival drastically (77.7% for 5-year and 61.9% for 10-year survival) compared to a 5- and 10-year survival of 105.5% and 107.5% in N0. Nonetheless, prostate cancer patients benefit from radical prostatectomy in the situation with lymph node metastases [10].

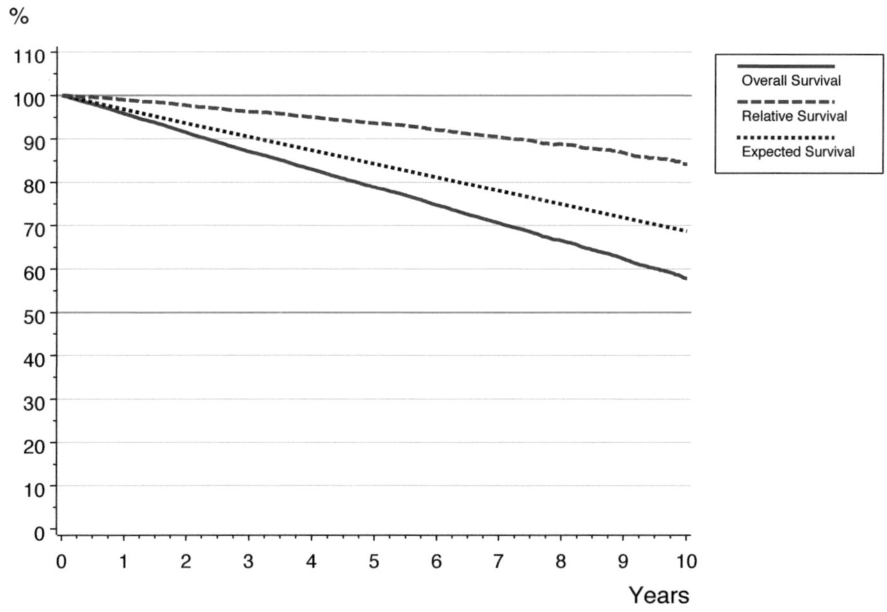

Figure 7. Overall, relative and expected survival of the complete collective (1998-2008, n = 25773) [4]. Relative survival is the quotient of overall survival and expected survival and thus an estimator for the cancer specific survival.

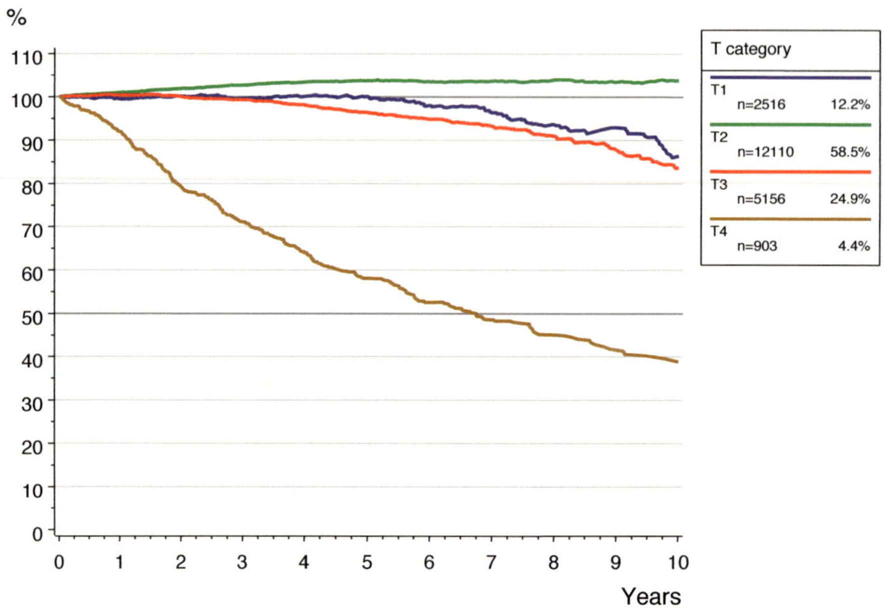

Figure 8. Relative Survival by T category (1998-2008, n = 20685) [4]. T category is a combination of cT and pT.

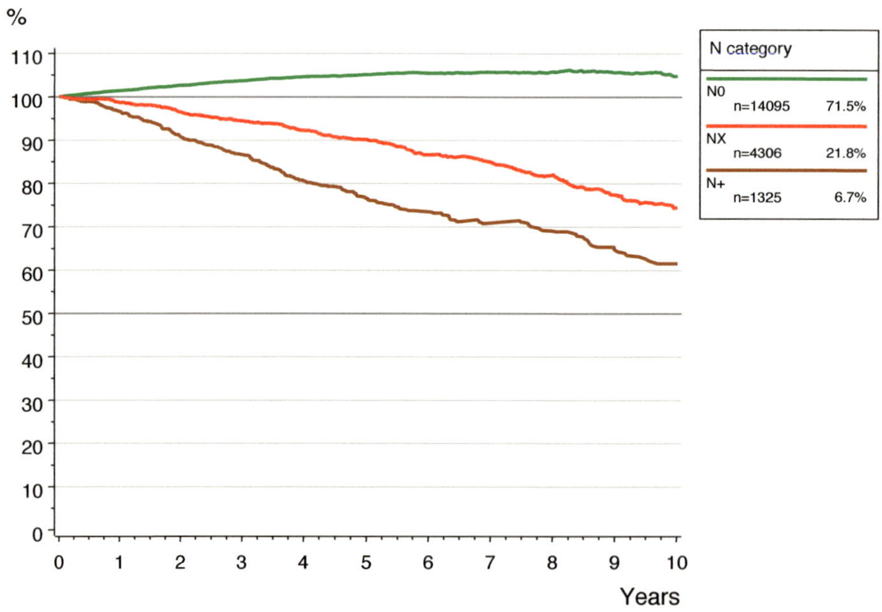

Figure 9. Relative Survival by N category (1998-2008, n = 19726) [4]. N category is a combination of cN and pN.

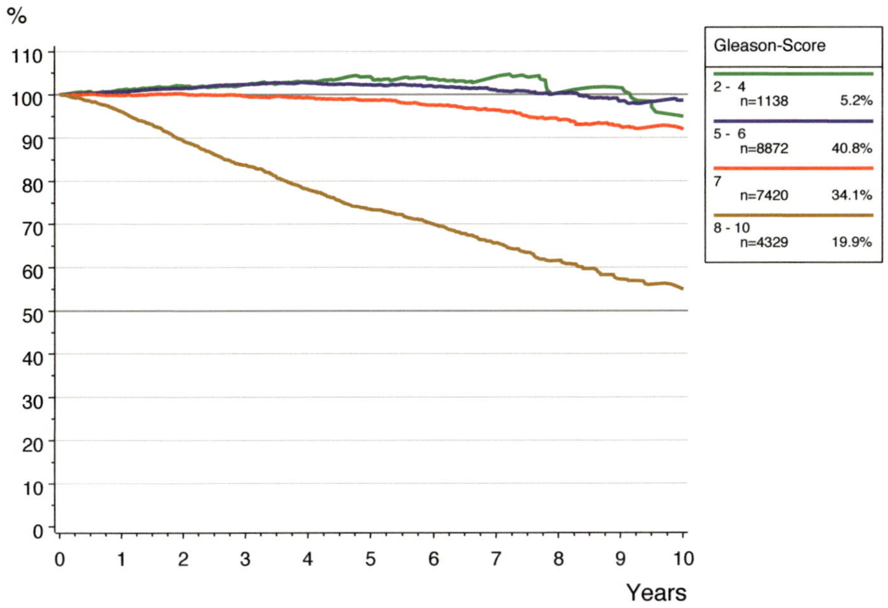

Figure 10. Relative survival by Gleason Score (1998-2008, n = 21759) [4]

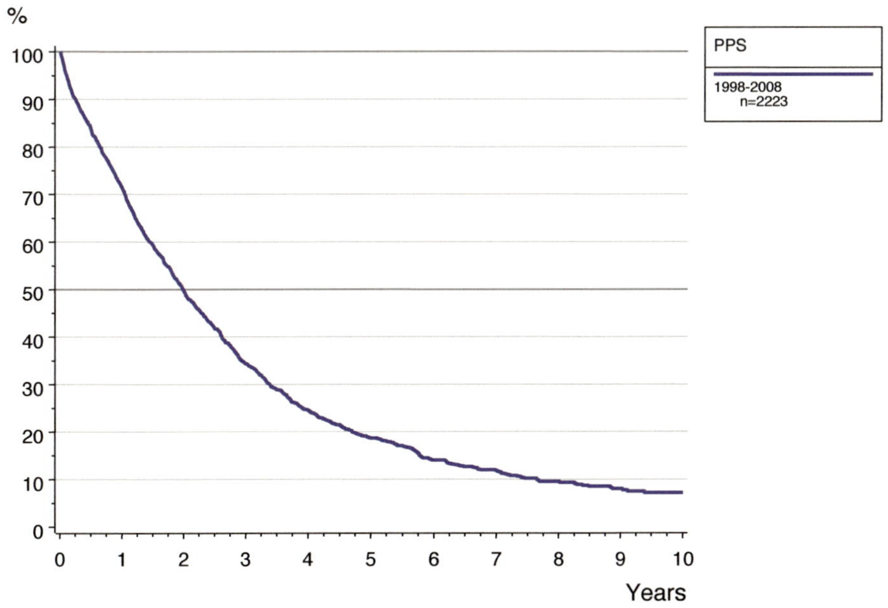

Figure 11. Post Progression Survival (1998-2008, n = 2223) [4]. Starting point of progression is from date of locoregional relapse or distant metastasis (primary M1 or metastases in further course of disease).

According to Figure 10 patients with the worst Gleason Score category (8 – 10) have a much poorer survival (73.4% for five year and 55.0% for ten year survival) than patients with a scoring of 7 and better, which does not discriminate very much (104.1% and 94.8% for Gleason Score 2 - 4, 102.2% and 98.6% for Gleason Score 5 – 6 and 98.6% and 91.8% for Gleason Score 7).

If the tumour has metastasised or locoregional recurrence has occurred, only 18.2% of the patients survive 5 years and 7.2% of the patients survive 10 years. The median survival is about two years (Figure 11).

Nomenclature

WHO→World Health Organization

SEER→"Surveillance, Epidemiology and End Results" Program of the National Cancer Institute of the USA

NCHS→National Center for Health Statistics

RKI→Robert Koch Institut

MCR→Munich Cancer Registry

PSA→Prostate specific antigen

RPE→Radical prostatectomy

XRT→Radiation therapy

HIFU→High-intensity focused ultrasound

Hormone→Hormon therapy

TUR→Transurethral resection of the prostate

AS→Active surveillance

WW→Watchful waiting

ASR (W)→Age-standardised rate, using the proposed world standard population of Segi (1960)

ASIR→Age-specific incidence rate

ASMR→Age-specific mortality rate

Author details

Martin Dörr, Anne Schlesinger-Raab and Jutta Engel

Munich Cancer Registry (MCR), Clinic Großhadern / IBE, Ludwig-Maximilians-University (LMU), Germany

References

[1] Ferlay, Shin, Bray et al., Globocan 2008: Cancer Incidence and Mortality Worldwide; 2011. http://globocan.iarc.fr.

[2] National Cancer Institute: "Surveillance, Epidemiology and End Results" (SEER) Program. http://www.seer.cancer.gov.

[3] Robert Koch Institut (RKI). http://www.rki.de.

[4] Munich Cancer Registry (MCR). http://www.tumorregister-muenchen.de.

[5] IARC Scientific Publications, Cancer Incidence in Five Continents, Volume IX, 2009. http://ci5.iarc.fr/.

[6] Siegel, Naishadham and Jemal, Cancer statistics, 2012. CA: A Cancer Journal for Clinicians 2012; 62(1):10–29.

[7] Cancer in Germany 2005/2006. Incidence and Trends. Seventh edition Robert Koch Institut (ed) and Association of Population-based Cancer Registries in Germany (ed). Berlin, 2010.

[8] Cancer in Germany 2007/2008. Eighth edition. Robert Koch Institut (ed) and Association of Population-based Cancer Registries in Germany (ed). Berlin, 2012.

[9] National Institute for Health and Clinical Excellence. www.nice.org.uk.

[10] Engel, Bastian et al., Survival benefit of radical prostatectomy in lymph node-positive patients with prostate cancer. Eur Urol 2010; 57(5):754-61.

Chapter 2

Is There an Infectious Agent Behind Prostate Cancer?

Ugo Rovigatti

Additional information is available at the end of the chapter

http://dx.doi.org/10.5772/54054

1. Introduction

This CHAPTER deals with a more defined and specified issue: whether we can already identify, point our fingers toward a specific infectious agent or infectivity pathway most likely targeting and lurking behind prostate cancer (PCa). This issue became quite evident in the past 5-6 years, in view of the heated debate on the possible role of a what was considered a novel retrovirus: Xenotropic Murine Related Virus, or XMRV, in the aetiology of PCa and subsequently also of Chronic Fatigue Syndrome (CFS). Over two years ago, the same issue was discussed by the author at the International Congress on Muscle Fatigue held in Pisa in July 2010. That presentation has been now transformed in a paper, which is in press in the journal Neuro Muscolar Disease (NMD, Springer Verlag) [1]. The reader is therefore referred to that article -most likely already published by the time of this book printing- for aetiological considerations on CFS [1]. In this section, I will more extensively discuss the association of XMRV with PCa. Such an association was the first one to be discovered and this finding was the basis for also searching XMRV in CFS. In CFS, the potential association with an infective agent doesn't appear to be trivial, since "fatigue" has been widely associated with several types of cancer in the so called Cancer Related Fatigue (CRF), also discussed more extensively in the NMD paper [1] [2].

2. Discovery and falsification of XMRV

2.1. Linkage RNASEL – HPC-1

XMRV isolation was not a sudden or isolated finding, but it rather stemmed out of approximately twenty years of research by several groups, with a leading role by the group of R. Silverman [3] [4]. This work, as well, has even older roots, since it was initiated by deciphering the antiviral response triggered by Interferon (IFN). Robert Silverman's work was pioneering and seminal in this effort: together with Ian Kerr, he clarified the Interferon (IFN) response to viral infection, initially by characterizing the 5'-triphosporylated, 2',5'-linked oligoadenylates or 2-5A, a second messenger in the IFN response and its synthesizing enzyme (oligo-2',5'-A synthethase, or OAS) and finally discovering that 2-5A is the activator of an endogenous RNase activity, called RNase L [5] [3]. This is ubiquitously distributed but inactive inside cells, but it becomes strongly activated by binding 2-5A. By using radiolabelled 2-5A as probe, Silverman was able to identify and clone the gene *RNASEL* and to map later its location on chromosome 1q25 [5]. After approximately ten years, these studies intersected a totally different discovery path. Linkage studies on families with increased hereditary risk of prostate cancer, identified in 2002 the prostate carcinoma susceptibility gene (*Hereditary Prostate Carcinoma 1, HPC-1*) on chromosome 1q25, the same of *RNASEL* location [6]. Different alleles on this locus were associated with higher risk of PCa, such as the R462Q variant, which appeared to provide a 50% risk increase, while homozygosity doubled the risk [7]. This association between a locus behaving as a Tumor Suppressor Gene (*TSG*) and an Anti-Viral Response (*AVR*) gene is strongly suggestive of viral involvement in PCa. In the July 2010 presentation at the International Meeting on Muscle Fatigue -which was very critical of the XMRV identification- the sound evidence for viral involvement was emphasized. A logical-inference analysis showed that –most likely- a wrong viral candidate was chosen [1], Fig.1. Subsequent work has vindicated our first prediction (XMRV falsification), but additional work is required to strength the association with another candidate Virus that we propose: MFV (see later) [1]. Several studies have confirmed the RNASEL-HPC1 association [7] [8] [9] [4], but not all [10] [4] of them.

2.2. XMRV discovery

For another five years at the turn of the century, these discoveries on HPC-1 remained just suggestive of a viral involvement in PCA, for a locus –RNASEL- which behaves as a Tumor Suppressor Gene (TSG) –as already indicated by an interesting Editorial by Lengyel, in 1993 [11] and as suggested by others [12] [13]. Then Silverman with colleagues DeRisi and Ganem utilized a micro-array approach (*viro-chip*) [14], in order to try identifying the responsible virus [3, 15]. The first papers on XMRV appeared at the end of 2006/ beginning of 2007: they showed that XMRV was present at high frequency in patients homozygous for the R462Q allele (i.e., 8/20 or 40%) and that it is a xenotropic retrovirus with similarities with murine leukaemia viruses (MuLV) [16] [15]. Xenotropic retroviruses are endogenous viruses, which cannot infect cells of the original species, while ecotropic viruses do. Typically, endogenous murine retroviruses have been divided into two large families: ecotropic and non-ecotropic retroviruses [17] [18]. Ecotropic retroviruses -being still capable of active infection in the same species, i.e. mouse, cells- are present in only one or just a few copies (0-6) per genome. Their genetics is rather well clarified by several years of research [19]. The structure/genetics of the non-ecotropic retroviruses is more complex, also in view of the fact that they are present in a considerable (40-60) number of copies/genome. In recent years, particularly thanks to the work of J. Coffin and J. Stoye [20], non-ecotropic retroviruses have been clarified and subdivided into three subfamilies: xenotropic (XMP), not capable of replicating inside cells of the same species, polytropic (PMV), which are capable of replicating inside cells of several species including the original (mouse) and modified-polytropic (MPMV), which display altered properties in terms structure/function of the *env* gene [21] [17] [18]. The experiments, which distinguish among different subfamilies of non-ecotropic mouse retroviruses are: 1. infectivity/replication assays; 2. characterization of their structure by restriction enzyme and/or Southern blotting analysis; 3. complete sequencing [20, 21]. For a more detailed overview of this fascinating but rather complex scientific area, the reader is referred to two excellent review articles by J. Coffin and J. Stoye [17] [18].

2.3. Positive evidence

XMRV was also found integrated inside mesenchimal/stromal cells -rather than in tumour cell genomes- in proximity of genes of cell cycle or hormonal control, which could provide a reasonable link to carcinogenesis [16] [4]. Indeed, such mechanisms variably defined as "promoter insertion" or "insertional mutagenesis" appear to be the most likely involved in chronically (or non-acutely) transforming Retroviruses [22] [23]. This initial report by the discoverer group was followed up a few months later by another PNAS paper, by Schlaberg et al., in which XMRV was associated to approximately 23% of cases by immuno-histochemistry (IHC), while detection of viral DNA by PCR was quite lower (6%) [24]. Beside this rather surprising finding (since the opposite would be typically expected), this report also slightly contradicted the previous ones, since 1. XMRV was directly identified in the carcinoma cells and not in surrounding mesenchimal/stromal cells, 2. there was no evidence of an association between XMRV positive cases in PCa and RNAse-L involvement by mutation/ lower function, as previously described in the Urisman et al. paper [15, 24]. In that report, 40% of cases which were homozygous for the R462Q variant in RNAse-L were XMRV+ [15]. In the following months of 2010, another group from Emory University in Atalanta (GA) also reported an association between XMRV and PCa, by employing three different and complementary technologies [25]: a) a very sensitive "nested" PCR assay, b) chromosomal fluorescence hybridisation (FISH) and c) very sensitive technology for detection of neutralizing antibodies (the same group and others had previously developed this technique for detecting anti-HIV antibodies) [26] [27] [25]. Also in this report, the serologic assay was the most sensitive, detecting XMRV antibodies in 27.5 % of cases (11/40), while positivity increased in carriers of the R462Q allele (8/20 –also in this study- or 40% of cases, which were RNASEL R462Q homozygous) [25]. Finally, this report confirmed, as in the original paper by Urisman et al., the presence of XMRV in stromal/mesenchimal and not in carcinoma cells [25]. In the same year, another group from Baylor College in Houston (TX) also detected an association between XMRV and PCa in 22% of cases [28]. However, virus was strangely detected in both tumour and normal cells of affected patients and there was no correlation –as in Schlaberg et. al - with RNaseL status [28].

2.4. Negative findings

Together with the appearance of such positive reports, however, a series of studies presenting negative findings started to appear in the literature. Many of these negative reports came from European laboratories, although an initial negative study –often ignored- was from Johns Hopkins University (JHU) in the US [29]: see below. While the issue of XMRV detection in PCa was getting more controversial, another "XMRV-front" opened with the publication in October 2009 of a paper in Science, where Lombardi et al. reported detection of XMRV in 67% (68/101) of Chronic Fatigue Syndrome (CFS) cases [30]. While controls showed much lower detection rates, i.e. 3.7% (8/218), such value (as well as previous ones) was alarming, since it suggested that a few million people may be infected in the general "healthy" population in the US and probably elsewhere [31]. The initial Lombardi et al. paper was followed by larger numbers of negative reports, appearing in the months immediately after its publication: they will not be reviewed extensively in this chapter and the reader is referred instead to the NMD paper [1], with only one exception. In September 2010, Lo et al. published a PNAS paper describing rather frequent association between CFS and a retrovirus different from XMRV: indeed this virus appeared to be polytropic (P-MLV) instead of xenotropic (X-MLV) [32]. While some scientists applauded this novel discovery [33], the PNAS paper was accompanied by an editorial by Andrew Mason's group, in which perplexities about these very findings were expressed [34]. Indeed, despite the relationship between the two viruses, it was extremely difficult to reconcile these findings or even to explain the discovery of XMRV as due to presence of P-MLV instead. In fact, the two viruses are clearly distinguishable by sequencing. Therefore, the idea presented at that time [33]: that the real culprit in CFS would be P-MLV and that the previous detection of XMRV should *de facto* be considered P-MLV detection, or that either virus could cause the same disease, was simply wrong.

The very first negative report for XMRV in PCa was from Hamburg, DE and was authored (1st) by one of the first co-authors of the original paper by Urisman: Nicole Fischer [35]. This suggests that very similar detection methods were employed in Germany: XMRV was detected only in one non-familiar PCa (of 87) and one control (of 70) sample. Neither one of these cases was homozygous for the R462Q allele [35]. An even more striking negative result was obtained by Hohn and collaborators in Berlin [36], who did not detect a single positive case among 589 PCa patients tested: this study employed a sensitive nested PCR detection, RT-PCR for *gag* sequences as well as serology for XMRV-specific antibodies [36]. A number of patients (76) were studied for the RNASEL allele and 12.9% scored positive [36]. Similar negative results were published in additional studies from Ireland (139 cases) [37], Holland (74 sporadic cases) [38], Mexico (55 cases) [39], USA (over 800 patients from a collaborative effort between Baylor, Johns Hopkins etc.) [40] and UK (437 patients from UK, Korea and Thailand) [41]. In the last study, a few patients scored positive: for example 2 out of 6 of Thailand's patients were positive, potentially reaching a score of 33%. However, evidence of contamination started emerging in this British International study: some of the amplified DNA did not contain a 24 bp deletion which is a hallmark of XMRV and other evidence suggested instead presence of P-MLV (as in the previous paper by Lo et al. on CFS) [41] [32]. A few assays, specific for contamination by mouse DNA, were therefore run to confirm identity of specimens. A very sensitive assay for Intracisternal A-type particles (IAPs) and mouse mitocondrial DNA was completely concordant with XMRV presence, clearly indicating presence of contamination [41]. Therefore, this 2010 paper by Robinson should have already signalled a red-flag warning for XMRV research [41].

2.5. Strength of RNASEL – HPC-1 paradigm

At the International Congress on Muscle Fatigue in 2010, I strongly criticized the association between *PCa* and *XMRV,* on the basis of such negative findings, most of which had been already published in the literature (July 2010). My analysis at the congress extended to the technology employed, thus suggesting that the *viro-chip* assay was –most likely- the source of error [1]. Still, data on the *RNase-L* association with *HPC-1* were indicative of viral involvement. Contrary to the situation in *PCa,* in which a few independent reports confirmed XMRV presence, while they were contradicted by a limited number of studies, CFS association with this virus was essentially based upon the unique paper by Lombardi et al. in 2009, somehow overwhelmed by a plethora of negative reports [1]. However, also in CFS, the case for the likely presence of an infectious agent, most probably a virus, can be made. This is particularly clear, in view of the presence of "micro-epidemics", often associated with CFS onset [1]. The rather strong evidence for a previous virus infection accompanied by the dramatic personal histories of CFS onset in thousands of patients could explain, but certainly NOT justify, the attachment of some patient-groups to the XMRV hypothesis, sometimes referred in the media as mass-hysteria [224]. We will later discuss whether the viral hypothesis should be completely dismissed in view of XMRV falsification or whether additional viral candidates should be investigated (see section 3).

2.6. XMRV controversy: looking back through 3 major Editorials

After 2010, the majority of XMRV reports documented negative results either in PCa or in CFS cases. Yet, the heated debate could have continued much longer, with some extreme defence of the XMRV hypothesis (J. Mikovitz) and with a more balanced overview of the criticisms by R. Silverman (see for example, his excellent review in Nature Reviews of Urology, extensively discussing criticisms) [4]. Examples of debates on possible infectious agents present in human cancers are abundant in the literature: for PCa, HPVs are still extensively discussed as potential etiological agents or onset-cofactors see discussion in Sections 4.3 (3) and 4.3.1 (c). What or who was capable of rescinding the "Gordian Knot" of XMRV cancer/CFS association ? If we want to name a single scientist this is certainly John Coffin, although he extensively collaborated with other groups, especially with the group of S. Pathak. And yet, Coffin himself had written with J. Stoye in *Science,* accompanying one of the first papers on XMRV discovery -that of Lombardi et al. on the CFS association [30]- a positive editorial comment, which emphasized the future potential of such discovery [31].

i. It may be instructive in this respect to re-analyse –so to speak: *after the facts-* the three major editorials, which accompanied the three major discovery-articles associated with XMRV. The first is the article by Dong et al. in PNAS at the beginning of 2007 [16], therefore immediately after publication of the Urisman et al. paper (December 2006). This article really gave credibility to the XMRV hypothesis, by showing that the virus was: 1. capable of replication in human cells, once a complete copy of the provirus was cloned and reconstructed; 2. responsive to the IFN pathway, as it had been predicted in view of the RNase L mutations; 3. uses a specific receptor, XPR-1 (therefore capable of mediating entrance for both xenotropic and polytropic retroviruses) for infecting human cells; 4. in three cases analysed, XMRV was integrated in tumour cells in regions surrounding potentially interesting/important genes, in two cases next to transcription factor genes (CREB and NFAT) and in the third, next to a hormone response gene, causing inhibition of androgen receptor trans-activation (APPB2/PAT1/ARA67). The accompanying editorial, by retro-virologist Hung Fan, is certainly the most cautious and critical of the three editorials [43]. Although underlying the potential importance of these findings, Fan clearly indicated that they were generating more questions than answers and that only by answering such questions could the XMRV hypothesis be strengthened or proven [43]. In one sentence, his cautionary criticism was particularly evident: *"However, another possibility is that XMRV is not causal to PC, but reflective of the reduced antiviral status of RNase L QQ individuals; another novel virus whose sequences were not detectd by the ViroChip might be the relevant agent"* (bold characters are my additions) [43].

ii. The second fundamental paper for the XMRV hypothesis was the one by Lombardi et al. (2009), in which an astonishing 67% XMRV presence was documented in Chronic Fatigue Syndrome samples [30]. The paper was already briefly described, as well as the strong critical reaction it has generated, although this section is covered in more depth in the NMD review (see [1]) [30]. Surprisingly, the accompanying editorial written by John Coffin and Jonathan Stoye, appears to emphasize the positive aspects of these findings, rather than caution the readers about potential pitfalls, such as contaminations/artefacts [31]. It is apparent that the two Editorialists, among the major experts in mouse retro-virology, believed in 2009 that XMRV had strong connection to CFS, although it should be reminded that other viral infections have been previously associated with CFS (EBV, HHSV-6, HTLV etc., see [1]) [31]. And yet Coffin's with Pathak's groups eventually *"put the nails into the XMRV coffin one by one"* [44]. Far from being a "changing party" episode, reassessment of scientific data and even of personal believes is an essential and intrinsic process of scientific endeavour. One of the greatest epistemologists of past century, Karl Popper, has identified in the process of empirical *falsification* one of the essential logical characters of science in western world. In his *"All Life is Problem Solving"* Popper suggests that our scientific theories develop as an evolutionary (almost *Darwinian*) process, in which it is however *falsification* rather than *verification* the discriminating instrument (*Occam's razor*). Therefore, it is just natural and physiological that today in science, hypotheses and theories are continuously re-evaluated and reassessed, although in this process strong intellectual honesty and courage are also needed. Most likely, in 2009 Coffin/Stoye positively reacted and were convinced by 1. the fact that XMRV demonstrated a clear homology to MLV endogenous sequences, but different enough and with constant/homologous difference (approximately 10% throughout the viral genome) to let us believe that this was a totally new isolate. 2. The fact that all XMRV isolates detected showed strong homology among each other (less than 30 nucleotide variations in a genome of over 8000 bp.s), could be again evidence of an exogenous infecting agent (but also a contaminating virus). 3. Somehow, the general homology of XMRV with endogenous MLVs of approx. 90% may have been misleading still in 2009, since it might have suggested a mechanism of constant mutation accrual, as in phylogenetic analysis, of which the two editorialists are great experts [31]. In XMRV, however, recombination plays a major and determining role, as it was initially suggested in a PNAS editorial one year later, by Andrew Mason and colleagues (accompanying the third XMRV/MLV paper by Lo et al.) [34] [32].

iii. Lo's paper initially appeared (or it was presented as) confirmatory of the infection hypothesis in CFS, since a murine retroviral sequence was detected in 86.5% of cases and only 7% of controls [32] [34]. The viral sequences however were not identical or very similar to XMRV, as previously reported, and appeared to be related to endogenous Polytropic retroviruses (PMLV). This generated some scepticism, as in previous work the viral sequences had little difference from the prototype retrovirus -XMRV. In his editorial, Mason underlines some discrepancies and yet does not clearly indicate that the finding of one xenotropic and one polytropic retroviruses are incompatible [34]. In other words, a general misconception could be –and apparently was- generated: there is an endogenous-like mouse retrovirus infecting cells in prostate carcinoma and CFS. In this scenario, *apparently* it didn't really matter whether it was marked with a P or with a X (for Polytropic and Xenotropic): the relevant and important point was that some type of murine endogenous-like retrovirus was infecting *Homo sapiens* in such disorders [34]. The paper by Ila Singh was also in line with such (mis-)interpretation [33]. On the other hand, as also pointed out in the previous editorial by Coffin and Stoye, the strength of the original XMRV hypothesis laid in the fact that all the isolates were similar to each other, although the prototype of XMRV appeared to be unique, different from any retrovirus known at that time [31]. Furthermore, Mason group's editorial suggested that, while the issue of which retrovirus exactly is present in PCa and/or CFS was being solved, a realistic and effective strategy could have been to test already potential therapeutic approaches with antiretroviral agents [34]. Again, such attitude is logically biased by the *caveat* that there was no firm evidence at that time for the real involvement of a retrovirus in both human conditions: this has been completely confirmed now by XMRV falsification. In fact, the paper by Lo et al. was rather good evidence *against* involvement of a retrovirus in both human conditions, since it suggested that contamination could be the cause [32]. Contamination, although denied in Lo's paper by a series of counter evidences, could explain the association with an endogenous murine polytropic retrovirus and, by extension, also with XMRV [32]. Andrew Mason group's editorial also emphasized the fact XMRV sequences appeared to be the result of recombinatory events [34]. They observed that in XMRV, while the 5′ portion of its genome shares great homology to polytropic murine retroviruses, the 3′ end is most similar to endogenous xenotropic MLV [34].

2.7. XMRV falsification

This observation, that inescapably leads to presence of recombination, was further developed approximately one year later in a seminal article by the groups of J. Coffin and S. Pathak [45]. In this Science paper in May 2011, Paprotka et al. convincingly showed that XMRV was generated by recombination during passage of the original tumor cells in nude mice [45]. The creation of human cell line 22 Rv1 was reported in 1999 after several passages by xenotransplantation, starting from 1993. The late passages /established cell line display presence of several copies of integrated XMRV provirus as well as high titers of virus production (10^{10}-10^{11} PFU/ml). However, Paprotka et al. established a few essential and undermining criticisms: 1. First of all, fully infectious XMRV could not be detected in the original tumor explant (less than 1 copy/200 cells). 2. Second, two regions of strong homology with endogenous viruses could be detected: the 5′-end (called preXMRV-2) displays strong homology to PMLV endogenous sequences, while the 3′-end region (called PreXMRV-1) is most similar to an endogenous xenotropic retrovirus (XMLV). 3. Third, highly infectious "recombinant" XMRV started to appear in xenografts passaged in nude mice since 1996, i.e., three years after initial establishment of this tumour xenografts. This strongly suggests that infectious XMRV was created or has infected these cells between 1993 and 1996. 4. Fourth, the original nude mice strains utilized in xenotransplantation experiments did contain as endogenous viruses both the endogenous xenotropic virus (pre-XMRV-1, present in 6 out of 48 tested and typical of European mouse strains) as well as the endogenous PMLV (preXMRV-2, present in 25 out of 48 tested and typical of Asian mouse strains). 5. Fifth, the overall structure of the infectious XMRV could be explained by six recombinatory events between the two viruses: preXMRV-2 and preXMRV-1. Indeed, recombination is known to frequently occur during retrovirus replication, due to a polymerase (i.e., reverse transcriptase) switching between two different templates, therefore a mechanism of *"copy-choice"* as compared to the classical mechanism of *"cut-and-paste"* typical of general recombination [45] [46]. 6. Finally, the presence of a unique XMRV structure after so many recombinatory events strongly indicates that this *"creation"* occurred only once, most likely during xenograft passaging into nude mice [45]. The paper by Poprotka et al. therefore concluded the "XMRV Odyssey" with a most logical and well proven explanation and XMRV-falsification [45].

Additional evidence against XMRV as an exogenous virus infecting the human species were also obtained by the group of Jay Levy, who analysed some of the same CFS samples initially studies by Lombardi et al. Since these patients, initially reported as XMRV-positive, were found devoid of this retrovirus, this finding once more strengthened the evidence for contamination in positive samples [47]. A series of subsequent papers then reported evidence for contamination [45] [44] [48] [49] [50] in: 1. PCR reagents (even Taq polymerase) employed for XMRV detection; 2. microtomes or blades for tumours sections (even one year after the initial experiment); 3. contamination of several cell lines, beside the original 22Rv1. Prostate carcinoma cells lack the APOBEK-GA3 activity and are therefore susceptible to XMRV infection, while other human cells –for example human lymphocytes- appear to be highly resistant in view of the strong mutagenic activity of APOBEK-GA3.

3. MFV as potential candidate in PCa

Together with criticism of XMRV as potential candidate for CFS, we presented data in July 2010 [1] related to a novel viral candidate for both PCa and CFS: Micro-Foci inducing Virus or MFV. While the more specific aspects related to CFS association are presented elsewhere [1], MFV properties which link this virus to PCa will be here described.

3.1. Cancer Cluster Genetic Data

Micro-Foci inducing Virus was initially discovered in a paediatric tumor diagnoses-association generally defined as *"Cancer-Cluster"* (CC). A CC of neuroblastoma (NB) cases was diagnosed in Southern Louisiana in 1987-88 in the small town of Morgan City, while also the surrounding area appeared to be affected. A 12 fold increased NB incidence was recorded for a period of 18 months, while diagnoses then decreased to none [51]. This is a typical epidemiological behaviour of CCs, as it has been also recorded in other instances, such as paediatric leukaemia/lymphoma clusters [52]. Most of the tumours of this CC were conveyed to the Ochsner Foundation Research Center for further genetic analysis. The majority of them (66%) displayed elevated MYCN amplification, a well-known marker of aggressive NB. In one tumour with extremely elevated MYCN amplification (1000X the diploid value of controls), we started witnessing an elevated genetic instability in cultured tumor cells (see Fig. 1) [51]. This was accompanied by appearance of very small foci (Micro-Foci, MF) of rounded and refractile cells growing on top of the mesenchimal cells which typically grew up slowly and as monolayer in the initial tumor cultures (1ary cultures) [51] [53]. Furthermore, the initial dramatic amplification of MYCN seemed to disappear in growing primary cultures, apparently diluted out by the growth of mesenchimal flat cells (Fig. 1).

3.2. Isolation of MFV/MFRVs, partial cloning/sequencing

In order to find an explanation for this phenomenon, it was also noticed that the number of MFs was extremely variable, with some cultures having hundreds while others being devoid of them. An assay was therefore established by utilizing supernatants from cultures with hundreds MFs, with which we infected cells devoid of them. Since MF formation could be reproducibly transmitted even after ultra-filtration of such supernatants (through 100 μm filters), presence of a virus was hypothesized and confirmed by Electron Microscopy (EM). Transmission EM detected cytoplasmic particles of 65-73 nm for MFV (Fig. 2), while similar particles of larger size (85-92 nm) were identified in samples of paediatric lymphoma cases (MFV related Virus or MFRV), studied a few years later in Switzerland [51] [53] (Fig. 3).

Molecular cloning and partial sequencing of MFV/MFRV genome convincingly demonstrated that they share strong homology with members of the Reoviridae family, particularly Reovirus-3 (Dearing Strain) (Fig. 4).

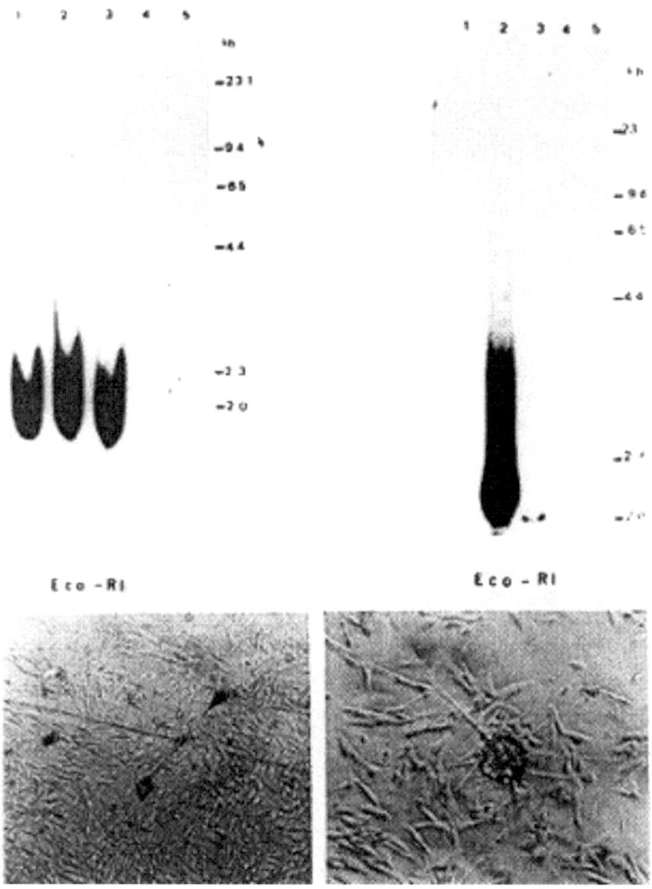

Figure 1. Top-left: Southern-blotting analysis shows high level of MYCN amplification in the original NB tumour from a Cancer-Cluster in Southern Louisiana. Lanes 1-3 contain DNA extracted from the original NB tumour, while lanes 4-5 two control DNAs (patient and normal blood donor peripheral leukocytes). Amplification was evaluated as 1000X fold by dilution experiments (not shown). Top-right: Southern-blotting analysis of DNA from the original tumour (lane 2) and from tumour cells passaged in culture for 2 weeks (lane 3) and 4 weeks (lanes 4-5). Bottom left: two microfoci, composed by small, rounded neuronal cells growing on top of a monolayer of large flat mesenchimal cells with Schwann cell markers. Lower magnification (40 X). Microfocus shown at higher magnification (100X).

http://dx.doi.org/10.5772/54054

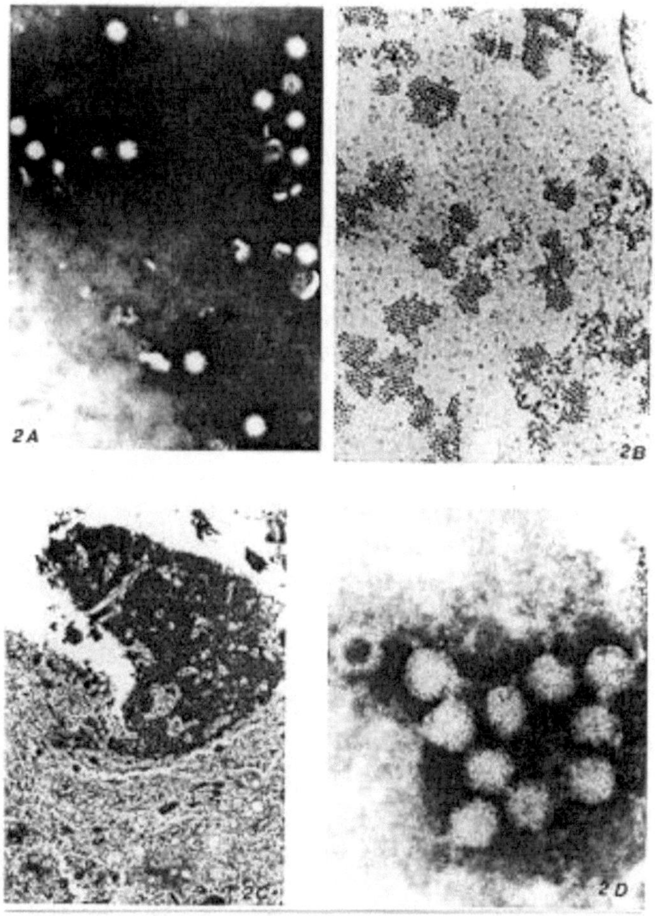

Figure 2. Electron Microscopy of MFV particles. 2A: negative staining of MFV particles (magnification = 100.000X). 2B and 2C: MFV viral "factories" in the cytoplasms of infected and transforming cells (magnifications: 15.000 and 10.000 respectively). 2D: Negative staining of MFV highest magnification (350.000X).

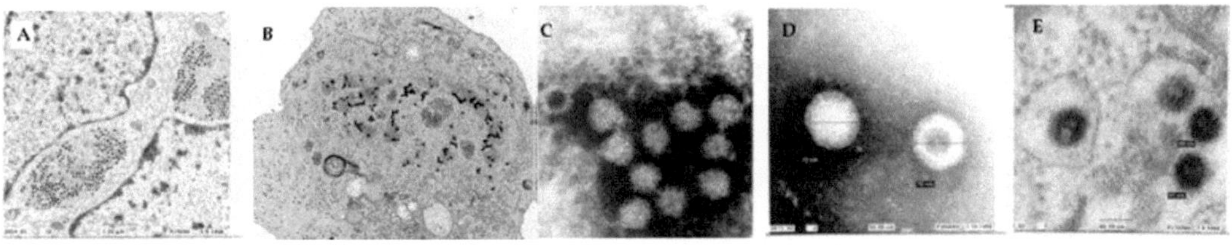

Figure 3. Electron Microscopy of MFV and MFRV particles. In 3A: MFV particles display a more localized pattern (15K X magnification), while in 3B, MFRV are spread through cell cytoplasm (5K X magnification). Fig.s 3C displays MFV at 350K X magnification (as in 2D) and Fig.s 3D-E MFRVs at 300K X and 175K magnification, respectively).

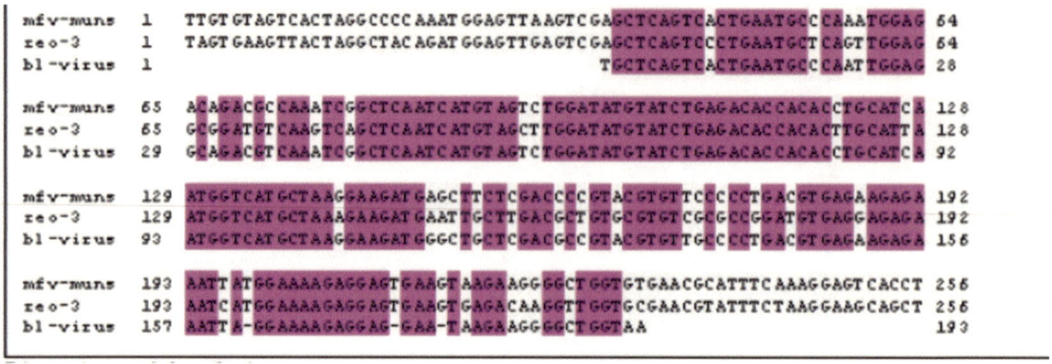

Figure 4. Comparison of sequences for Micron-NS –μNS- gene from MFV, a classical Reoviridae (Reovirus-3) and one isolate from Burkitt's Lymphoma (BL). Divergence from Reo-3 is approximately 20%.

3.3. MFV-transformed cells growth *in vitro* and *in vivo*

Furthermore, extensive work *in vitro* and *in vivo* has convincingly shown that MFV causes malignant transformation in vitro and tumours in animals (see Fig.s 5-8) [51] [53].

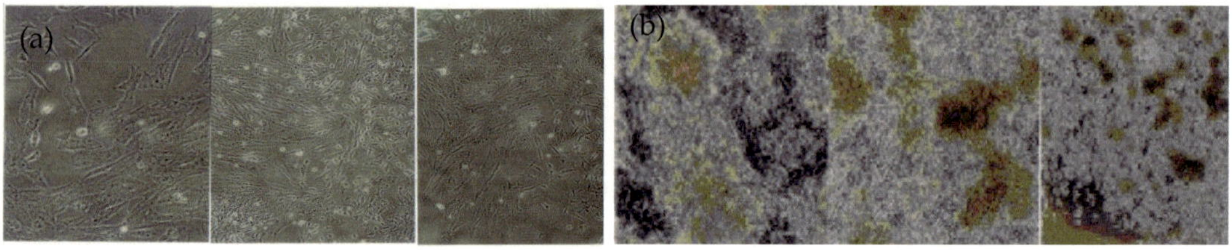

Figure 5. As shown in Fig. 5A normal, quasi-diploid SK-N-SH cells grow as mesenchimal cell (or Schwann-Cells) monolayers, but after MFV infection they transform (Fig. 5B) into aggressively growing NB cells. Transformed cells extensively grow in these *in vitro* conditions in the presence of low serum (2%), forming masses of rounded, small and packed cells (similar to MFs), which are loosely attached to the mesenchimal cell monolayer, othen floating in the medium supernatant.

Fig. 5 shows the different patterns of growth of uninfected neuroblastic SK-N-SH cells (a) and MFV-infected/transformed SK-N-SH (b). While the original SK-N-SH cells grow slowly in low serum conditions (Fig. 6), MFV-transformed cells are undistinguishable in their growth properties from cells obtained from aggressive NB tumours -for example, SK-N-BE cells (Fig. 6).

3.4. Carcinogenesis Mechanism(s)

The molecular mechanism of carcinogenesis induced by MFV has been partially clarified when it became evident that normal non-tumorigenic diploid neuroblasts are rapidly destroyed by MFV infection: most monolayers are "wiped-out" in 36-72 hrs [54] [53] [55]. The only cells, which appear to sustain MFV infection without extensive apoptosis, have ampli-

http://dx.doi.org/10.5772/54054

fied the *MYCN* locus [54]. In Fig. 7, in the left panel, Southern blotting analysis (employing a *MYCN* specific probe) of the cell line *SK-N-AS* shows that the *MYCN* is diploid in mock-infected cells (-), but becomes highly amplified (approx. 100X) upon MFV infection and relative transformation (line 2: *SK-N-AS* +). A similar result was obtained with cell line *VA-N-BR* (3rd lane) [51]. Similar results were also obtained with cell line *SK-N-SH* (which is also initially diploid and non-tumorigenic in nude mice) by Q-PCR analysis. Upon MFV infection, these cells acquire a *MYCN* DNA level intermediate between the mock-infected cells (yellow, green lines) and cell line *IMR-32* (MYCN amplification approx. 20X: black line): SH-10 cells (i.e., MFV-infected *SK-N-SH)* display an amplification level –by comparison- of approximately 10X (blue line).

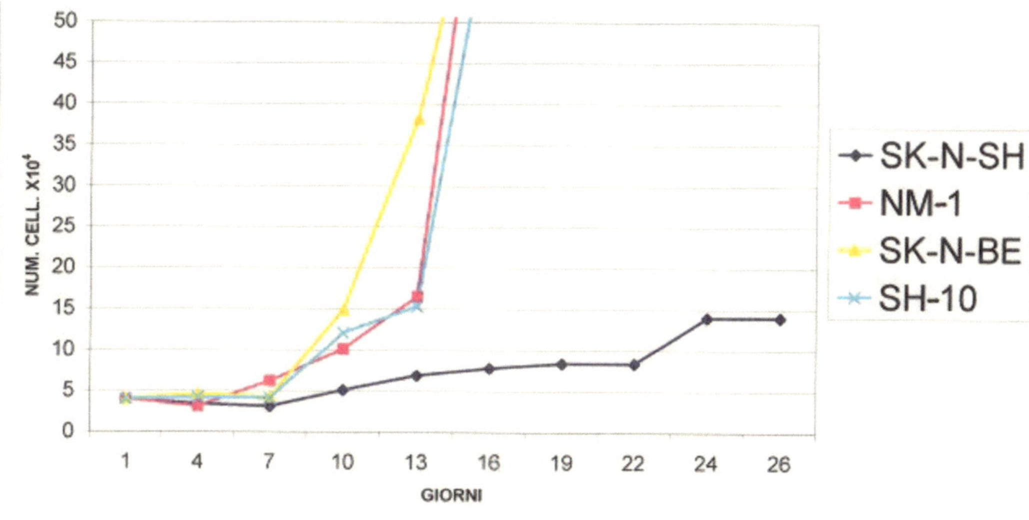

Figure 6. All cells were grown in Dulbecco's Modified MEM with the addition of 2 % Foetal Bovine Serum (FBS). NM-1 and SH-10 are two different clones of MFV- transformed SK-N-SH cells, while SK-N-BE is a a Neuroblastoma cell line established from an aggressive tumour with MYCN amplification.

The same MFV-infected/transformed *SK-N-SH* cells -, shown in previous page [53]- were also employed in *in vivo* experiments of nude mice inoculation and relative tumour growth. Inoculation of MFV-transformed SK-N-SH cells into the left flank of a nude mouse causes the appearance of large tumoral masses of NB cells (uninfected SK-N-SH cells were injected in the contra-lateral flank as control, Fig. 8).

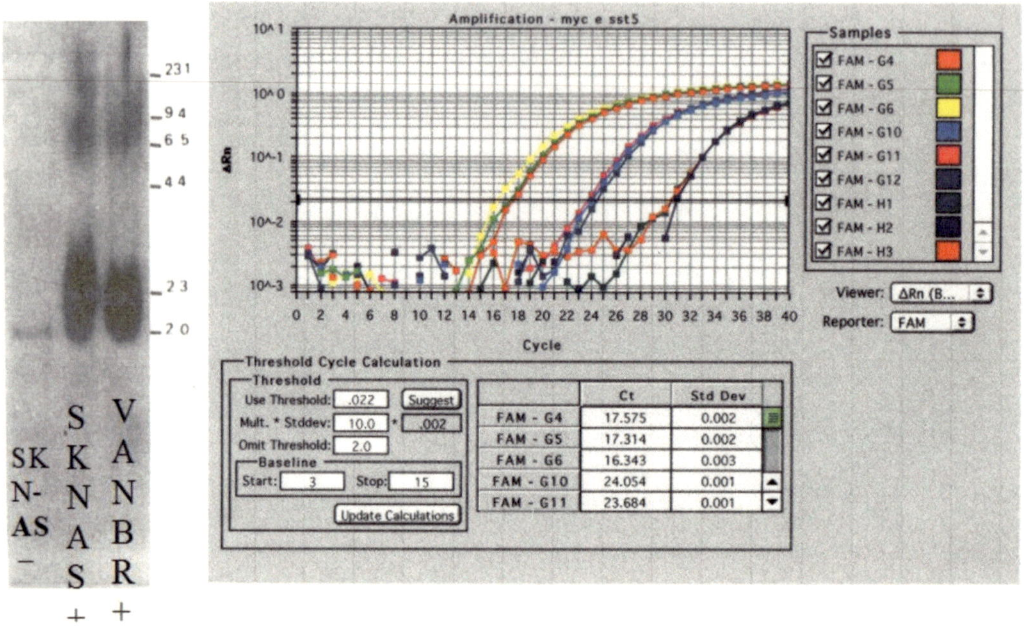

Figure 7. Southern Blotting and Q-PCR analysis of genomic DNA from cells infected/transformed by MFV. Left panel: Southern blotting analysis of cell line SK-N-AS before (lane 1) and after (lane 2) MFV infection; in lane 3, cell line SK-N-VR after infection/transformation with MFV (see also text description). Right panel: Q-PCR analysis of SK-N-SH cell DNA, DNA from SH-10 (the same line infected/transformed by MFV) and DNA from IMR-32 a cell line from aggressive neuroblastoma with MYCN amplification (approximately 20X). The relative level of MYCN amplification in SH-10 cells is estimated –by comparison- in the order of 10X.

4. Evidence for the association between MFV/MFRVs and prostate cancer

4.1. The Interferon (IFN) pathway

Evidence presented so far indicate that 1. in prostate carcinoma, an interferon-sensitive pathway appears to be affected. Attempts to identify an infectious agent (also on the basis of these observations), had led to identification of XMRV, a candidate virus, which has been eventually falsified by several groups (see part 1). However, as it has been emphasized in this chapter, evidence for viral involvement in PCa are rather strong and independent from the particular isolate XMRV. Indeed, as previously underlined, XMRV isolation is based upon usage of *viro-chip* technology and logical inference analysis predicts that this step is most error-prone [1]. In order to list and underline numerous elements indicating MFV as a strong candidate, the general IFN pathway is here considered and RNase-L as next point.

Although RNase-L is also an essential part of IFN pathway, it will be discussed separately, since it is prominent in view of numerous evidence and studies performed in PCa and other pathologies. Furthermore, the fact that transgenic animals *knockouts* for *RNASEL* gene do not develop tumours at higher frequency, suggests that additional elements in the IFN pathway may also be relevant [56] [57]. Since several years ago, the IFN pathways has been extensively dissected: beside RNase-L, two additional pathways are prominent: a) the PKR signal transduction and b) the Adenosine-Deaminase of RNA (ADAR) mechanism.

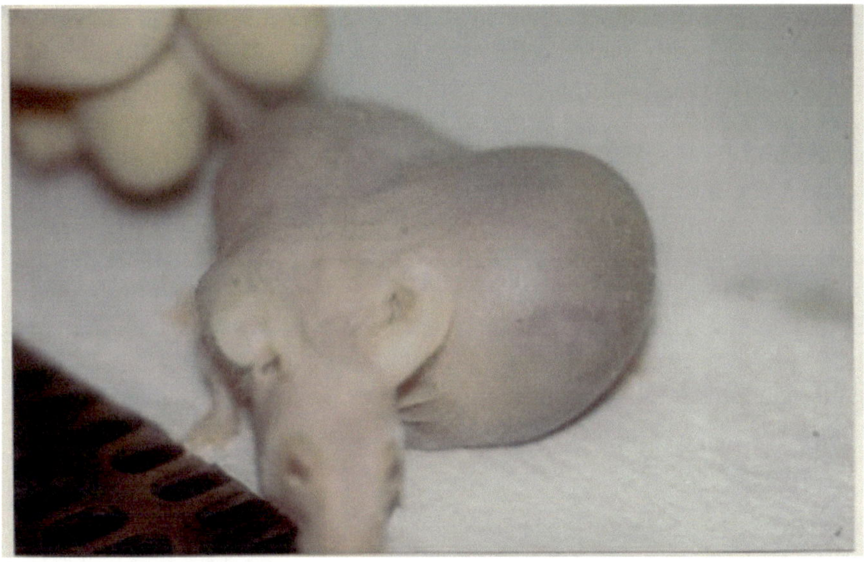

Figure 8. Tumorigenesis in nude-mice of SK-N-SH cells infected/transformed by MFV. Injection of 10^7 SK-N-SH cells (right flank) or SH-10 clone (left flank) with the same number of MFV-transformed SK-N-SH cells shows the outgrowth 3 weeks later of large tumoral masses in the case of MFV-infected/transformed cells (SH-10). Histological analysis confirmed the presence of human neuroblastoma cells after xenotransplantation [53].

4.1.1. PKR

PKR was one of the best characterized pathways in the IFN signal transduction, starting from pioneering work of Isaacs and Lindenman, who initially characterized the IFN activity [58] [59]. One of the first enzymatic activities induced by IFN and its inducers (i.e., dsRNAs) is the dsRNA dependent Protein Kinase or PKR. PKR conveys the IFN message in several ways but especially by phosphorylation of: 1. PKR itself (autocatalysis); 2. the α subunit of eIF-2a ; 3. the inhibitor of transcription factor NFkB, IkB, thus releasing such inhibition; 4. the TAT transcription factor, essential activator of HIV; 5. the NFAT protein and 6. the phosphoprotein MPP4, which binds dsRNA and is activated during the M phase of cell cycle [58] [59] [60]. Among the different activities elicited by PKR activation, the best studied and known is certainly the inhibitory effect on protein synthesis (eIF-2a) [61]. Ser-51 Phosphorylation in this case blocks initiation of protein synthesis, by inhibiting the exchange of guanine nucleotide [61] [62] [63]. There are some discussions and discrepancies on the regulation of PKR from different portions of the gene/structure: two knockout transgenic mice were generated by the groups of Karomillas/Bell [64] and Ch. Weissmann [65] [66].

The first one has been targeted in the carboxy-terminal of PKR, where is present the kinase activity, and doesn't show impairment of antiviral response or TNF-α responses, thus indicating the redundant role of PK activity [60, 64]. To the contrary, Weissmann's lab ko mouse and its MEFs are strongly inhibited in view of the deletion of the NH2- portion of the protein, where the dsRNA-binding domain of PKR resides [65] [66] [60]. Effectors of PKR are several types of dsRNA molecules, both artificial and natural [67]. In this respect, the genome of MFV is a strong/ideal inducer of PKR in acutely infected cells, as we have documented in both mouse and human cells. Most likely, PKR induction also contributes to the strong apoptotic effects we have documented 36-72 hours post-infection [53]. In particular, MFV-infected cells completely block protein synthesis and strongly impair rRNA production (see later) and these effects seem to be mediated by PKR and RNase-L respectively. In prostate cancer, the same pathway of PKR appears to be downstream of another essential regulator and also Tumor Suppressor function of prostate cells: PTEN [68]. Therefore, typically the deletion of PTEN (which is extremely common in prostate cancer [69]) will lead to ablation of the TSG function of PKR by phosphorylation of eIF-2a and block of protein synthesis [68] [69]. In view of the MFV/MFRV connection hypothesis, it is speculated that infection by this family of viruses will eventually cause/select for PTEN deletion, as this will inhibit cellular apoptosis, which would otherwise be inescapable [53] [55] [69].

4.1.2. ADAR

The additional and last form of IFN response here considered is the RNA-specific Adenosine Deaminase or ADAR, which is strongly induced after viral infection [70] [71]. Although such RNA editing was initially considered a rare phenomenon, almost a curiosity of RNA regulation and fine tuning, extensive genomic sequencing by NGS and high-throughput technologies have allowed to discern considerable editing in several DNA genomic sequences by a related Deaminase activity which targets DNA, called APOBEC, as well as ADAR activity on expressed mRNAs [72] [73] [74]. It is still not clear how efficient such mechanism may be at the RNA level, since ADAR activity may protect cells but also favour virus aggression or persistence inside infected cells [70]. DNA deaminase activity as well is still poorly understood, but new phenomena discovered in human cancer cells through Next Generation Sequencing (NGS) technology suggest that genome modulation and plasticity by APOBEC could also play a major role in carcinogenesis [73] [75].

Could the ADAR activity induced by Interferon (ADAR-1) be responsible for important antiviral effects in human and other cells ? Although the question is still open and there are also examples of opposite regulation as previously mentioned –for example in Hepatitis Delta Virus (HDV) [70]-, important inhibitory effects were documented, with Measles Virus [76] [77] and with Influenza Virus in mouse cells [78]. Furthermore, a specific gene of the Adenovirus genome is responsible for counteracting the RNA-editing activity of ADAR: the VAI gene [79]. In the case of Reoviridae, little is still known but there is at least one animal model in which ADAR was induced by both artificial dsRNA and reoviridae genome (which obviously is dsRNA), although the response modality of ADAR appeared quite different [80] [81].

Among human cancer as well very little is known, particularly in the case of prostate carcinoma [82] [73]. More data have been obtained in the case of brain tumours, since ADAR is known to effect important editing in brain neurons. In at least two tumour examples, hypoediting seems to characterize cancer cells. In *glioblastoma multiforme*, rectification of a mutated permeable glutamate receptor to Ca++-impermeable receptor suppressed proliferation [83] [84], while in hypo-editing astrocytoma cells, re-balancing editing expression induced regression [85]. Additional work on ADAR/APOBEC in prostatic cancer and reoviridae is certainly warranted.

4.2. RNase-L, an essential pathway

The clearest evidence for viral involvement in prostate carcinoma and in human cancer in general was obtained through studies of the IFN response leading to RNase-L activation. The general scheme of IFN genes activation has been clarified through years of intense studies with several models, cell lines, laboratory and transgenic animals, in vitro assays and molecular/biochemical systems [60] [86]. Without getting into too many details –and referring instead the readers to some excellent review articles on this subject [60] [86] [87] [88] - two general types of IFN molecules are known: viral IFN and immune IFN. Both IFN-α and IFN- β (as well as IFN-omega) belong to the viral form, induced by viral infection [60], while the immune form is essentially composed by IFN−γ and is induced by immune stimulation. Focusing on viral genes, this is a rather large family in humans, since 13 genes for IFN-α, 1 for IFN-β and one for IFN-omega were mapped on the short arm of human chromosome 9 [89] [90]. None of these genes contains introns, while the only IFN gene with introns is the IFN-γ form with 3, on the long arm of chromosome 12. Two types of IFN receptors, IFNAR-1 and IFNAR-2 are known on human chromosome 21: they must heterodimerize for activation by IFN-α/β [91] [92] [93]. The following signalling is today understood mostly in the JAK-STAT transduction pathway, thanks to the work of several molecular biologists, first and foremost the group of Jim Darnell at Rockefeller University [94] [95] [96]. STATs are "signal transducers and activator of transcription" molecules: at least seven of them are known, i.e. Stat-1, Stat-2, Stat-3, Stat-4, Stat-5a, Stat-5b and Sta-6. STATs are activated by members of the Janus family of Tyrosine kinases (JAKs), of which 4 members are known, i.e. Jak-1, Jak-2, Jak-3 and Tyk-2. Various combinations of Jak's and Stat's elements are active in transducing both viral and immune IFN signalling [87] [88]. Additional important elements are the IRFs, (IFN Regulatory Factor) family [97], which cooperate in the activation of IFN-responsive genes. These are characterized by presence of regulatory elements: ISRE or IFN-stimulated Response elements [98], usually for viral IFNs and the GAS (gamma IFN activation sites) [99]. In conjunction with Stat's, IRFs constitute the so called ISGF (IFN stimulated gene factor's) [100]. Having clarified this terminology, ds-RNA activation of IFN pathway does not always or only use Jak-Stat elements. The transcription factor IRF-3 (IFN response Factor 3) acts as subunit of a complex called ds-RNA activated transcription factor complex (DRAF) by sereine/threonine phosphorylation, translocation to the nucleus, association with p300/CBP and gene activation [101]. Among the activated genes, the Oligo Adenylate Synthetase gene family, or OAS, is one of the most important, because it conveys the anti-viral signal to the next and final effector: RNase-L. In humans, three OAS genes of different sizes (proteins of 40-46 kDa -OAS1-, of 69 kDa –OAS2- and of 100 kDa -OAS3-) have been mapped on the long arm of chromosome 12 (12q24.2), thus suggesting genome duplications in *H. sapiens* [102]. Similarly to the effectors previously considered –PKR and ADAR-, OAS proteins do contain regions for binding dsRNA, the signalling and activating effector [103] [104] [105]. However, all three effectors contain separate regions with peculiar enzymatic activities: kinase, deaminase, synthethase [60]. The exact nature of dsRNA activators is not always completely clear, but hypothesized to be formed by or to contain dsRNA elements. In the case of interest, i.e. MFV/MFRVs infection, since these belong to Reoviridae family, it is clearly fragments or segments of viral genome (dsRNA) [53] [55]. Great variation has been documented in the extent/level of OAS activation and 2-5 A production [80].

Last element, RNase-L, is activated by 2-5 A signal molecules, typically oligomers with >2 elements for optimal induction, while RNase-L must dimerize for activation [106] [107]. This endoribonuclease is typically present as monomer in a latent form, essentially in every cell (tested so far), but -after 2-5 A interaction- it homodimerizes and is activated [107], although heterodimers with RLI (RNase-L inhibitor) have been also described. As previously mentioned, RNase-L gene, called RNS4, has been mapped on the long arm of chromosome 1 (1q25), on a location corresponding to the chromosomal site for the Human Prostate Carcinoma susceptibility (HPC-1) [108], as mapped with linkage studies by Jeff Trent and others [108] [6].

In view of the coincident chromosomal location of RNASEL and HPC-1 [6] [108] and the initial speculations by Lengyel and others that this gene may behave as a bona fide Tumor Suppressor [109] [12] [13], Silverman with DeRisi and Ganem undertook the described *viro-chip* high-throughput search for potential viral candidates, leading to XMRV isolation [15]. As previously described and discussed in Section 1, XMRV identification has been clearly falsified as a recombination artefact arising during xenograft transplantation in nude mice [45].

In view of the coincidental chromosomal localization of HPC-1 and RNASEL, what are the evidence for RNase-L involvement after MFV/MFRV infection ? The acute phase of infection by these viruses is accompanied by a very high activation of RNase-L [53]. An assay, detecting ribosomal RNA (rRNA) degradation in infected and transforming cells was developed (U. Rovigatti, unpublished), thus confirming the extremely high levels of RNase-L induction, often leading to block of cell proliferation and apoptosis [53] [55]. In the past several years, groups in USA, France and Belgium have also documented a strong deregulation of this endoribonuclease in patients affectd by Chronic Fatigue Syndrome. Pioneering work by Suhadolnick et al at Temple Univ. initially disclosed that 2-5 A activated RNase-L is upregulated in CFS patients [110] [111] [112]. This finding was followed up by description of a lower molecular weight form (37 kDa) of the same enzyme in CFS patients by the same group [113]. The French-Belgian group of De Meirleir et al. then showed that the 37 kDa fragment is proteolytically cleaved from the original enzyme of 87 kDa, by human elastase and/or calpain [114]. The same authors also speculated that the levels of 2–5 A molecules with structures larger than dimers (trimers/tetramers) protect the 83 kD moiety from degradation [115] [116]. Presence of the 37 kD RNase-L could also explain the higher enzymatic activity (associated with the low MW form) and the ratio between the two forms was proposed as potential marker for CFS [117] [111] [118].

In conclusion, the extremely elevated levels of RNase-L in every cell type infected by MFV indicate that this could be an important parameter to be evaluated. Analysis is being performed for addressing the question of whether cells with impaired/mutated alleles of RNase-L (such as the R462Q allele) may be more resistant to the apoptogenic effect(s) of MFV/MFRV and could become better targets for carcinogenesis [53] [55] [1].

4.3. Inflammation - ubiquitous in PCa

Inflammation has been estimated as being somehow responsible for 20% of human cancers: these are typically linked to infectious agents, causing chronic infections as well as by other environmental factors [119] [120] [121]. While it appears to be an essential component of carcinogenesis –being defined as "the seventh hallmark of cancer" [122]– inflammatory processes are particularly prominent in PCa [121] [119]. Furthermore, inflammation in PCa adds an enigmatic component, which could be or become one of the best clue for deciphering its aetiology [55]. This enigmatic nature is however rather complex, as it can be distinguished by several elements:

1. The **paradox of a rather common disease** (most common cancer among men), afflicting this year over 300.000 people and killing more than 33.000 patients, only in the US [123]. For comparison, it has been observed that there is just a handful of cases described in the literature for Primary Seminal Vesicle Carcinoma, essentially in the same anatomical location [124]. This shows a peculiar and striking difference between two very close histological sites: PCa is diagnosed only in the prostate peripheral zone, rarely in the transition zone and almost never in the central zone [125]. This pattern is accompanied by typical phenomena of inflammation which is almost never of acute type (at time of diagnosis) and is characterized in the described zones by: a. chronic inflammation, b. benign prostatic hyperplasia (BPH), d. focal atrophy, e. a new type of inflammatory response defined as prostatic inflammatory atrophy (PIA) and finally developing into f. prostatic intraepithelial neoplasia (PIN) and/or g. prostatic carcinoma (PCa) [125] [126] [127] [128]. This pattern associates with an extremely common disease, the most common form of cancer in men, again suggesting a rather "common" causality [55]. As we will also consider other clues (see 2,3,4), the best explicatory mechanism is that of a common infection, in particular an infectious agent which is "endogenous" or "persitent" in *H. sapiens* and apparently much more frequent in certain human populations or races [129] [130] (see below)

2. **Variation in epidemiological data** for Chinese, Japanese or Arab men in comparison with the male population in Western Countries: for example, men born in South East Asia who then migrated to the US acquire a higher incidence within the first two gener-

ations [130] [131] [132]. In Shri-Lanka men, the incidence was recently assessed as 5.7 per 100.000 males, while such incidence rose up by twenty folds in immigrants to the Western Countries (for example, UK) [133]. This is again indicative of "life-style" rather than genetic factors being responsible for prostate carcinogenesis. Similar data are also present in Japanese men who migrate to the US [134]. Using similar epidemiological approaches, Hsing has recently divided different nations into three risk groups for incidence and mortality of PCa. The high risk group includes USA and several European Countries; to medium risk group belong European Nations such as UK, Italy and Spain, while Asian Countries are mostly included in the third, low risk group [130]. There is a general trend of increasing incidence, which the authors attribute to westernisation of life-style in the low-risk nations, but to TUR (trans-uretral resection) and PSA-testing in the high risk Nations [130, 134]. Interestingly, the incidence in US black males is 50-60 fold higher that that in Shanghai, China [130] [135]. The data by Julian Peto and others have confirmed these trends and the rapid changes in incidence/mortality in migrant populations (often within the first generation), thus emphasizing the concept that factors different from genetics (i.e. environmental, such as infectious agents) may be responsible [129].

3. The fact that inflammation, BPH and PCa **typically occur in the prostate peripheral area**, with almost no tumours in the central zone. This led initially LM Franks to hypothesize that in prostate cancer, the inflammatory effects are always accompanied by hyperproliferation and/or atrophy/necrosis [126]. Later, McNeal et al. have elaborated the same concept, by noticing in 1988 that in the whole gland, there is a clear-cut zonal distribution [125]. Out of 88 tumours studied, the majority (68%) arose in the peripheral gland, while 24% in the transitional zone and only 8% in the central gland zone. As mentioned, this suggests that infection through ascending urethra could be a responsible/associated factor [125] [136] [119]. Although bacteria have been initially suspected as responsible for inflammatory phenomena and as causes of carcinogenesis (*Neisseria Gonorrhoeae, Clamydia Trachomatis, Trichomonas Vaginalis,* and *Treponema Pallidum*), such intepretation has been reconsidered in post-antibiotics era, since prostatic persistant bacterial infections have dramatically dropped [137]. Still, bacteria can be often grown even from expressed fluids of asymptomatic men [138]. The possible causality by viruses is still an open question, as extensively discussed in the first section on XMRV discovery and refusal. Among viruses, several have been extensively investigated throughout the years and particularly: **i.** *Cytomegalovirus (CMV)* has been investigated in view of its association with malignant transformation in vitro. Seven studies on tissues and 2 on serology do not support an association with PCa. [139] [140, 141] **ii.***Epsten Barr Virus (EBV)* levels were shown to be not significantly different in PCa/BPH by Ab's, PCR and IHC; [142] **iii.** *HHV-8* was initially detected by Chang and Moore in *Kaposi Sarcoma (KS)* by subtractive hybridisation [143]. Initial positive results in PCa by Monini et al. [144] were later explained by infiltration with lymphocytes, most likely in *HIV-1* positive (and therefore *HHV-8+*) patients [145, 146]. Also, the strongly positive findings by Hoffman in men from Trinidad and Tobago can be probably explained by bias of selected controls [147] [148]. **iv.** *Polyoma* **Viruses** have been also associated with PCa: an ini-

tial report by Monini et al. [149] was followed by an interesting paper by Das et al., since they found *BKV* DNA positivity more frequently in malignant tissue [150]. However, also these studies were not confirmed [151] [152]. **v.** *Human Papilloma Viruses (HPVs)* : Extensive work has focused on these viruses throughout the years. Their relevance was also surmised from studies on women cervical/uterine cancer –pioneered by Harald zur Hausen (Nobel Prize for Medicine in 2008)- where *HPVs* are clearly involved in >90% of cases [153]. However: i) even Zur Hausen in reviewing this subject in his Nobel lecture dismisses the role of HPVs in PCa: in this sense, men would be some kind of "healthy carriers" of the viral carcinogen [154]; ii) Several studies have been published, some of which with positive results (for example, in an Argentinean study, 42% PCa were positive versus 0% BPH samples) [155]. However, in 24 studies from other Countries, there is no evidence of different *HPV* involvement between cancer specimens and controls [156]. Furthermore, the most recent meta-analysis didn't show significant OR for PCa associated with *HPV-16* (OR = 1.09) or with *HPV-18* (OR = 1.08) infections [157]. Similar results were obtained by a recent review article (in press) [156]. iii) Another element which does not fit *HPVs* as potential carcinogens in PCa is the observation –initially made by Woodsworth [158] - that *HPV* infections do not elicit high inflammation or inflammation at all ([158], see also later discussion). As already mentioned, inflammation –most likely associated with a prostatic infection- is one of the Hallmarks of Cancer, particularly in this tumor type, PCa [122] [121].

4. Several reports (Platz; Mahmoud; Chan; Jacobs) have documented that **assumption of aspirin or Non-Steroidal Anti-Inflammatory Drugs (NSAIDs)** for different periods could considerably lower PCa risk [159] [160] [161] [162]. These studies have been expanded in recent years, particularly by the work of Mahmud with several Meta-Analyses [163] [164, 165] [166] [167]. A positive correlation has been detected for aspirin usage (protection) with OR in the range of 0.81- 0.83 and this is confirming what was already known from animal studies, which typically display stronger and clear-cut protective effects (also with NSAID). In the case of NSAID, the effect is less apparent, or maybe diluted out [166]. In most recent nested case-control studies, Mahmud has confirmed a modest but significant effect with all propionates, ie. Ibuprofen, Naproxen etc., but not with other NSAIDs [167]. The question is somehow connected also to the relationship between BPH and PCa, since the former has been often considered a precursor and initial inflammatory response leading to the latter [168] [169] [170]. Additional findings hower do not lend support to this hypothesis [171] [172]. Finally, a very recent study by Sutcliffe and others also does not show any effect for NSAID treatment in BPH as well as LUTS (Low Urinary Tract Symptoms) [173]. In either cases and also in view of the Mahmud meta-analyses, there may be a positive (protective) effect, but too small and/or diluted out [173].

4.3.1. How can this Inflammation-Scenario fit the proposed role of MFV/MFRVs

a. First of all, this family of viruses infects the human population in the first years of life. By age 5, >95% of human population displays antibodies against Reoviridae and this type of viruses have been shown to be capable of persisting in infected patients and animals for several months/years [174]. Furthermore and as discussed in the next section, MFV/MFRVs display all the features of a "Stem Cell Virus" (SCV), with features of interaction in early childhood with a developing immune system [53, 175]. That a prostate cancer stem cell may be present in PCa and targeted in the first phase of carcinogenesis has been longly hypothesized and recently confirmed [176] [177] [178]. Further studies are certainly warranted in order to assess presence of MFV/MFRVs in early childhood and during ontogeny [55].

b. Different levels/types of MFV/MFRVs appear to be present in different human populations worldwide. However, a clear picture of the specific subtypes involved is still missing, particularly for what concerns MFV/MFRVs. This should be clarified experimentally (by viral nucleic acid and specific protein detection, presence of antibodies etc.) [174]. Furthermore, essential aspects of these viruses features are still missing as we do not have full knowledge of these viruses genome sequence/structure [53]. Patterns of infections and micro/mini-epidemics in different populations could be deduced and mirrored by what is happening with Rotaviruses (another member of Reoviridae) in the paediatric population, where dominance of one particular genotype was shown to dramatically change from year to year, at least in Central and Eastern Europe [179].

c. The question of inflammation in PCa leads to the search of a causing agent in both affected patients and experimental systems. This chapter has dwelled trough different aspects of this essential question. The presented appraisal of potential responsible agents clearly indicates today a lack of credible candidates among bacterial infections. Even for viral candidates, the previous discussion showed that Herpes Viruses (CMV, EBV, and HHV-8), Polyoma Viruses and Papilloma Viruses lack some of the essential features as triggering agents [157] [156]. For all these viruses, extensive detection studies were performed for years without reaching any consensus nor obtaining evidence for their presence but in a limited percentage of cases [157] [156]. Same negative result was finally obtained for a Retrovirus, XMRV, after much controversy and discussion [4] [45] [44] [48] [49] [180], while a previously retroviral candidate (HTLV-II) had been previously falsified in the case of CFS [181] [1]. It must be stressed that the essential feature discussed here is inflammation and the two most likely candidates in the previous list, i.e. Retroviruses and Papillomaviruses do not appear to induce inflammation as expected from analysis of PCa: I) Retroviruses are known to be capable of replicating inside cells, even without causing cytopathic effects or transformation for that matter [182]; II) for HPVs, the quoted work by Woodworth has clarified this point. He wrote [158]: "*A hallmark of HPV infection is absence of an inflammatory response. Basal cells express low levels of HPV early proteins, they don't undergo lysis, and they are not rapidly recognized and destroyed by resident leukocytes such as NK cells and tissue macrophages.....HPV infections can persist and remain latent for long periods and may induce tolerance to HPV antigens..*"

To the contrary and as described in Section II, MFV/MFRVs are strongly apoptogenic and capable of inducing strong/very strong inflammatory responses in several experimental systems [53] [1]. In preliminary experiments, we have established primary cultures from approximately 20 cases of PCa. In the majority of cases, cultured cells displayed extensive cytopathic effects and did not survive for extensive passages, with three exceptions. While these results confirm previous descriptions by Frank, McNeal and by De Marzo's group [125] [126] [127] [128], they also suggest that whatever factor elicited strong inflammatory mechanisms in the prostate, with cycles of hyperplasia and of necrosis, the same factor may increase its effects during in vitro culturing [55]. We are presently testing this set of PCa tumors and relative cultures (different passages) for presence of MFV/FMRVs.

d. Although never specifically tested, sialycilic acid and similar salts have been shown to be effective for the containment/ replication-inhibition of this family of viruses (reoviridae) [183] [184]. Any strategy or molecule capable of reducing their inflammatory responses would probably elicit similar results.

4.4. Stemness in PCa: MFV as a "Stem Cell Virus"

4.4.1. Prostate Cancer stem Cell or Cells ?

Essential aspects of PCa have been here discussed with emphasis on viral models [55] [1]. In this last section of the chapter and also in dealing with peculiar aspects of PCa carcinogenesis in connection with an infecting virus (with MFV/MFRVs as potential candidates), the issue of Cancer Stem Cells (*CSC*) or *stemness* will be discussed. The concept of Cancer Stem Cell dates back to much ground work in the past two centuries, with several pioneers such as Julius Cohnheim and Rudolf Virkow already in the 19th century: they predicted the existence of *"embryonic rests"* at the origin of tumor formation [185] [186]. At the beginning of XXth century, Pappenheim hypothesized the existence of embryonic stem cells, but it was only in the second half of '900 that experimental evidence was provided for them [187]. In Toronto, in the '60s and '70s, the research of Ernest McCulloch and James Till demonstrated that only a minute fraction of myeloma cells grew in *in vitro* assays in order to form colonies in semisolid media [188, 189]. The Toronto school settled the basis for further work by John Dick (see later). In the same years, similar work was carried on by Robert Bruce, showing that only 1-4% of lymphoma cells did transplant into recipients [190], and by Jim Griffin, who demonstrated low clonogenic potential for Acute Myelogenous Leukaemia cells growing in methylcellulose [191]. Three additional lines of research paved the way for the final development of CSC hypothesis. 1. Mutations or translocations were discovered in cells at birth, which became markers of leukaemia-precursor cells (i.e., TEL-AML1, MLL-AF4, AML-ETO, OTT-MAL): these cells behave as leukaemia stem cells, since they could differentiate into several lineages/compartments, while additional mutations were required for achievment of full-leukemogenesis [192] [193] [194] [52], 2. the work of Peter Fialkow clearly indicated clonal expansions of leukaemia stem cells in specific diseases such as CML, AML and Myelodisplastic Syndromes (MDS) [195] [196]. Most of this work was carried on using genetic markers such as G6PD, present on the X chromosomes: in females, one of the X is silenced by the so-called lyonization phenomenon (from Mary Lyon's work) [197], thus allowing to distinguish the expansion of individual clones in cases of heterozygosity (for ex., A/B alleles for G6PD) [198] [199]; 3. The work of A. Hamburger and S. Salmon in Tucson,

AZ, who also showed low frequency ($1/10^{-3}$ to $1/10^{-4}$) of colony formation from solid tumours [200, 201]. These experiments were, however only partly convincing or reproducible (for example, in S. Salmon's work) and further ethical questions and concern were raised by experiments of C. Sautham and A. Brunschwig who injected harvested cancer cells into the same cancer patients, again discovering that only large numbers (i.e., 10^6) were capable of tumor iniriation [42]. Only at the end of the 80's and with the advent of authomated high-speed Fluresecence Activated Cell Sorting (FACS) [202], the group of John Dick in Toronto was capable of convincingly and reproducibly demonstrating the existence of Leukemic Stem Cells (LSCs). This was accomplished by xenotransplantation assays, in which LSCs from AML were transplanted into Severe Combined Immunodeficient (SCID) mice, often crossed with Non-Obese Diabetic (NOD) mice, in which also the natural immune response (NK cells) is defective [203] [204]. In order to demonstrate stemness, these experiments had to prove the three essential features of stem cells, i.e. a. their capability of remaining dormant, b. their pluripotency, being capable of reproducing the full spectrum of cancer (i.e. leukaemia) phenotype; c. their capability of self-renewal by asymmetric division, thus, giving rise to both bulk tumour cells and their immature precursors [205] [206]. The paper by Bonnet and Dick in 1997 is considered the first clear-cut demonstration of the LSC concept by xenotransplantation [207]. Subsequently, the same concept (Cancer Stem Cell or CSC) was also proven in solid tumours, initially in breast cancer by Al-Hajj et al. in 2003, where the CSC was shown to be CD44+CD24-/low lineage [208]. However, additional markers were subsequently identified in breast cancer, one of the most interesting ones being Aldehyde Dehydrogenase (ALDH), which appears to affect the phenotype of cancer cells, being associated to capacity of detoxification and a more aggressive behaviour also in other types of CSC [209] [210]. ALDH however doesn't seem to be an universal marker, as it is not, for example, associated with a more aggressive phenotype in melanoma cells [211]. Another controversial issue in recent years has concerned the frequency of Cancer Stem Cells (CSC) in different tumours. For example, a recent paper by Quintana et al. calculated that with an assay employing NOD/SCID IL2Rg mice, up to 25% of melanoma cells were tumorigenic [212]. Similar controversies are also present for the identification of prostate CSC [176] [177] [178]. In fact, two different populations of SC and prospective CSC were isolated in PCa [213] [214]. An initial paper in Nature described regeneration of the whole prostate from a single basal cell, which in addition to classical markers of prostate cell differentiation (Sca-1+, CD133+, CD44+) also displayed presence of c-KIT receptor (CD117+) [215]. However, a subsequent paper by the group of Michael Shen convincingly showed that among luminal cells, rare precursors exist which display presence of the homeobox gene NKx3-1 in absence of androgens and are therefore called castration-resistant Nkx3-1 expressing cells (CARNs) [216]. These cells can reconstitute prostate ducts after transplantation and, upon deletion of the suppressor gene PTEN, rapidly form carcinomas *in vivo* [216]. Finally, the group of Owen Witte has recently shown that it is also a basal cell which can initiate tumorigenesis in nude mice through cooperation of AKT, ERG and androgen receptor [217]. It is therefore possible that more than one precursor stem cell is the target of malignant transformation in prostate cancer. Furthermore, this could also fit with the described PCa carcinogenesis, in which a rather diffuse "field effect" has been known for some time [218] [219].

4.4.2. Evidence for MFV as Stem Cell Virus, possibly involved in PCa Carcinogenesis.

a. In initial preliminary experiments, we have shown that dilutions of MFV/MFRVs for several log.s (from 10^{-2} to 10^{-8} FFU/ml) will cause a similar number of transformants, thus indicating that the limiting factor was not the virus itself, but rather its target. Since an equal number of precursor stem cells are believed to be present in such cultures, it is hypothesized that the target is indeed a SC [1].

b. The Micro-Foci induced by MFV have several features of deranged stem cells, in which genetic aberrations took place, such as MYCN amplification in neuroblasts and t(8;14) / t(2;8) in paediatric lymphomas (BL-type). Even the so-called organoids or tumorspheres of PCa (prostaspheres) have similar fetures of MFs: we are now performing experiments in order to convert normal prostate tissue/cell lines into prostaspheres by MFV infection [53].

c. As mentioned, PCa is characterized by an initial oligoclonality, which underlines carcinogenesis through a "field-effect" (FE). Evidence of oligoclonality were also obtained by molecular biology studies (see next point). However a molecular explanation for FEs is still lacking [218] [219]: MFV/MFRVs could explain FE alterations in view of the slowly progressing infection, mostly through cell-to-cell contacts [53] [55].

d. In approximately 50% of PCa, peculiar translocations TMPRSS2-ERG have been detected, which join together an androgen regulated gene: the transmembrane protease serine 2 gene, TMPRSS2, with at least 26 different genes for transcription factors [220] [221, 222]. Although data on association of translocations with PCa aggressiveness are controversial, the translocation is an excellent marker of clonality (individual breakpoints): they have shown initial existence of oligoclonal disease, further evolving into monoclonality during metastatic disease [223].

e. We have shown in several experiments –and previously discussed in section 2- that MFV/MFRVs infection is associated or causing peculiar genetic aberrations such as MYCN amplification (I.E., Fig. 7) or t(8;14) / t(2;8) translocations in paediatric lymphoma [53]. Similarly, we hypothesize that the associated translocations induced by MFV/ MFRVs in prostate cells are TMPRSS2-ERG translocations, which would confer resistance to virus-induced apoptosis [55]. Experiments are being carried out in several PCa biopsies already characterized for presence of translocations (in 25% of cases).

5. Summary and conclusion

In this chapter, a review of general literature, as well as data previously published or unpublished by the author, was presented with the specific aim of fostering an ongoing debate on prostate cancer aetiology. This debate was particularly spurred in the past six years by the controversy arising after isolation of a new retrovirus, highly homologous to endogenous xenotropic and polytropic murine retroviruses, called XMRV [55] [1].

The first part of the chapter has focused on XMRV, its isolation and eventual falsification, also as a "parable" of scientific trajectories and behaviours in science. The most heated episodes are probably missing (but the reader could easily find them in some well-written editorials, for example the one in Science: *False Positive,* [224]), but the scientific rationale should be easily followed from isolation to falsification. In this first section, I underlined the difference between RNASEL – HPC-1 association and XMRV identification. While the first is rather logically strong and corroborated by several evidence and years of research, the second was essentially based on just one high-throughput technology –kind of *shot-in-the-dark*- experiment. It is easily biased and prone to artefacts, as it happened in this instance. However, the idea of an infecting agent in PCa is strengthened by several other elements, of which RNASEL involvement is only one (also: IFN, PKR, etc are affected; presence of inflammation, involvement of peripheral prostate, field cancerization effects, etc.).

In the second part, the candidate MFV virus was presented, in view of its affinity with PCa (IFN involvement, RNase-L strong induction, generation of inflammatory mechanisms). For RNase-L, evidence was also coming from CFS studies, again pointing toward similarities between the two conditions (and cancer related fatigue –CRF ? [2] [1]). Furthermore, MFV was isolated from a cancer-cluster (NOT through PCR enrichment) in view of its strong/powerful biological activity. This is exemplified by its very strong apoptogenic mechanisms (entire cultures wiped-out in 36-72 hours) or its capability of inducing strong genetic instability, leading to genomic aberrations, such as MYCN amplification and t(8;14) or t(2;14) [53].

Finally, in the third section, the elements of PCa carcinogenesis, where MFV/MFRVs could show more clearly its effects, were underlined: they included IFN pathways, RNASEL, inflammation and MFV capability of infecting/transforming stem-like cells [53] [55].

What are then the MFV/MFRVs properties which should be emphasized or taken home as messages? Or how we should rationalize them in this ongoing debate on PCa carcinogenesis ? As mentioned, the RNASEL – HPC-1 paradigm is logically strong and also in CFS numerous evidence point toward infections (micro-epidemics, virus-infection symptoms, IFN pathway etc.) [3] [1].

One essential property of MFV/MFRVs is its biological power, which could lead to strong and persistent infections and long-lasting inflammations in affected hosts. This could easily explain cycles of necrosis/regeneration, which we witness in BPH, PIA, PCa [53] [119].

A second important question -not addressed by this review for limited space- regards the nature of these viruses and whether they have been isolated before. In view of the persistent/ long-lasting infections they can initiate, an easy comparison/association is with EBV, which infects *H. sapiens* in early childhood/youth (depending from geographic areas), then remaining latent, and has been also associated with lymphomagenesis and other human cancers. Indeed, in the *hospital-safari's* expeditions of Dennis Burkitt, there was a second type and non-Herpes virus (not EBV) constantly isolated [225] [226] [227] [228] [229] [230] [231] [232] (also: Jay Levy/ Thomas Bell, personal communications). All the data available today point toward a virus similar to MFV/MFRVs: in this sense and in view of our MFRVs data,

http://dx.doi.org/10.5772/54054

these viruses could be the missing link to malignancy in BL (EBV does not cause malignancy, it just immortalizes lymphoblasts) [53] [233].

A final question, in view of the close relationship of these viruses in terms of persistence in the human population, is what justifies this proximity, which –at least for its "*cousin* EBV"- resembles parasitism. Several authors and M. Greaves among them, have introduced elements of "*Darwinian-medicine*" analysis in our interpretation of carcinogenesis [234] [235] [52] [175] [236] [237] [53] [55] [1]. The *take-and-give* of MFV/MFRVs with *H. sapiens* infections could certainly be associated to some of their properties. For example, to their strong apoptogenic effects, leading to inflammatory reactions in BPH/PIA/PCa, but also possibly to useful tissue modelling/reshaping in other instances. The described strong relationship of these viruses with stem-like cells further suggests a closer partnership of MFV/MFRVs with *H. sapiens* in *Darwinian-medicine* terms. With all possible consequences.

Author details

Ugo Rovigatti

Address all correspondence to: profrovigatti@gmail.com

University of Pisa Medical School, Pisa, Italy

References

[1] Rovigatti, U., Chronic Fatigue Syndrome (CFS) and Cancer Related Fatigue (CRF): two "fatigue" syndromes with overlapping symptoms and possibly related aetiologies. Neuro-Muscolar Disorders, 2012. In the Press.

[2] MEEUS, M., et al., Immunological Similarities between Cancer and Chronic Fatigue Syndrome: The Common Link to Fatigue? . Anticancer Research November 2009 29 (11): p. 4717-4726

[3] Silverman, R., A scientific journey through the 2-5A/RNase L system. Cytokine Growth Factor Rev, 2007. 18: p. 381 - 388.

[4] Silverman, R.H., et al., The human retrovirus XMRV in prostate cancer and chronic fatigue syndrome. Nature Reviews of Urology, 2010. 7(7): p. 392-402.

[5] Silverman, R.H., Viral encounters with OAS and RNase L during the IFN antiviral response. 2007. J. Virol., 81: p. 12720-12729.

[6] Carpten, J., et al., Germline mutations in the ribonuclease L gene in families showing linkage with HPC1. Nature Genetics, 2002. 30(2): p. 181-184.

[7] Casey, G., et al., RNASEL Arg462Gln variant is implicated in up to 13% of prostate cancer cases. Nature Genetics, 2002. 32(4): p. 581-583.

[8] Roekman, A., et al., Germline Alterations of the RNASEL Gene, a Candidate HPC1 Gene at 1q25, in Patients and Families with Prostate Cancer. The American Journal of Human Genetics, 2002. 70(5): p. 1299-1304.

[9] Noonan-Wheeler, F.C., et al., Association of hereditary prostate cancer gene polymorphic variants with sporadic aggressive prostate carcinoma. The Prostate, 2006. 66(1): p. 49-56.

[10] Wiklund, F., et al., Genetic Analysis of the RNASEL Gene in Hereditary, Familial, and Sporadic Prostate Cancer ClinCanRes 2004 10 (21): p. 7150-56

[11] Lengyel, P., Tumor-suppressor genes: news about the interferon connection Proceedings of the National Academy of Sciences 1993 90 (13): p. 5893-5895

[12] Hassel, B.A., et al., A dominant negative mutant of 2-5A-dependent RNase suppresses antiproliferative and antiviral effects of interferon. EMBO J., 1993. 12: p. 3297-3304.

[13] Zhou, A., Interferon action and apoptosis are defective in mice devoid of 2-5 A- oligoadenylate-dependent RNase L. EMBO J., 1997. 16: p. 6355-6363.

[14] Wang, D., et al., Microarray-based detection and genotyping of viral pathogens Proceedings of the National Academy of Sciences 2002 99 (24): p. 15687-15692

[15] Urisman, A., et al., Identification of a novel Gammaretrovirus in prostate tumors of patients homozygous for R462Q RNASEL variant. PLoS Pathog, 2006. 2: p. e25.

[16] Dong, B., et al., An infectious retrovirus susceptible to an IFN antiviral pathway from human prostate tumors. Proc Natl Acad Sci USA, 2007. 104: p. 1655 - 1660.

[17] Stoye, J.P. and J.M. Coffin, The four classes of endogenous murine leukemia virus: structural relationships and potential for recombination. . Journal of Virology 1987 61 (9): p. 2659-2669

[18] COFFIN, J.M., J.P. STOYE, and W.N. FRANKEL, Genetics of Endogenous Murine Leukemia Virusesa. Annals of the New York Academy of Sciences, 1989. 567(1): p. 39-49.

[19] Jenkins, N.A., et al., Organization, distribution, and stability of endogenous ecotropic murine leukemia virus DNA sequences in chromosomes of Mus musculus. . Journal of Virology 1982 43 (1): p. 26-36

[20] Stoye, J.P. and J.M. Coffin, Polymorphism of murine endogenous proviruses revealed by using virus class-specific oligonucleotide probes. . Journal of Virology 1988 62 (1): p. 168-175

[21] Dorner, A.J., J.P. Stoye, and J.M. Coffin, Molecular basis of host range variation in avian retroviruses. . Journal of Virology 1985 53 (1): p. 32-39

[22] Hayward, W.S., B.G. Neel, and S.M. Astrin, Activation of a cellular onc gene by promoter insertion in ALV-induced lymphoid leukosis. NATURE, 1981. 290(5806): p. 475-480.

[23] Varmus, H.E., Retroviruses and Oncogenes I (Nobel Lecture). Angewandte Chemie International Edition in English, 1990. 29(7): p. 707-715.

[24] Schlaberg, R., et al., XMRV is present in malignant prostatic epithelium and is associated with prostate cancer, especially high-grade tumors. Proc Natl Acad Sci USA, 2009. 106: p. 16351-16356.

[25] Arnold, R.S., et al., XMRV Infection in Patients With Prostate Cancer: Novel Serologic Assay and Correlation With PCR and FISH. Urology, 2010. 75(4): p. 755-761.

[26] Montefiori, D.C., et al., Demographic Factors That Influence the Neutralizing Antibody Response in Recipients of Recombinant HIV-1 gp120 Vaccines Journal of Infectious Diseases 2004 190 (11): p. 1962-1969

[27] Li, B., et al., Evidence for Potent Autologous Neutralizing Antibody Titers and Compact Envelopes in Early Infection with Subtype C Human Immunodefic. Virus Type 1 Journal of Virology, 2006. 80(11): p. 5211-5218.

[28] Danielson, B.P., G.E. Ayala, and J.T. Kimata, Detection of Xenotropic Murine Leukemia Virus-Related Virus in Normal and Tumor Tissue of Patients from the Southern United States with Prostate Cancer Is Dependent on Specific Polymerase Chain Reaction Conditions Journal of Infectious Diseases 2010 202 (10): p. 1470-1477

[29] Sfanos, K., et al., A molecular analysis of prokaryotic and viral DNA seq.s in prost. tissue from patients with prostate cancer indicates the presence of multiple and diverse microorganisms. Prostate, 2008. 68: p. 306 - 320.

[30] Lombardi, V.C., Detection of an infectious retrovirus, XMRV, in blood cells of patients with chronic fatigue syndrome. SCIENCE, 2009. 326: p. 585-589.

[31] Coffin, J.M. and J.P. Stoye, A New Virus for Old Diseases? Science 2009 326 (5952): p. 530-531

[32] Lo, S.-C., Detection of MLV-related virus gene sequences in blood of patients with chronic fatigue syndrome and healthy blood donors Proceedings of the National Academy of Sciences 2010 107 (36): p. 15874-15879

[33] Singh, I.R., Detecting Retroviral Sequences in Chronic Fatigue Syndrome. Viruses, 2010. 2(11): p. 2404-2408.

[34] Courgnaud, V., et al., Mouse retroviruses and chronic fatigue syndrome: Does X (or P) mark the spot? Proceedings of the National Academy of Sciences 2010 107 (36): p. 15666-15667

[35] Fischer, N., et al., Prevalence of human gammaretrovirus XMRV in sporadic prostate cancer. J Clin Virol, 2008. 43: p. 277 - 283.

[36] Hohn, O., et al., Lack of evidence for xenotropic murine leukemia virus-related virus(XMRV) in German prostate cancer patients. Retrovirology, 2009. 6(1): p. 92.

[37] D'Arcy, F., et al., No evidence of XMRV in Irish prostate cancer patients with the R462Q mutation. European Urology Supplements, 2008. 7: p. 271.

[38] Verhaegh, G.W., et al., Prevalence of human xenotropic murine leukemia virus-related gammaretrovirus (XMRV) in dutch prostate cancer patients. The Prostate, 2011. 71(4): p. 415-420.

[39] Martinez-Fierro, M., et al., Identification of viral infections in the prostate and evaluation of their association with cancer. BMC Cancer, 2010. 10(1): p. 326.

[40] Aloia, A.L., et al., XMRV: A New Virus in Prostate Cancer? Cancer Research 2010 70 (24): p. 10028-10033

[41] Robinson, M., et al., Mouse DNA contamination in human tissue tested for XMRV. Retrovirology, 2010. 7(1): p. 108.

[42] Brunschwig, A., C. M. Southam, et al. (1965). "Host resistance to cancer. Clinical experiments by homotransplants, autotransplants and admixture of autologous leucocytes." Ann Surg 162(3): 416-25.

[43] Fan, H., A new human retrovirus associated with prostate cancer Proceedings of the National Academy of Sciences 2007 104 (5): p. 1449-1450

[44] Groom, H.C.T. and K.N. Bishop, The tale of xenotropic murine leukemia virus-related virus Journal of General Virology 2012

[45] Paprotka, T., et al., Recombinant Origin of the Retrovirus XMRV Science 2011 333 (6038): p. 97-101

[46] Coffin, J.M., S.H. Hughes, and H.E. Varmus, Retroviruses. 1997.

[47] Knox, K., et No Evidence of Murine-Like Gammaretroviruses in CFS Patients Previously Identified as XMRV-Infected Science 2011 333 (6038): p. 94-97

[48] Cingoz, O. and J.M. Coffin, Endogenous Murine Leukemia Viruses: Relationship to XMRV and Related Sequences Detected in Human DNA Samples. Adv Virol. 2011: p. 940210.

[49] Kang, D.E., et al., XMRV Discovery and Prostate Cancer-Related Research. Adv Virol, 2011. 2011: p. 432837.

[50] Sfanos, K.S., et al., XMRV and prostate cancer[mdash]a 'final' perspective. Nature Reviews Urology, 2012. 9(2): p. 111-118.

[51] Rovigatti, U., Isolation and initial characterization of a new virus: Micro-Foci inducing virus or MFV. C R Acad Sci III, 1992. 315(5): p. 195-202.

[52] Greaves, M., Infection, immune responses and the aetiology of childhood leukaemia. Nature Reviews of Cancer, 2006. 6(3): p. 193-203.

[53] U. Rovigatti, A.T., A. Piccin, R. Colognato amd B. Sordat. Preliminary Characterization of a New Type of Viruses Isolated from Paediatric Neuroblastoma and Non-Hodgkin's Lymphoma: potential Implications for Aetiology. in Intn. Conference Childhood Leukaemia. Section P1-18 pp I-IV, September 2004. 2004. London, United Kingdom: Editor: CwL.

[54] Rovigatti, G.B.a.B.S.M. MFV Virus unduces MYCN DNA amplification and transforms benign neuroblastsinto cells tumorigenic in nude mice. in 18th International Congress of Biochemistry and Molecular Biology "Beyond the Genome". 2000. London, UK.

[55] Rovigatti, U., C. Selli, and R. Bartoletti, Of Mice and Men - Viruses and Prostate Cancer: What Is the Next Step? European Urology, 2010. 58(5): p. 684-686.

[56] Liu, W., et al., Tumour suppressor function of RNase L in a mouse model. European Journal of Cancer, 2007. 43(1): p. 202-209.

[57] Zhou, A., et al., Interferon action and apoptosis are defective in mice devoid of 2[prime],5[prime]-oligoadenylate-dependent RNase L. EMBO Journal, 1997. 16(21): p. 6355-6363.

[58] Garcia, M.A., E.F. Meurs, and M. Esteban, The dsRNA protein kinase PKR: Virus and cell control. Biochimie Interferons 1957-2007: from discovery to mechanism of action and clinical applications, 2007. 89(6â€"7): p. 799-811.

[59] Garcia, M.A., et al., Impact of Protein Kinase PKR in Cell Biology: from Antiviral to Antiproliferative Action. Microbiology and Molecular Biology Reviews, December 2006. 70(4): p. 1032-1060.

[60] Samuel, C.E., Antiviral Actions of Interferons Clinical Microbiology Reviews 2001 14 (4): p. 778-809

[61] Williams, B.R., PKR; a sentinel kinase for cellular stress. Oncogene., 1999. 18(45): p. 6112-20.

[62] Pathak, V.K., D. Schindler, and J.W. Hershey, Generation of a mutant form of protein synthesis initiation factor eIF-2 lacking the site of phosphorylation by eIF-2 kinases. Molecular and Cellular Biology 1988 8 (2): p. 993-995

[63] Samuel, C.E., Mechanism of interferon action: Phosphorylation of protein synthesis initiation factor eIF-2 in interferon-treated human cells by a ribosome-associated kinase processing site specificity similar to hemin-regulated rabbit reticulocyte kinase Proceedings of the National Academy of Sciences 1979 76 (2): p. 600-604

[64] Abraham, N., et al., Characterization of Transgenic Mice with Targeted Disruption of the Catalytic Domain of the Double-stranded RNA-dependent Protein Kinase, PKR Journal of Biological Chemistry 1999 274 (9): p. 5953-5962

[65] Yang, Y.L., et al., Deficient signaling in mice devoid of double-stranded RNA-dependent protein kinase. Embo J., 1995. 14(24): p. 6095-106.

[66] Balachandran, S., et al., Essential Role for the dsRNA-Dependent Protein Kinase PKR in Innate Immunity to Viral Infection. Immunity, 2000. 13(1): p. 129-141.

[67] Li, X.-L., et al., A central role for RNA in the induction and biological activities of type 1 interferons. Wiley Interdisciplinary Reviews: RNA, 2011. 2(1): p. 58-78.

[68] Mounir, Z., et al., Tumor Suppression by PTEN Requires the Activation of the PKR-eIF2{alpha} Phosphorylation Pathway SciSig., 2009. 2(102): p. ra85-.

[69] Squire, J.A., et al., Prostate Cancer as a Model System for Genetic Diversity in Tumors Advances in Cancer Research, D. Gisselsson, Editor. 2011, Ac. Press. p. 183-216.

[70] Samuel, C.E., Adenosine deaminases acting on RNA (ADARs) are both antiviral and proviral. VirologySpecial Reviews 2011, 2011. 411(2): p. 180-193.

[71] George, C.X., et al., Adenosine deaminases acting on RNA, RNA editing, and interferon action. J Interferon Cytokine Res. 31(1): p. 99-117.

[72] Galeano, F., et al., A-to-I RNA editing: The "ADAR" side of human cancer. Developmental Cell Behavior, 2012. 23(3): p. 244-250.

[73] Dominissini, D., et al., Adenosine-to-inosine RNA editing meets cancer Carcinogenesis 2011 32 (11): p. 1569-1577

[74] Li, J.B., et al., Genome-Wide Identification of Human RNA Editing Sites by Parallel DNA Capturing and Sequencing Science 2009 324 (5931): p. 1210-1213

[75] Zaranek, A.W., et al., A Survey of Genomic Traces Reveals a Common Sequencing Error, RNA Editing, and DNA Editing. PLoS Genet, 2010. 6(5): p. e1000954 EP -.

[76] Cattaneo, R., et al., Accumulated measles virus mutations in a case of subacute sclerosing panencephalitis: Interrupted matrix protein reading frame and transcription alteration. Virology, 1986. 154(1): p. 97-107.

[77] Cattaneo, R., et al., Biased hypermutation and other genetic changes in defective measles viruses in human brain infections. Cell, 1988. 55(2): p. 255-265.

[78] tenOever, B.R., et al., Multiple Functions of the IKK-Related Kinase IKKÎµ in Interferon-Mediated Antiviral Immunity Science 2007 315 (5816): p. 1274-1278

[79] Lei, M., Y. Liu, and C.E. Samuel, Adenovirus VAI RNA Antagonizes the RNA-Editing Activity of the ADAR Adenosine Deaminase. Virology, 1998. 245(2): p. 188-196.

[80] Samuel, C.E., Reoviruses and the interferon system. Curr Top Microbiol Immunol., 1998. 233(Pt 2): p. 125-45.

[81] Yang, C., et al., Identification and expression profiles of ADAR1 gene, responsible for RNA editing, in responses to dsRNA and GCRV challenge in grass carp (Ctenopharyngodon idella). Fish & Shellfish Immunology, 2012. 33(4): p. 1042-1049.

[82] Paz, N., et al., Altered adenosine-to-inosine RNA editing in human cancer Genome Research 2007 17 (11): p. 000

[83] Ishiuchi, S., et al., Blockage of Ca2+-permeable AMPA receptors suppresses migration and induces apoptosis in human glioblastoma cells. Nature Medicine, 2002. 8(9): p. 971-978.

[84] Ishiuchi, S., et al., Ca2+-Permeable AMPA Receptors Regulate Growth of Human Glioblastoma via Akt Activation The Journal of Neuroscience 2007 27 (30): p. 7987-8001

[85] Cenci, C., et al., Down-regulation of RNA Editing in Pediatric Astrocytomas Journal of Biological Chemistry 2008 283 (11): p. 7251-7260

[86] Stark, G.R., et al., How Cells Respond To Interferons. Annual Review of Biochemistry, 1998. 67(1): p. 227-264.

[87] Darnell, J.E., Jr., Interferon research: impact on understanding transcriptional control. Curr Top Microbiol Immunol., 2007. 316: p. 155-63.

[88] Stark, G.R. and J.E. Darnell Jr., The JAK-STAT Pathway at Twenty. Immunity, 2012. 36(4): p. 503-514.

[89] Roberts, R.M., et al., The evolution of the type I interferons. Journal of Interferon and Cytokine Research, 1998. 18(10): p. 805-816.

[90] Deonarain, R., et al., Impaired Antiviral Response and Alpha/Beta Interferon Induction in Mice Lacking Beta Interferon Journal of Virology 2000 74 (7): p. 3404-3409

[91] Bach, E.A., M. Aguet, and R.D. Schreiber, THE IFNÎ³ RECEPTOR:A Paradigm for Cytokine Receptor Signaling. Annual Review of Immunology, 1997. 15(1): p. 563-591.

[92] Prejean, C. and O.R. Colamonici, Role of the cytoplasmic domains of the type I interferon receptor subunits in signaling. Seminars in Cancer Biology, 2000. 10(2): p. 83-92.

[93] Malmgaard, L., Induction and regulation of IFNs during viral infections. J Interferon Cytokine Res., 2004. 24(8): p. 439-54.

[94] Darnell, J., I. Kerr, and G. Stark, Jak-STAT pathways and transcriptional activation in response to IFNs and other extracellular signaling proteins Science 1994 264 (5164): p. 1415-1421

[95] Schindler, C. and J.E. Darnell, Transcriptional Responses to Polypeptide Ligands: The JAK-STAT Pathway. Annual Review of Biochemistry, 1995. 64(1): p. 621-652.

[96] Darnell, J.E., Jr., Studies of IFN-induced transcriptional activation uncover the Jak-Stat pathway. J Interferon Cytokine Res., 1998. 18(8): p. 549-54.

[97] Nguyen, H., J. Hiscott, and P.M. Pitha, The growing family of interferon regulatory factors. Cytokine & Growth Factor Reviews, 1997. 8(4): p. 293-312.

[98] BraganÃ§a, J. and A. Civas, Type I interferon gene expression: Differential expression of IFN-A genes induced by viruses and double-stranded RNA. Biochimie, 1998. 80(8â€"9): p. 673-687.

[99] Decker, T., P. Kovarik, and A. Meinke, GAS elements: a few nucleotides with a major impact on cytokine-induced gene expression. J Interferon Cytokine Res., 1997. 17(3): p. 121-34.

[100] Copeland, K.F., Modulation of HIV-1 transcription by cytokines and chemokines. Mini Rev Med Chem., 2005. 5(12): p. 1093-101.

[101] Daly, C. and N.C. Reich, Characterization of Specific DNA-binding Factors Activated by Double-stranded RNA as Positive Regulators of Interferon /-stimulated Genes Journal of Biological Chemistry 1995 270 (40): p. 23739-23746

[102] Rebouillat, D., et al., Characterization of the Gene Encoding the 100-kDa Form of Human 2â€²,5â€²Oligoadenylate Synthetase. Genomics, 2000. 70(2): p. 232-240.

[103] Clemens, M.J. and B.R. Williams, Inhibition of cell-free protein synthesis by pppA2[prime]p5[prime]A2[prime]p5[prime]A: a novel oligonucleotide synthesized by interferon-treated L cell extracts. Cell, 1978. 13: p. 565-572.

[104] Floyd-Smith, G., E. Slattery, and P. Lengyel, Interferon action: RNA cleavage pattern of a (2[prime]-5[prime])oligoadenylate-dependent endonuclease. Science, 1981. 212: p. 1030-1032.

[105] Zhou, A., B.A. Hassel, and R.H. Silverman, Expression cloning of 2-5A-dependent RNAase: a uniquely regulated mediator of interferon action. Cell, 1993. 72: p. 753-765.

[106] Dong, B., et al., Intrinsic molecular activities of the interferon-induced 2-5A-dependent RNase. . Journal of Biological Chemistry 1994 269 (19): p. 14153-14158

[107] Dong, B. and R.H. Silverman, 2-5A-dependent RNase Molecules Dimerize during Activation by 2-5A Journal of Biological Chemistry 1995 270 (8): p. 4133-4137

[108] Smith, J., et al., Major susceptibility locus for prostate cancer on chromosome 1 suggested by a genome-wide search. Science, 1996. 274: p. 1371 - 1374.

[109] Lengyel, P., Tumor-suppressor genes: news about the interferon connection. Proc. Natl Acad. Sci. USA, 1993. 90: p. 5893-5895.

[110] Suhadolnik, R.J., et al., Upregulation of the 2-5A Synthetase/RNase L Antiviral Pathway Associated with Chronic Fatigue Syndrome Clinical Infectious Diseases 1994 18 (Supplement 1): p. S96-S104

[111] Shetzline, S.E., et al., Structural and functional features of the 37-kDa 2-5A-dependent RNase L in chronic fatigue syndrome. J Interferon Cytokine Res, 2002. 22(4): p. 443-56.

[112] De Meirleir, K., et al., Antiviral Pathway Activation in Chronic Fatigue Syndrome and Acute Infection Clinical Infectious Diseases 2002 34 (10): p. 1420-1421

[113] Suhadolnik, R.J., et al., Biochemical evidence for a novel low molecular weight 2-5A-dependent RNase L in chronic fatigue syndrome. J Interferon Cytokine Res, 1997. 17(7): p. 377-85.

[114] Demettre, E., et al., Ribonuclease L Proteolysis in Peripheral Blood Mononuclear Cells of Chronic Fatigue Syndrome Patients Journal of Biological Chemistry 2002 277 (38): p. 35746-35751

[115] Nijs, J., et al., Chronic fatigue syndrome: intracellular immune deregulations as a possible etiology for abnormal exercise response. Medical Hypotheses, 2004. 62(5): p. 759-765.

[116] Frémont, M., et al., 2-5 A Oligoadenylate size is critical to protect RNase L against proteolytic cleavage in chronic fatigue syndrome. Experimental and Molecular Pathology, 2005. 78(3): p. 239-246.

[117] NIJS, J. and K. DE MEIRLEIR, Impairments of the 2-5A Synthetase/RNase L Pathway in Chronic Fatigue Syndrome In Vivo November-December 2005 19 (6): p. 1013-1021

[118] MEEUS, M., et al., Unravelling Intracellular Immune Dysfunctions in Chronic Fatigue Syndrome: Interactions between Protein Kinase R Activity, RNase L Cleavage and Elastase Activity, and their Clinical Relevance In Vivo January-February 2008 22 (1): p. 115-121

[119] De Marzo, A., et al., Inflammation in prostate carcinogenesis. Nat Rev Cancer, 2007. 7(4): p. 256 - 269.

[120] Nelson, W., et al., The role of inflammation in the pathogenesis of prostate cancer. J Urol, 2004. 172(5 Pt 2): p. S6 - 11.

[121] Nelson, W., A. De Marzo, and W. Isaacs, Prostate cancer. N Engl J Med, 2003. 349: p. 366 - 381.

[122] Colotta, F., et al., Cancer-related inflammation, the seventh hallmark of cancer: links to genetic instability Carcinogenesis 2009 30 (7): p. 1073-1081

[123] Siegel, R., et al., Cancer statistics, 2011. CA: A Cancer Journal for Clinicians, 2011. 61(4): p. 212-236.

[124] Bostwick, D.G., Urologic Surgical Pathology. 1997. p. 423-456.

[125] McNeal, J.E., et al., Zonal distribution of prostatic adenocarcinoma. Correlation with histologic pattern and direction of spread. Am. J. Surg. Pathol., 1988. 12: p. 897-906.

[126] Franks, L.M., Atrophy and hyperplasia in the prostate proper. J. Pathol. Bacteriol., 1954. 68: p. 617-621.

[127] De Marzo, A., et al., Proliferative inflammatory atrophy of the prostate: implications for prostatic carcinogenesis. Am J Pathol, 1999. 155: p. 1985 - 1992.

[128] Putzi, M.J. and A.M. De Marzo, Morphologic transitions between proliferative inflammatory atrophy and high-grade prostatic intraepithelial neoplasia. Urology, 2000. 56: p. 828-832.

[129] Peto, J., Cancer epidemiology in the last century and the next decade. Nature, 2001. 411: p. 390-395.

[130] Hsing, A.W., L. Tsao, and S.S. Devesa, International trends and patterns of prostate cancer incidence and mortality. Int J Cancer, 2000. 85: p. 60-67.

[131] Cook, L.S., Et Al., Incidence Of Adenocarcinoma Of The Prostate In Asian Immigrants To The United States And Their Descendants. The Journal of urology, 1999. 161(1): p. 152-155.

[132] Sion-Vardy, N., et al., Ethnicity and its significance in the pathobiology of prostatic carcinoma in Southern Israel. Urologic oncology, 2008. 26(1): p. 31-36.

[133] Ranasinghe, W.K.B., et al., Incidence of prostate cancer in Sri Lanka using cancer registry data and comparisons with the incidence in South Asian men in England. BJU International, 2011. 108(8b): p. E184-E189.

[134] Shiraishi, T., et al., The frequency of latent prostatic carcinoma in young males: the Japanese experience. In Vivo, 1994. 8(3): p. 445-7.

[135] Zhu, Y.P., et al., Prevalence of incidental prostate cancer in patients undergoing radical cystoprostatectomy: data from China and other Asian countries. Asian J Androl, 2009. 11(1): p. 104-8.

[136] McNeal, J.E., Normal histology of the prostate. Histology for Pathologists (Ed. Sternberg), 1988. 12: p. 619-633.

[137] Pelouze, P.S., Gonorrhea in the male and female: a book for practitioners. 1935, W B Sounders Company: Philadelphia.

[138] Handsfield, H.H., et al., Asymptomatic gonorrhea in men. Diagnosis, natural course, prevalence and significance. New England Journal of Medicine, 1974. 290: p. 117-123.

[139] Boldogh, I., et al., Human cytomegalovirus and herpes simplex type 2 virus in normal and adenocarcinomatous prostate glands. Journal of the National Cancer Institute, 1983. 70(5): p. 819-826.

[140] Eizuru, Y., et al., Herpesvirus RNA in human urogenital tumors. Proceedings of the Society for Experimental Biology and Medicine, 1983. 174(2): p. 296-301.

[141] Bergh, J., et al., No link between viral findings in the prostate and subsequent cancer development. Br J Cancer, 2006. 96(1): p. 137-139.

[142] Berrington de Gonzalez, A., et al., Antibodies against six human herpesviruses in relation to seven cancers in black South Africans: A case control study. Infectious Agents and Cancer, 2006. 1(1): p. 2.

[143] Chang, Y., et al., Identification of herpesvirus-like DNA sequences in AIDS-associated Kaposi's sarcoma. Science, 1994. 266(5192): p. 1865-9.

[144] Monini, P., et al., Kaposi's Sarcomaâ€"Associated Herpesvirus DNA Sequences in Prostate Tissue and Human Semen. New England Journal of Medicine, 1996. 334(18): p. 1168-1172.

[145] Corbellino, M., et al., Absence of HHV-8 in prostate and semen [2]. New England Journal of Medicine, 1996. 335(16): p. 1237-1239.

[146] Diamond, C., et al., Human herpesvirus 8 in the prostate glands of men with Kaposi's sarcoma. Journal of Virology, 1998. 72(7): p. 6223-6227.

[147] Hoffman, L.J., et al., Elevated Seroprevalence of Human Herpesvirus 8 among Men with Prostate Cancer Journal of Infect. Diseases 2004 189 (1): p. 15-20

[148] Sutcliffe, S., et al., Plasma Antibodies against Chlamydia trachomatis, Human Papillomavirus, and Human Herpesvirus Type 8 in Relation to Prostate Cancer: A Prospective Study Cancer Epidemiology Biomarkers & Prevention 2007 16 (8): p. 1573-1580

[149] MONINI, P., et al., DNA Rearrangements Impairing BK Virus Productive Infection in Urinary Tract Tumors. Virology, 1995. 214(1): p. 273-279.

[150] Das, D., R.B. Shah, and M.J. Imperiale, Detection and expression of human BK virus sequences in neoplastic prostate tissues. Oncogene, 2004. 23(42): p. 7031-7046.

[151] Newton, R., et al., Antibody levels against BK virus and prostate, kidney and bladder cancers in the EPIC-Oxford cohort. Br J Cancer, 2005. 93(11): p. 1305-1306.

[152] Das, D., K. Wojno, and M. Imperiale, BK virus as a cofactor in the etiology of prostate cancer in its early stages. J Virol, 2008. 82: p. 2705 - 2714.

[153] zur Hausen, H., Papillomaviruses in the causation of human cancers - a brief historical account. Virology, 2009. 384: p. 260 - 265.

[154] zur Hausen, H., The search for infectious causes of human cancers: Where and why. Virology, 2009. 392(1): p. 1-10.

[155] Leiros, G., et al., Detection of human papillomavirus DNA and p53 codon 72 polymorphism in prostate carcinomas of patients from Argentina. BMC Urology, 2005. 5(1): p. 15.

[156] Hrbacek, J., et al., Thirty years of research on infection and prostate cancer: No conclusive evidence for a link. A systematic review. Urologic Oncology: Seminars and Original Investigations, In the Press (0).

[157] Hrbacek, J., et al., Serum antibodies against genitourinary infectious agents in prostate cancer and benign prostate hyperplasia patients: a case-control study. BMC Cancer, 2011. 11(1): p. 53.

[158] Woodworth, C.D., HPV innate immunity. Front Biosci, 2002. 7: p. d2058-71.

[159] Platz, E.A., Nonsteroidal anti-inflammatory drugs and risk of prostate cancer in the Baltimore Longitudinal Study of Aging. Cancer Epidemiology Biomarkers Prevention, 2005. 14: p. 390-396.

[160] Mahmud, S., E. Franco, and A. Aprikian, Prostate cancer and use of nonsteroidal anti-inflammatory drugs: systematic review and meta-analysis. Br. J. Cancer, 2004. 90: p. 93-99.

[161] Chan, J.M., et al., The epidemiology of prostate cancer [mdash] with a focus on nonsteroidal anti-inflammatory drugs. Hematl Oncol Clin. North Am., 2006. 20: p. 797-809.

[162] Jacobs, E.J., A large cohort study of aspirin and other nonsteroidal anti-inflammatory drugs and prostate cancer incidence. J. Natl. Cancer Inst., 2005. 97: p. 975-980.

[163] Mahmud, S., E. Franco, and A. Aprikian, Prostate cancer and use of nonsteroidal anti-inflammatory drugs: systematic review and meta-analysis. Br J Cancer, 2004. 90(1): p. 93-99.

[164] Mahmud, S.M., et al., Non-steroidal anti-inflammatory drug use and prostate cancer in a high-risk population. Eur J Cancer Prev, 2006. 15(2): p. 158-64.

[165] Dasgupta, K., et al., Association between nonsteroidal anti-inflammatory drugs and prostate cancer occurrence. Cancer J, 2006. 12(2): p. 130-5.

[166] Mahmud, S.M., E.L. Franco, and A.G. Aprikian, Use of nonsteroidal anti-inflammatory drugs and prostate cancer risk: A meta-analysis. International Journal of Cancer, 2010. 127(7): p. 1680-1691.

[167] Mahmud, S.M., et al., Use of Non-Steroidal Anti-Inflammatory Drugs and Prostate Cancer Risk: A Population-Based Nested Case-Control Study. PLoS ONE, 2011. 6(1): p. e16412 EP -.

[168] Chokkalingam, A.P., et al., Prostate carcinoma risk subsequent to diagnosis of benign prostatic hyperplasia. Cancer, 2003. 98(8): p. 1727-1734.

[169] Dennis, L.K., C.F. Lynch, and J.C. Torner, Epidemiologic association between prostatitis and prostate cancer. Urology, 2002. 60: p. 78-83.

[170] Sarma, A.V., Sexual behavior, sexually transmitted diseases and prostatitis: the risk of prostate cancer in black men. J. Urol., 2006. 176: p. 1108-1113.

[171] Sondergaard, G., M. Vetner, and P.O. Christensen, Prostatic calculi. Acta Pathol. Microbiol. Immunol. Scand., 1987. 95: p. 141-145.

[172] Sutcliffe, S., Gonorrhea, syphilis, clinical prostatitis, and the risk of prostate cancer. Cancer Epidemiol Biomarkers Prev, 2006. 15: p. 2160-2166.

[173] Sutcliffe, S., et al., Non-steroidal anti-inflammatory drug use and the risk of benign prostatic hyperplasia-related outcomes and nocturia in the Prostate, Lung, Colorectal, and Ovarian Cancer Screening Trial. BJU International, 2012. 110(7): p. 1050-1059.

[174] Ogilvie, I., et al., Burden of community-acquired and nosocomial rotavirus gastroenteritis in the pediatric population of Western Europe: a scoping review. BMC Infectious Diseases, 2012. 12(1): p. 62.

[175] Greaves, M., Darwinian medicine: a case for cancer. Nature Reviews of Cancer, 2007. 7(3): p. 213-221.

[176] Wang, Z.A. and M.M. Shen, Revisiting the concept of cancer stem cells in prostate cancer. Oncogene, 2011. 30(11): p. 1261-1271.

[177] Kasper, S., Identification, characterization, and biological relevance of prostate cancer stem cells from clinical specimens. Urologic oncology, 2009. 27(3): p. 301-303.

[178] Li, H. and D.G. Tang, Prostate cancer stem cells and their potential roles in metastasis. Journal of Surgical Oncology, 2011. 103(6): p. 558-562.

[179] Ogilvie , I., et al., Burden of rotavirus gastroenteritis in the pediatric population in Central and Eastern Europe: Serotype distribution and burden of illness. vaccines, 2011. 7(5) 2164-5515): p. 523-533.

[180] Sfanos, K.S., et al., XMRV and prostate cancer[mdash]a 'final' perspective. Nature Reviews of Cancer, 2012. 9(2): p. 111-118.

[181] DeFreitas, E., et al., Retroviral sequences related to human T-lymphotropic virus type II in patients with chronic fatigue immune dysfunction syndrome Proceedings of the National Academy of Sciences 1991 88 (7): p. 2922-2926

[182] John Coffin, S.H.H.a.H.V., Retroviruses. 1997: Cold Spring Harbor Laboratory Press.

[183] Daniel, P. and R. Morin, [Effect of sodium salicylate on the "in vitro" development of RNA viruses (author's transl)]. Ann Microbiol (Paris), 1975. 126(3): p. 381-7.

[184] Ward, R.L., D.S. Sander, and D.R. Knowlton, In vitro activities of bismuth salts against rotaviruses and other enteric viruses. Antimicrobial Agents and Chemotherapy 1985 27 (3): p. 306-308

[185] Cohnheim, J., Ueber entzundung und eiterung. Path. Anath. Physiol. Klin., 1867. 40: p. 1-79.

[186] Virchow, R.E., Editorial. Virchows. Path. Anath. Physiol. Klin., 1855. 3: p. 23.

[187] Pappenheim, A., Prinzipen der neuren morphologischen haematozytologie nach zytogenetischer grundlage. Folia Hematol., 1917. 21: p. 91-101.

[188] McCulloch, E.A. and J.E. Till, Perspectives on the properties of stem cells. Nature Medicine, 2005. 11(10): p. 1026-1028.

[189] BECKER, A.J., E.A. McCULLOCH, and J.E. TILL, Cytological Demonstration of the Clonal Nature of Spleen Colonies Derived from Transplanted Mouse Marrow Cells. Nature, 1963. 197(4866): p. 452-454.

[190] Bruce, W.R. and H. Van Der Gaag, A quantitative assay for the number of murine lymphoma cells capable of proliferation in vivo. nature, 1963. 199: p. 79-80.

[191] Sabbath, K.D., et al., Heterogeneity of clonogenic cells in acute myeloblastic leukemia. J. Clin. Invest., 1985. 75: p. 746-753.

[192] Greaves, M., Childhood leukaemia. Bmj, 2002. 324(7332): p. 283-7. 2.

[193] Greaves, M.F., et al., Leukemia in twins: lessons in natural history. Blood, 2003. 102: p. 2321-2333.

[194] Greaves, M.F. and J. Wiemels, Origins of chromosome translocations in childhood leukaemia. Nature Reviews Cancer, 2003. 3: p. 639-649.

[195] Fialkow, P.J., S.M. Gartler, and A. Yoshida, Clonal origin of chronic myelocytic leukemia in man. Proc Natl Acad Sci U S A, 1967. 58(4): p. 1468-71.

[196] Fialkow, P.J., et al., Leukaemic transformation of engrafted human marrow cells in vivo. Lancet, 1971. 1(7693): p. 251-5.

[197] Fialkow, P.J., Is lyonisation total in man? Lancet, 1970. 2(7667): p. 315.

[198] Fialkow, P.J., et al., 6-Phosphogluconate Dehydrogenase: Hemizygous Manifestation in a Patient with Leukemia Science 1969 163 (3863): p. 194-195

[199] Fialkow, P.J., Use of genetic markers to study cellular origin and development of tumors in human females. Adv Cancer Res, 1972. 15: p. 191-226.

[200] Hamburger, A. and S. Salmon, Primary bioassay of human myeloma stem cells. J Clin Invest, 1977. 60: p. 846 - 854.

[201] Hamburger, A. and S. Salmon, Primary bioassay of human tumor stem cells. Science, 1977. 197: p. 461 - 463.

[202] Herzenberg, L.A., et al., The history and future of the fluorescence activated cell sorter and flow cytometry: a view from Stanford. Clin. Chem., 2002. 48: p. 1819-1827.

[203] McCune, J.M., The SCID-hu mouse: murine model for the analysis of human hematolymphoid differentiation and function. Science, 1988. 241: p. 1632-1639.

[204] Kamel-Reid, S., A model of human acute lymphoblastic leukemia in immune-deficient SCID mice. Science, 1989. 246: p. 1597-1600.

[205] Sirard, C., et al., Normal and leukemic SCID-repopulating cells (SRC) coexist in the bone marrow and peripheral blood from CML patients in chronic phase, whereas leukemic SRC are detected in blast crisis. Blood, 1996. 87(4): p. 1539-48.

[206] Lapidot, T., et al., A cell initiating human acute myeloid leukaemia after transplantation into SCID mice. Nature, 1994. 367(6464): p. 645-8.

[207] Bonnet, D. and J.E. Dick, Human acute myeloid leukemia is organized as a hierarchy that originates from a primitive hematopoietic cell. Nat Med, 1997. 3(7): p. 730-7.

[208] Al-Hajj, M., et al., Prospective identification of tumorigenic breast cancer cells. Proc Nat Acad Sci, 2003. 100: p. 3983-3988.

[209] Moreb, J.S., Aldehyde dehydrogenase as a marker for stem cells. Curr Stem Cell Res Ther, 2008. 3(4): p. 237-46.

[210] Marcato, P., et al., Aldehyde dehydrogenase: Its role as a cancer stem cell marker comes down to the specific isoform. Cell Cycle, 2011. 10(91538-4101): p. 1378-1384.

[211] Prasmickaite, L., et al., Aldehyde Dehydrogenase (ALDH) Activity Does Not Select for Cells with Enhanced Aggressive Properties in Malignant Melanoma. PLoS ONE, 2010. 5(5): p. e10731 EP -.

[212] Quintana, E., et al., Efficient tumour formation by single human melanoma cells. Nature, 2008. 456: p. 593 - 598.

[213] La Porta, C.A., Thoughts about cancer stem cells in solid tumors. World J Stem Cells. 4(3): p. 17-20.

[214] Tu, S.-M. and S.-H. Lin, Prostate Cancer Stem Cells. Clinical Genitourinary Cancer, 2012. 10(2): p. 69-76.

[215] Leong, K.G., et al., Generation of a prostate from a single adult stem cell. Nature, 2008. 456(7223): p. 804-808.

[216] Wang, X., et al., A luminal epithelial stem cell that is a cell of origin for prostate cancer. Nature, 2009. 461(7263): p. 495-500.

[217] Goldstein, A.S., et al., Identification of a Cell of Origin for Human Prostate Cancer Science 2010 329 (5991): p. 568-571

[218] Mackinnon, A.C., et al., Molecular Biology Underlying the Clinical Heterogeneity of Prostate Cancer: An Update. Archives of Pathology & Laboratory Medicine, 2009. 133(7): p. 1033-1040.

[219] Nonn, L., V. Ananthanarayanan, and P.H. Gann, Evidence for field cancerization of the prostate. The Prostate, 2009. 69(13): p. 1470-1479.

[220] Tomlins, S.A., et al., Recurrent fusion of TMPRSS2 and ETS transcription factor genes in prostate cancer. Science, 2005. 310(5748): p. 644-648.

[221] Kumar-Sinha, C., S.A. Tomlins, and A.M. Chinnaiyan, Recurrent gene fusions in prostate cancer. Nature Reviews of Cancer, 2008. 8(7): p. 497-511.

[222] Tomlins, S.A., et al., ETS Gene Fusions in Prostate Cancer: From Discovery to Daily Clinical Practice. European Urology, 2009. 56(2): p. 275-286.

[223] Clark, J.P. and C.S. Cooper, ETS gene fusions in prostate cancer. Nat Rev Urol, 2009. 6(8): p. 429-39.

[224] Cohen, J. and M. Enserink, False Positive Science 2011 333 (6050): p. 1694-1701

[225] Bell, T.M., et al., Isolation of a Reovirus from a Case of Burkitt's Lymphoma. Br Med J., 1964. 1(5392): p. 1212-3.

[226] Bell, T.M., et al., Further isolations of reovirus type 3 from cases of Burkitt's lymphoma. Br Med J., 1966. 1(5502): p. 1514-7.

[227] Bell, T.M. and M.G. Ross, Persistent latent infection of human embryonic cells with reovirus type 3. Nature., 1966. 212(5060): p. 412-4.

[228] Bell, T.M., G.M. Munube, and D.H. Wright, Malignant lymphoma in a rabbit inoculated with reovirus. Lancet., 1968. 1(7549): p. 955-7.

[229] McCrae, A.W., et al., Trans-stadial maintenance of reovirus type 3 in the mosquito Culex (C) pipiens fatigans Weidmann and its implications. East Afr Med J., 1968. 45(10): p. 677-86.

[230] Munube, G.M., et al., Sero-epidemiology of reovirus type 3 infections in four areas of Uganda with varying incidence of Burkitt's tumour. East Afr Med J., 1972. 49(5): p. 369-75.

[231] Levy, J.A., E. Tanabe, and E.C. Curnen, Occurrence of reovirus antibodies in health African children and in children with Burkitt's lymphoma. Cancer., 1968. 21(1): p. 53-7.

[232] Levy, J.A., et al., Effect of reovirus type 3 on cultured Burkitt's tumour cells. Nature., 1968. 220(5167): p. 607-8.

[233] Macsween, K.F. and D.H. Crawford, Epstein-Barr virus-recent advances. Lancet Infect Dis., 2003. 3(3): p. 131-40

[234] Maley, C.C., Cancer: The Evolutionary Legacy. Heredity, 2002. 88(3): p. 219.

[235] Greaves, M., Cancer causation: the Darwinian downside of past success? The Lancet Oncology, 2002. 3(4): p. 244-251.

[236] Greaves, M., Darwin and evolutionary tales in leukemia ASH Education Program Book 2009 2009 (1): p. 3-12

[237] Greaves, M. and C.C. Maley, Clonal evolution in cancer. Nature, 2012. 481(7381): p. 306-313.

Section 2

Supporitve Care

Chapter 3

Psychological and Social Factors influencing Patients' Treatment Selection for Localised Prostate Cancer

Luke A Robles, Shihning Chou, Owen J Cole,
Akhlil Hamid, Amanda Griffiths and Kavita Vedhara

Additional information is available at the end of the chapter

http://dx.doi.org/10. 5772/52641

1. Introduction

Prostate cancer is the most common form of cancer in men in the United Kingdom (UK). A quarter of all new cases of cancer diagnosed in men are prostate cancers. In 2009, over 40,000 cases of prostate cancer were reported in the UK and more than 10,000 men die from the disease each year [1]. Prostate cancer is also a major concern worldwide. Its highest incidence rates are found in Australia and New Zealand with its lowest in South-Central Asia [2].

The rate of men being diagnosed with prostate cancer has significantly increased worldwide in recent decades [3]. This is likely due to the prostate-specific antigen test being performed among younger men and resulting in the majority of men being diagnosed with localised prostate cancer (LPCa) [4, 5]. These men are usually presented with treatment options, which most commonly include: (1) active surveillance (i. e. , regular monitoring of disease activity for those intended to be treated with subsequent curative treatment), (2) radical prostatectomy, (3) external beam radiation therapy, and (4) brachytherapy, and are asked to consider and select their preferred treatment. The situation that patients with LPCa face is somewhat unique. They have to decide between treatments because there is no substantial evidence to suggest that one treatment modality differs from other treatments, in terms of overall survival rate [6, 7]. However, there are considerable differences in the side-effects associated with each treatment option.

2. Treatment side-effects and their psychological impact

Men confronted with this treatment decision often need to take into consideration a range of factors, including the potential physical side effects of treatments and their psychological, social and emotional consequences. For example, patients being treated with radical therapies can experience severe side-effects, such as urinary incontinence (UI) and erectile dysfunction (ED), as a result of treatment. UI symptoms can persist years after treatment [8] and this can have an impact on all aspects of an individual's functioning. Men with UI often avoid social situations due to the risk of their incontinence becoming apparent to other people. They can feel embarrassed by their inability to self-control their bodily functions and by the lack of empathy from other people within social situations [9].

Relatively little research has been conducted to examine the relationship between ED and psychological morbidity among men with prostate cancer. Nevertheless, ED has been reported to have a profound effect on a patient's quality of life post-treatment. Nelson et al. [10] examined the relationship between depressive symptoms and erectile function. A group of men, who did not receive any treatment for their prostate cancer, completed self-report questionnaires measuring anxiety and depression symptoms and erectile function approximately 4-years post-diagnosis. Erectile dysfunction was found to be a significant predictor of depression independent of other influential factors of depression, such as anxiety and marital status. This finding suggests that men can experience lasting psychological effects from their disease. Another study by Nelson et al. [11] examined men's responses to ED affecting their sexual function and their adjustment to diminished erections after having undergone a radical prostatectomy. These men completed self-report questionnaires measuring erectile function and sexual satisfaction pre-operatively, 12 and 24 months post-operatively. The findings revealed that sexual satisfaction decreased after surgery with patients feeling ashamed and embarrassed by their difficulty to perform sexually with their partners. Sexual dissatisfaction persisted over the period of 24-months, even in men who reported good erectile function post-operatively. Thus, it appears that men do not seem to adjust well to the consequences of their treatment.

ED is a condition which not only affects the individual but also affects couples. There have been differences in the perceptions held by men with ED due to treatment for prostate cancer and their partners. Men with ED have reported an "all or nothing" approach to their sexual relationship with their partner; in that if they are unable to 'perform' sexually then it is pointless to engage in sexual contact. This can lead to men withdrawing from intimate contact with their partners causing strain on the relationship [12]. Women partners have reported to be less concerned about treatments to help the physical functioning of their partners with ED, and are more focused on finding alternative ways to maintain intimacy and sexual stimulation [13].

The option of active surveillance as a management plan for LPCa can also affect the quality of life of men diagnosed with the disease. Although no active treatment is administered, active surveillance can have a psychological impact. Qualitative studies have provided some insight into the experiences of living with prostate cancer. For instance,

Hedestig et al. [14] conducted interviews with patient with untreated LPCa and analysed the interview transcripts using in-depth qualitative narrative analysis. Their findings revealed that men perceived their disease as life-threatening, experienced uncertainty, fear and worry about their cancer progression, and a repressed sense of manhood due to sexual dysfunctions.

3. Personal beliefs and treatment selection

The decision on a treatment modality for LPCa could, therefore, be described as a challenging one requiring patients to weigh up a range of physical and psychological outcomes of treatments. Indeed, it has been shown that patients can experience decision-related distress at diagnosis, which can persist over time and lead to poorly informed treatment decisions [15]. The difficulties associated with making a treatment choice can be further magnified by patients making their decisions based on their personal beliefs. These personal beliefs can help patients construct a mental representation about their disease and its treatment, which can guide their adjustment to their disease. Such beliefs are of particular importance to treatment decisions when there is great uncertainty around the long-term effects of treatment.

Extensive research has found that personal beliefs can predict a range of outcomes, including quality of life, help-seeking behaviour and treatment adherence [16-18]. These beliefs have also been shown to affect treatment choice, mainly by way of selecting between conventional treatment and complementary and alternative medicines (CAM) for conditions, such as chronic pain, hypertension, and both localised and advanced prostate cancer [19-22]. These studies reported that patients who used CAM were more likely to hold negative beliefs about their illness (i. e. , that their illness was chronic and that they had little personal control over its management); and about conventional treatments (i. e. , believed the treatments would result in significant undesirable side-effects). In contrast, patients who were less likely to favour CAM held positive beliefs about their illness and its treatment (i. e. , believed the condition was not severe and would easily be controlled with conventional treatment). Indeed, patients' positive beliefs about their illness were also shown to increase the likelihood of choosing generic rather than branded medicines, as well as reduce the amount of drugs they consumed to manage their conditions [20, 23].

It is not well-understood how patients, who are diagnosed with LPCa and offered conventional treatments, make sense of their disease and their treatment decisions through examining personal beliefs. Patients with LPCa can make treatment decisions that may not necessarily be in accordance with the treatment-related information provided by urologists [24]. Thus, patients may choose a treatment based on confounding information derived from their own experience and from other sources available to them. By gaining a better understanding of patients' personal beliefs may help both patients and urologists make more informed decisions about treatments.

4. A systematic review of the literature

An initial scope for existing literature reviews in prostate cancer research yielded two reviews [25, 26]. The more recent review [26] was conducted five years ago and restricted its search period to a 14 year time span, used a small number of literature databases and only searched for original, peer-reviewed studies to explore broadly the personal (not just beliefs specifically) and external factors pertaining to the decision-making process of patients. It concluded that there is a general lack of understanding about the role of patients' beliefs in treatment selection and that this was an area worthy of enquiry. Our aim was, therefore, to provide an updated review on factors influencing treatment selection for LPCa, as well as specifically examine the literature pertaining to patients' personal beliefs about LPCa and/or its treatments.

A systematic search of the literature was conducted in electronic databases to retrieve relevant published papers from 1980 – 2010, which included: MEDLINE (1950-present); CINAHL; ScienceDirect and CancerLIT (PubMed). Searches were conducted by exploding and combining the medical subject term 'prostate cancer' and free-text words, such as 'beliefs, cognitions, choices, treatment options'. A language restriction was not set whilst searching for the papers.

Non-scholarly literature was searched using the following charity databases: The Prostate Cancer Charity (Jan-April 2010) and Cancer Research UK. The following Government websites were also searched: World Health Organisation (WHO) and the National Institute of Health and Clinical Excellence (NICE). The Networked Digital Library of Theses and Dissertations was searched for theses discussing relevant work and studies.

The reference lists of literature reviews were hand-searched and key authors identified from the search procedure were contacted for any other relevant studies.

The studies retrieved from the literature searches were screened against the inclusion criteria, which included: (i) samples of men diagnosed with, and being treated for, LPCa, and (ii) studies examining patients' beliefs about their LPCa and treatment options. All study designs except reviews, opinion papers and single case studies, were considered for inclusion into the present review.

The titles and abstracts of the references yielded from the search procedure were screened against the inclusion criteria. The full text of the potentially relevant papers were retrieved and read for consideration into the review. The papers that met the inclusion criteria were assessed for their methodological quality.

5. Synthesis of findings

The search procedure yielded ten papers, which are summarised in Tables 1 and 2. It was inappropriate to combine findings statistically to produce meaningful outcomes. This was partly due to the small number of quantitative studies identified for inclusion into the review. Primarily, the assessment of the included studies revealed there to be many methodological differences that existed between the studies. This made it difficult to pool studies to determine the effect of perceptions on treatment selection. Therefore, a qualitative synthesis of the findings was undertaking with studies being grouped according to treatment modality and those factors affecting decision-making. Statistical findings from the quantitative studies were used to support the observed findings from the qualitative studies.

5.1. Beliefs underpinning treatment selection for localised prostate cancer

5.1.1. Radical prostatectomy

Patients' beliefs and other influences in selecting to undergo a radical prostatectomy were clearly reported in nine of the studies [27-35]. Many of the patients perceived their cancer as a localised problem and that the most tangible and definitive method of curing or preventing the disease from spreading was to remove the tumour [27-29, 31, 35]. These findings were also replicated in three of the quantitative studies, which reported that beliefs about the effectiveness of surgery and complete tumour removal were statistically associated with selecting surgery [33-35]. Surgery would also allow for surgeons to be more informed about the nature and extent of the cancer and would provide the patients with more information about their disease [27, 28]. Surgery was considered to have the best evidence base in terms of its efficacy in combating cancer compared to other curative treatment options [31, 32]. Overall, patients believed surgery to be the best and most effective form of treatment. This corresponds with current treatment rates, which show that the majority of patients with LPCa opt for surgery [36].

5.1.2. External beam radiation therapy and brachytherapy

External beam radiation therapy (EBRT) was regarded by most patients as being an inferior treatment option to a radical prostatectomy. This was based on their belief that EBRT provided uncertainty surrounding its ability to cure their cancer [27, 28, 30, 31] through treatment administered externally to the body. Unlike a radical prostatectomy, EBRT was believed to disadvantage the patient by being time-consuming and disruptive to daily life with severe consequential side-effects [27, 28]. Interestingly, some of these side-effects were mistaken for side-effects associated with chemotherapy (e. g. , hair loss, weight loss, vomiting) [27, 28, 30]. It appeared that when patients selected EBRT as their preferred treatment, it was to avoid the negative effects of surgery, i. e. , being less invasive and resulting in fewer side-effects [31, 35]. These beliefs were similar to those held by patients who selected brachytherapy as their preferred treatment. However, like a radical prostatectomy, brachytherapy was believed to provide a 'direct' and, therefore, more effective and convenient form of treatment to cure their cancer [31, 34].

5.1.3. Active surveillance / watchful waiting

The terms 'watchful waiting' were used in some of the papers along with the other active treatment options. Watchful waiting usually refers to a less intense management plan where palliative care is usually provided. These options were rarely considered by patients as a management option for their cancer. They were typically rejected due to patients' fear about the cancer spreading [31, 33] and their need to be "doing something" active to combat their prostate cancer [28, 31]. Holmboe and Concato [31] suggested that other possible explanations for patients rejecting watchful waiting included fear of death or the inability to monitor cancer progression. Patients who opted for active surveillance perceived their cancer as 'a very small growth' and a common disease among men as they get older. These men were accepting of the uncertainty surrounding their disease progression and believed it would be best to endure the severe side-effects of curative treatment only when it was evident that treatment was required [37]. However, this willingness to accept active surveillance as a management option appeared to occur in men whose urologists advocated the view that the disease was not severe and would progress slowly [37].

Study Ref	Authors, year, & study location	Design	Characteristics of sample	Major findings
[27]	Denberg et al. (2006) Denver, USA	Perspective cohort (follow-up 6-8 months) using semi-structured interviews	20 men newly diagnosed with LPCa considering treatment options Age range 53-80 years 70% (white); 25% (African American); 5% (Latino)	40% perceived surgery as a definitive treatment Surgery offered crucial knowledge about tumour 55% perceived surgery as undesirable regarding invasiveness
[28]	O'Rourke (1999) North Carolina, USA	Perspective cohort (follow-up 3 & 12 months) using couple & individual semi-structured interviews	18 men newly diagnosed with LPCa who have made a treatment decision 18 spouses recruited Mean age 67.6 (range 52-78 years) (patient) Mean age 62.1 (range 49-74 years) (partner) 13% white (patient), 5% African American; 72% white, 28% African American (spouse)	Couples believed cancer is only curable through surgery Perceived uncertainty about radiotherapy regarding efficacy & outcome Men more concerned about side-effects than wives

http://dx.doi.org/10. 5772/52641

Study Ref	Authors, year, & study location	Design	Characteristics of sample	Major findings
[29]	O'Rourke & Germino. (1998) North Carolina, USA	Retrospective cross-sectional study using unstructured focus groups	11 men diagnosed with LPCa, who have made a treatment decision 6 spouses recruited Age range 58-72 years (patients) Age range 51-64 years (spouses) 99% white; 1% African American	Surgery perceived as a first line choice Prior bias toward surgery due to perceived association with cure Radiotherapy perceived inferior to surgery due to its efficacy & side-effects
[30]	Steginga et al. (2002) Queensland, Australia	Cross-sectional study using semi-structured interviews	108 men diagnosed with LPCa considering curative treatment options Mean age 62 years (range 39-80 years) Ethnicity not specified	47% described other patients' treatment experiences used in their decision-making 34% held lay belief that surgery was the best way to cure their cancer 12% were uncertain about radiotherapy as a way to cure their cancer
[31]	Holmboe & Concato. (2000) New Haven, USA	Cross-sectional study using interviews with open-ended questions	102 men newly diagnosed with LPCa, who have made a treatment decision Mean age 66.4 years Majority white (89%)	Majority influenced by external information (i.e., 30% for physician recommendation) Classified likes & dislikes of treatments Removal of tumour & evidence of efficacy as main likes for surgery Fear of future consequences was the most common reason to reject watchful waiting
[37]	Davison et al. (2009) Vancouver, Canada	Retrospective cross-sectional study using interviews with semi-structured interviews	25 men with low-risk prostate cancer on active surveillance Mean age 66 years (range 48-77 years) Majority white (92%); 8% South Asian	Men perceived their cancer as a common disease & exaggerated the potential incidence Realised treatment might be necessary, but viewed as "a grey zone"

Table 1. Description of the Qualitative Studies included in the Systematic Review

Study ID reference	Authors, year, & study location	Design	Characteristics of sample	Major findings
[32]	Hall et al. (2003) Virginia, USA	Retrospective cross-sectional study using self-report questionnaires developed from literature review & clinical impressions	351 men with LPCa treated with surgery or brachytherapy Mean age 62±5 years (radical prostatectomy); 66±8 years (brachytherapy); 70±7 years (combination of brachytherapy & radiotherapy) Ethnicity not specified	42.9% brachytherapy patients & 97.5% radical prostatectomy patients chose treatment based on evidence shown to cure the cancer Side-effects were an important motivator Urologists were the most important source of information and a major factor in decision-making process
[33]	Zeliadt et al. (2010) USA	Cross-sectional study using self-report questionnaires developed from preliminary focus groups & cognitive interviews	198 newly diagnosed patients considering surgery only & patients considering other treatment options Mean age 63 years 72% white, 11% black, 16% Hispanic/Asian (surgery); 68% white, 26% Black, 6% Hispanic/ Asian (other options)	Treatment efficacy influenced preference for surgery Personal burden influenced nonsurgical options
[34]	Gwede et al. (2005) Florida, USA	Cross-sectional study using questions derived from previous study	69 men diagnosed with LPCa, who have made a decision about treatment Mean age: 57.7 years (range 39.6-71.1) (surgery); 65.2 years (range 45.7-89.2) (brachytherapy) 86.5% (surgery); 97% (brachytherapy) white	Cure and complete tumour removal were the main motivations for surgery (74%) Brachytherapy related to quality-of-life issues
[35]	Teramoto et al. 2006 Kamogawa, Japan	Cross-sectional study using self-report questionnaires	51 men diagnosed with LPCa treated with radical prostatectomy or external beam radiation therapy Overall mean age: 68.2 (range 56–75 years) Japanese sample	Physician was the major factor influencing treatment decisions in both treatment groups (>90%) Family and others was a more important factor for patients undergoing surgery than patients undergoing radiation therapy Surgery was desired for cancer control Radiation therapy favoured concerning side-effects

Table 2. Description of the Quantitative Studies included in the Systematic Review

5.1.4. The role of urologists and partners in informing patient beliefs

The recommendations made by urologists emerged in many of the papers [28, 29, 31-33, 37] as being influential in shaping patients' beliefs regarding their treatment choice. A high percentage of patients (48-65%) said they would selected the treatments recommended by their urologist [30, 32]. Consequently, seeking a second opinion was unnecessary serving only to delay treatment and provide potentially more conflicting information to process [27, 28].

Partners, who often experience considerable emotional distress themselves on hearing the diagnosis [25, 38], have also been found to exert an important influence on patients' beliefs. Three studies reported the role of the partners to be a source of information or a mediator in helping men to process their treatment information [27, 32, 34]. However, it was also reported in two studies that, ultimately, it is the patients themselves who reported ownership of their treatment decision [29, 37].

5.1.5. The role of patients' information seeking behavior in informing beliefs

Another major factor influencing patients' beliefs was their own information-seeking behaviour. Patients and their partners are often actively engaged in learning about their treatment options, side-effects and the background of their urologists [29]. The evidence suggested that they made use of a variety of resources, including health care professions (HCPs) (i. e. , urologists, radiation oncologist), the internet, books, magazines, friends and family [27, 29, 30, 32, 34, 37]. Processing such large amounts of advice and potential contradictory information was suggested to be an explanation for the misconceptions about treatments reported by the patients (i. e. , associating the effects of chemotherapy with radiotherapy) [27, 30].

5.1.6. The role of other patients' treatment experiences in informing patient beliefs

In four studies, there was evidence that patients [27, 28, 30, 33] and their partners used the experiences of other people with cancer in their decisions about treatment. Denberg et al. [27] described that these experiences influenced patients' beliefs regarding LPCa, its treatment and treatment side-effects. Steginga et al. [30] reported that 47% of men described considering other people they knew (not just those with prostate cancer), who had negative experiences with cancer or cancer treatment, in their decision-making. O'Rourke [28] reported that comparisons with other patients, who had a positive outcome from treatment, were mostly related to surgery and that comparisons were usually made between friends and family members, who had undergone surgery and were making a good recovery. It has been suggested that patients may pay more attention to the experiences of other patients with cancer than to the risk information presented to them by their urologists and specialist nurses [27]. The reliability of their findings was supported by the quantitative findings of Zeliadt et al. [33], who reported a statistically significant association between the experiences from other patients and treatment selection for patients who only considered surgery as a viable treatment.

6. Discussion

The findings synthesised in the present review have demonstrated that patients select a treatment or management option based on their beliefs about their cancer, the perceived effectiveness of the treatment and their beliefs regarding the side-effects of the treatment. With regards to the present findings, the majority of patients select active surveillance because of their belief that their cancer was not aggressive, selected to undergo a radical prostatectomy because they believed it to be most effective at curing their cancer, and selected EBRT because of the reduced risk of side-effects. A range of factors external to the patient, which inform these beliefs, were also identified. These included the patients' high regard of the urologists' treatment recommendation, the emotional distress experienced by partners, the various modes of seeking information about treatments, and other peoples' experiences of treatment.

It is, however, also very clear that the evidence base on patients' beliefs in the context of LPCa remains limited. This is an area in need of high quality prospective studies to gain a greater understanding of the factors that influence treatment decisions. This understanding could help develop interventions designed to support men in these decisions and to assist with their long-term adjustment to prostate cancer and its treatment.

The limited evidence that has been synthesised in this review does, however, enable some clear recommendations to be made how this area of research and, ultimately, clinical practice may move forward. In particular, it is clear that the existing findings relate well to two theoretical frameworks, which have been developed to understand patients' beliefs regarding illness and treatment; and which have also been the basis of therapeutic interventions [39, 40]. These are the self-regulatory model (SRM) [41, 42] and the Necessity Concerns Framework (NCF) [17, 43]. The SRM describes that individuals' personal beliefs allow them to make sense of their disease and enable them to reach their illness goals (e. g. , in LPCa these could be survival, reducing the risk of side effects, etc.). These beliefs cluster around 5 domains: (1) identity (the way patients describe their disease and its symptoms); (2) cause (what caused the disease); (3) timeline (how long the disease is going to last); (4) consequence (how will the disease and/or its treatment affect me?); and (5) controllability (whether the disease is believed to be preventable, curable, or controllable). Similarly, the NCF also focuses on personal beliefs, but those specifically related to treatment. Previous research has shown that patients' beliefs regarding treatment tend to focus on two domains: beliefs regarding how necessary/important the treatment is to their future well-being and beliefs regarding concerns (i. e. , what are the potential adverse consequences of the treatment?).

There was clear evidence in the studies included in this review of the beliefs specified by both the SRM and NCF. For example, patients believed their cancer to be a mass within the body (akin to identity beliefs) and that removing this mass would cure their cancer (akin to controllability beliefs). Similarly, patients believed curative treatment would offer them the best outcome in terms of survival (akin to necessity beliefs) because their cancer could potentially re-occur (akin to concern beliefs). Furthermore, the importance of factors external to the patient in shaping their beliefs is also specified by the SRM. Thus, it was suggested that the results of this review provide strong evidence to support the use of these theoretical frameworks in future research.

7. Recommendation for health care

It is clear that the use of patients' beliefs in their decisions on a treatment modality has led them to base their decisions on misconceptions rather than on evidential information. HCPs may need to challenge misinformed beliefs held by patients to help them make more informed decisions regarding their treatment. In order to make more conclusive recommendations for health care practice, further research is required to establish the extent to which personal beliefs alter treatment selection.

8. Recommendations for further research

The majority of the studies included in this review used a qualitative approach. Such methods explore a topic area in-depth and provide a descriptive account of findings. While this approach can provide very rich data in specific domains, these data are not intended to be generalisable. Thus, quantitative studies (preferably with prospective designs) are required in the future to ascertain, not only the salient beliefs influencing treatment choices but also, how these beliefs affect long-term adjustment to the disease and its treatment.

With regards to the studies which employed quantitative methodologies, none used standardised and validated measures for examining illness or treatment beliefs. Two of the quantitative studies [32, 34] developed their measures of beliefs from previous published work. The remaining study developed its measure from preliminary focus groups and interviews [33]. It could be suggested that further validation of these measures is required before any strong conclusions can be drawn.

The time at which illness and treatment beliefs were measured is another shortcoming of the included studies. Some of the studies included those patients who had already made a treatment decision or who had already started treatment. This may have affected the reliability of the findings due to the potential bias of patients recalling what they believed about their illness and its treatment at these times in the treatment process. Prospective designs involving the assessment of beliefs before a treatment choice is made would offer a more robust approach.

A further limitation concerned the majority of the patient samples being predominantly white and from North America. Therefore, the experiences of other groups, such as men of Afro-Caribbean origin in whom the risk of prostate cancer is greater, were not represented. Further research is required across a range of ethnic and cultural groups.

9. Conclusion

The present review has revealed that our understanding of the role played by the personal beliefs of men regarding their LPCa and its treatment is still limited. The existing evidence has been dominated by qualitative methods, cross-sectional designs and the use of non-validated instruments. However, it is also clear from existing findings that the adoption of the SRM and NCF, with their associated validated instruments, could provide a greater understanding of the factors that influence treatment decisions. Further research using psychological frameworks could also help develop interventions to support men in their treatment decisions, and assist with their long-term adjustment to LPCa and its treatment.

Acknowledgements

The authors would like to thank Dr Chris Bridle for his help and support with this review.

Author details

Luke A Robles[1], Shihning Chou[1], Owen J Cole[2], Akhlil Hamid[3], Amanda Griffiths[1] and Kavita Vedhara[4]

*Address all correspondence to: lwxlar@nottingham. ac. uk

1 Institute of Work, Health & Organisation, The University of Nottingham, Nottingham, UK

2 Department of Urology, The Medical Specialist Group, Guernsey

3 Department of Urology and University of Western Australia, Royal Perth Hospital, Western Australia

4 Division of Primary Care, The University of Nottingham, Nottingham, UK

References

[1] Cancer Research UK. *Prostate cancer key Facts.* http://info.cancerresearchuk.org/cancerstats/keyfacts/prostate-cancer/cancerstats-key-facts-on-prostate-cancer (accessed 23 July 2012).

[2] World Cancer Research Fund International. *The incidence of prostate cancer is 25 times higher in Australia and New Zealand then in South-Central Asia.* http://www.wcrf.org/cancer_facts/prostate-cancer-worldwide.php (accessed 23 July 2012).

[3] Albertsen PC. When is active surveillance the appropriate treatment for prostate cancer? *Acta Oncologica* 2011; 50(1): 120-6.

[4] Moore AL, Dimitropoulou P, Lane A, Powell PH, Greenberg DC, Brown CH, et al. Population-based prostate-specific antigen testing in the UK leads to a stage migration of prostate cancer. *British Journal of Urology International* 2009; 104(11): 1592-8.

[5] McGregor M, Hanley J, Boivin J, McLean R. Screening for prostate cancer: estimating the magnitude of overdetection. *Canadian Medical Association Journal* 1998; 159(11): 1368-72.

[6] O'Rourke ME. Choose wisely: therapeutic decisions and quality of life in patients with prostate cancer. *Clinical Journal of Oncology Nursing* 2007; 11(3): 401-8.

[7] Neal DE, Donovan J. Prostate cancer: to screen or not to screen. *Lancet Oncology* 2000; 1: 17-24.

[8] Ponholzer A, Brössner C, Struhal G, Marszalek M, Madersbacher S. Lower urinary tract symptoms, urinary incontinence, sexual function and quality of life after radical prostatectomy and external beam radiation therapy: real life experience in Austria. *World Journal of Urology* 2006; 24(3): 325-30.

[9] Palmer MH, Fogarty LA, Somerfield MR, Powel LL. Incontinence after prostatectomy: coping with incontinence after prostate cancer surgery. *Oncology Nursing Forum* 2003; 30(2): 229-38.

[10] Nelson C, Mulhall J, Roth A. The association between erectile dysfunction and depressive symptoms in men treated for prostate cancer. *Journal of Sexual Medicine* 2011; 8(2): 560-6.

[11] Nelson C, Deveci S, Stasi J, Scardino P, Mulhall J. Sexual bother following radical prostatectomyjsm. *Journal of Sexual Medicine* 2010; 7(1): 129-35.

[12] Sand MS, Fisher W, Rosen R, Heiman J, Eardley I. Erectile dysfunction and constructs of masculinity and quality of life in the multinational Men's Attitudes to Life Events and Sexuality (MALES) study. *Journal of Sexual Medicine* 2008; 5(3): 583-94.

[13] Chambers SK, Schover L, Halford K, Clutton S, Ferguson M, Gordon L, et al. ProsCan for Couples: randomised controlled trial of a couples-based sexuality intervention for men with localised prostate cancer who receive radical prostatectomy. *BMC Cancer* 2008; 8: 226.

[14] Hedestig O, Sandman PO, Widmark A. Living with untreated localized prostate cancer: a qualitative analysis of patient narratives. *Cancer Nursing* 2003; 26(1): 55-60.

[15] Steginga S, Turner E, Donovan J. The decision-related psychosocial concerns of men with localised prostate cancer: targets for intervention and research. *World Journal of Urology* 2008; 26: 469-74.

[16] Karamanidou C, Clatworthy J, Weinman J, Horne R. A systematic review of the prevalence and determinants of nonadherence to phosphate binding medication in patients with end-stage renal disease. *BMC Nephrology* 2008; 9: 2.

[17] Horne R, Weinman J. Patients' beliefs about prescribed medicines and their role in adherence to treatment in chronic physical illness. *Journal of Psychosomatic Research* 1999; 47(6): 555-67.

[18] Petrie KJ, Jago LA, Devcich DA. The role of illness perceptions in patients with medical conditions. *Current Opinion in Psychiatry* 2007; 20(2): 163-7.

[19] Brown M, Dean S, Hay-Smith EJC, Taylor W, Baxter GD. Musculoskeletal pain and treatment choice: an exploration of illness perceptions and choices of conventional or complementary therapies. *Disability and Rehabilitation* 2010; 32(20): 1645-57.

[20] Figueiras M, Marcelino DS, Claudino A, Cortes MA, Maroco J, Weinman J. Patients' illness schemata of hypertension: The role of beliefs for the choice of treatment. *Psychology & Health* 2010; 25(4): 507-17.

[21] Boon H, Brown JB, Gavin A, Westlake K. Men with prostate cancer: making decisions about complementary/alternative medicine. *Medical Decision Making* 2003; 23(6): 471-9.

[22] Porter MC, Diefenbach MA. Pushed and Pulled: The Role of Affect and Cognition in Shaping CAM Attitudes and Behavior among Men Treated for Prostate Cancer. *Journal of Health Psychology* 2009; 14(2): 288-96.

[23] Al Anbar NN, Dardennes RM, Prado-Netto A, Kaye K, Contejean Y. Treatment choices in autism spectrum disorder: The role of parental illness perceptions. *Research in Developmental Disabilities* 2010; 31(3): 817-28.

[24] Berry D, Ellis W, Woods N, Schwien C, Mullen K, Yang C. Treatment decision-making by men with localized prostate cancer: the influence of personal factors. *Urologic Oncology* 2003; 21(2): 93-100.

[25] O'Rourke ME. Decision Making and Prostate Cancer Treatment Selection: A Review. *Seminars in Oncology Nursing* 2001; 17(2): 108-17.

[26] Zeliadt SB, Ramsey SD, Penson DF, Hall IJ, Ekwueme DU, Stroud L, et al. Why do men choose one treatment over another?: a review of patient decision making for localized prostate cancer. *Cancer* 2006; 106(9): 1865-74.

[27] Denberg TD, Melhado TV, Steiner JF. Patient treatment preferences in localized prostate carcinoma: The influence of emotion, misconception, and anecdote. *Cancer* 2006; 107(3): 620-30.

[28] O'Rourke ME. Narrowing the options: the process of deciding on prostate cancer treatment. *Cancer Investigation* 1999; 17(5): 349-59.

[29] O'Rourke ME, Germino BB. Prostate cancer treatment decisions: a focus group exploration. *Oncology Nursing Forum* 1998; 25(1): 97-104.

[30] Steginga SK, Occhipinti S, Gardiner RA, Yaxley J, Heathcote P. Making decisions about treatment for localized prostate cancer. *British Journal of Urology International* 2002; 89(3): 255-60.

[31] Holmboe ES, Concato J. Treatment decisions for localized prostate cancer: asking men what's important. *Journal of General Internal Medicine* 2000; 15(10): 694-701.

[32] Hall JD, Boyd JC, Lippert MC, Theodorescu D. Why patients choose prostatectomy or brachytherapy for localized prostate cancer: results of a descriptive survey. *Urology* 2003; 61(2): 402-7.

[33] Zeliadt SB, Moinpour CM, Blough DK, Penson DF, Hall IJ, Smith JL, et al. Preliminary treatment considerations among men with newly diagnosed prostate cancer. *American Journal of Managed Care* 2010; 16(5): 121-30.

[34] Gwede CK, Pow-Sang J, Seigne J, Heysek R, Helal M, Shade K, et al. Treatment decision-making strategies and influences in patients with localized prostate carcinoma. *Cancer* 2005; 104(7): 1381-90.

[35] Teramoto S, Ota T, Itaya N, Maniwa A, Matsui T, Nishimura Y, et al. [Survey of factors underlying treatment choice for patients with localized prostate cancer (radical prostatectomy vs extrabeam radiotherapy)]. *Nippon Hinyokika Gakkai Zasshi - Japanese Journal of Urology* 2006; 97(7): 823-9.

[36] McVey GP, McPhail S, Fowler S, McIntosh G, Gillatt D, Parker CC. Initial management of low-risk localized prostate cancer in the UK: analysis of the British Association of Urological Surgeons Cancer Registry. *British Journal of Urology International* 2010; 106(8): 1161-4.

[37] Davison BJ, Oliffe JL, Pickles T, Mroz L. Factors influencing men undertaking active surveillance for the management of low-risk prostate cancer. *Oncology Nursing Forum* 2009; 36(1): 89-96.

[38] Kirby R, Holmes K, Amoroso P. Supporting the supporter: helping the partner of patients newly diagnosed with prostate cancer. *British Journal of Urology International* 2010; 105(11): 1489-90.

[39] Petrie KJ, Cameron LD, Ellis CJ, Buick D, Weinman J. Changing illness perceptions after myocardial infarction: an early intervention randomized controlled trial. *Psychosomatic Medicine* 2002; 64(4): 580-6.

[40] Petrie KJ, Jago LA, Devcich DA. The role of illness perceptions in patients with medical conditions. *Current Opinion in Psychiatry* 2007; 20(2): 163-7.

[41] Leventhal H, Brissette I, Leventhal EA. The common-sense model of self-regulation of health and illness. In: Cameron LD, Leventhal, H. (ed.) *The self-regulation of health and illness behaviour.* New York: Routledge; 2003. p42-65.

[42] Meyer D, Leventhal H, Gutmann M. Common-sense models of illness: the example of hypertension. *Health Psychology* 1985; 4(2): 115-35.

[43] Horne R, Cooper V, Gellaitry G, Date HL, Fisher M. Patients' perceptions of highly active antiretroviral therapy in relation to treatment uptake and adherence: the utility of the necessity-concerns framework. *Journal of Acquired Immune Deficiency Syndromes* 2007; 45(3): 334-41.

Chapter 4

The Role of Physiotherapy in the Pre and Post Treatment Interventions in Prostate Cancer Patients

Mario Bernardo Filho and
Mauro Luis Barbosa Júnior

Additional information is available at the end of the chapter

http://dx.doi.org/10.5772/52441

1. Introduction

1.1. Cancer and physiotherapy

Cancer is the common term for all malignant tumours and its consequences are a concern for people worldwide. Advances in health and medical science procedures (early diagnosis, improved chemotherapy and radiotherapy) and surgical techniques, and their utilization in the field of oncology, have significantly improved survival and have thus strongly influenced the practice of physiotherapy [1, 2, 3, 4].

People are living longer with their cancers, which in many cases are treated as chronic disease, due to the early detection and advances in treatment options. Thus, physiotherapists require greater knowledge of the clinical conditions and improved skill in managing patients with cancer, before, during and after the specific medical procedures. They also have the responsibility of managing and treating patients during the pre and postoperative periods with the provision of the best particular physiotherapeutic intervention to each patient [5, 6].

Besides the knowledge about clinical interventions, the physiotherapist needs to be in contact with the recent advances in the scientific literature in general. Moreover, this professional must know about the risk factors to cancer and participate in actions to aid in the prevention of this disease [5, 6, 7].

In oncology, for example, there is increasing evidence, initially only from epidemiological studies but increasingly from individuals case studies, that risk of some cancers, such as prostate, may be reduced in people living in areas of high ambient solar radiation or with high sun exposure than in those where the converse is the case. Naturally, the information about the protection against the unnecessary exposition of the sunlight is also very important [8, 9].

Images are suitable tools to aid in the early diagnosis of several types of cancer. However, some modalities of images, as the positron emission tomography (PET) dependenting on the radiopharmaceutical, and in some clinical condition, false negative information can be obtained. As a profisssional of an interdisciplinar team, the physiotherapist must have enough knowledge to suggest a modality of image and to know about the limitations of each procedure [4, 10, 11]

Epidemiological researches have put in evidence the benefits of physical activity in relation to the risk of cancer. Moreover, the physical activity has been considered as a modifiable lifestyle risk factor that has the potential to reduce the risk of the majority of the types of diseases, as the cancer. The physiotherapist must be also involved in public and private actions to guide the Society to have correct style of the life also related to adequate exercise (kinesiotherapy) and physical activities in general. Naturally, these actions must consider the individual characteristic of each subject [5, 12].

Undesirable clinical conditions due to the use of some techniques to treat cancer can bring bothersome that can comprise the sexual health and the quality of life. It is important that the interprofessional team be prepared to discuss these questions [13, 14].

2. Role of physiotherapy

Physiotherapeutic procedures have an important role in the healthcare of people of all ages and with different types of clinical status. These procedures are relevant in the treatment, in the prevention of diseases or complications and in the management or treatment of undesirable pathological conditions to thus minimize the impact these may have in the quality of life of the patient [7].

Physiotherapy is a profession defined by great diversity in areas of clinical practice with the purpose of developing, maintaining and restoring the maximum movement and functional ability of each person, considering the specific limitations of the individual. The role of the physiotherapist within the interdisciplinary group (physician, nurse, nutritionist, occupational therapy, social worker, psychologist, speech therapist) is well defined in various clinical conditions, as with the patient with cancer [5, 7].

The pressing need arises for the existence of a differentiated care system with the purpose to cater for the particular needs of the patients and their families. It is desirable that the physiotherapist working in oncology has a broad knowledge of other clinical areas, such as neurology, the musculoskeletal and cardiopulmonary systems and in rehabilitation and kinesiotherapy in general, as well as in services along the entire spectrum of patient care. There is also a considerable role for the physiotherapists in the evaluation of the clinical conditions and management of the patients, as well as in assisting people's return to work and normal life following treatment [6, 14].

It is often the fatigue and weakness caused by the disease and/or its treatment that delay this return to normal functions and limit the quality of life of a specific individual. An important aspect related to cancer and its treatment is the typically induced muscle atrophy. Probably this clinical condition is due to perturbations in different pathways of the muscle protein metabolism, including decreased muscle protein synthesis, increased muscle protein degradation, or a combination of both [5, 12, 15].

The most prevalent symptom in cancer is fatigue, which has now overtaken pain as the most common distressing symptom of the disease. The intensity of the fatigue varies from patient to patient and it is a complex and subjective phenomenon. Non-pharmacological fatigue cares are desirable. There is much evidence to suggest that appropriately prescribed physical exercises (kinesiotherapy) play an important role in the decrease of cancer fatigue and the improvement of the quality of life of the patient. The reduction of fatigue is highly relevant and desirable for the patient to (i) have the ability to continue or return to work; (ii) develop daily activities at home; and (iii) participate in social activities, all of which are clear parts of the overall quality of life of the patient [2-4, 15, 16]

It is thus essential that physiotherapists working with cancer patients have a clear and comprehensive understanding of the individual cancers and their staging and development, as well as the techniques that are being used in the diagnosis and treatment of the patient. The physiotherapist must have knowledge of the consequences and complications of clinical procedures, such as surgery, chemotherapy and radiotherapy, and their potential side effects such as neuropathies and cardiomyopathies. Moreover, the physiotherapist must be informed about the specific procedures that were used in the patient during medical intervention. A discussion about these procedures and the possible complications and occurrences are relevant to the management of the patient before and after the surgery. In addition, the physiotherapist must also know how these medical procedures can affect the physiotherapeutic interventions and thus select the best and convenient procedure for each patient [5, 7, 14]

The physiotherapist also needs to know more about individual medications as patients can survive longer using new cancer treatments, but often with severe side effects, which leave them weaker and often feeling quite unwell during the process. Hormonal therapy, for example, has an important effect on the muscle mass. The decrease in muscle mass, leading to muscle weakness and general debility, can be minimized by specific kinesiotherapyprogrammes. These appropriated exercises are established and implemented by physiotherapists considering the anatomical area of the disease and specific capabilities and limitations of each patient [5, 6, 7, 14].

Whole body vibration exercises (WBV) performed in oscillating platform could be a good option to aid the patient with cancer. The vibrations generated in these platforms can be transmitted to body of the patient, and, it is suggested that, in appropriated conditions, these vibrations could improve walking function, muscle strength, bone mineral density, cardiovascular fitness and body balance. Moreover, the health-related quality of life is increased and the fall risk is decreased. The frequency and the amplitude of the vibration can be totally controlled by the physiotherapist that is supervising the clinical procedure. The duration of the work, as well as, the time to rest, the number of sets in a session and the number of sessions are also controlled. All these conditions depend on, mainly, the clinical and physical conditions of the patient. The mechanisms responsible for the WBV benefits are not fully understood, however it is hypothesized that these effects are probably related to direct and indirect actions. The direct effects would be related with the transmission of energy of the vibration, for example, to a muscle that would be stimulated. The indirect effects might to be associated with the neuroendocrine system. Whole body mechanical vibration on the muscle performance would be due to the induction of a myotatic reflex contraction referred as the tonic vibration reflex [17, 18, 19].

Normally, the person is standing on the platform, but other positions are possible, as it is shown in the Figure 1. It is possible to see in the Figure 1.c that the man has bent knees.

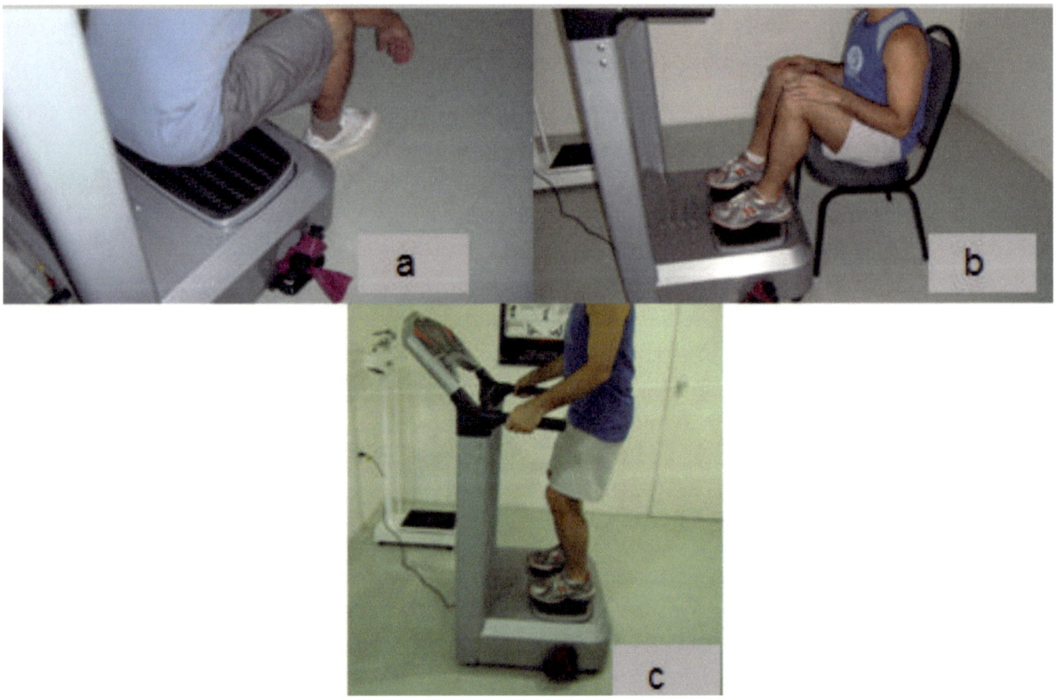

Figure 1. Some of the positions of the person in the oscillating platform. (a) sitting, (b) sitting in a chaise and the feet in the platform, (c) standing.

Physiotherapists utilize physical agents, such as therapeutic exercises (kinesiotherapy), electrotherapy and manipulative therapy to provide a holistic approach to the prevention, diagnosis and therapeutic management of clinical disorders, as well as possible future complications [5, 7]. Involving the movements of the body and the optimization of the functions of the tissues, they aim to enhance the health, welfare and quality of life and thus they can play an important role in the management and rehabilitation of patients with prostate cancer (PCa). In patients with PCa, the physiotherapist will also guide the patient in relation to the knowledge and understanding of the anatomic structures related directly with the pelvic floor, the correct breathing and the perception of the muscles of the pelvic floor, as other muscles of the pelvis. Specific attention is given to the comprehension of the functions of these muscles, especially to the levatorani muscle [20-26]

Sexual health is a state of physical, emotional, mental and social well-being in relation to sexuality; it is not merely the absence of disease, dysfunction or infirmity. Sexuality is considered as a personal and human dimension that is characterized as a strong aspect of the human personality and it is an aspect of the emotional and physical intimacy that men and women experience through their lives. Moreover, sexuality is experienced and expressed in thoughts, fantasies, desires, beliefs, attitudes, values, behaviours, practices, roles and relationships [27, 28, 29]

Sexuality is influenced by the interaction of biological, psychological, social, economic, political, cultural, ethical, legal, historical, religious and spiritual factors. Sexuality is present from the conception up to the dead and it consists of three interrelated and inseparable aspects, that are biological, psychological and social. In consequence, particular attention must be done to the relevance and hole of the organs related to the biological components involved in the sexuality [29, 30]. The importance of the comprehension of the possible undesirable consequences of the clinical procedures used to treat the PCa must be discussed with the patient and/or with the partner. The physiotherapist must have also knowledge about the sexuality to define specific exercises and techniques available to aid the patient with PCa in different steps of his life, as well as the limitations of these and other procedures. [6, 14]

Figure 2 shows some tools used to explain the patient about the anatomic structures directly and indirectly involved with the prostate and the structures that can be damaged in the surgery for the treatment of the PCa.

During the final stages of cancer treatment, the palliative care becomes paramount and the participation of the physiotherapist is also desirable in the interdisciplinary team. The care with the patient with cancer will contribute to minimize the progression of secondary symptoms [5, 6, 26].

The correct and appropriated mobilization of the scars to avoid adherence and important alterations in the posture of the patient is also highly relevant. This procedure contributes to the improvement of the quality of life of the patient immediatly and in the future [5].

Procedures of the physiotherapy in palliative care is also used for pain, lymphoedema, dyspnoea and other symptom assessment and treatment, as well as for the education on safe transfer and mobility management of the patient. Constipation, nausea, sleep disturbance (insomnia), anxiety, fatigue, dyspnoea, pain scores and appetite are all improved by physiotherapeutic intervention. Some of these clinical complications can be also prevented or minimized. Along the time, the lymphoedema management in the terminally diseases has developed more effectively, with evidence supporting the complex physiotherapy treatment and the integration with other professionals [5, 7, 16].

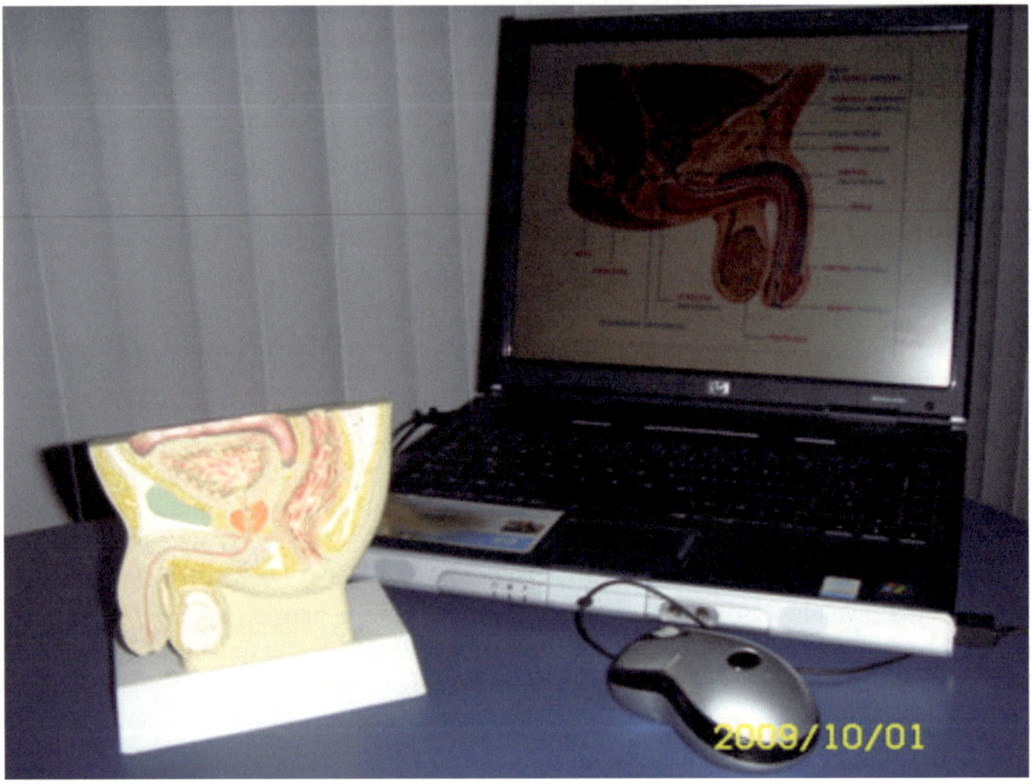

Figure 2. Tools used to explain to the patient about the anatomic structures of the pelvic floor

3. Prostate cancer in the world

Cancer is an important public problem and is considered a national health priority area in several countries due to the burden that it places on the individual, families and the community [1, 2, 31].

The World Health Organization (WHO) develops strategies towards the prevention, research, education and control of the cancer. Important medical developments and relevand scientific findings have permitted that people with cancer can survive with their disease and with the side effects of their disease and its treatment for longer [31].

The high relevance of the cancer in public health and research activity can also be demonstrated by the number of scientific research identified in the database system PubMed (a service of the National Library of Medicine and the National Institutes of Health) [32].

It is possible to see in the Table I, the number of publications in the PubMed related to cancer and cancer and some organs. It is possible to identify in the Table I approximately 2 700

000 full papers in this databank with the keyword cancer and 2.22% of these publications are related with PCa.

The mainly risk factors for PCa are (a) age (it is the strongest risk factor for PCa andthe probability of developing this disease is 1 in 12,833 for men aged birth to 39, 1 in 44 for men aged 40 to 59, and 1 in 7 for men aged 60 to 79 years), (b) family history (greater risk if father or brother had the disease and slightly higher for men whose mothers or sisters have had breast cancer), (c) Race/Ethnicity (greater risk among African American men compared with white, Asian, and American Indian men), (d) prostate changes (abnormal cells described as high-grade prostatic intraepithelial neoplasia), and (e) diet (food with high animal fat and low in fruits and vegetables).Moreover, between 5 to 10% of the PCa cases are believed to be due primarily to high-risk inherited genetic factors or PCa susceptibility genes. Genetic testing has been a reality and it has been well documented that genetic factors might increase the risk of cancer onset [33, 34].

Keyword	Number of publications
Cancer	2 656 222
“Breast cancer”	49 804
“Prostate cancer”	59 245
“Colorectal cancer”	47 010

Table 1. Number of publications in the PubMed with keywords related to cancer

PCa is the most common solid cancer in men worldwide and is the most common of all cancers in the North America. In an epidemiological study was reported that the estimated PCa incidence rates remain most elevated in North America, Oceania, and Western and Northern Europe. Mortality rates tend to be higher in less developed regions of the world including parts of South America, the Caribbean, and sub-Saharan Africa. Increasing PCa incidence rates were observed in 32 of the 40 countries examined, which clearly demonstrates the increasing problem related to this disease, that it would be not desirable. However, PCa mortality rates decreased in 27 of the 53 countries under study, whereas rates increased in 16 and remained stable in 10 countries [2, 15, 33, 34].

4. The importance of the early diagnosis of the prostate cancer

The early diagnosis of PCa has been facilitated by the determination of the prostate specific antigen (PSA), rectal touch and ultrasonography, which has subsequently led to a high cure rate in the early stages (stage I/II) of the disease. However, it is important to have in mind, that these current diagnostic techniques have not, in several cases, sufficient specificity and sensitivity to determine the stage and aggressiveness of the PCa and to identify appropriate treatment [2, 6, 35-37].

International guidelines support opportunistic PSA screening in well-informed patients and recommend a baseline PSA at 40 years of age. Although some relevant controversies continue about the real benefit of the screening program, the undisputable finding is that an increasing percentage of young men have an early PCa diagnosis and this condition has the advantage to permit curative interventions [2, 35-37].

When a man has the PCa early diagnosed, he has a number of treatment options, which carry similar success rates. Surgery, brachytherapy or external beam radiotherapy in combination with several months of initial hormone treatment all carry the same chance of cure but they all have very different recovery times, or number of visits to the hospital to consider [4, 6].

Concerning to the recurrent PCa, a key treatment decision is based on whether the disease is only localized in the prostate fossa. If the sites of cancer in the early phase of recurrent disease were known, patients would be treated properly, leading to fewer side effects, a better prognosis with curative approache, and reduced treatment cost. Nuclear medicine imaging has been considered a reliable technique to be used with this purpose and an important aspect of the nuclear imaging that should be understood is that this type of imaging demonstrates physiology rather than anatomy [4, 6, 10, 11].

PET is a nuclear medicine technique for tumor imaging. The radiopharmaceutical 18F-FDG was firstly introduced to image brain tumors. Along the time, this radiopharmaceutical has been widely accepted and it was considered a highly effective and successfully way to image several types of cancers. In consequence, investigations using 18F-FDG were performed to evaluate the use of this radiopharmaceutical in the diagnosis of the PCa. Unfortunately, in general, the PCacan not be imaged with this radiopharmaceutical. This poor performance of 18F-FDG is mainly related to the low glucose metabolic rate in the PCa, as well as, a relevant excretion of the radiopharmaceutical into the adjacent urinary bladder. Moreover, it is well known that the ability of FDG-PET to detect cancer is based on an increased expression of cellular membrane glucose transporter and enhanced hexokinase II enzyme activity within the tumor cells, where the 18F-FDG undergoes enzymatic transformation to FDG-6 phosphate [10, 11].

Due to the limitations to use the 18F-FDG to detect PCa, other molecules to be labeled with a radionuclide, to be utilized as PET-radiopharmaceuticals, have been investigated with this purpose. Choline is a substrate for phosphatidylcholine, which is incorporated into cell membrane phospholipids, and is not dependent on cell proliferation and this molecule can be labeled with 11C or 18F for detection. 11C-choline has been shown to be superior to 18F-FDG to detect PCa, in part due to its negligible urinary secretion. 11C-choline PET has been shown to be able to localize primary PCa to the fossa of the prostate gland in up to 86.5% of patients and localize lymph node spread in up to 81.8% of patients [10, 11].

http://dx.doi.org/10.5772/52441

Another molecule, acetate, as 18F or 11C-labeled acetate, which is involved in cytoplasmic lipid synthesis, has been investigated to detect PCa. The retention of radiolabeled acetate in PCa cell lines has been shown to be related to fatty acid metabolism and enhanced beta-oxidation pathway. As PET-labeled acetate has minimal urinary activity, it is considered very suitable for evaluation of local prostatic disease with a high sensitivity for PCa lesions. When compared with 18F-FDG-PET for detection of primary tumors, there is a markedly increased sensitivity of 11C-acetate PET compared with 18F-FDG-PET, and the uptake of 11C-acetate is higher if the PSA is >3 ng/mL [10, 11].

The considerations about the early detection of the PCa is necessary, due to, there is considerable variation in the likely side effects and risks of long-term consequences such as urinary incontinence (UI) and erectile dysfunction (ED) in patients with PCa. With the early diagnosis there is an expectation of curing cancer, minimizing the risk of UI and ED and increasing the quality of life of the patient [38-41].

In general, radical prostatectomy (RP) is a curative and appropriated therapy for any patient whose tumour is clinically confined to the prostate, has a life expectancy of 10 years or more, and has no serious co-morbid conditions that would contraindicate surgery. Other factors affecting treatment decisions include patient factors, such as (i) Current symptoms (International Prostate Symptom Score, urinary flow rate), (ii) Current age (preference under the age of 70 years), (iii) Concurrent illnesses may determine suitability or not for surgery, (iv) Patient preference (psychological factors including patients ideas, concerns and expectations). Tumor/cancer factors, such as (a) Grade of tumour (the "aggressiveness" determines the risk of relapse), (b) Stage of tumour (determines radical of palliative approach), (c) Chance of response to treatment, (d) Chance of recurrence, and (e) Possibility of second curative treatment modalities if the first treatment fails must be also considered [6, 34, 38-41].

It is also important to consider that the risk of death under the anaesthetic for a RP is about 1 in 250 patients. The procedures used in the surgery become technically more challenging when the patient is overweight or obese and the risks of surgery increase. Improved knowledge about the anatomy of the organs of the pelvis and the muscles of the pelvic floor and the functions related to them had resulted in major improvements in this surgical technique [38-41].

Radiation therapy (RT) is another option for treatment of PCa. RT uses high-energy X-rays or other types of ionizing radiation to try to kill the cancer cells in various organs/tissues. There are mainly two types of radiotherapy: (i) External radiotherapy that uses a source of ionizing radiation that is outside of the body and (ii) Internal radiotherapy that uses a radioactive substance sealed in needles, seeds, wires, or catheters that are placed directly into or near the cancer (brachytherapy). The external radiotherapy is a complex procedure and requires the patient to make a number of steps, as (i) positioning and immobilization of the patient, (ii) localization of the tumor, (iii) determination of the size of the tumor, (iv) delineation of the target (tumor) and critical tissues structures in the neighborhood, (v) dose prescription, (vi) type of ionizing radiation, (vii) treatment planning, (viii) simulation and verification of the treatment and (ix) evaluation.Concerning to the brachytherapy to the PCa, several radioactive seeds (in general with iodine-125] are implanted into the prostate gland with the aim to irradiate the tumor. These seeds are not removed and will be permanently in the prostate. As the iodine-125 emits low level energy electromagnetic radiation, the energy of the radiation is deposited in the prostate, treating locally the tumor [4].

Various severe complications following RT can occur and these complications depend on the type of the procedure used in the treatment. In addition, clinical complications, such as UI and ED have also been associated with the RT [6, 14, 40, 42].

In Figure 3 is shown some modalities of treatment for PCa and possible adverse effects associated with some of these treatments.

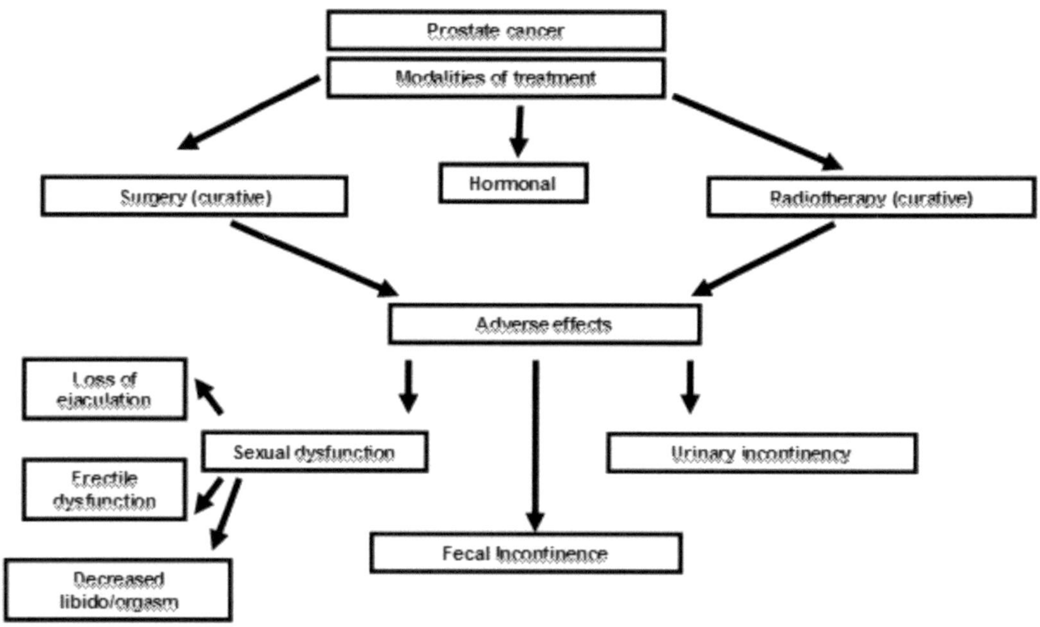

Figure 3. Modalities of treatment for the prostate cancer and possible adverse effects associated.

As presented before, UI and ED are undesirable side effects normally associated with the RP and RT due to the damage of the muscles of the pelvic floor. [26, 38, 39, 43]

UI has a prevalence ranging from 5 to 60 per cent. UI after RP is the most bothersome complication of this operation and has a major impact on the quality of life and it is therefore of the utmost importance to minimize its prevalence after this kind of surgery. In the clinical routine with the patient that was submitted to treatment to PCa, it is verified that the UI is an unpleasant condition [21, 24, 26].

The types and characteristics of UI secondary to PCa are (a) Stress UI, which is mainly associated with RP; (b) Urge incontinence, which is associated with RT and consists of a strong, unpleasant and sudden urge to urinate, with burning sensation or irritation in the bladder; and (c) Mixed incontinence, which affects mainly older patients on radiation and/or hormone therapy [21, 24]

In addition to the functional problem of the UI, this clinical condition causes a psychosocial disorder characterized by distress. Moreover, this is potentialised and augmented by the inability of the patient to perform habitual activities. Furthermore, the impossibility of controlling leakage and the resulting feeling of regression, and the inability to overcome the fatigue resulting from the interruption in the number of hours and the quality of sleep in the case of nocturia and anxiety increase dissatisfaction. In consequence, a restrictive social situation can be usually observed, characterized by shyness, shame from the leakage, and social stigmatization and isolation. Additionally, UI may trigger an undesirable, obsessive and strong psychological behavior related to the control of leakage of urine and of associated odors. These factors can increase the anxiety and to cause a reduction of the social life of the patient. Additionally, UI may trigger an obsessive and strong psychological behavior related to the control of leakage and odors. These factors can contribute to cause a reduction of the social life of the patient [6, 14, 20, 24, 42].

The impact of UI on the quality of life of the PCa patient is determined by the self-perception of the severity and the disruption of daily activities caused by the symptoms. An important consideration is that the cases of UI and ED (and other sexual dysfunctions, see Figure 3] recorded in clinics seem to be much higher than the number described in the publications. This discrepancy could be attributed to the great variability of definitions, measurement instruments, and manners of assessing UI. If a good interview with the patient before the treatment of the PCa is not performed, it is also difficult to determine whether the symptom is a result of the treatment of the disease or of the natural involution that would occur with age. Moreover, there is a fatalistic and resigned attitude that makes the patients hide or mask the symptom from the professional or the professional is not prepared to obtain the informations that are relevant to the clinical conditions of the patient [6, 20, 24, 42].

ED, in general, is usually due to a multifactorial etiology, comprising organic, psychological, or mixed aspects, and may often require a multidisciplinary approach for assessment and treatment. Organic causes encompass vascular, neurologic, hormonal, as a result of medications, pelvic surgery (mainly RP), RT, diabetes or mixed factors. In general, any condition that can cause damages to the nerves or impair blood flow in the penis may lead to ED. Pelvic surgery (especially RP and bladder surgery for cancer) might damage cavernous nerves and arteries near the penis, causing ED [23, 30, 39].

Penile erection is the consequence of a complex neurovascular process in which nerves, endothelium of sinusoids and blood vessels, and smooth muscle cells are involved. Several central nervous and peripheral transmitters and transmitter systems participate in the process and the nitric oxide (NO) is the main mediator of penile erection. It is produced by a group of enzymes called nitric oxide synthase (NOS) which utilizes the amino acid L-arginine and molecular oxygen as substrates to produce NO and L-citrulline. The endothelial NOS is constitutively expressed within the vascular system, it is tightly regulated and produces physiologically relevant levels of NO.The investigations about the NO, that can readily cross plasma membranes to enter target cells, and its functions as a mediator synthesized and released from the vascular endothelium and as a neurotransmitter in inhibitory nerves innervating the penis represented a breakthrough in the comprehension of the neurophysiological basis of erection. Moreover, the synthesis of NO and the consequences of NO binding to soluble guanylylcyclase is essential for the erectile process [44, 45, 46].

Impaired erectile function, or the total inability to maintain or achieve sufficient penile rigidity for satisfactory sexual intercourse performance, it was firstly used as a definition of impotence. On 1992, it was recommended that the term "erectile dysfunction" replace the term "impotence," but, sometimes, the two terms have been used interchangeably. The term ED is more precise and eliminates the confusion of multiple meanings and connotations associated with the word impotence. ED is defined as a “consistent or recurrent inability of a man to attain and/or maintain penile erection sufficient for sexual activity”. The condition must be present for a minimum of 3 months to establish the diagnosis. The exception to this is when ED is preceded by trauma or pelvic surgery [47, 48, 49]

In addition, penile erection involves a complex interaction between the central nervous system and local factors. The penis is innervated and regulated by autonomic (sympathetic and parasympathetic) and somatic (sensory and motor) nerve fibers. Overall, erection is a neurovascular event modulated by psychological and hormonal factors. The economic burden of ED is not just limited to the cost of diagnosis and treatment. Subtle impacts on the society that are difficult to quantify are (i) lost time at work, (ii) decreased productivity of the patient due to distress, (iii) impact on the partner and family and (iv) alteration of the social interactions. The comprehensive knowledge and the understanding of these conditions have also reflected in the number of papers published in important scientific journals that have increased along of the years [27, 38, 39, 41, 46].

Reports of studies describing ED after RP have shown a range from 29% to 97.5% with less ED occurring in younger men. Men with ED may suffer from depression and low self-esteem, and experience difficulties establishing and maintaining relationships. Treatment regimens currently available for ED include psychotherapy, sex therapy, oral pharmacological agents, androgen replacement therapy, intraurethral therapy, intracavernosal injections, several procedures related to the physiotherapy and surgery [27, 38, 39, 41, 50].

The pelvic floor muscles, besides other functions, play an important role in sexual activity and contractions of the ischiocavernosus and bulbocavernosus muscles produce an increase in the intracavernous pressure and influence penile rigidity. The bulbocavernosus muscle compresses the deep dorsal vein of the penis to prevent the outflow of blood from an engorged penis. The procedures of the physiotherapy, associated with a interdisciplinar team, including exercises for the muscles of the pelvic floor muscle only or associated with manometric biofeedback, electrotherapy, vaccum pumps can be used successfully in various patients with ED [20-26]

In addition, it is highly desired to consider that beneficial effects of pre- and postoperative pelvic floor interventions (RT or RP) using physiotherapy procedures, since both the duration and degree of UI after RP decrease in these case [24, 51-53].

When a patient with PCa is referred to undertake physiotherapy procedures before the surgery or radiotherapy, it is possible to teach him about the perception of the muscles of the pelvic foor, facilitating the performance of exercises involving these muscles associated with an ideal breathing, just after the RP or RT [6, 22-24].

As it is possible to see in the Figure 3, besides the ED, another clinical conditions related to the sexual functions can appear in the patient submitted to a RP, as the loss of ejaculation and the decrease of the libido and orgasm [6, 27, 39, 41].

The interventions related to the physiotherapy will contribute to aid the patient to live your sexuality. Moreover, it is important to show to the patient that sexuality is not only genitality, but it goes beyond the limits of genital impulse and is characterized as a strong experience of human personality [6, 13, 27, 39, 41].

Several options of treatment are available to treat ED, as psychosexual counseling, medication, use of physiotherapy (exercises to the pelvic floor muscles, electrotherapy, acupuncture and external vacuum devices), intracavernous injection therapy, vascular surgery, and use of a penile prosthesis. The etiology of the ED, the acceptability for the patient, the available information about methods and the success rate have been used to determine the choice of intervention. The clinical interventions used in the physiotherapy provide noninvasive methods that are easy to perform, painless, and inexpensive [6, 39, 41, 50, 51].

5. Physiotherapy procedures in the management of the patient with prostate cancer

The physiotherapist, from his assessment, can also help the patient with PCa in the presurgical period in which the exercises for the pelvic floor and for the respiration that will be performed in the post-surgical period can be learned early by the patient. Moreover, the knowledge and the perception of the muscles of the pelvic floor by the patient will be very important. As these muscles are located inside the pelvis, they are considered a continence muscle group giving structural support for the pelvic organs and the pelvic sphincters (urethra and anus, for exemple in men). Based on urethral continence maintained by muscles of the pelvic floor, the procedures of the physiotherapy of this muscle group can retake the control of the urinary continence or maximize it, also by nerve stimulation, according to the consensus, which can inhibit the detrusor muscle, increasing the quality of life of patients with Pca [20-26].

Patient assessment by the physiotherapist is accomplished through the anamnesis, voiding diary, pad test, data collection of the urodynamic study and/or other complementary examinations, if any, physical examination and specific maneuvers to assess urine leakage [24].

In the interview, beyond identifying the main complaint and history of the patient, issues inherent in urination are of utmost importance to be addressed. The voiding diary is a useful tool because it allows the physiotherapist to objectively quantify the volume of urine loss, as well as the frequency of the urination. As the voiding diary is fully performed by the patient over a period of about two to three days, with notes of drinking water, the type of the drink, volume voided, urgency severity, quantification of loss and its association to carry out some activity at the time,he is leding to observe his behavior voiding, generating his self-knowledge [20-26].

The completion of the pad test lasts one hour, and after that the pad is weighed, depicting the severity of UI. When the weigth is less than 3g, the UI is considered light. The UI is moderated to 3 up to 10 g, and over 10g is considered severe incontinence [20-26].

Urodynamic investigations involve the evaluation of the dynamic function of the lower urinary tract. The urodynamic study, an examination of the gold standard, evaluates the morphology, pressure (urethral, vesical and abdominal under static and dynamic conditions), physiology and hydrodynamic transport urine of the voiding mechanism, thus detailing the stages of filling and emptying as well as the sphincter behavior. Common urodynamic findings in post-RP patients are (a) internal sphincter deficiency and (b) bladder dysfunction (detrusor instability and decreased compliance) [20-26].

On physical examination is evaluated the strength and the tone of the pelvic floor muscles through the anal sphincter, perineal sensation and bulb-cavernosum reflex. Maneuver effort, such as coughing, can evaluate the sphincter function, which can be performed with the patient standing, with the bladder full, and where he is asked to simulate cough. From this assessment is given the goal of treatment [20-23].

One of the objectives of the intervention of the physiotherapy is to re-train the muscles of the pelvis by improving the active retention strength of the striated muscles of the pelvic floor in order to overcome the insufficiency of the injured sphincters and improve the continence of men with PCa. This level includes the awareness of the pelvic floor musculature and the coordination of the contraction-relaxation process to improve the control and the quality of the muscle contraction. Specific attention is given to the muscles of the deep plane of the pelvic floor [5, 24, 25].

To facilitate the perception of the muscles of the pelvic floor, electrotherapy is often used. This technique beyond to guide the patient to correct the contraction of muscles, depending on the type of electrical current, it also can be used other responses. Two types of electrodes can be used in the electrotherapy; internal (anal) and external electrodes [20-26].

In the case of functional electrical stimulation, which is an alternating current of low frequency, it generates muscle contractions and an increase of muscle function. In the pelvic floor muscles, electrode stimulation in the perineal body, the contraction is perceived by the patient and the physiotherapist with the apparent anal contraction. This contraction also acts by stimulating the sacral nerve roots, or specifically the pelvic and pudendal nerves, suppressing the (hyper) detrusor activity [24]

In figure 4, a patient that is undergone electrotherapy with external electrodes is shown. A correct frequency is choosen, following international studies and the intensity of electric current is selected considering the sensibility of the patient.

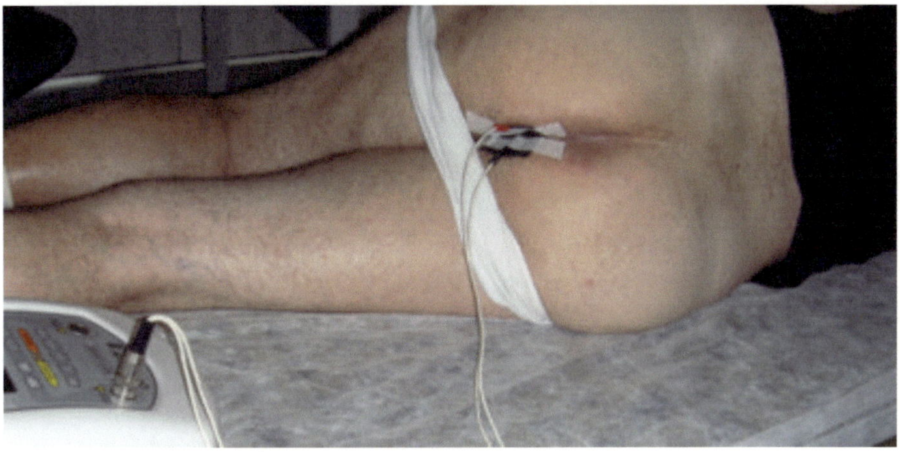

Figure 4. Patient after prostate cancer surgery undergoing electrotherapy

Physiotherapy also assists with postoperative respiratory recovery, early mobilization, lymphoedema prevention, education and garments if required, as well as the later management of pelvic floor re-education, continence advice and lymphoedema treatment if necessary. Men undergoing RP under a general anaesthetic will be off work for about 6 weeks. Moerover, they will stay in hospital for 5-7 days and have a urinary catheter for 2 weeks. The sphincter "valve" has gone and the urine leaks without control, day and night until the patient has learned again to use his muscles of the pelvic floor to regain his continence. Concerning ED, when a man wakes up from a RP he will almost certainly have ED initially. If there is going to be a recovery of erectile function, it may take 18-24 months to occur. Approximately 30% of men will recover erectile function and medication (Viagra or Cialis) will usually boost this recovery. However, physiotherapy procedures could be another suitable option without contraindications. In figure 3 is possible to see a man that has previously been submitted to RP and is undergoing external electrotherapy. In addition, the patient that has learned about the exercises involving the muscles of the pelvic floor can start these exercises immediately just after the surgery or after the catheter removal [20-26, 52, 53].

In the figure 5 are shown men doing exercises using a ball to increase the perception of the pelvic floor muscles, as well as to work these muscles.

In figure 5.a, the man relaxed and in 6.b, he has raising the hips and contracting the pelvic floor muscles. In figure 5.c, the man is sitting on the ball to increase the perception of the pelvic floor muscles and in 6.d, the man puts the hands together and begins to lift up the hands and feeling the contraction of the pelvic floor muscles to upward movement.

Beneficial effects of pre- and postoperative pelvic floor re-education are clear, since both the duration and degree of UI after RP can be distinguishably decreased [5, 43, 51].

Physiotherapy has responded to the improved outcomes and patient demand for quality of life improvements by instituting new treatments and education, such as informing about the possible importance of the sunlight in the prevention of the PCa and the equal need to protect against the harmful effects of the ultraviolet radiation, or about the options of physiotherapy for rehabilitation and re-integration to normal life [5, 6, 8, 9].

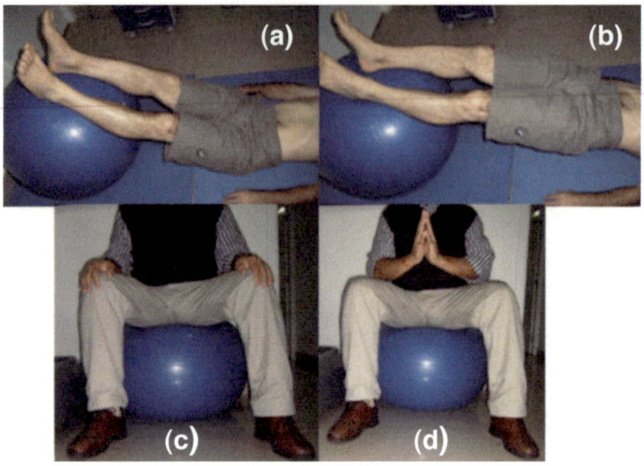

Figure 5. Men doing exercises with a ball to perception and to work the pelvic floor muscles.

Alternative and complementary techniques have also been considered as an option to be used for treating ED. One of these techniques that is related to the physiotherapy is the acupuncture. Acupuncture is safe and involves the insertion of thin needles into different areas of the body known as acupuncture points. Traditionally, acupuncture has been often used to restore and maintain health through the stimulation of these specific points on the body. As this stimulation could modulate the NO, it is possible to consider that acupuncture might be effective for treating ED. Although, in some studies the acupuncture has been used successfully to treat ED, there is sufficient evidence that acupuncture is an effective intervention for treating ED [55].

Mechanical vacuum devices cause erection by creating a partial vacuum, which draws blood into the penis, engorging and expanding it. The devices have three components. A plastic cylinder, into which the penis is placed; a pump, which draws air out of the cylinder; and an elastic band, which is placed around the base of the penis to maintain the erection after the cylinder is removed and during intercourse by preventing blood from flowing back into the body.One variation of the vacuum device involves a semirigid rubber sheath that is placed on the penis and remains there after erection is attained and during intercourse [27, 28, 50].

In general, physiotherapy management in the area of oncology have relevant contributions to patient care, including: (i) Decreasing length of stay in acute facilities (early discharge planning, outpatient follow up and education, involvement in palliative care facilities and physiotherapy services in home care); (ii) Improving functional capacity (early mobilization, management of complications of surgery, convenient manipulations of the areas submitted to RT and other treatments, as treating lymphoedema and scars); (iii) Improving lymphoedema management that has lead to decreased hospital admissions for cellulitis (a feature of poorly controlled lymphoedema and/or orientation of the patient) and decreased need for costly and at times uncomfortable pressure garments; (iv) Improving local and general exercise capacity (prevention of loss of body weight and managing the side effects of the disease, medication and surgery); (v) Shortening the period of time of UI after RP; and (vi) Affecting quality of life factors for all patients with cancer and their carers and families. These all provide examples where physiotherapy intervention contributes considerably to the health care provision and demonstrate how the various disciplines allied to medicine are working together to either bring the now healthy individual back to normal life and re-integration to the society, or improve the quality of life of patients that have to live with cancer as a chronic disorder and those that are in the terminal stages of the disease and life [5-7, 43, 53].

6. Considerations about the various prostate cancer treatments and their associated side effects

A number of side effects are associated with the various treatments available for PCa. As it was presented before, associated side effects include ED and UI amongst others, and a number of palliative care treatments and exercises have been proposed to counteract these effects [24, 52, 53]

A very important and unquestionable point is that pelvic floor muscle exercises are relevant to the treatment of ED in patients with PCa that will be submitted to RP. Most physiotherapy treatments for ED focus also on pelvic floor muscles. It is relevant to consider also the arrangement of the muscles at the base of the penis, as well as the other local structures that, with the time without erection, can lead to veno-occlusive ED. This undesirable condition is the result of a sequence of penile morphologic alterations post-RP. The physiotherapist will guide the patient to do exercises for the muscles direct related to the pelvic floor and also to the muscles indirectly related with the pelvis, such as abdominal and gluteal muscles. When they are contracted an increase of the local blood flow to the pelvic region is verified. This process seems to lead to a release of NO to the penis, acting on endothelium vasodilation and dependent on the flow, increasing in oxygen supply to the penile tissue and keeping the erectile tissue healthy [22, 24, 54].

On this same point of view about the treatment of the ED with physiotherapy, the vaccum therapy could also provide oxygen supply generated by negative pressure that distends the corporal sinusoids and increases the blood inflow to the penis. This system reduces apoptosis minimizing fibrosis of the corpora cavernosa which directly influences in the maintaining of the penile length. Differently, the use of the vacuum device (figure 6) for intercourse, the vaccum therapy does not use the ring constrictor, since it would keep in the corpora cavernosa a poorly oxygenated blood. The vaccum therapy could be combined with anothers therapies for ED, as pelvic floor muscles exercices (kinesiotherapy) and oral therapies (medications) [27, 40, 50].

UI has been also treated with the various exercises (kinesiotherapy) involving the muscles of the pelvic floor in patients submitted to RP. Prior to a pelvic floor muscle exercise program, an anal assessment is performed to grade the strength, endurance and speed of the anal sphincter and the puborectalis muscle. Pelvic floor muscle exercises are individually taught to ensure that they are being performed correctly [52],

In consequence, a number of pertinent considerations arise from the treatments and their associated side effects, which can related directly to personal circumstances and situations, clinical conditions after treatment or laboratory determinations (PSA) and medications/procedures used after treatment [40, 41, 46, 47].

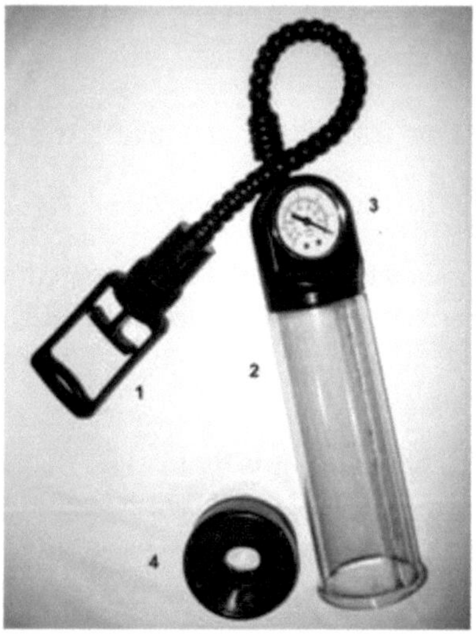

(1)Suction syringe, (2) Plexiglass cylinder, (3) Barometer,
(4) Sealing ring of silicone cylinder

Figure 6. A model of a vacuum device

Personal situations related with the possible treatments for PCa must be considered, as bladder irritation is common after RT, bowel complications might occur in the long-term and have high incidence during external beam RT, ED can be early in the surgery in comparison with RT, and penile shortening or fibrosis might occur after RP [6, 14].

Clinical conditions after the RP, such as pelvic pain, is common mainly in young men, UI will occur in the post operative period, erectile functioning might return slowly over years after the surgery. All these must be considered and must be explained to the patient and his family [6, 14].

The decline of the quality of the sexual activity can lead to a complicated pattern of change in quality of life and also negatively affect the psychosocial wellbeing of men and of the couple [6, 14].

Concerning the laboratory determinations as well as the medications used after the RP, it is important to consider that phosphodiesterase-5 inhibitors have limited actions in the cases of ED and the velocity is a more reliable indicator of recurrence than an isolated PSA measurement. When the available procedures to minimize the clinical complications of the RP or of the RT are considered, it is highly relevant to emphasize that the decrease of the appearance of complications occurs in patients thar have undergone physiotherapy before the RP and the improvement of the symptoms is observed due to the procedures of the physiotherapy just after the RP [6, 14].

Due to the high occurence of the PCa in the world, the high cost involved in the treatment and its impact in the quality of life of the patients with this disease, considerations about the different kinds of treatment as well as the possible complications of the treatments available are desirable [6, 14].

In addition, the questions associated with the personal situations related with the possible treatments for PCa would be relevant for a better understanding of the clinical situations of each patient [6, 14].

Finally, the knowledge of the patient about his situation as well as the involvement of the family and partner must be strongly considered. Moreover, it is also important to explain and present all the possibilities involving the treatment of the PCa. In addition, it is highly desired thal all the modalities of procedures that are available to aid in the prevention of undesirable clinical conditions. Furthermore, it is suggested that is necessary to consider the techniques related to the physiotherapy before and after the treatment of choice to the PCa.

Acknowledgements

We. would like to acknowledge the assistance of Dr Sotiris Missailidis in the proof reading of this manuscript. We thank the support of the CNPq (Conselho Nacional de Desenvolvimento Científico e Tecnológico - "National Counsel of Technological and Scientific Development") and UERJ (Universidade do Estado do Rio de Janeiro).

Author details

Mario Bernardo Filho[1*] and Mauro Luis Barbosa Júnior[2*]

*Address all correspondence to: bernardofilhom@gmail.com

*Address all correspondence to: maurolbarbosajr@gmail.com

1 Coordenadoria de Pesquisa, Instituto Nacional de Câncer and Departamento de Biofísica e Biometria, Instituto de Biologia Roberto Alcântara Gomes, Universidade do Estado do Rio de Janeiro, Rio de Janeiro, RJ, Brasil

2 Departamento de Medicina de Integral Familiar e Comunitária, Hospital Universitário Pedro Ernesto, Universidade do Estado do Rio de Janeiro, Rio de Janeiro, RJ, Brasil

References

[1] Instituto Nacional do Câncer. Available: http://www2.inca.gov.br/wps/wcm/connect/inca/portal/home. Accessed 2012 July 11th.

[2] National Cancer Institute, Available: http://www.cancer.gov/cancertopics/types/prostate. Accessed 2012 July 11th.

[3] Boulikas T, Alevizopoulos N (2008) Representative Cancers, Treatment and Market. In: Missailidis S (editor) Anticancer Therapeutics.UnitedKingdon: Wiley & Sons. pp. 377-386.

[4] Perkins AC (2007) Tumour imaging and therapy. In: Missailidis S (editor) The Cancer Clock. UK: Wiley & Sons. pp. 135- 157

[5] Bernardo-Filho M, Bergmann A, Tavares A (2007) Physiotherapy in cancer patients. In: Missailidis S (editor) The Cancer Clock. United Kingdon: Wiley & Sons. pp. 245-263.

[6] Bernardo-Filho M, Missailidis S, Santos-Filho S, Fonseca A (2009) Prostate cancer therapies, complications and sixteen questions that the patients and the multidisciplinary team are interested in. Gene Ther. Mol. Biol. 13: 254-263

[7] Bennett CJ, Grant MJ (2004). Specialisation in physiotherapy: a mark of maturity. Aust. J. Physiother. 50: 3-5.

[8] Moon SJ, Fryer AA, Strange RC (2005) Ultraviolet radiation, vitamin D and risk of prostate cancer and other diseases. Photochem. Photobiol. 81: 1252–1260.

[9] Kricker A, Armstrong B (2006) Does sunlight have a benefificial influence on certain cancers? Prog. Biophys. Mol. Biol. 92: 132-139.

[10] Oyama N, Miller TR, Dehdashti F, Siegel BA, Fischer KC, Michalski JM, Kibel AS, Andriole GL, Picus J, Welch MJ (2003) 11C-Acetate PET Imaging of prostate cancer: detection of recurrent disease at PSA Relapse. J. Nucl. Med. 44: 549–555.

[11] Lee ST, Lawrentschuk N, Scott AM (2012) PET in Prostate and bladder tumors. Semin. Nucl. Med. 42: 231-246.

[12] Friedenreich CM, Neilson HK, Lynch BM (2010) State of the epidemiological evidence on physical activity and cancer prevention. Eur. J. Cancer. 46: 2593-2604

[13] Johnson BK (2004) Prostate Cancer and Sexuality: Implications for Nursing. Geriatr. Nurs. 25: 341-347.

[14] Katz A, Katz A (2008) The top 13: what family physicians should know about prostate cancer. Can. Fam. Physician. 54: 198-203.

[15] Wolin KY, Schwartz AL, Matthews CE, CourneyaKS, Schmitz KH (2012) Implementing the Exercise Guidelines for Cancer Survivors. J. Support. Oncol. May 10

[16] Sternberg CN, Krainer M, Oh WK, Bracarda S, Bellmunt J, Ozen H, Zlotta A, Beer TM, Oudard S, Rauchenwald M, Skoneczna I, Borner MM, Fitzpatrick JM (2006) The medical management of prostate cancer: a multidisciplinary team approach. BJU Int. 99: 22-27.

[17] Pinto NS, MonteiroMB, Santos-FilhoSD, Paiva D, Tavares A, Missailidis S, Marin PJ, Bernardo-Filho M (2010) Postmenopausal/menopause, bone mineral density and whole body vibration: a short review. J. Med. Med. Sci. 1: 516-525.

[18] Santos-Filho SD, PintoNS, MonteiroMB, Arthur AP, Misssailidis S, Marín PJ, Bernardo-Filho M (2011) The ageing, the decline of hormones and the whole-body vibration exercises in vibratory platforms: a review and a case report. J. Med. Med. Sci. 2: 925-931.

[19] Cardinale M, Wakeling J (2005) Whole body vibration exercises: are vibrations good for you? Br. J. Sports Med. 39: 585-589.

[20] Cornel EB, de Wit R, Witjes JA (2005) Evaluation of early pelvic floor physiotherapy on the duration and degree of urinary incontinence after radical retropubic prostatectomy in a non-teaching hospital. World J. Urol. 23: 353-355.

[21] Dorey G, Speakman M, Feneley R, Dunn C, Swinkels A, Ewings P. (2004a) Randomised controlled trial of pelvic floor muscle exercises and manometric biofeedback for post-micturition dribble. Urol. Nurs. 24: 490-512

[22] Dorey G, Speakman M, Feneley R, Dunn C, Swinkels A, Ewings P (2004b) Randomised controlled trial of pelvic floor muscle exercises and manometric biofeedback for erectile dysfunction. Br. J. Gen. Pract. 54: 819-825

[23] Dorey G, Speakman MJ, Feneley RCL, Swinkels A, Dunn CDR (2005) Pelvic floor exercises for erectile dysfunction. BJU Int. 96: 595-597.

[24] Dorey G (2006) Pelvic Dysfunction in men: Diagnosis and Therapy of Male Incontinence and Erectile Dysfunction.Chichester: John Wiley & Sons. pp. 1-221.

[25] Dorey G (2007) Why men need to perform pelvic floor exercises? Nurs. Times. 103: 40-43.

[26] Feys H, Baert L (2000) Effect of physiotherapy on duration and degree of incontinence after radical prostatectomy: a randomised controlled study. Lancet. 355: 98-102.

[27] Miner MM, Seftel AD (2007) Centrally Acting Mechanisms for the Treatment of Male Sexual Dysfunction. Urol. Clin. North Am. 34: 483-496.

[28] Mulhall JP, Morgentaler A (2007) Penile rehabilitation should become the norm for radical prostatectomy patients. J. Sex. Med. 4: 538-543.

[29] World Health Organization, Defining sexual health, Sexual health document series, Available: http://www.who.int/reproductivehealth/topics/gender_rights/defining_sexual_health.pdf, 2006. Accessed 2012 July 24th

[30] Mello AS, Carvalho EC, PeláNT (2006) The sexuality of patients with onco-hematological diseases. Rev. Lat. Am. Enfermagem.14: 227-232.

[31] World Health Organization (WHO), http://www.who.int/cancer/en/, accessed 2012 July 24th

[32] PubMed, http://www.ncbi.nlm.nih.gov/pubmed/, accessed 2012 July,

[33] Center MM, Jemal A, Lortet-Tieulent J, Ward E, Ferlay J, Brawley O, Bray F (2012) International Variation in Prostate Cancer Incidence and Mortality Rates. Eur. Urol. 61: 1079-1092.

[34] National Institutes of Health. Publication No. 06-3923 December 2005, National Kidney and Urologic Diseases Information Clearinghouse

[35] Wolf AMD, WenderRC, Etzioni RB, Thompson IM, D'Amico AV, Volk, RJ,Brooks DD, Dash C, Guessous I, Andrews K, DeSantis C, Smith RA (2010). American Cancer Society Guideline for the Early Detection of Prostate Cancer Update 2010. CA: Cancer J. Clin. 60: 70–98.

[36] Greene KL, Albertsen PC, Babaian RJ, Carter HB, Gann PH, Han M, Kuban DA, Sartor AO, Stanford JL, Zietman A, Carroll P (2009) Prostate specific antigen best practice statement. J. Urol. 182: 2232–2241.

[37] Imamura T, Yasunaga H (2008) Economic evaluation of prostate cancer screening with prostate-specific antigen. Int. J. Urol. 15: 285-288.

[38] Kendirci M, Bejma J, Hellstrom WJ (2006) Update on erectile dysfunction in prostate cancer patients. Curr. Opin. Urol. 16: 186-195.

[39] McCullough AR (2008) Rehabilitation of erectile function following radical prostatectomy. Asian J. Androl.10: 61-74.

[40] Seftel AD, Mohammed MA, Althof SE (2004) Erectile dysfunction: etiology, evaluation, and treatment options. Med. Clin. North. Am. 88: 387-416.

[41] Sivalingam S, Hashim H, Schwaibold H (2006) An overview of the diagnosis and treatment of erectile dysfunction. Drugs. 66: 2339-2355.

[42] Weber BA, Roberts BL, Yarandi H, Mills TL, Chumbler NR, Algood C (2007). Dyadic support and quality-of-life after radical prostatectomy. J. Mens. Health Gend. 4: 156–164.

[43] Filocamo MT, Marzi VL, Del Popolo G, Cecconi F, Marzocco M, Tosto A, Nicita G (2005) Effectiveness of early pelvic floor rehabilitation for post-prostatectomy incontinence. Eur. Urol. 48: 734-738.

[44] Musicki B, Burnett AL (2006) eNOS Function and Dysfunction in the Penis. Exp. Biol. Med. 231: 154-165.

[45] Priviero FBM, Leite R, Webb RC, Teixeira CE (2007) Neurophysiological basis of penile erection. ActaPharmacol. Sin. 28: 751-755.

[46] Andersson KE (2011). Mechanisms of penile erection and basis for pharmacological treatment of erectile dysfunction. Pharmacol. Rev. 63: 811-859.

[47] National Institutes of Health (2003) Consensus Development Panel on Impotence. JAMA.270:83-90.

[48] Ribeiro CG, Moura R, Neves RF, Spinosa JP, Bernardo-Filho M (2007) Nuclear medicine imaging technique in the erectile dysfunction evaluation: a mini-review. Braz. Arch. Biol. Technol. 50: 91-96.

[49] Santos-Filho SD, Paoli S, Vicentini SC, Pinto NS, Oliveira MP, Tavares A, Bernardo-Filho M (2012) Erectile dysfunction: The interest of the scientific community. J. Med. Med. Sci. 3: 70-76.

[50] Yuan J, Hoang AN, Romero CA, Lin H, Dai Y, Wang R (2010) Vacuum therapy in erectile dysfunction - Science and clinical evidence. Int. J. Impot. Res. 22: 211-219.

[51] Burgio KL, Goode PS, Urban DA, Umlauf MG, Locher JL, Bueschen A, Redden DT (2006) Preoperative biofeedback assisted behavioral training to decrease post-prostatectomy incontinence: a randomized controlled trial. J. Urol. 175: 196-20.1

[52] Parekh AR, Feng MI, Kirages D, Bremner H, Kaswick J, Aboseif S (2003) The role of pelvic floor exercises on postprostatectomy incontinence. J. Urol. 170: 130-133.

[53] Serdà BC, Vesa J, del Valle A, Monreal P (2010) Urinary incontinence and prostate cancer: A rehabilitation program design. Actas Urol. Esp. 34: 522-530.

[54] Claes H, Van Kampen M, Lysens R, Baert L (1995) Pelvic floor exercises in the treatment of impotence. Eur. J. Phys. Rehabil. Med. 5: 135-140.

[55] Lee MS, Shin B, Ernst E (2009) Acupuncture for treating erectile dysfunction: a systematic review. BJU Int. 104: 366-370.

Section 3

Surgical Care and Radiation Therapy

Chapter 5

Abdominoperineal Resection: Consideration and Limitations of Prostate Cancer Screening and Prostate Biopsy

Zachary Klaassen, Ray S. King, Kelvin A. Moses,
Rabii Madi and Martha K. Terris

Additional information is available at the end of the chapter

http://dx.doi.org/10.5772/52291

1. Introduction

Prostate cancer and colorectal malignancies are the most common cancers in men, contributing to 15% and 9% of new cancer cases, respectively [1]. Furthermore, it is not uncommon to encounter patients with synchronous or metachronous colorectal and prostate cancers [2-3]. Abdominoperineal resection (APR) is often performed for surgical treatment of rectal cancer in addition to treatment of ulcerative colitis and familial polyposis coli. The technical aspects of an APR include a combined perineal and abdominal approach to resecting the rectum and mesorectum, in addition to the anus, perineal soft tissue and pelvic floor musculature [4].

The screening and treatment of patients with prostate cancer after an APR is challenging and unique. Enblad et al. [5] found a relative risk of 2.2 for the diagnosis of a second primary neoplasm in the prostate within 1 year after the diagnosis of rectal malignancy. After APR for colorectal pathologic features, however, there is no rectum for access to the prostate. This precludes the use of digital rectal examination (DRE) or transrectal ultrasound (TRUS)-guided prostate biopsies to diagnose primary tumors of the prostate [6-10].

Several methods have been described to evaluate the prostate in the patient with elevated prostate-specific antigen (PSA) levels who have undergone APR, including transperineal ultrasound (TPUS)-guided biopsy, transurethral ultrasounded guided perineal biopsy and computed tomography (CT)/magnetic resonance imaging (MRI) guided techniques. The aim of this chapter is to review the screening for prostate cancer in patients preparing for an APR and discuss post-APR screening and prostate biopsy techniques, limitations and practical considerations.

2. Abdominoperineal resection

Abdominoperineal resection is a surgery for carcinoma of the rectum and/or anus, performed through incisions in the abdomen and perineum. APR involves the removal of the anus, rectum, and the distal portion of the sigmoid colon along with regional lymph nodes. Without an anal opening, the patient has a permanent end-colostomy from the proximal sigmoid colon created through the anterior abdominal wall, typically placed in the left lower quadrant [11-12].

2.1. Diagnosis of rectal carcinoma

In patients with rectal cancer, the most common initial presenting symptom or complaint is bleeding, followed by changes in bowel habits, diarrhea, and lower abdominal pain. A DRE may detect rectal masses located within the distal 1/3 of the rectum. A potential source of confusion from a standard DRE may arise from carcinoma of the prostate encroaching on the nearby rectum, causing similar obstructive symptoms [11]. Flexible sigmoidoscopy or colonoscopy allow for a more thorough visual characterization, location, and size of the mass, and provides an opportunity for biopsy and histological examination. Endoluminal ultrasonography has recently been shown to be a diagnostic tool for characterizing the depth of invasion of the rectal mass. Pre-operative evaluation using colonoscopy and CT and/or MRI is indicated to rule-out synchronous lesions and/or metastatic disease [13].

2.2. Indications for treatment

Classic surgical dogma throughout the 20th century states that the standard treatment for rectal tumors located less than 8cm from the anal verge is to perform an APR. Careful surgical technique must be utilized to avoid complications such as recurrence of disease due to inadequate surgical margins, anastomotic breakdown, obstruction, and re-operation. Tumors located more proximally are generally treated successfully using the standard low anterior resection with restoration of bowel continuity. Absolute contraindications for anastomosis following resection of rectal cancer are invasion of the sphincter mechanism or the anal canal. The decision to preserve the anal sphincter can be affected by several factors including: level of the tumor, depth of invasion, extent of circumferential involvement, tumor fixation, local and metastatic invasion, age, and the ability to manage a colostomy. However, advances in instrumentation and techniques often allow for some tumors in the distal rectum to be resected and anastomosis performed [13-14].

2.3. Technique

APR can be performed by a single surgeon or with a two-surgeon (abdominal and perineal) team approach. Once the patient is prepped and draped, the anus is closed using a purse-string suture. A site for the colostomy should be selected prior to incision. The surgeon may consider preoperative ureteral stent placement to aid in identification of the ureters and to facilitate repair in case of inadvertent injury. A midline infra-umbilical incision is made, and the abdomen is explored for evidence of metastatic and/or synchronous disease. Once the tumor is deemed resectable, the surgeon on the perineal side can begin dissection simultaneously. In the abdominal compartment, the sigmoid colon and rectum is mobilized by incision of the left lateral mesentery, paying careful attention to avoid the left ureter as it courses over the bifurcation of the iliac vessels. Identification and control of the inferior mesenteric artery is followed by its ligation distal to the first branch to maintain adequate blood supply to the colon segment used for the stoma. The rectum is then bluntly dissected posterior along the presacral space and mobilized to the tip of the coccyx. Anteriorly, the rectum is retracted away from the bladder and Denonvillier's fascia is incised to free the rectum away from the prostate to its posterior margin. The lateral ligaments that contain the middle rectal arteries are controlled and ligated. At this point the proximal sigmoid colon is divided using a stapling device and brought through the anterior abdominal wall. The colostomy is then matured.

On the perineal side, an elliptical incision is made around the anus. Dissection is then made through the sphincters and the ischiorectal fossa is entered. The presacral space is entered from below and the rectum is mobilized circumferentially. Careful dissection is performed to avoid perforation of the rectum and compromise the containment of the malignancy. The perineal dissection is completed by dividing the levator muscle on each side. The distal sigmoid and rectum can be delivered through the perineal opening. The perineal wound is closed primarily, with a closed drain left in place. The peritoneum is repaired above and the floor of the pelvis is closed [12, 14-16].

3. Concomitant prostate cancer screening in the patient preparing for an APR

Patients scheduled to undergo APR represent a patient population in which prostate cancer screening may be indicated. Most cases of rectal cancer are diagnosed after 50 years of age [17], and are in the same age category of men at risk for prostate cancer diagnosis. However, the stage of rectal cancer should be taken into consideration when considering screening the same individual for prostate cancer: Stage T1 and T2 rectal tumors treated with APR have a ~90% 5-year survival, while stage T3 and T4 tumors are generally treated with neoadjuvant chemotherapy and/or radiation and generally have a 5-year survival of 50% and 25%, respectively [17]. Thus, prostate cancer screening in patients with advanced disease should be avoided.

Terris and Wren previously described a prostate cancer-screening program for 19 consecutive men scheduled for APR for colorectal carcinoma with no history of prostate cancer [18]. Screening included serum PSA and DRE and those with suspicious findings underwent TRUS-guided sextant biopsy. Six patients (31%) had a PSA >4.0 ng/mL (range 4.4 to 32.4 ng/mL, mean 9.3 ng/mL) of which two patients also had an abnormal DRE. TRUS-guided biopsy revealed prostate cancer in three individuals (50%). These patients included an individual with clinical stage T1c, Gleason 3+3=6 adenocarcinoma of the prostate treated with radiation, a second patient with clinical stage T2a, Gleason 3+4=7 adenocarcinoma of the prostate treated with radiation, and a third individual with a PSA of 32.4 ng/mL and DRE consistent with extracapsular extension of prostate cancer (clinical stage T3, Gleason 4+4=8 adenocarcinoma of the prostate) managed with androgen deprivation therapy. Concomitant prostate cancer screening for patients planning an APR should be a multi-disciplinary decision between the General Surgeons and Urologist in the male patient older than 50 years of age with clinical stage T1 or T2 rectal cancer and a life expectancy of more than 10 years.

4. Post-APR prostate cancer screening and modalities for prostate biopsy

The clinical scenario of a patient with an elevated PSA and no access to the rectum precludes the urologist from performing a DRE or a TRUS biopsy of the prostate. Other approaches to the prostate to allow a biopsy include CT and MRI guided techniques, transurethral ultrasound guided perineal biopsy and TPUS-guided biopsy.

4.1. CT and MRI-guided prostate biopsy

Transgluteal CT-guided prostate biopsy involves imaging the lower pelvis at 10-mm intervals and with a 10-mm slice thickness. The transgluteal approach allows sampling of both sides of the midline at the base, midgland and apical levels. When one entry site is used, the angle of the needle is projected to the contralateral side of the prostate; entry sites are chosen 3-4cm off the midline to avoid paraspinal ligaments and potential post-APR fibrosis around the tip of the coccyx (Figure 1) [19].

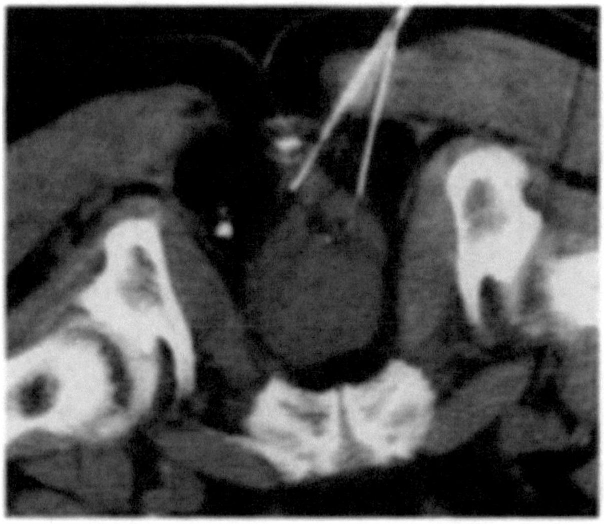

Figure 1. CT-guided percutaneous transgluteal biopsy of the prostate. Two needles are inserted at different angles to ensure adequate sampling of both sides of the prostate (Reprinted from American Journal of Roentgenology, Volume 166/Issue 6, Papanicolaou N, Eisenberg PJ, Silverman SG, McNicholas MM, Althausen AF. 1996, 1332-1334, with permission from The American Roentgen Ray Society).

Papanicolaou et al. [19] described this technique in 10 patients with a mean age of 67 years and mean PSA of 33.9 diagnosing prostate cancer in 6 patients (60%). While CT scan offers limited anatomical detail of the prostate, it does allow visualization of the peripheral zones to facilitate biopsy in patients without rectal access.

Limited experience with MRI-guided transperineal biopsy [20] and CT-MRI fusion to guide radiotherapy [21] has been described but is not widely available.

4.2. Transurethral ultrasound guided perineal prostate biopsy

The patient undergoing a transperineal biopsy guided by transurethral ultrasound is placed in the lithotomy position and a 26F resectoscope sheath is passed into the urethra. Subsequently, a 5.5 MHx transurethral ultrasound probe is passed through the sheath for visualization of the prostate. The width and height of the prostate are measured on the sagittal image and withdrawing the probe from the base to the apex of the prostate assesses length [22]. The advantage of this modality is that direct prostate imaging allows for precise guidance of transperineally placed biopsy needles. However, the major limitation is that one is only able to view the prostate in the sagittal plane. Seaman et al. [22] utilized this technique to perform 7 biopsies in 5 patients with a history of APR and elevated PSA (two patients had repeat biopsy secondary to increasing PSA), diagnosing prostate cancer in three patients (60%).

4.3. Transperineal Ultrasound (TPUS) guided prostate biopsy

The TPUS guided prostate biopsy is performed in the lithotomy position. A Foley catheter may be inserted to delineate the prostate anatomy and avoid the urethra with the biopsy needle [23]. The scrotum is then retracted anteriorly and the perineum is prepared in a sterile fashion. Then 1% Lidocaine is applied to the perineum for anesthesia. The transrectal ultrasound probe is adjusted to a frequency of 5-6 MHz and the prostate is visualized after traversing the course of the urethral catheter. The 18-guage biopsy needle is then directed at a 45-degree angle and biopsy specimens are obtained through the posterior aspect of the prostate. The needle forms an acute angle with the long axis of the prostate apex is nearly parallel with the long axis of the prostate base and mid-gland (Figure 2). Biopsy specimens are then obtained from the medial and lateral aspect of the prostate apex, mid-gland and base as is performed for TRUS biopsy. A "fan technique" for obtaining a six-core TPUS guided biopsy has also been described (Figure 3) [24].

A number of studies have compared the efficacy of TPUS-guided biopsies compared to TRUS-guided biopsies in patients with a rectum [8, 24]. Shinghal and Terris [8] prospectively identified 20 patients with prostate cancer diagnosed by TRUS-guided biopsies to evaluate the accuracy of TPUS prostate biopsies. Six TPUS-guided biopsies were obtained, followed by sextant TRUS-guided biopsies prior to radical prostatectomy. Final pathology demonstrated that all 20 patients had adenocarcinoma of the prostate. TPUS-guided biopsies identified cancer in only 2 of 20 patients (10%) compared to 13 of 20 patients (65%) for TRUS-guided biopsies. The positive TPUS-guided biopsy specimens were higher Gleason grade, and were found in patients with larger volume prostates and higher PSA. Emiliozzi et al. [24] performed a prospective study comparing TPUS versus TRUS-guided prostate biopsy in 107 patients with PSA > 4.0 ng/mL. The patients underwent TPUS-guided six core biopsy, followed by TRUS-guided six core biopsy. Prostate cancer was found in 43 of 107 patients (40%): 41 (95%) were found via the TPUS approach compared to 34 (79%) via the TRUS approach (p = 0.012).

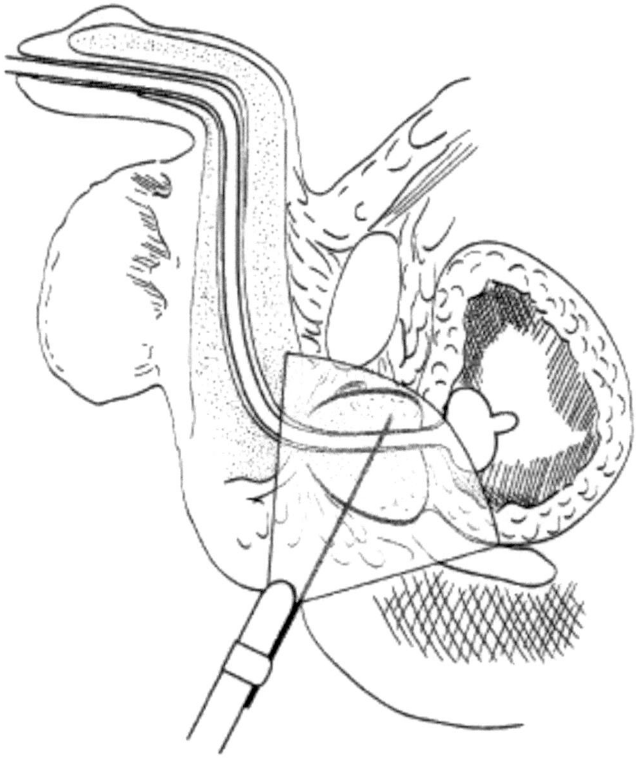

Figure 2. Transperineal prostate biopsy. There is a relatively acute angle of the needle in regard to the long axis of the prostate. The needle becomes almost parallel with the long axis of the prostate middle and base (Reprinted from The Journal of Urology, Volume 169/Issue 1, Shinohara K, Gulati M, Koppie TM, Terris MK. 2003, 141-144, with permission from American Urological Association).

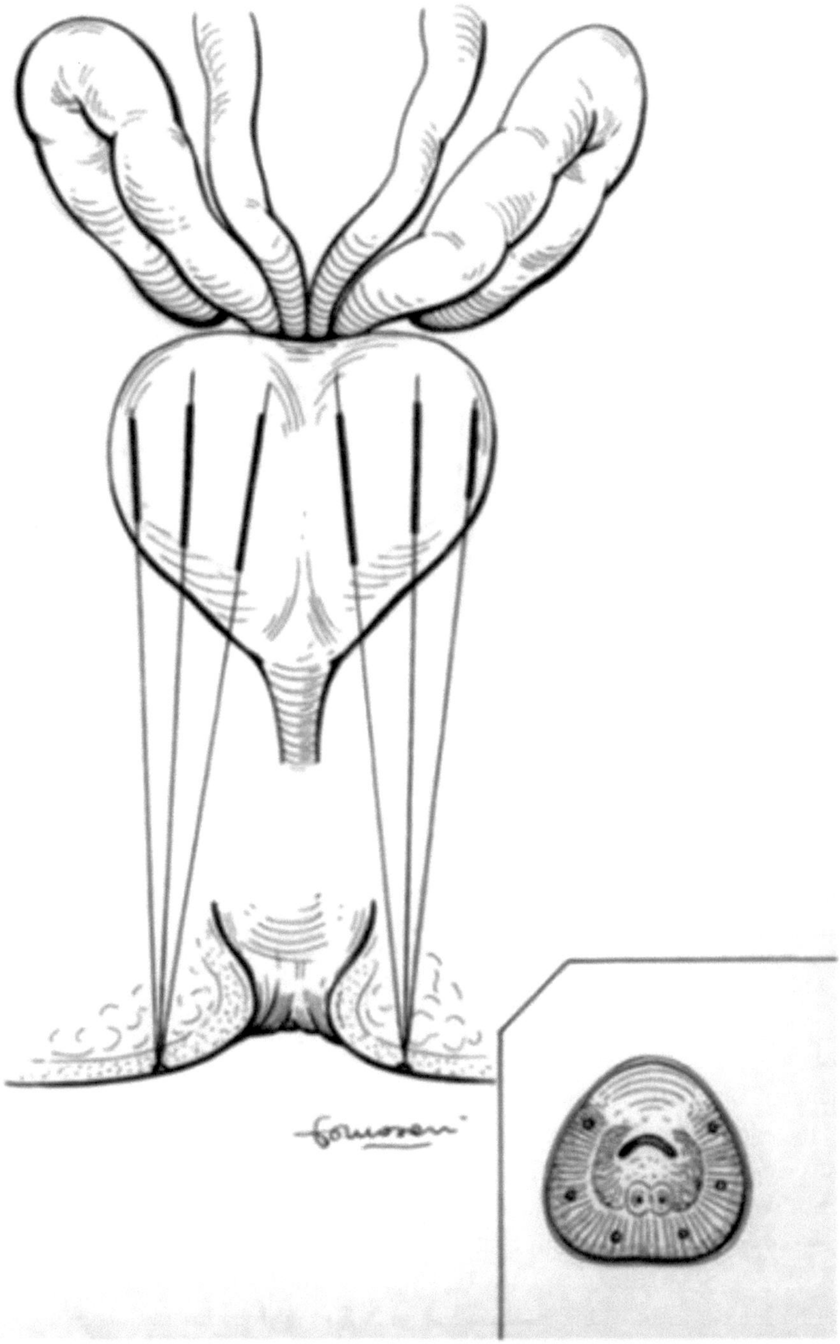

Figure 3. Scheme of the transperineal six-core fan biopsy. Cores are also taken from the far lateral aspect of the prostate (Reprinted from Urology, Volume 61/Issue 5, Emiliozzi P, Corsetti A, Tassi B, Federico G, Martini M, Pansadoro V. 2003, 961-966, with permission from Elsevier).

A number of studies have reported TPUS-guided biopsy in patients after APR [6, 9, 23] (Table). Shinohara et al. [23] reported the largest experience analyzing 28 patients with a history of APR who were referred for biopsy with a mean PSA of 22 ng/mL (median 9.5, range 4.1 to 237). The mean time from APR to referral was 14 years (range 1 to 33 years) and five patients had previously undergone radiation therapy as part of the treatment for colorectal cancer. Of the 28 patients, 23 were diagnosed with prostate cancer (82.1%), with a mean Gleason score of 6.6 (range 3 to 9). Twenty-two of the 23 patients (95.7%) elected for treatment, including prostatectomy (n=8), androgen deprivation therapy (n=7), external radiation therapy (n=6) and high dose radiation therapy (n=1).

Study	Patients (N)	Median Age (Yrs)	Mean PSA (ng/mL)	Median PSA (ng/mL)	Mean Interval From APR to Biopsy (Yrs)	Biopsy Proven Prostate Cancer, N= (%)
Shinohara et al. [23]	28	65	22	9.5	14	23 (82%)
Twidwell et al. [6]	10	67	NR	NR	12	2 (20%)
Filderman et al. [99]	5	62	16.5	NR	NR	2 (40%)

Table 1. A comparison of studies analyzing transperineal ultrasound-guided prostate biopsy results in patients after abdominoperineal resection. (NR - not reported)

4.4. Practical considerations for TPUS-guided prostate biopsy

4.4.1. Image quality

The image quality of TPUS of the prostate compared to TRUS has been previously described by Terris et al. [7]. In a prospective study of 50 patients who had not undergone APR, TPUS was performed with a 4-MHz abdominal probe at a frequency of 5 - 7 MHz and TRUS at 7 MHz (Figure 4). TPUS allowed good visualization of the prostate in 48 (96%) patients in the coronal plane and in 45 (90%) patients in the sagittal plane. Prostate volume, as calculated by the prolate spheroid method, correlated well with TRUS calculations (r = 0.876). Prostatic calcifications were seen in 12 patients (24%), identified by both TRUS and TPUS, however 29 patients (58%) with hypoechoic lesions identified by TRUS were not visualized by TPUS. Furthermore, six patients (12%) with cystic lesions visualized by TRUS were seen in half of the patients by TPUS (3/6). Image quality of TPUS is inadequate for staging purposes secondary to poor transverse and longitudinal visualization of the prostatic capsule. While the imaging quality of TPUS may be inferior to TRUS, it likely represents the most reliable modality in patients without access to the rectum and has been proposed as a diagnostic modality in patients at high risk for prostate cancer with previous negative TRUS-guided biopsies [25].

http://dx.doi.org/10.5772/52291

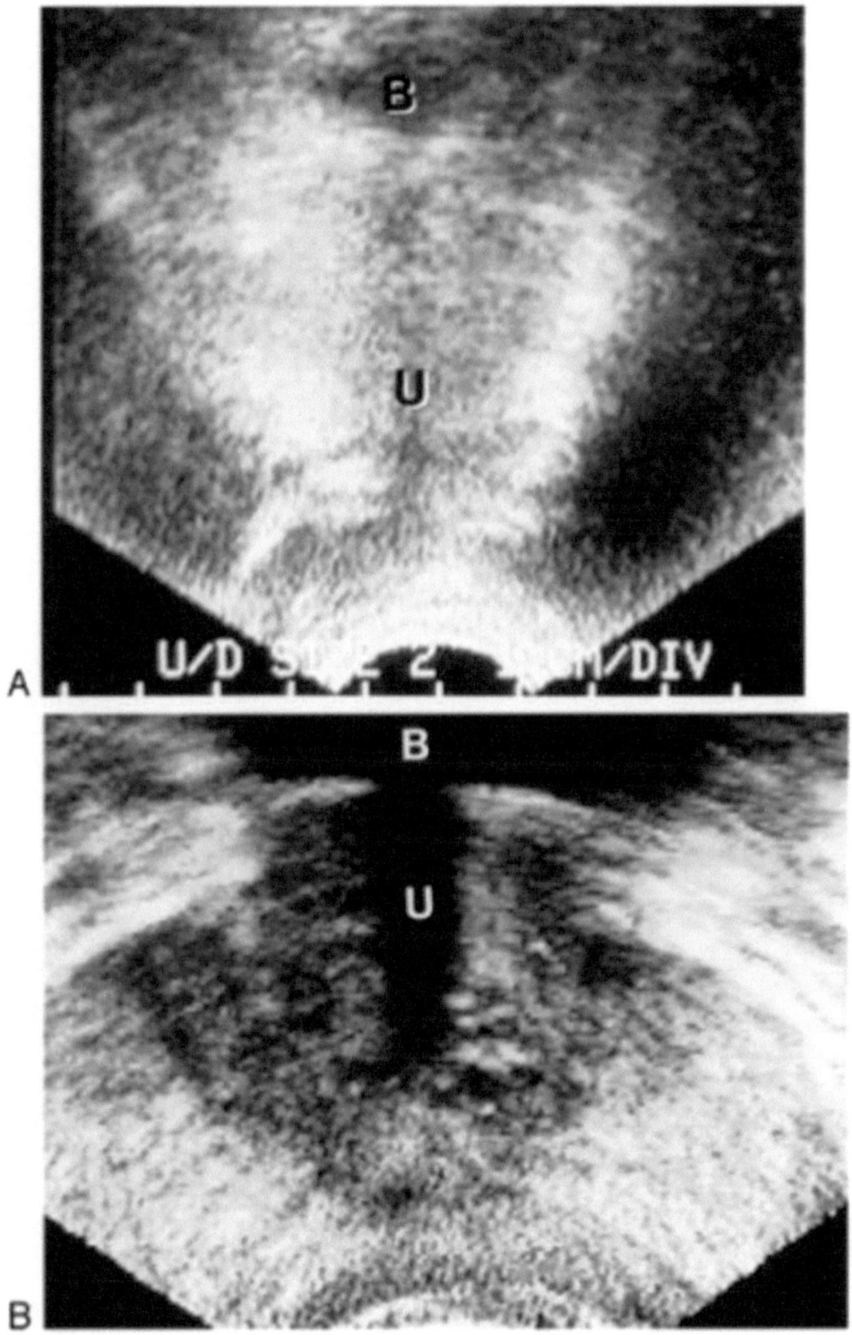

Figure 4. A) Transperineal image showing vague outline of the prostate in the coronal plane. (B) Transverse image of the prostate in the transverse plane. B = bladder; U = urethra (Reprinted from Urology, Volume 52/Issue 6, Terris MK, Hammerer PG, Nickas ME. 1998, 1070-1072, with permission from Elsevier).

4.4.2. *Improved sampling of the far lateral peripheral zone*

When performing TPUS-guided biopsy, the needle forms an acute angle with the long axis of the prostate apex before becoming nearly parallel with the long axis of the prostate base and mid-gland. Geometrically, this allows sampling of more peripheral zone tissue, notably the far lateral peripheral zone [23, 25]. Eskew et al. [26] performed sextant biopsies in addition to cores taken from the far lateral and mid regions of the prostate in 119 patients, diagnosing prostate cancer in 48 patients (40.3%). Among these 48 patients, 17 (35%) had carcinoma only in the far lateral and mid regions of the prostate.

5. Conclusions

Evaluation of the prostate in men with an elevated PSA who have undergone APR is challenging due to inability to perform DRE and TRUS-guided prostate biopsy. TPUS-guided prostate biopsy is the most cost effective and feasible modality for diagnosing prostate cancer in these patients. However, given that men aged 50-75 are at increased risk for both prostate cancer and colorectal cancer, preoperative prostate cancer screening in men who are planning APR allows for proper assessment of the prostate before access to the rectum is compromised, provides a baseline PSA to compare with further testing after the APR, and may detect synchronous malignancies. A multidisciplinary approach is ideal when considering prostate cancer screening in men 50 years of age or older with reasonable life expectancy who are planning APR.

Author details

Zachary Klaassen[1], Ray S. King[2], Kelvin A. Moses[1], Rabii Madi[1] and Martha K. Terris[1*]

1 Department of Surgery, Section of Urology, Georgia Health Sciences University, Augusta, Georgia

2 Department of Surgery, Georgia Health Sciences University, Augusta, Georgia

References

[1] Siegel R, Naishadham D, Jemal A. Cancer Statistics, 2012. CA – A Cancer Journal for Clinicians 2012;62(1) 10-29.

[2] Lee T, Barringer M, Myers RT, Sterchi JM. Multiple primary carcinomas of the colon and associated extracolonic primary malignant tumors. Annals of Surgery 1982;195(4) 501-507.

[3] Weir JA. Colorectal cancer: metachronous and other associated neoplasm. Diseases of the Colon and Rectum 1975;18(1) 4-5.

[4] Park J, Guillem JG. Chapter 47 – Rectal Cancer. In: Cameron JL, Cameron AM (eds). Current Surgical Therapy, 10th ed. Philadelphia, PA: Elsevier Health Sciences; 2011.

[5] Enblad P, Adami H, Glimerlius B, Krusemo U, Pahlman L. The risk of subsequent primary malignant diseases after cancers of the colon and rectum. Cancer 1990;65(9) 2091-2100.

[6] Twidwell JJ, Matthews RD, Huisam TK, Sands JP. Ultrasound evaluation of the prostate after abdominoperineal resection. The Journal of Urology 1993;150(3) 902-904.

[7] Terris MK, Hammerer PG, Nickas ME. Comparison of ultrasound imaging in patients undergoing transperineal and transrectal prostate ultrasound. Urology 1998;52(6) 1070-1072.

[8] Shinghal R, Terris MK. Limitations of transperineal ultrasound-guided prostate biopsies. Urology 1999;54(4) 706-708.

[9] Filderman PS, Jacobs SC. Prostatic ultrasound in the patient without a rectum. Urology 1994;43(5) 722-724.

[10] Koppie TM, Presti JC, Shinohara K, Terris MK, Carroll PR. Transperineal biopsy after abdominoperineal resection: A two center experience. J Urol 2000;163(1) 260.

[11] Corman ML. Colon and Rectal Surgery, 5th Ed. Philadelphia: Lippincott Williams & Wilkins; 2005.

[12] Perry WB, Connaughton JC. Abdominoperineal resection: how is it done and what are the results? Clinics in Colon and Rectal Surgery 2007;20(3) 213-220.

[13] Murrell ZA, Dixon MR, Vargas H, Arneel TD, Kumar R, Stamos MJ. Contemporary indications for and early outcomes of abdominoperineal resection. American Surgeon 2005;71(10) 837-840.

[14] Reshef A, Lavery I, Kiran R. Factors associated with onocologic outcomes after abdominoperineal resection compared with restorative resection for low rectal cancer: patient and tumor related or technical factors only? Diseases of the Colon and Rectum 2012;55(1) 51-58.

[15] Simorov A, Reynoso J, Dolghi O, Thompson J, Oleynikov D. Comparison of perioperative outcomes in patients undergoing laparoscopic versus open abdominoperineal resection. The American Journal of Surgery 2011;202(6) 666-672.

[16] Marr R, Birbeck K, Garvican J, Macklin CP, Tiffin NJ, Parsons WJ, Dixon MF, Mapstone NP, Sebag-Montefiore D, Scott N, Johnston D, Sagar P, Finan P, Quirke P. The modern abdominoperineal excision: the next challenge after total mesorectal excision. Annals of Surgery 2005;242(1) 74-82.

[17] Surveillance, Epidemiology, and End Results (SEER) Program (www.seer.cancer.gov). Research Data (1973-2009), National Cancer Institute, DCCPS, Surveillance

Research Program, Surveillance Systems Branch, released April 2012, based on the November 2011 submission.

[18] Terris MK, Wren SM. Results of a Screening Program for Prostate Cancer in Patients Scheduled for Abdominoperineal Resection for Colorectal Pathologic Findings. Urology 2001;57(5) 943-945.

[19] Papanicolaou N, Eisenberg PJ, Silverman SG, McNicholas MM, Althausen AF. Prostatic biopsy after proctocolectomy: a transgluteal, CT-guided approach. AJR American Journal of Roentgenology 1996;166(6) 1332-1334.

[20] D'Amico AV, Tempany CM, Cormack R, Hata N, Jinzaki M, Tuncali K, Weinstein M, Richie JP. Transperineal magnetic resonance image guided prostate biopsy. The Journal of Urology 2000;164(2) 385-387.

[21] Lau HY, Kagawa K, Lee WR, Hunt MA, Shaer AH, Hanks GE. Short communication: CT-MRI image fusion for 3D conformal prostate radiotherapy: use in patients with altered pelvic anatomy. The British Journal of Radiology 1996;69(828) 1165-1170.

[22] Seaman EK, Sawczuk IS, Fatal M, Olsson CA, Shabsigh R. Transperineal prostate needle biopsy guided by transurethral ultrasound in patients without a rectum. Urology 1996;47(3) 353-355.

[23] Shinohara K, Gulati M, Koppie TM, Terris MK. Transperineal prostate biopsy after abdominoperineal resection. The Journal of Urology 2003;169(1) 141-144.

[24] Emiliozzi P, Corsetti A, Tassi B, Federico G, Martini M, Pansadoro V. Best approach for prostate cancer detection: A prospective study on transperineal versus transrectal six-core prostate biopsy. Urology 2003;61(5) 961-966.

[25] Igel TC, Knight MK, Young PR, Wehle MJ, Petrou SP, Broderick GA, Marino R, Parra RO. Systematic transperineal ulatrasound guided template biopsy of the prostate in patients at high risk. The Journal of Urology 2001;165(5) 1575-1579.

[26] Eskew LA, Bare RL, McCullough DL. Systematic 5 region prostate biopsy is superior to sextant method for diagosing carcinoma of the prostate. The Journal of Urology 1997;157(1) 199-202.

Chapter 6

Radiation Therapy for Prostate Cancer

Shinji Kariya

Additional information is available at the end of the chapter

http://dx.doi.org/10.5772/53180

1. Introduction

Public concern on the radiation therapy for prostate cancer has increased recently. The leading causes of this phenomenon are thought of as popularization of prostate-specific antigen (PSA) measurement and having been able to tell the curable patients apart by means of the accomplished risk classifications. Massive development of radiation therapy technology also seems to be one of the leading causes. This chapter focuses on the variety of curative radiation therapy for clinically localized prostate cancer.

2. External beam radiation therapy

2.1. Conventional External Beam Radiation Therapy (EBRT)

In the 1970s, the treatment field size and portal configuration for radiation therapy were based on estimations of the anatomic boundaries of the prostate defined by plain-film radiography and by the digital rectal examination. At that time, a variety of treatment techniques were used. In general, four fields were used to treat the pelvis and prostate to an initial dose of 45 Gy, with a boost to 70 Gy to the prostate only [1, 2]. Early conventional external beam radiation therapy used total doses in the range of 60 to 70 Gy, because it was believed that this dose was close to the maximum dose allowed by the surrounding normal tissues, especially rectum. Today, it is obvious that this dose is not sufficient to get an adequate local control rate.

2.2. Three-Dimensional Conformal Radiation Therapy (3D-CRT)

In the early to mid-1908s, three-dimensional conformal treatment techniques became increasingly available. Although these techniques vary in some aspects, they share certain common principles that offer significant advantages over conventional external beam radiation therapy techniques. CT-based images referenced to a reproducible patient position are used to localize the prostate and normal organs and to generate high resolution 3D reconstructions of the patient. Treatment field directions are selected using beam`s-eye-view techniques and the fields are shaped to conform to the patient`s CT-defined target volume, thereby minimizing the volume of normal tissue irradiated. Compared with treating a patient by conventional external beam radiation therapy technique, 3D-CRT is associated with a nearly 30% reduction in the dose received by 50% of the rectum. Based on this kind of analysis, it greater than or equal to 10% should be possible without an increase in acute or chronic toxicity [3].

2.3. Intensity Modulated Radiation Therapy (IMRT)

IMRT is a relatively recent refinement of three-dimensional conformal techniques that uses treatment fields with highly irregular radiation intensity patterns to deliver exquisitely conformal radiation distributions. These intensity patterns are created using special inverse and optimization computer planning systems. Rather than define each shape and weight as is done in conventional treatment planning, planners of IMRT treatment specify the desired dose to the target and normal tissues using mathematical descriptions referred to as constraints or objectives [4]. Sophisticated optimization methods are then used to determine the intensity pattern for each treatment field that results in a dose distribution as close to the user-defined constraints as possible. IMRT delivery is significantly more complex than conformal delivery as well. Delivery of an IMRT intensity pattern requires a computer-controlled beam-shaping apparatus on the linear accelerator known as a multi-leaf collimator (MLC). The MLC consists of many small individually moving leaves or fingers that can create arbitrary beam shapes. The MLC is used for IMRT delivery in either a static mode referred to as step and shoot, which consists of multiple small, irregularly shaped fields delivered in sequence, or a dynamic mode with the leaves moving during treatment to create the required irregular intensity patterns [5]. Since its inception, IMRT has become a common and important method for treating prostate cancer and has facilitated an escalation in dose.

2.4. Clinical results of EBRT

2.4.1. Clinical results of conventional EBRT

The results of several large single-institution comparison between radical prostatectomy (RP) and EBRT were reported.

Investigators from Cleveland Clinic Foundation, USA analyzed 1,682 patients with clinical stage T1 and T2 disease treated with either RP or RT. They reported that the 8-year biochemical relapse free survival (bRFS) rates for RP and conventional EBRT less than 72 Gy were 72% and 34%, respectively, and conventional EBRT less than 72 Gy was inferior to RP in the 8-year bRFS rate (Fig 1)[6].

http://dx.doi.org/10.5772/53180

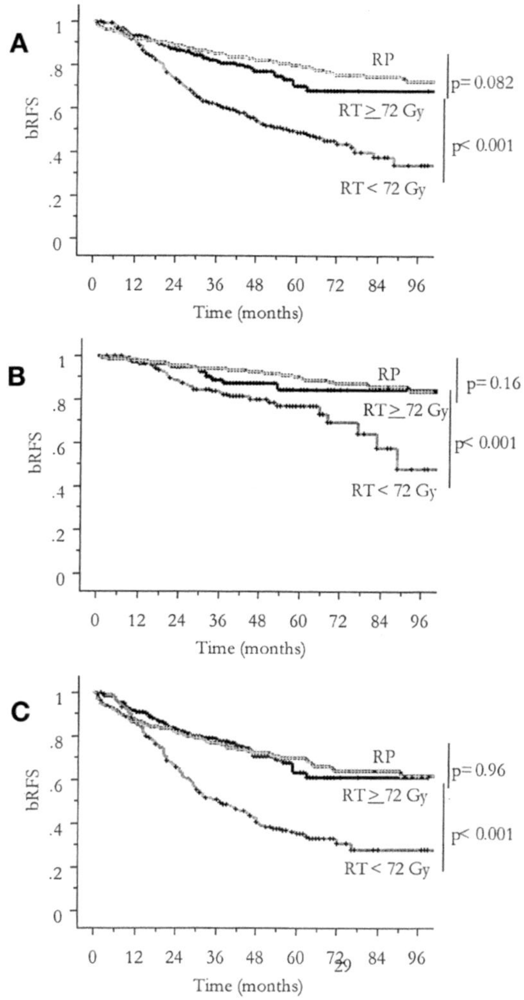

(Cited from Kupelian PA et al.[5])

Figure 1. Biochemical relapse-free survival by treatment modality: RT to doses < 72 Gy, RT to doses > or = 72 Gy, and RP for all (A), favorable (B), and unfavorable patients(C).

D'Amico et al. reported a retrospective cohort study of 2635 patients with either RP or RT of median dose to 70.4 Gy (95% CI, 69.3-70.4 Gy) [7]. Eight-year bRFS rates for low-risk (T1c, T2a, PSA < or = 10 ng/ml, and Gleason score (GS) < or = 6) patients were 88% and 78% for RP and RT, respectively. Eight-year bRFS rates for intermediate-risk (T2b or GS 7 or PSA > 10 and < or = 20 ng/ml) patients with < 34% positive prostate biopsies were 79% and 65% for PR and RT, respectively. Eight-year bRFS rates were 36% versus 35% for intermediate-risk patients with at least 34% positive prostate biopsies and 33% versus 40% for high-risk (T2c or PSA > 20ng/ml or GS > or = 8) patients treated with RP versus those treated with RT, respectively. In conclusion, in their retrospective cohort study, intermediate-risk and low-risk patients with a low biopsy tumor volume who were treated with RP appeared to fare significantly better compared with patients who were treated using conventional-dose RT. For the meanwhile, Intermediate-risk and high-risk patients with a high biopsy tumor volume who were treated with RP or RT had long-term estimates of bRFS that were not found to be significantly different.

2.4.2. Clinical results of 3D-CRT

Above-mentioned investigators from Cleveland Clinic Foundation reported that 3D-CRT more than 72 Gy was superior to Conventional EBRT less than 72 Gy and very similar to RP in the 8-year bRFS (6). Eight-year bRFS rate were 86% versus 86% (p=0.16) for favorable-risk (T1 to T2a, GS<or=6, PSA<or=10 ng/ml) patients and 62% versus 61% (p=0.96) for unfavorable-risk (T2b to T2c, GS>or=7, PSA>10 ng/ml) patients with RP versus those treated with RT>or=72 Gy (Fig 1). Several study also have demonstrated that doses in excess of 70 to 72 Gy are associated with a reduction in the risk of recurrence compared with lower doses [8-12].

2.4.3. Clinical results of IMRT

Investigators from Memorial Sloan Kettering Cancer Center (MSKCC) reported their experience in 1002 patients treated with IMRT of 86.4 Gy [13]. They reported 7-year bRFS rates for low, intermediate, and unfavorable risk group patients as 98.8%, 85.6%, and 67.9%, respectively. In this report, they concluded that high dose IMRT to 86.4 Gy for localized prostate cancer resulted in excellent clinical outcomes with acceptable toxicity.

2.4.4. Clinical results of combined with Androgen Deprivation Therapy (ADT) and EBRT

Thus far, there have been five phase III randomized controlled trials for high-risk prostate cancer that compared radiotherapy alone with radiotherapy and ADT [14-18]. In all of these trials, ADT improved bRFS. In three of these four trials, ADT improved both overall survival (OS) and cause-specific survival (CSS).

From above-mentioned results, combining ADT with radiotherapy should be recommended in the high-risk group.

For intermediate-risk prostate cancer, two studies were published. Investigators from Brigham and Women's Hospital reported their randomized trial that consisted of 206 patients [19]. Two months each of total androgen blockade given before, during, and after radiotherapy for a total of 6 months. After a median follow-up of 4.52 years, ADT had improved 5-year bRFS, CSS, and OS. The Trans-Tasman Radiation Oncology Group (TROG) 96.01 study consisted of 802 patients, who were randomized to radiotherapy alone, 3 months, or 6 months of neoadjuvant hormones with radiotherapy. Five-year bRFS was significantly improved in the 3-month and 6-month arms as compared to the control arm. Although the 6-months arm showed significantly improved 5-year CSS, the 3-month arm was not significantly improved.

The thing to note is that these trials used doses less than 72 Gy that would be considered suboptimal by today's standard. Whether the benefit of ADT remains in the current era of dose escalation is currently unclear.

2.5. Acute and late adverse events

2.5.1. *Acute and late adverse events of conventional EBRT*

EBRT delivered with conventional techniques is fairly well tolerated, although grade 2 or higher acute rectal morbidity (discomfort, tenesmus, diarrhea) or urinary symptoms (frequency, nocturia, urgency, dysuria) requiring medication occur in approximately 60% of patients. Symptoms usually appear during the third week of treatment and resolve within days to weeks after treatment is completed. The incidence of late complications that develop > or = 6 months after completion of treatment is significantly lower, whereas serious complications that require corrective surgical intervention are rare. An analysis of 1,020 patients treated in two large Radiation Therapy Oncology Group (RTOG) trials 7506 and 7706 demonstrated an incidence of chronic urinary sequelae, such as cystitis, hematuria, urethral stricture, or bladder contracture, requiring hospitalization in 7.7% of cases, but the incidence of urinary toxicities requiring major surgical interventions such as laparotomy, cystectomy, or prolonged hospitalization was only 0.5% [20]. More than half of chronic urinary complications were urethral strictures, occurring mostly in patients who had undergone a previous transurethral resection of the prostate (TURP). The incidence of chronic intestinal sequelae, such as chronic diarrhea, proctitis, rectal and anal stricture, rectal bleeding or ulcer, requiring hospitalization for diagnosis and minor intervention was 3.3%, with 0.6% of patients experiencing bowel obstruction or perforation. Fatal complications were rare (0.2%). Most complications attributed to radiation therapy are observed within the first 3 to 4 years after treatment, and the likelihood of complications developing after 5 years in low. The risk of complications is increased when radiation doses exceed 70 Gy. The risk of rectal toxicity has been correlated with the volume of the anterior wall exposed to the higher doses of irradiation

2.5.2. *Acute and late adverse events of CRT*

Michalski et al. reported the toxicity outcomes of Stages T1-T2 prostate cancer in RTOG 9406, a phase I-II dose escalation study [21]. Two hundred twenty five patients were treated to 78 Gy (2 Gy fractions). The median follow-up was 2.2 years. Only 3% of patients had grade 3 acute toxicity. No grade 4 or 5 acute toxicity was reported. The late grade 2 and 3 bowel toxicity rates were 18% and 2%, respectively. 2 had grade 4 bowel toxicity. The late grade 2 and 3 bladder toxicity rates were 17% and 4%, respectively. No grade 4 or 5 late bladder toxicity was reported.

Zietman et al. reported acute and late genitourinary (GU) and gastrointestinal (GI) toxicity among patients treated on a randomized controlled trial [22]. The median follow-up was 5.5 years. The acute GU grade 3 toxicity for both the 70.2 Gy (1.8 Gy fractions) and 79.2 Gy dose arms in 2 Gy per fraction were 1%. The acute GI grade 3 toxicity for the 70.2 Gy and 79.2 Gy dose arms were 1% and 0%, respectively. The late GU grade 2 and 3 toxicity were 18% and 2%, respectively, for the 70.2 Gy dose arm, and 20% and 1%, respectively, for the 79.2 Gy dose arm (difference not significant between two arms). The late GI grade 2 for the 70.2 Gy and 79.2 Gy arms were 8% and 17%, respectively ($p = 0.005$). The late GI grade 3 toxicity, however, was 1% for both arms.

Zelefsky et al. reported the long-term tolerance of high-dose 3D-CRT at MSKCC [23]. The 5-year actuarial rate of grade 2 rectal toxicity for patients receiving 64.8 to 70.2 Gy was 7%, compared with 16% for those treated to 75.6 Gy and 15% for those who treated to 81 Gy (70.2 vs. 75.6 or 81 Gy, p <0.001). The 5-year actuarial rate of grade 3 or higher rectal toxicity was 0.85%, and no correlation between dose and the development of grade 3 complications was found within the range of 64.8 to 81 Gy. Multivariable analysis demonstrated the following variables as predictors of late grade 2 or higher GI toxicity: prescription doses >75.6 Gy (p < 0.001), history of diabetes mellitus (p = 0.01), and the presence of acute GI symptoms during treatment (p = 0.02). The 5-year actuarial likelihood of Grade 2 or higher late GU toxicity for patients who receiving 75.6 to 81 Gy was 15%, compared with 8% for those treated to 64.8 to 70.2 Gy (p = 0.008). The 5-year actuarial likelihood of the development of a urethral stricture (Grade 3 toxicity) for patients who had a prior TURP was 4%, compared with 1% for those who did not have a prior TURP (p = 0.03). No correlation was observed between higher radiation doses and the development of a urethral stricture. Multivariable analysis demonstrated the following variables as predictors of late Grade 2 or higher GU toxicity: prescription doses >75.6 Gy (p = 0.008) and the presence of acute GU symptoms during treatment (p <0.001).

Peeters et al. reported on the incidence of acute and late complications in a multicenter randomized trial comparing 68 Gy to 78 Gy 3D-CRT [24]. The median follow-up was 31 months. For acute toxicity, no significant differences were seen between the two arms. GI toxicity Grade 2 and 3 was reported as the maximum acute toxicity in 44% and 5%, respectively. For acute GU toxicity, these figures were 41% and 13%. The 3-year in incidence of grade 2 and higher GI and GU toxicities for the 68 Gy dose arm was 23.2% and 28.5%, respectively. The 3-year incidence of grade 2 and higher GI and GU toxicities for the 78 Gy dose arm was 26.5% and 30.2%, respectively. The differences were not significant. However, the authors did note a significant increase in grade 3 rectal bleeding at 3 years was 10% for the 78 Gy arm, compared to 2% for the 68 Gy arm (p = 0.007), and in nocturia (p = 0.05). The factors related to acute GI toxicity were hormone therapy (HT) (p < 0.001), a higher dose-volume group (p = 0.01), and pretreatment GI symptoms (p = 0.04). For acute GU toxicity, prognostic factors were: pretreatment GU symptoms (p < 0.001), ADT (p = 0.003), and prior TURP (p = 0.02). The following variables were found to be predictive of late GI toxicity: a history of abdominal surgery (p <0.001), and the presence of pretreatment GI symptoms (p = 0.001). The following variables were predictive of late GU toxicity: pretreatment urinary symptoms (p <0.001), the use of neoadjuvant ADT (p <0.001), and prior TURP (p = 0.006).

Sabdhu et al. reported that urethral strictures for 1,100 patients treated with 3D-CRT [25]. The 5-year actuarial likelihood of developing urethral stricture was 4% for 120 patients with a prior history or TURP compared to 1% for 980 patients with no history of TURP (p = 0.01). Other late urinary toxicities were not observed among patients with a prior history of a TURP. Lee et al. observed a 2% incontinence rate among patients with a prior history of TURP who were treated with EBRT compared with a 0.2% rate in patients without a prior TURP[26].

2.5.3. Acute and late adverse events of IMRT

In an attempt to improve further the conformality of the high-dose therapy plans and decrease the rate of grade 2 and higher toxicity, an IMRT approach was introduced for the treatment of clinically localized disease.

Zelefsky et al. reported their experience in 1571 patients treated with 3D-CRT or IMRT with dose raging from 66 to 81 Gy [27]. The median follow-up was 10 years. In this experience, IMRT significantly reduced the risk of grade 2 and higher late GI toxicities compared with conventional 3D-CRT (5% vs. 13%, $p < 0.001$), although IMRT delivered higher dose than 3D-CRT. However, IMRT increased the risk of acute and late grade 2 and higher GU toxicities and acute grade 2 and higher GI toxicities compared with conventional 3D-CRT (37% vs. 22%, $p = 0.001$, 20% vs. 12%, $p = 0.01$, and 3% vs. 1%, $p = 0.04$, respectively).

According to the latest report from MSKCC, actuarial 7-year grade 2 or higher late GI and GU toxicities with the use of IMRT to 86.4 Gy were 4.4% and 21.1%, respectively. Late grade 3 GI and GU toxicities were 0.7% and 2.2%, respectively [13].

Mamgani et al. compared the toxicity of 41 prostate cancer patients treated with IMRT to 78 Gy with that of 37 patients treated with the 3D-CRT approach at the same dose level within the Dutch dose-escalation trial [28]. They reported that IMRT significantly reduced the incidence of acute grade 2 or higher GI toxicity compared with 3D-CRT (20% vs. 61%, $p = 0.001$). For acute GU toxicity and late GI and GU toxicities, the incidence was lower after IMRT, although these differences were not statistically significant (53% vs. 69%, $p = 0.3$, 21% vs. 37%, $p = 0.16$, and 43% vs. 45%, $p = 1.0$, respectively).

3. Low-Dose-Rate (LDR) brachytherapy (Permanent implants)

3.1. Introduction to permanent implants

Interstitial prostate brachytherapy was first performed by Barringer in 1915 [29-31]. Its first widespread adoption occurred in the 1970s, when the retropubic method was popularized [32]. A laparotomy was done for lymph node dissection and exposure of the prostate. Iodine-125 sources were implanted under direct visualization. The procedure was technically difficult to perform, in part because of limited working space in the pelvis. As a result, retropubic implantation lost popularity in the 1980s [33]. Instead, ultrasound-guided permanent prostatic implantation emerged in the early 1980s and has spread all over the world. The ultrasound-guided transperineal technique was initially described by Holm and coworkers in 1983 [34]. Transrectal ultrasound (TRUS) allowed visualization of the needle location within the prostate, facilitating real-time read-justments of needle position as necessary. Implants could be computer preplanned using transverse ultrasound images. Transperineal implants also could be done percutaneously on an outpatient basis, without laparotomy. Combined with modern, computer-based treatment planning, technological advances allowed for higher quality outpatient prostate brachytherapy [35].

Brachytherapy offers substantial biologic advantages over EBRT in terms of dose localization and higher biologic doses. A modification of the time, dose, and fractionation tables has been made to allow interconvertability between beam radiation and low-dose-rate brachytherapy [36]. There are also substantial practical advantages of brachytherapy, including vastly shorter treatment times and lower costs. These practical advantages have helped maintain widespread interest in brachytherapy, despite continuous improvements in beam radiation. Although enthusiasm remains high in some quarters, there are still vexing discrepancies in reported cure rates and morbidities. It is becoming clearer that such discrepancies result partly from different technical expertise and patient management policies [37]. Brachytherapy, like surgery, is operator-dependent and outcomes vary with skill and experience.

3.2. Patient selection

Contraindications to brachytherapy include metastatic disease (including lymph node involvement), gross seminal vesicle involvement because that radioactive seeds are unlikely to be capable of sterilizing more than the most proximal 1 cm of seminal vesicle tissue, or large T3 disease that cannot be adequately implanted because of geometrical impediments to adequate tumor mass implantation (an unusual presentation).

Large prostate size can be often contraindication to brachytherapy because that the anterior and lateral portion of the gland may be inadequately covered because of pubic arch interference of needle placement. When a patient has a prostate > 60 cc, and pubic arch interference is a concern, a short course of ADT will reduce prostate volume by an average of approximately 30% in 3-4 months [38, 39]

Patients with a high International Prostate Symptom Score (IPSS) for urinary irritative and obstructive symptoms are at increased risk of developing postimplant urinary retention [40-43]. Terk et al. [44] and Gutman et al. [45] reported that patients with IPSS had a high risk of urinary retention.

Patients with prior pelvic radiotherapy may be at increased risk of developing late GI or GU toxicity. In such patients, the dose delivered to the prostate, rectum, and bladder should be considered.

In patients with prior TURP, a large TURP defect may disturb implantation of seed throughout the entire gland, resulting in unacceptable dosimetry.

Early-stage prostate cancer with T < or = 2a, initial PSA < or = 10ng/ml, and GS < or = 6 is suitable for brachytherapy without supplemental EBRT. Meanwhile, the generally accepted policy has been to add EBRT for the prostate cancer with T > 2a, initial PSA > 10ng/ml, or GS > 6. However, patients with intermediate-risk disease (T = 2b, GS = 7, or PSA > 10 and < or = 20 ng/ml) represent a heterogeneous patient population some of whom may benefit from monotherapy. Some investigators reported their experiences to perform monotherapy for patients with intermediate- and high-risk disease [46 – 51].

3.3. Treatment techniques

3.3.1. Preplanned transperineal implantation techniques

First of all, TRUS imaging is obtained before planned procedure to assess the prostate volume. A computerized plan is generated from the ultrasound images, producing isodose distributions and the ideal location of seeds within the gland to deliver the prescription dose to the prostate. Several days to weeks later, the implantation procedure is performed. Needles are then placed under ultrasonographic guidance through a perineal template according to the coordinates determined by the preplan. Radioactive seeds are individually deposited in the needle with the aid of an applicator or with preloaded seeds on a semirigid strand containing the preplanned number of seeds. In the latter case, this is accomplished by stabilizing the needle obturator that holds the seed column in a fixed position while the needle is withdrawn slowly, depositing a row or series of seeds within the gland.

In general most brachytherapists use a modified peripheral loading technique for permanent interstitial implantation. This approach can reduce the urethral doses more than a homogenous loading technique. The portion of the urethra receiving 150% dose (UV_{150}) should be limited [52]. Likewise, the volume of the rectum (RV_{100}) receiving the prescription dose ideally should be < 1 cc [53].

3.3.2. Intraoperative planning techniques

Intraoperative planning takes advantage of the opportunity of using real-time measurements of the prostate during the procedure while preplanning is often preformed several weeks before implantation, frequently under different conditions than the actual operative procedure. Subtle changes in the position of the ultrasound probe as well as the distortion of the prostate associated with needle placement and subsequent edema can result in profound changes in the shape of the gland compared with the preplanned prostatic contour.

3.4. Dose selection

Numerous studies have confirmed D_{90} (the minimum dose received by 90% of the prostate volume) and V_{100} (percentage of the prostate volume receiving 100% of the prescribed dose) are correlated with outcome [54-56].

Prescription doses for I-125 or palladium-103 (^{103}Pd) are typically 140 to 160 Gy or 110 to 130 Gy, respectively. In practice, many brachytherapists plan a dose higher than the above mentioned doses to compensate for edema, seed misplacement, and so on. Merrick et al. [57] examined variability in permanent prostate brachytherapy preimplant dosimetry among eight experienced brachytherapy teams. A range of D_{90} values from 112% to 151% of the prescription dose was planned. Several investigations suggest that an acceptable dose range for postimplant D_{90} for I-125 may be 130 to 180 Gy as long as normal structures are not overdosed. Zelefsky et al. [58] reported that D_{90} < 130 Gy was associated with and increased risk of failure. Meanwhile, Gomez-Iturriaga Pina et al. [59] reported that D_{90} from 180 Gy to 200 Gy was associated with excellent biochemical disease-free survival and acceptable toxicity.

When combined EBRT and brachytherapy, a wide variety of implant and beam radiation dose combinations are used. Implant prescription doses area generally dropped to approximately 70% to 80% of monotherapy doses, ranging from 110 to 120 Gy with I-125 and 90 to 100 Gy with Pd-103. External beam doses of 40 to 50 Gy area typically used. No studies have investigated either the sequencing of EBRT and brachytherapy, or the time interval between the two.

A wide variety of seed activities, seed numbers, or total activities have been used because of no clinical evidence of any effect outcome. Seed activities typically vary from 0.3 to 0.6 mCi for I-125 and 1.2 to 2.2 mCi for Pd-103.

3.5. Clinical results

3.5.1. Clinical results of LDR brachytherapy as monotherapy

It is generally accepted that patients with low-risk disease are excellent candidate for LDR monotherapy. There is no randomized data comparing therapeutic outcomes between LDR monotherapy, surgery, and EBRT. However, multiple reports of low-risk patients treated with LDR monotherapy have demonstrated excellent long-term biochemical control rates of 80 – 95% (Table 1).

Patients with intermediate-risk disease represent a heterogeneous patient population. Some of them seem to benefit from LDR monotherapy, whereas others may require combined modality approaches with EBRT and/or ADT. D'Amico et al [65] reported that percentage of positive prostate biopsy cores is a predicting factor of biochemical outcome following EBRT, particularly for intermediate-risk patients. In their report, patients with > 50% of biopsy cores positive had PSA relapse rates comparable to those of high-risk patients, whereas patients with < 34% of biopsy cores positive had favorable biochemical outcomes similar to those of low risk patients. Long-term biochemical control rate for intermediate-risk patients treated with LDR monotherapy is also favorable, ranging from 70% to 90% (Table 1).

Authors	N	Mean/Median Follow-up	Adjuvant Hormone Therapy	bRFS rate		
				Low-risk	Intermediate-risk	High-risk
Sylvester et al [60]	215	11.7 years	NO	15-year		
				85.90%	79.90%	62.20%
Prade et al [61]	734	55 months	YES	10-year		
				92.00%	84%	65%
Henry et al [62]	1298	4.9 years	YES	10-year		
				86.40%	76.70%	60.60%
Zelefsky et al [63]	2693	63 months	NO	8-year		
				82%	70%	48%
Zelefsky et al [64]	367	63 months	YES	5-year		
				96%	89%	-

Table 1. LDR brachytherapy as monotherapy

http://dx.doi.org/10.5772/53180

For patients with high-risk disease, the use of supplemental beam radiation to cover the periprostatic prostate tissue has been widely practiced. However, LDR monotherapy has been good results comparable to combination of monotherapy and EBRT even in patients with high-risk disease.

3.5.2. Clinical results of combination of LDR brachytherapy and EBRT

Outcomes (bRFS rates) for a combination of LDR brachytherapy and EBRT are shown in Table 2.

Authors	N	Mean/Median Follow-up	Adjuvant Hormone Therapy	bRFS rate		
				Low-risk	Intermediate-risk	High-risk
Critz et al [66]	1469	6 years	NO		10-year	
				93%	80%	61%
Merrick et al [67]	204	7 years	YES		10-year	
						86.60%
Sylvester et al [68]	223	9.43 years	NO		15-year	
				85.60%	80.30%	67.80%
Stock et al [69]	181	65 months	YES		8-year	
						73%
Wernicke et al [70]	242	10 years	NO		10-year	
					77.30%	-

Table 2. Combination of LDR brachytherapy and EBRT

3.6. Acute and late adverse events of LDR brachytherapy

3.6.1. Urinary toxicity

Almost all patients after LDR brachytherapy develop some kind of acute urinary symptoms, for example, urinary frequency, urgency, and occasional urge incontinence. These symptoms often peak at about 3 months after brachytherapy, subsequently gradually decline over the ensuing 3 to 6 months, and resolve with in 1 year (71). Most patients benefit with the use of an

α-blocker. However, Brown et al [71] reported that 22% of patients experienced persistent urinary symptoms even after 12 months.

Acute urinary retention (AUR) is a common complication of modern brachytherapy, but can occur immediately after LDR brachytherapy. Crook et al. [72] demonstrated on the basis of a multivariate analysis that larger prostate volumes and prior hormone therapy were each independent predictors of AUR. AUR should be managed by intermittent or continuous bladder drainage. If AUR persists more than a few days, clean intermittent self-catheterization is preferred to continuous drainage by a Foley catheter. The use of transurethral incision of prostate should be avoided in the first 6 months, but if retention persists, transurethral incision of prostate or minimal TURP may be considered, recognizing the risk of urinary incontinence after these procedures [73-75].

3.6.2. Rectal toxicity

Grade 2 rectal toxicity symptoms, which manifest as rectal bleeding or increased mucous discharge, occur in 2 to 10% of patients, nearly always manifests between 6 and 18 months of implantation [76]. It is partly related to rectal dose and its volume exposed to a particular dose. The incidence of grade 3 or 4 rectal toxicity, which symptoms manifest rectal ulceration or fistula, is unusual (< 1.0%), providing that the volume of rectal wall receiving the prescription dose is kept below 0.5 cc on day 0 or 1 cc on day 30 dosimetry [77]. Most cases of rectal bleeding do not progress to rectal ulceration or fistula and are self-limited in nature. However, healing is typically slow. With the ineffectiveness of medical therapies, more invasive therapies with argon plasma coagulation or topical formalin have been highly effective therapy for rectal bleeding [78]. Invasive therapies, however, might exacerbate radiation damage, so they should be undertaken with caution. Rectal wall biopsy in the course of evaluation for rectal toxicity should avoid as much as possible because it may result in the development of rectal ulceration or fistula.

3.6.3. Sexual dysfunction

Erectile impotence occurs from 20% to 80% after implantation. According to Zelefsky et al [79], whereas the incidence of impotence at 2 years after implantation was 21%, the rate increased to 42% at 5 years after. Merrick et al. [80] reported that there is a strong correlation between radiation-induced impotence and the dose to the penile bulb and proximal penis. They recommend that with day 0 dosimetric evaluation, the minimum dose delivered to 50% and 25% of the bulb should be maintained below 40% and 60% of prescribed minimum peripheral dose, respectively, whereas the minimum dose delivered to 50% and 25% of the crura should be maintained below 40% and 28% of prescribed minimum peripheral dose, respectively, to maximize posttreatment potency.

Several reports suggest that sildenafil citrate have good response to impotence after implantation[81, 82]. Potters et al. [83] reported that the addition of neoadjuvant androgen deprivation had a significant impact on the potency preservation rate after implantation.

The response to sildenafil was significantly better in those patients not treated with neo-adjuvant ADT.

4. High-Dose-Rate (HDR) brachytherapy (Temporary implants)

4.1. Introduction to HDR brachytherapy

HDR brachytherapy has been used as the brachytherapy component in combination with EBRT for the treatment of prostate cancer [84-90]. In general, for this approach patients undergo transperineal placement of afterloading catheters in the prostate under ultrasonographic guidance. After CT-based treatment planning, several high-dose fractions are administered during an interval of 24 to 36 hours using ^{192}Ir. This treatment is followed by supplemental EBRT directed to the prostate and periprostatic tissues to a dose of 40 to 50.4 Gy using conventional fractionation. Recently, dose-escalation studies have been implemented to increase gradually the dose per fraction delivered with the HDR boost [91]. Improved outcomes with higher HDR boost doses were observed compared with outcomes achieved using lower dose level. Single higher dose fraction also becomes used for dealing with the issue of needle displacement between each fraction [92]. More recently, several institutes have used HDR brachytherapy as monotherapy without the addition of EBRT, largely for low-risk, but also for intermediate- and high-risk patients [93-99].

HDR brachytherapy offers several potential advantages over other techniques. Taking advantage of an afterloading approach, the radiation oncologist and physicist can more easily optimize the delivery of radiation therapy to the prostate and compensate for potential regions of underdosage that may be present with permanent interstitial implantation. Further, this technique reduces involved in the procedure compared with permanent interstitial implantation. Finally, HDR brachytherapy boosts may be radiobiologically more efficacious in terms of tumor cell kill for patients with increased tumor bulk or adverse prognostic features compared with low-dose-rate boost such as ^{125}I or ^{103}Pd.

4.2. Clinical results of HDR brachytherapy

The reported outcomes of combination of HDR brachytherapy and EBRT are favorable (Table 3). Multiple reports of low- and intermediate-risk patients treated with combination of HDR brachytherapy and EBRT have demonstrated excellent long-term biochemical control rates of 90-100% and 87-98%, respectively (Table 3). Long-term biochemical control rate for high-risk patients treated with combination of HDR brachytherapy and EBRT is also favorable.

Yoshioka et al. [99] have performed HDR brachytherapy as monotherapy for localized prostate cancer since 1996. The 5-year bRFS rate for low-, intermediate-, and high-risk patients was 85%, 93%, and 79%, respectively.

Authors	N	Mean/Median Follow-up	HDR dose	bRFS rate		
				Low-risk	Intermediate-risk	High-risk
Boost						
Astrom et al. [100]	214	4 years	10 Gy x 2	5-year		
				92%	88%	61%
Bachand et al. [101]	153	44 months	9 Gy x 2/ 10 Gy x 2	5-year		
				95.9%		95.5%
Chen et al. [84]	85	40 months	5.5 Gy x 3	4-year		
				100%	91%	81%
Demanes et al. [85]	209	6.4 years	5.5 Gy x 4/ 6.0 Gy x 4	10-year		
				92%	87%	63%
Yamada et a.l [86]	105	44 months	5.5 Gy x 3/ 7.0 Gy x 3	5-year		
				100%	98%	92%
Phan et al. [89]	309	59 months	6 Gy x 4	5-year		
				98%	90%	78%
Prada et al. [102]	313	71 months	11.5 Gy x 2	10-year		
				100%	91%/88%	79%
Monotherapy						
Yoshioka et al. [99]	112	5.4 years	6 Gy x 9	5-year		
				85%	93%	79%
Rogers CL et al. [103]	284	35.1 months	6.5 Gy x 6	5-year		
				94.40%		

Table 3. HDR brachytherapy

4.3. Acute and late adverse events of HDR brachytherapy

4.3.1. Urinary toxicity

Acute urinary symptoms such as urinary urgency and frequency are common and usually resolve within a few months. Urinary retention occurs in less than 5% of patients treated with combination of HDR brachytherapy and EBRT [89, 94, 104, 105]. Urinary strictures are reported in up to 15% of patients, and most commonly seen in the bulbomembranous urethra [106, 107]. Urinary incontinence is extremely rare, and seen in less than 2% of patients [107, 108].

4.3.2. Rectal toxicity

Transient rectal symptoms such as rectal urgency or frequency often occur. Late rectal bleeding may occur and is usually not clinically significant. Rectal fistula is extremely rare, and seen in less than 1% of patients[89].

4.3.3. Sexual toxicity

Erectile dysfunction has been reported in up to 40% of patients, but approximately 80% will respond to phosphodiesterase-5 inhibitors (86).

5. Particle beam radiation therapy

Particle beam radiation therapy is the cancer therapy to deliver the ions accelerated by means of a cyclotron or synchrotron. Nowadays, protons and carbon ions (heavy particles) are in clinical use.

For protons and heavy particles, unlike electrons or X-rays, the dose increases while the particle penetrates the tissue and loses energy continuously. Hence the dose increases with increasing thickness up to the Bragg peak that occurs near the end of the particle's range. Beyond the Bragg peak, the dose drops to zero (for protons) or almost zero (for heavy particles). The advantage of this energy deposition profile is that less energy is deposited into the healthy tissue surrounding the target tissue.

Although proton beams have approximately the same biological effectiveness as X-rays or electrons, carbon ions have 1.2 to 3.5 times as much effectiveness as X-rays. Carbon ions many other biological features, which X-rays don`t have, as follows; 1) having their reduced ability to repair damage DNA, 2) having smaller oxygen enhancement ratio, 3) effectiveness even against the hypoxic cancer cells, 4) effectiveness even against S-late phase cancer cells because of their being less of cell cycle dependence.

Investigators from National Institute of Radiological Sciences, Japan reported their experience in 927 patients treated with hypofractionated conformal carbon-ion radiation therapy between April 2000 and December 2010 [109]. Of 927 patients, 250, 216, and 461 patients were treated with 66 GyE (Gray equivalent (a measure of carbon-ion radiation dose base on an relative biological effectiveness (RBE) ratio of 3 with respect to photon radiation)) in 20 fractions (Fr), 63 GyE in 20 Fr, and 57.6 GyE in 16 Fr, respectively. Neoadjuvant ADT was given to the patients in the intermediate- and high-risk groups for 2 to 6 months. Adjuvant ADT was continued for a duration of 6 months for intermediate-risk patients and for 2 years for the high-risk patients. They reported the 5-year cause specific survival rates for the low-, intermediate-, and high-risk group patients as 100%, 100%, and 97.9%, respectively. The 5-year bRFS rates of the low-, intermediate-, and high-risk groups were 89.4%, 96.8%, and 88.4%, respectively. They reported that grade 2 rectal bleeding developed in 15 patients (1.6%), but no grade 3 or worse morbidities at the rectum were observed in all groups. They also reported that late grade 2 and grade 3 GU toxicities were observed in 57 (6.1%) and one (0.1%) of 927 patients, respectively. These incidences of late morbidities, especially of rectal bleeding are favorable compared with other RT methods (Table. 4).

Authors	Method	Dose fractionation (Gy/Fr)	No. patients	Morbidity rate	
				GI	GU
Coote et al. [110]	IMRT	60.0/20	60	9.5%	4.0%
Martin et al. [111]	IMRT	60.0/20	92	6.3%	10.0%
Kupelian et al.[112]	IMRT	70.0/28	770	4.4%	5.2%
King et al. [113]	SRT	36.25/5	41	15.0%	29.0%
Madsen et al. [114]	SRT	33.5/5	40	7.5%	22.5%
Michalski JM et al. [115]	3DCRT	68.4-79.2/38-41	275	7-16%	18-29%
	3DCRT	78.0/39	118	25-26%	23-28%
Schulte RW [116]	Proton	75.0/39	901	3.5%	5.4%
Ishikawa et al. [109]	Carbon-ion	57.6-66.0/16-20	927	1.9%	6.3%

(Cited from Ishikawa et al [109])

Table 4. Comparison of Grade 2 or worse late morbidity rates according to RT method

6. Postoperative radiotherapy

6.1. Adjuvant radiotherapy (ART)

The results of three large phase III trials, which evaluated the merits of adjuvant versus expectant management in postoperative patients with positive surgical margins and/or pT3 disease, were reported.

EORTC 22911 confirmed the value of ART, which reduced the risk of biochemical failure and prolongs the time to clinical progression [117]. Patients eligible for this study had pT2-3N0M0 tumors and one or more pathologic risk factors (extracapsular extension (ECE), positive surgical margins (PSM), seminal vesicles invasion (SVI)). After a median follow-up of 5 years, biochemical and clinical progression-free survivals were significantly improved in the radiotherapy group ($P < 0.0001$ and $P = 0.0009$, respectively). The rate of local regional failure was also lower in the radiotherapy group ($P = 0.07$). Severe toxicity (grade 3 or higher) was similar, being 2.6% versus 4.2% at 5 years in the postoperative radiotherapy group ($P = 0.07$).

SWOG 8794 randomly assigned 473 node-negative patients initially treated with radical prostectomy, but found to have either PSM or pT3 (ECE and/or SVI) disease to ART or observation [118]. ART consisted of 60 to 64 Gy. ART resulted in an improvement in metastasis-free and overall survival compared with deferred therapy (HR 0.71; $P = 0.016$ and HR 0.72; $P = 0.023$, respectively). Although adverse effects were more common with radiotherapy versus observation, by 5 years there were no differences in health-related QOL, and a subset analysis suggests that earlier treatment is better than delayed treatment [119].

From the German Cancer Society, ARO 96-02/AUO AP 09/95 randomized 385 patients with pT3 or PSM to either ART (60Gy in 2 Gy fractions) or observation [120]. Although this study had the short median follow-up of 40 months, ART significantly improved progression-free survival ($P < 0.0001$) with a low incidence of late complications from radiotherapy.

6.2. Salvage radiotherapy (SRT)

A multi-institutional study suggests that early intervention with radiotherapy is better than delayed intervention for patients with biochemical failure [121, 122]. This analysis included patients with pT3-4N0 disease who received either SRT or early ART. Early ART for pT3-4N0 disease significantly reduces the risk of long-term biochemical progression after radical prostatectomy compared with SRT.

Stephenson et al. [123] reported on the outcomes and prognostic factors of 501 men who had salvage radiotherapy after a biochemical recurrence. In the entire cohort, the 4-year progression-free survival (PFS) was 45%, and 67% attained a PSA nadir of <0.1 ng/mL. Multivariate analyses demonstrated that Gleason score of 8 to 10, preradiotherapy PSA >2 ng/mL, negative margins, PSA-doubling time <10 months, and seminal vesicle invasion were associated with PSA progression. Supporting earlier intervention, preradiotherapy PSA <0.6 ng/mL had significantly improved PFS than a PSA of 0.61 to 2 ng/mL ($P = 0.006$) and >2 ng/mL ($P = 0.001$).

Author details

Shinji Kariya*

Address all correspondence to: kariyas@kochi-u.ac.jp

Department of Diagnostic Radiology and Radiation Oncology, Kochi Medical School, Kohasu, Oko-town, Kochi, Japan

References

[1] Bagshaw MA, Cox RS, Ray GR. Status of radiation treatment of prostate cancer at Stanford University. NCI Monogr 1988;(7) 47-60.

[2] Pilepich MV, Krall JM, Sause WT, et al. Prognostic factors in carcinoma of the prostate —analysis of RTOG study 75-06. Int J Radiat Oncol Biol Phys 1987; 13(3) 339-349.

[3] Roach M 3rd, Pickett B, Weil M, et al. The "critical volume tolerance method" for estimating the limits of dose escalation during three-dimensional conformal radiotherapy for prostate cancer. Int J Radiat Oncol Biol Phys 1996; 35(5) 1019-1025.

[4] Webb S. The physical basis of IMRT and inverse planning. Br J Radiol 2003; 76(910) 678-689.

[5] Spirou SV, Chui CS. Generation of arbitrary intensity profiles by dynamic jaws or multileaf collimators. Med Phys 1994; 21(7) 1031-1041.

[6] Kupelian PA, Elshaikh M, Reddy CA, et al. Comparison of the efficacy of local therapies for localized prostate cancer in the prostate-specific antigen era: a large single-institution experience with radical prostatectomy and external-beam radiotherapy. J Clin Oncol 2002; 20(16) 3376-3385.

[7] D'Amico AV, Whittington R, Malkowicz SB, et al. Biochemical outcome after radical prostatectomy or external beam radiation therapy for patients with clinically localized prostate carcinoma in the prostate specific antigen era. Cancer 2002; 95(2) 281-286.

[8] Roach M, Meehan S, Kroll S, et al. Radiotherapy for high grade clinically localized adenocarcinoma of the prostate. J Urol 1996; 156(5) 1719-1723.

[9] Zelefsky MJ, Leibel SA, Gaudin PB et al. Dose escalation with three-dimensional conformal radiation therapy affects the outcome in prostate cancer. Int J Radiat Oncol Boil Phys 1998; 41(3) 491-500.

[10] Fiveash JB, Hanks G, Roach M, et al: 3D conformal radiation therapy (3DCRT) for high grade prostate cancer: a multi-institutional review. Int J Radiat Oncol Biol Phys 2000; 47(2) 335-342.

[11] Pollack A, Hanlon AL, Horwitz EM, et al. Prostate cancer radiotherapy dose response: an uptake of the fox chase experience. J Urol 2004; 171(3) 1132-1136.

[12] Kupelian PA, Buchsbaum JC, Reddy CA, et al. Radiation dose response in patients with favorable localized prostate cancer (Stage T1-T2, biopsy Gleason < or = 6, and pretreatment prostate-specific antigen < or = 10). Int J Radiat Oncol Biol Phys 2001; 50(3) 621-625.

[13] Spratt DE, Pei X, Yamada J, et al. Long-term survival and toxicity in patients treated with high-dose intensity modulated radiation therapy for localized prostate cancer. Int J Radiat Oncol Biol Phys 2012, in press.

[14] Bolla M, Collette L, Blank L, et al. Long-term results with immediate androgen suppression and external irradiation in patients with locally advanced prostate cancer (an EORTC study): A phase III randomized trial. Lancet 2002; 360(9327) 103-106.

[15] Pilepich MV, Winter K, Lawton CA, et al. Androgen suppression adjuvant to definitive radiotherapy in prostate carcinoma-long-term results of phase III RTOG 85-31. Int J Raiat Oncol Biol Phys 2005; 61(5) 1285-1290.

[16] Pilepich MV, Winter K, John MJ, et al. Phase III radiation therapy oncology group (RTOG) trial 86-10 of androgen deprivation adjuvant to definitive radiotherapy in locally advanced carcinoma of the prostate. Int J Radiat Oncol Biol Phys 2001; 50(5) 1243-1252.

[17] Laverdiere J, Nabid A, De Bedoya LD, et al. The efficacy and sequencing of a short course of androgen suppression on freedom from biochemical failure when administered with radiation therapy for T2-T3 prostate cancer. J Urol 2004; 171(3) 1137-1140.

[18] Granfors T, Modig H, Damber JE, et al. Combined orchiectomy and external radiotherapy versus radiotherapy alone for nonmetastatic prostate cancer with or without pelvic lymph node involvement: A prospective randomized study. J Urol 1998; 159(6) 2030-2034.

[19] D'Amico AV, Manola J, Loffredo M, et al. 6-months androgen suppression plus radiation therapy vs radiation therapy alone for patients with clinically localized prostate cancer: A randomized controlled trial. JAMA 2004; 292(7) 821-827.

[20] Lawton CA, Won M, Pilepich M, et al. Long-term treatment sequelae following external beam irradiation of adenocarcinoma of the prostate: analysis of RTOG studies 7506 and 7706. Int J Radiat Oncol Biol Phys 1991; 21(4) 935-939.

[21] Michalski JM, Winter K, Purdy JA, et al. Toxicity after three-dimensional radiotherapy for prostate cancer on RTOG 9406 dose level V. Int J Radiat Oncol Biol Phys 2005; 62(3) 706-713.

[22] Zietman AL, DeSilvio ML, Slater JD, et al. Comparison of conventional-dose vs high-dose conformal radiation therapy in clinically localized adenocarcinoma of the prostate. JAMA 2005; 294: 1233-1239.

[23] Zelefsky MJ, Cowen D, Fuks Z, et al. Long-term tolerance of high dose three-dimensional radiotherapy in patients with localized prostate carcinoma. Cancer 1999; 85(11) 2460-2468.

[24] Peeters ST, Heemsbergen WD, Koper PC, et al. Acute and late complications after radiotherapy for localized prostate cancer: results of a multicenter randomized phase III trial comparing 68 Gy to 78 Gy. Int J Radiat Oncol Biol Phys 2005; 61(4) 1019-1034.

[25] Sandhu AS, Zelefsky MJ, Lee HJ, et al. Long-term urinary toxicity after 3-dimensional conformal radiotherapy for prostate cancer in patients with prior history of transurethral resection. Int J Radiat Oncol Biol Phys 2000; 48(3) 643-647.

[26] Lee WR, Schulthesis TE, Hanlon AL, et al. Urinary incontinence following external-beam radiotherapy for clinically localized prostate cancer. Urology 1996; 48(1) 95-99.

[27] Zelefsky MJ, Levin EJ, Hunt M, et al. Incidence of late rectal and urinary toxicities after three-dimensional conformal radiotherapy and intensity-modulated radiotherapy for localized prostate cancer. Int J Raiat Oncol Biol Phys 2008; 70(4) 1124-1129.

[28] Mamgani AA, Heemsbergen WD, Peeters STH, et al. Role of intensity-modulated radiotherapy in reducing toxicity in dose escalation for localized prostate cancer. Int J Radiat Oncol Biol Phys. 2009; 73(3) 685-691.

[29] Barringer BS. Radium in the treatment of prostatic carcinoma. Ann Surg 1924; 80(6) 881-884.

[30] Aronowitz JN. Benjamin Barringer: originator of the transperineal prostate implant. Urol 2002; 60(4) 731-734.

[31] Aronowitz JN. Dawn of prostate brachytherapy: 1915-1930. Int J Radiat Oncol Biol Phys 2002; 54(3) 712-718.

[32] Whitemore WF, Hilaris B, Grabstald H. Retropubic implantation of Iodine 125 in the treatment of prostatic cancer. J Urol 1972; 108(6) 918-920.

[33] Fuks Z, Leibel SA, Wallner KE, et al. The effect of local control on metastatic dissemination in carcinoma of the prostate: Long term results in patients treated with 125-I implantation. Int J Radiat Oncol Biol Phys 1991; 21(3) 337-347.

[34] Holm HH, Juul N, Pedersen JF, et al. Transperineal 125iodine seed implantation in prostatic cancer guided by transrectal ultrasonography. J Urol 1983; 130(2) 283-286.

[35] Charyulu KKN. Transperineal interstitial implantation of prostate cancer: a new method. Int J Radiat Oncol Biol Phys 1980; 6(9) 1261-1266.

[36] Orton CG, Webber BM. Time-dose factor (TDF) analysis of dose rate effects in permanent implant dosimetry. Int J Radiat Oncol Biol Phys 1977; 2(1-2) 55-60.

[37] Merrik G, Butler WM, Wallner KE, et al. Variability of prostate brachytherapy preimplant dosimetry: a multi-institutional analysis. Brachytherapy 2005; 4(4) 241-251.

[38] Kucway R, Vicini F, Huang R, et al. Prostate volume reduction with androgen deprivation therapy before interstitial brachytherapy. U Urol 2002; 167(6) 2443-2447.

[39] Solhjem MC, Davis BJ, Pisansky TM, et al. Prostate volume before and after permanent prostate brachytherapy in patients receiving neoadjuvant androgen suppression. Cancer J 2004; 10(6) 343-348.

[40] Crook J, McLean M, Gatton C, et al. Factors influencing risk of acute urinary retention after TRUS-guided permanent prostate seed implantation. Int J Radiat Oncol Phys 2002; 52(2) 453-460.

[41] Keyes M, Schellenberg D, Moravan V, et al. Decline in urinary retention incidence in 805 patients after prostate brachytherapy: The effect of learning curve? Int J Radiat Oncol Biol Phys 2006; 64(3) 825-834.

[42] Terk M, Stock R, Stone N. Identification of patients at increased risk for prolonged urinary retention following radioactive seed implantation of the prostate. J Urol 1998; 160(4)1379-1382.

[43] Lee N, Wuu CS, Rrody R, et al. Factors predicting for postimplantation urinary retention after permanent prostate brachytherapy. Int J Radiat Oncol Biol Phys 2000; 48(5) 1457-1460.

[44] Terk MD, Stock RG, Stone NN. Identification of patients at increased risk for prolonged urinary retention following radioactive seed implantation of the prostate. J Urol 1998; 160(4) 1379-1382.

[45] Gutman S, Merrick GS, Butler WM, et al. Severity categories of the International Prostate Symptom Score before, and urinary morbidity after, permanent prostate brachytherapy. BJU Int 2006; 97(1) 62-68.

[46] Zelefsky MJ, Yamada Y, Cohen GN, et al. Five-year outcome of intraoperative conformal permanent I-125 interstitial implantation for patients with clinically localized prostate cancer. Int J Radiat Oncol Biol Phys 2007; 67(1) 65-70.

[47] Zelefsky MJ, Kuban DA, Levy LB, et al. Multi-institutional analysis of long-term outcome for stages T1-T2 prostate cancer treated with permanent seed implantation. Int J Radiat Oncol Biol Phys 2007; 67(2)327-333.

[48] Henry AM, Al-Qaisieh B, Gould K, et al. Outcome following iodine-125 monotherapy for localized prostate cancer: The results of leeds 10-year single-center brachytherapy experience. Int J Radiat Oncol Biol Phys 2010; 76(1) 50-56.

[49] Prada PJ, Juan G, Gonzalez-Suarez H, Fernandez J, et al. Prostate-specific antigen relapse-free survival and side-effects in 734 patients with up to 10 years of follow-up with localized prostate cancer treated by permanent ^{125}iodine implants. BJU Int 2010; 106(1) 32-36.

[50] Sylvester JE, Grimm PD, Wong J, et al. Fifteen-year biochemical relapse-free survival cause-specific survival, and overall survival following I125 prostate brachytherapy in clinically localized prostate cancer Seattle experience. Int J Radiat Oncol Boil Phys. 2011; 81(2) 376-381.

[51] Kinnen KA, Batterman JJ, van Roermung JG, et al. Long-term biochemical and survival outcome of 921 patients treated with i-125 permanent prostate brachytherapy. Int J Radiat Oncol Biol Phys 2010; 76(5) 1433-1438.

[52] Crook JM, Potters L, Stock RG, et al. Critical organ dosimetry in permanent seed prostate brachytherapy: Defining the organs at risk. Brachytherapy 2005; 4(3) 186-194.

[53] Snyder KM, Stock RG, Hong SM, et al. Defining the risk of developing grade 2 proctitis following 125-I prostate brachytherapy using a rectal dose-volume histogram analysis. Int J Radiat Oncol Biol Phys 2001; 50(2) 335-341.

[54] Papagikos MA, Deguzman AF, Rossi PJ, et al. Dosimetric quantifier for low-dose-rate prostate brachytherapy: Is V(100) superior to D(90)? Brachytherapy 2005; 4(4) 252-258.

[55] Orio P, Wallner K, Merrick G, et al. Dosimetric parameters as predictive factors for biochemical control in patients with higher risk prostate cancer treated with Pd-103 and supplemental beam radiation. Int J Radiat Oncol Biol Phys 2007; 67(2) 342-346.

[56] Morris WJ, Keyes M, Palma D, et al. Evaluation of dosimetric parameters and disease response after 125 iodine transperineal brachytherapy for low- and intermediate-risk prostate cancer. Int J Radiat Oncol Biol Phys 2009; 73(5) 1432-1438.

[57] Merrick GS, Butler WM, Wallner KE, et al. Variability of prostate brachytherapy pre-implant dosimetry: A multi-institutional analysis. Brachytherapy 2005; 4(4) 241-251.

[58] Zelefsky MJ, Kuban DA, Levy BJ, et al. Multi-institutional analysis of long-term outcome for stage T1-T2 prostate cancer treated with permanent seed implantation. Int J Radiat Oncol Biol Phys 2007; 67(2) 327-333.

[59] Gomez-Iturriaga Pina A, Crook J, Borg J, et al. Biochemical disease-free rate and toxicity for men treated with iodine-125 prostate brachytherapy with d(90) > 180 Gy. Int J Radiat Oncol Biol Phys 2010; 78(2) 422-427.

[60] Sylvester JE, Grimm PD, Wong J, et al. Fifteen-year biochemical relapse-free survival, cause-specific survival, and overall survival following I^{125} prostate brachytherapy in clinically localized prostate cancer: Seattle experience. Int J Radiat Oncol Biol Phys 2011; 81(2) 376-381.

[61] Prada PJ, Juan G, Gonzalez-Suarez H, et al. Prostate-specific antigen relapse-free survival and side-effects in 734 patients with up to 10 years of follow-up with localized prostate cancer treated by permanent ^{125}iodine implants. BJU Int 2010; 106(1) 32-36.

[62] Henry AM, Al-Qaisieh B, Gould K, et al. Outcome following iodine-125 monotherapy for localized prostate cancer: the results of leeds 10-year single-center brachytherapy experience. Int J Radiat Oncol Biol Phys 2010; 76(1) 50-56.

[63] Zelefsky MJ, Kuban DA, Levy LB, et al. Multi-institutional analysis of long-term outcome for stages T1-T2 prostate cancer treated with permanent seed implantation. Int J Radiat Oncol Biol Phys 2007; 67(2) 327-333.

[64] Zelefsky MJ, Yamada Y, Cohen GN, et al. Five-year outcome of intraoperative conformal permanent I-125 interstitial implantation for patients with clinically localized prostate cancer. Int J Radiat Oncol Biol Phys 2007; 67(1) 65-70.

[65] D'Amico AV, Schultz D, Silver B, et al. The clinical utility of the percent of positive prostate biopsies in predicting biochemical outcome following external-beam radiation therapy for patients with clinically localized prostate cancer. Int J Radiat Oncol Biol Phys 2001; 49(3) 679-684.

[66] Critz FA, Levinson K. 10-year disease-free survival rates after simultaneous irradiation for prostate cancer with a focus on calculation methodology J Urol 2004; 172(6 Pt 1) 2232-2238.

[67] Merrick GS, Butler WM, Wallner KE, et al. Androgen deprivation therapy does not impact cause-specific or overall survival in high-risk prostate cancer managed with brachytherapy and supplemental external beam. Int J Radiat Oncol Biol Phys 2007; 68(1) 34-40.

[68] Sylvester JE, Grimm PD, Blasko JC, et al. 15-year biochemical relapse free survival in clinical stage T1-T3 prostate cancer following combined external beam radiotherapy and brachytherapy; Seattle experience. Int J Radiat Oncol Biol Phys 2007; 67(1):57-64.

[69] Stock RG, Cesaretti JA, Hall SJ, et al. Outcomes for patients with high-grade prostate cancer treated with a combination of brachytherapy, external beam radiotherapy and hormonal therapy. BJU Int 2009; 104(11) 1631-1636.

[70] Wernicke AG, Shamis M, Yan W, et al. Role of isotope selection in long-term outcomes in patients with intermediate-risk prostate cancer treated with a combination of external beam radiotherapy and low-dose-rate interstitial brachytherapy. Urol 2012; 79(5) 1098-1104.

[71] Brown D, Colonias A, Miller R, et al. Urinary morbidity with a modified peripheral loading technique of transperineal ^{125}I prostate implantation. Int J Radiat Oncol Biol Phys 2000; 47(2) 353-360.

[72] Crook J, McLean M, Catton C, et al. Factors influencing risk of acute urinary retention after TRUS-guided permanent prostate seed implantation. Int J Radiat Oncol Biol Phys 2002; 52(2) 453-460.

[73] Blasko JC, Ragde H, Grimm PD. Transperineal ultrasound-guided implantation of the prostate: Morbidity and complications. Scand J Urol Nephrol Suppl 1991; 137 113-118.

[74] Hu K, Wallner K. Urinary incontinence in patients who have a TURP/TUIP following prostate brachytherapy. Int J Radiat Oncol Biol Phys 1998; 40(4) 783-786.

[75] Kollmeier MA, Stock RG, Cesaretti J, et al. Urinary morbidity and incontinence following transurethral resection of the prostate after brachytherapy. J Urol 2005; 173(3) 808-812.

[76] Snyder KM, Stock RG, Hong SM, et al. Defining the risk of developing grade 2 proctitis following ^{125}I prostate brachytherapy using a rectal dose-volume histogram analysis. Int J Radiat Oncol Biol Phys 2001; 50(2) 335-341.

[77] Tran A, Wallner K, Merrick G, et al. Rectal fistulas after prostate brachytherapy. Int J Radiat Oncol Biol Phys 2005; 63(1) 150-154.

[78] Smith S, Wallner K, Han B, et al: Argon plasma coagulation for rectal bleeding following prostate brachytherapy. Int J Radiat Oncol Biol Phys 2001; 51(3) 636-642.

[79] Zelfsky MJ, Yamada Y, Cohen G, et al. Comparison of the 5-year outcome and morbidity of three dimensional conformal radiotherapy versus transperineal permanent iodine-125 implantation for early stage prostate cancer. J Clin Oncol 1999; 17(2) 517-522.

[80] Merrick GS, Butler WM, Wallner KE et al. The importance of radiation doses to the penile bulb vs. crura in the development of postbrachytherapy erectile dysfunction. Int J Radiat Oncol Biol Phys 2002; 54(4) 1055-1062.

[81] Merrck GS, Butler WM, Wallner KE, et al. Erectile function after prostate brachytherapy. Int J Radiat Oncol Biol Phys 2005; 62(2) 437-447.

[82] Raina R, Agarwal A, Goyal KK et al. Long-term potency after iodine-125 radiotherapy for prostate cancer and role of sildenafil citrate. Urology 2003; 62(6) 1103-1108.

[83] Potters L, Torre T, Fearn PA et al. Potency after permanent prostate brachytherapy for localized prostate cancer. Int J Radiat Oncol Biol Phys 2001; 50(5) 1235-1242.

[84] Chen YC, Chuang CK, Hsieh ML, et al. High-dose-rate brachytherapy plus external beam radiotherapy for T1 to T3 prostate cancer: An experience in Taiwan. Urology 2007; 70(1) 101-105.

[85] Demanes DJ, Brandt D, Schour L, et al. Excellent results from high dose rate brachytherapy and external beam for prostate cancer are not improved by androgen deprivation. Am J Clin Oncol 2009; 32(4) 342-347.

[86] Yamada Y, Bhatia S, Zaider M, et al. Favorable clinical outcome of three-dimensional computer-optimized high-dose-rate prostate brachytherapy in the management of localized prostate cancer. Brachytherapy 2006; 5(3) 157-164.

[87] Ducchesne GM, Williams SG, Das R, et al. Patterns of toxicity following high-dose-rate brachytherapy boost for prostate cancer: Mature prospective phase I/II study results. Radiother Oncol 2007; 84(2) 128-134.

[88] Hiratsuka J, Jo Y, Yoshida K, et al. Clinical results of combined treatment conformal high-dose-rate iridium-192 brachytherapy and external beam radiotherapy using staging lymphadenectomy for localized prostate cancer. Int J Radiat Oncol Biol Phys. 2004; 59(3) 684-690.

[89] Phan TP, Syed AM, Puthawala A, et al. High dose rate brachytherapy as a boost for the treatment of localized prostate cancer. J Urol 2007; 177(1) 123-127.

[90] Zwahlen DR, Andrianopoulos N, Matheson B, et al. High-dose-rate brachytherapy in combination with conformal external beam radiotherapy in the treatment of prostate cancer. Brachytherapy 2010; 9(1) 27-35.

[91] Martinez AA, Gonzalez J, Ye H. Dose escalation improves cancer-related events at 10 years for intermediate- and high-risk prostate cancer patients treated with hypofractionated high-dose-rate boost and external beam radiotherapy. Int J Radiat Oncol Biol Phys 2011; 79(2) 363-370.

[92] Morton G, Loblaw A, Cheung P, et al. Is single fraction 15 Gy the preferred high dose-rate brachytherapy boost dose for prostate cancer? Radiother Oncol 2011; 100(3) 463-467.

[93] Demanes DJ, Martinez AA, Ghilezan M, et al. High-dose-rate monotherapy: Safe and effective brachytherapy for patients with localized prostate cancer. Int J Radiat Oncol Biol Phys 2011; 81(5) 1286-1292.

[94] Ghilezan M, Martinez AA, Gustason G, et al. High dose rate brachytherapy as monotherapy delivered in two fractions within one day for favorable/intermediate risk prostate cancer: Preliminary toxicity data. Int J Radiat Oncol Biol Phys 2012; 83(3) 927-932.

[95] Jabbari S, Weinberg VK, Shinohara K, et al. Equivalent biochemical control and improved prostate-specific antigen nadir after permanent prostate seed implant brachytherapy versus high-dose three-dimensional conformal radiotherapy and high-

dose conformal proton beam radiotherapy boost. Int J Radiat Oncol Biol Phys 2010; 76(1) 36-42.

[96] Grills IS, Martinez AA, Hollander M, et al. High dose rate brachytherapy as prostate cancer monotherapy reduces toxicity compared to low dose rate palladium seed. J Urol 2004; 171(3) 1098-1104.

[97] Rogers CL, Alder AS, Rogers RL, et al. High dose rate brachytherapy as monotherapy for intermediate risk prostate cancer. J Urol 2012; 187(1) 109-116.

[98] Prada PJ, Jimenez I, Gonzalez-Suarez H, et al. High-dose-rate interstitial brachytherapy as monotherapy in one fraction and transperineal hyaluronic acid injection into the perirectal fat for the treatment of favorable stage prostate cancer: Treatment description and preliminary results. Brachytherapy 2012; 11(2) 105-110.

[99] Yoshioka K, Konishi K, Sumida I, et al. Monotherapeutic high-dose-rate brachytherapy for prostate cancer: Five-year results of an extreme hypofractionation regimen with 54 Gy in nine fractions. Int J Radiat Oncol Biol Phys 2011; 80(2) 469-475.

[100] Astrom L, Pedersen D, Mercke C, et al. Long-term outcome of high dose rate brachytherapy in radiotherapy of localized prostate cancer. Radiother Oncol 2005; 74(2) 157-161.

[101] Bachand F, Martin AG, Beaulieu L, et al. An eight-year experience of HDR brachytherapy boost for localized prostate cancer: Biopsy and PSA outcome. Int J Radiat Oncol Biol Phys 2009; 73(3) 679-684.

[102] Prada PJ, Gonzalez H, Fernandez J, et al. Biochemical outcome after high-dose-rate intensity modulated brachytherapy with external beam radiotherapy: 12 years of experience. BJU Int 2011; 109(12) 1787-1793.

[103] Rogers CL, Alder SC, Rogers RL, et al. High dose brachytherapy as monotherapy for intermediate risk prostate cancer. J Urol 2012; 187(1) 109-116.

[104] Demanes DJ, Rodriguez RR, Schour L, et al. High-dose-rate intensity-modulated brachytherapy with external beam radiotherapy for prostate cancer. Int J Radiat Oncol Biol Phys 2005; 61(5) 1306-1316.

[105] Deger S, Boehmer D, Roigas J, et al. High dose rate (HDR) brachytherapy with conformal radiation therapy for localized prostate cancer. Eur Urol 2005; 47(4) 441-448.

[106] Sullivan L, Williams SG, Tai KH, et al. Urethral stricture following high dose rate brachytherapy for prostate cancer. Radiother Oncol 2009; 91(2) 232-236.

[107] Pellizzon AC, Salvajoli JV, Maia MA, et al. Late urinary morbidity with high dose prostate brachytherapy as a boost to conventional external beam radiation therapy for local and locally advanced prostate cancer. J Urol 2004; 171(3) 1105-1108.

[108] Duchesne GM Williums SG, Das R, et al. Patterns of toxicity following high-dose-rate brachytherapy boost for prostate cancer: Mature prospective phase I/II study results. Radiother Oncol 2007; 84(2) 128-134.

[109] Ishikawa H, Tsuji H, Kamada T, et al. Carbon-ion radiation therapy for prostate cancer. Int J Urol 2012; 19(4) 296-305.

[110] Coote JH, Wylie JP, Cowan RA, et al. Hypofractionated intensity-modulated radiotherapy for carcinoma of the prostate: analysis of toxicity. Int J Radiat Oncol Biol Phys 2009; 74(4) 1121-1127.

[111] Martin JM, Rosewall T, Bayley, et al. Phase II trial of hypofractionated image-guided intensity-modulated radiotherapy for localized prostate adenocarcinoma. Int J Radiat Oncol Biol Phys 2007; 69(4) 1084-1089.

[112] Kupelian PA, Thakkar VV, Khuntia D, et al. Hypofractionated intensity-modulated radiotherapy (70 Gy at 2.5 Gy per fraction) for localized prostate cancer: long-term outcomes. Int J Radiat Oncol Biol Phys 2005; 63(5) 1463-1468.

[113] King CR, Brooks JD, Gill H, et al. Stereotactic body radiotherapy for localized prostate cancer: interim results of a prospective phase II clinical trial. Int J Radiat Oncol Biol Phys 2009; 73(4) 1043-1048.

[114] Madsen BL, His RA, Pham HT, et al. Stereotactic hypofractionated accurate radiotherapy of the prostate (SHARP), 33.5 Gy in five fractions for localized disease: first clinical trial results. Int J Radiat Oncol Biol Phy 2007; 67(4) 1099-1105.

[115] Michalski JM, Bae K, Roach M, et al. Long-term toxicity following 3D conformal radiation therapy for prostate cancer from the RTOG 9406 phase I/II dose escalation study. Int J Radiat Oncol Biol Phy 2010; 76(1) 14-22.

[116] Shulte RW, Slater JD, Rossi CJ Jr, et al. Value and perspectives of proton radiation therapy for limited stage prostate cancer. Strahlenther Onkol 2000; 176(1) 3-8.

[117] Bolla M, van Poppel H, Collette L, et al. Postoperative radiotherapy after radical prostatectomy: a randomized controlled trial (EORTC trial 22911). Lancet 2005; 366(9485) 572-578.

[118] Thompson IM, Tangen CM, Paradelo J, et al. Adjuvant radiotherapy for pathological T3N0M0 prostate cancer significantly reduces risk of metastases and improves survival: long-term followup of a randomized clinical trial. J Urol 2009; 181(3) 956-962.

[119] Swanson GP, Hussey MA, Tangen CM, et al. Predominant treatment failure in post-prostatectomy patients is local: analysis of patterns of treatment failure in SWOG 8794. J Clin Oncol 2007; 25(16) 2225-2229

[120] Wiegel T, Bottke D, Steiner U, et al. Phase III postoperative adjuvant radiotherapy after radical prostatectomy compared with radical prostatectomy alone in pT3 prostate cancer with postoperative undetectable prostate-specific antigen: ARO 96-02/AUO AP 09/95. J Clin Oncol 2009; 27(18) 2924-2930.

[121] Trabulsi EJ, Valicenti RK, Hanlon AL, et al. A multi-institutional matched-control analysis of adjuvant and salvage postoperative radiation therapy for pT3-4N0 prostate cancer. Urology 2008; 72(6) 1298-1302.

[122] Trock BJ, Han M, Freedland SJ, et al. Prostate cancer-specific survival following salvage radiotherapy vs observation in men with biochemical recurrence after radical prostatectomy. JAMA 2008; 299(23) 2760-2769.

[123] Stephenson AJ, Scardino PT, Kattan MW, et al. Predicting the outcome of salvage radiation therapy for recurrent prostate cancer after radical prostatectomy. J Clin Oncol 2007; 25(15) 2035-2041.

Chapter 7

High-Dose-Rate Interstitial Brachytherapy as Monotherapy in One Fraction for the Treatment of Favorable Stage Prostate Cancer

Pedro J. Prada

Additional information is available at the end of the chapter

http://dx.doi.org/10.5772/51758

1. Introduction

Low dose rate (LDR) brachytherapy has rapidly gained popularity in the USA [1, 2] and Europe [3, 4] as an accepted, effective and safe therapy for localized prostate cancer. Many reports are now available which confirm good outcomes in selected patients with PSA relapse-free survivals that are equivalent to those achieved by surgery.

The potential for a therapy that is equally efficient but less harmful than other interventions is especially attractive for patients with early prostate cancer.

On the other hand, treatment with temporary high dose rate (HDR) brachytherapy with 192-Ir as monotherapy has a number of advantages compared to LDR. The overall treatment time is decreased from many months with LDR to several minutes with HDR. Besides, HDR improves the dose distribution because of the possibility of accurately controlling the source and vary the source dwell time during treatment. The intraoperative optimization used with HDR allows better source position targeting with the potential for limiting toxicity. There are also advantages in radiation safety for both staff and patient who leave the treatment room without any radioactive implants.

The purpose of this chapter was to determine the possibility to treat patients with favorable stage prostate cancer (5, 6) with HDR monotherapy in one fraction and transperineal hyaluronic acid injection into the perirectal fat.

2. Brachytherapy implant characteristics

Patients received one implant and one fraction of HDR. Fraction dose is 20.5 Gy because it is considered to correspond biologically (biologic effective dose) to > 90 Gy administered at 2 Gy/fraction according to the linear quadratic model, assuming an α/β of 1.2 Gy (7, 8, 9, 10).

Brachytherapy procedure is done under spinal anesthesia with the patient in the lithotomy position (Fig. 1). A Foley catheter is placed, and the bladder is partially filled with 100 cm^3 of sterile water. The needles are positioned (Fig. 2) by transperineal placement under real time TRUS guidance using a template. Axial cross-sections is captured in 5mm steps and transferred to the Treatment Planning Software. Prostate gland, normal structures (urethra and rectum) and needle positions are identified and mapped based on the ultrasound image. Dose optimization is done on the reconstructed applicator geometry using dose point and manual optimization algorithms to determine dwell positions and times (Fig. 3).

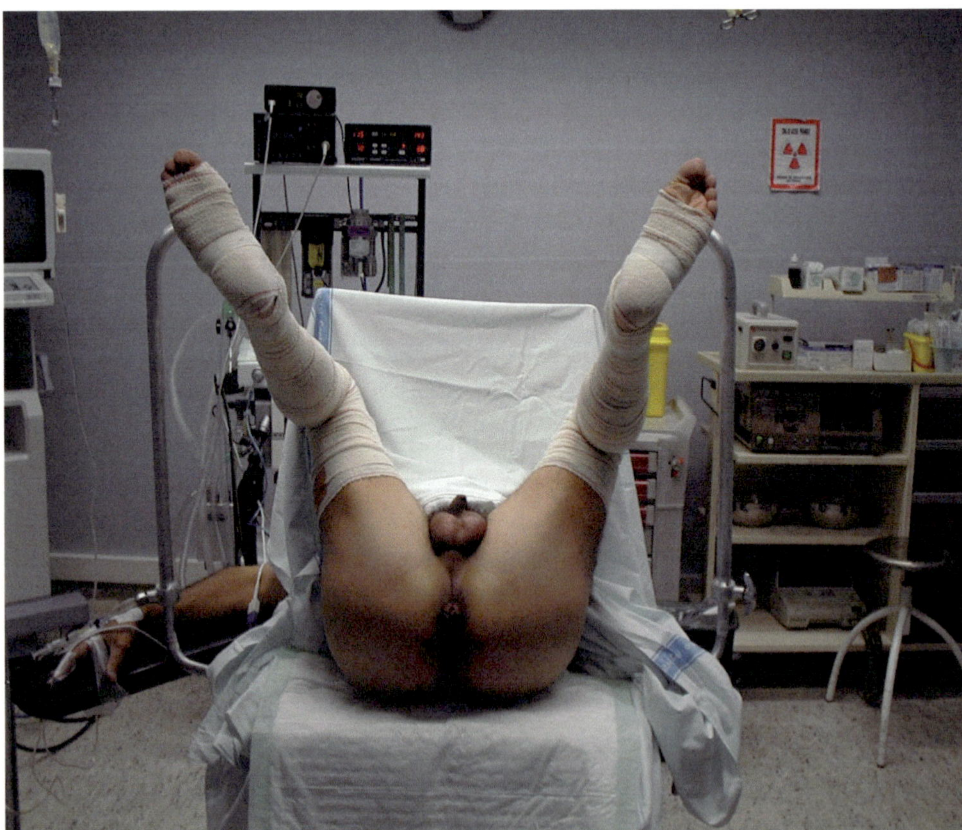

Figure 1. Lithotomy position

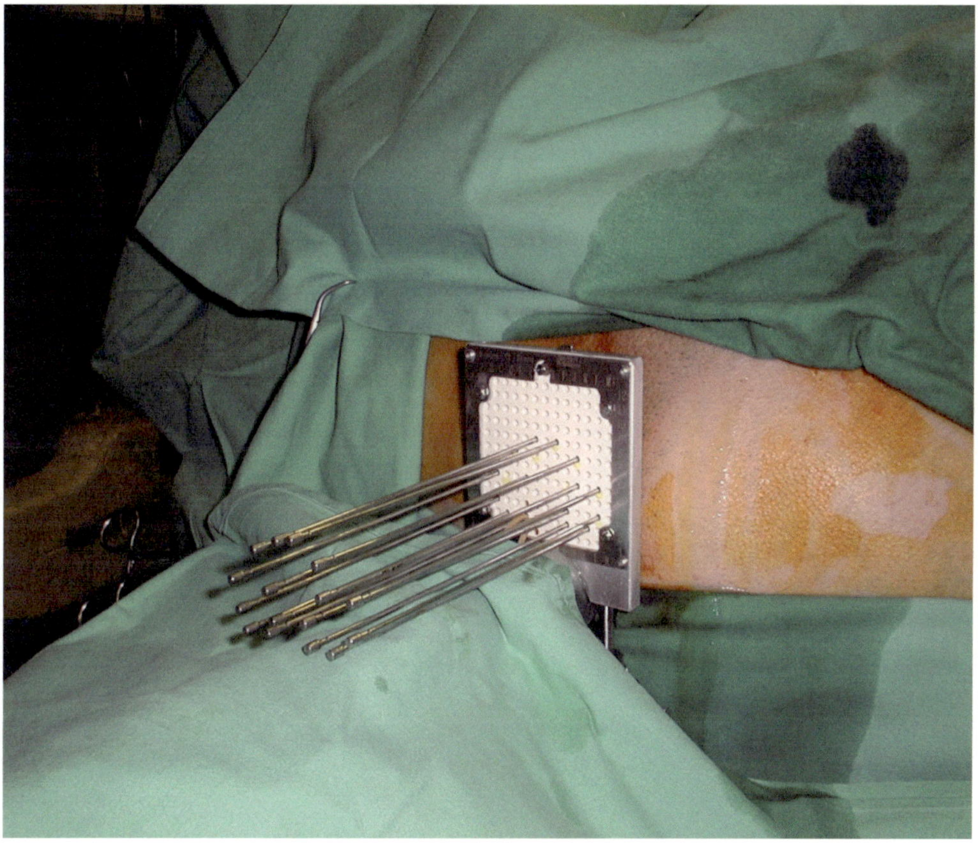

Figure 2. The needles are positioned

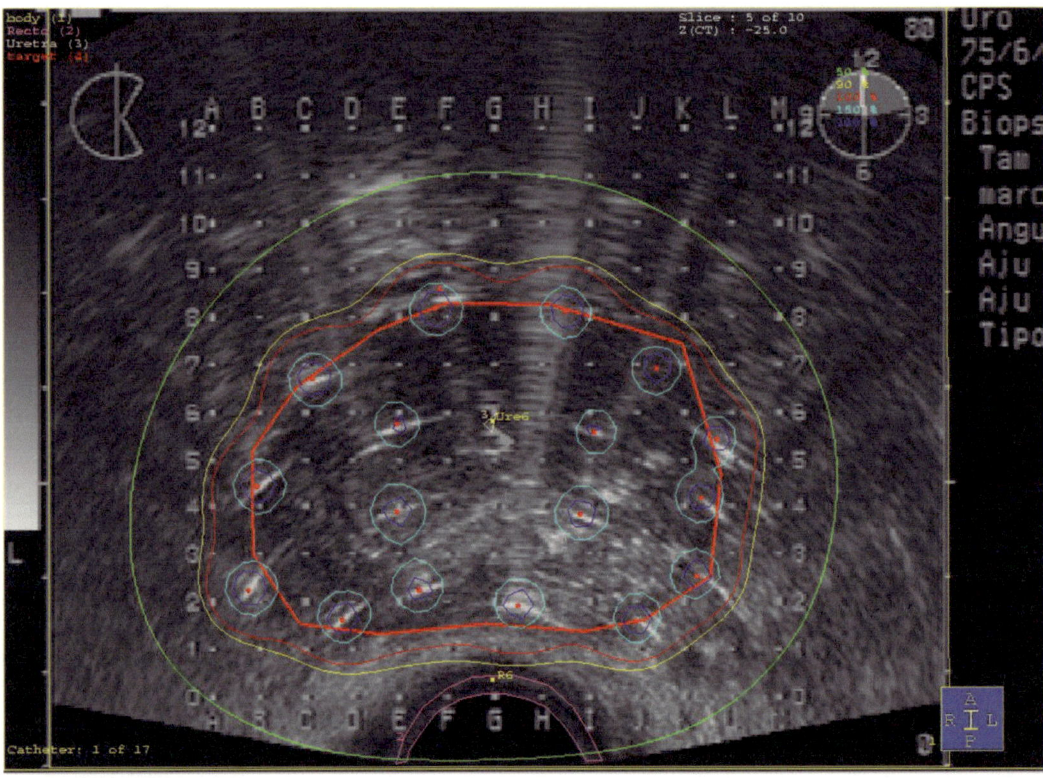

Figure 3. Dose optimization

The prostate without safety margins is then defined as the planning target volume (PTV) to be treated (Fig. 4) with the prescribed dose (PD).

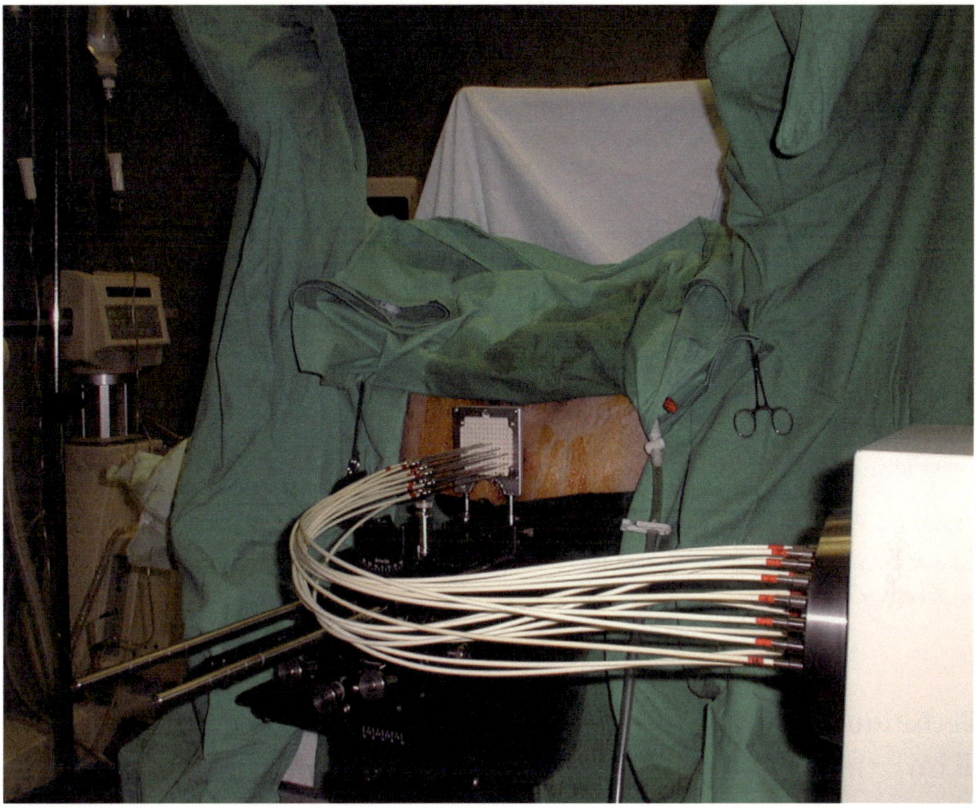

Figure 4. Treatment

Based on the dose volume histograms (DVH) data, the quality of plans and implants is evaluated using following indicators:

- The rectal dose is calculated at the anterior edge of the TRUS probe and is limited to ≤ 75% of the prescription dose.
- The dose to any segment of the urethra is limited to ≤ 110% of the prescription dose. V120 and D100 of the prostatic urethra are determined (volume that received a dose of 120% and dose delivered to 100% of the urethra).
- The PTV V90, V100, V150 and V200 (% of PTV receiving 90%, 100%, 150% and 200% of the PD) are recorded.
- D90 (dose delivered to 90% of the PTV) is calculated.

All patients are discharged from the center on the same day of the procedure between 6-8 hours of implantation.

To decrease rectal toxicity, transperineal hyaluronic acid (HA) injection into the peri-rectal fat is used to consistently displace the rectal wall away from the radiation sources in all patients. We believe that the increase in distance (mean 2 cm along the length of the prostate) will be enough to provide a significant radiation dose reduction from HDR brachytherapy [11, 12].

3. Hyaluronic acid

The Hyaluronic acid (HA) is a polysaccharide normally found in human tissues as a component of the connective tissue. Normally, it plays a vital role on the skin and in the synovial fluid of the joints. It is normally degradable by the normal enzymatic system in relative short time. However, to make it last for months when used for the treatment of skin wrinkles and osteoarthritis, the compound is modified making it stable for duration close to 1 year before it is reabsorbed by the body. Only one type of HA is used in our Department (Restylane sub-Q).

The total injected amount is related to the need for systematically creating a minimum of a 2 cm space between the prostate and rectum throughout this length. Usually, we use between 6 and 8 cc per patient

4. Technique of hyaluronic acid injection

The injection technique of HA in the perirectal fat occurs before all needles are in treatment position according to the following procedure.

- Step 1. The transrectal ultrasound (TRUS) probe with the transperineal template is placed and fixed in the standard fashion.
- Step 2. Using TRUS guidance, the needle tip is placed in the perirectal fat (Fig. 5), between the posterior prostate capsule and the anterior rectal wall, at the level of the maximum transverse diameter of the prostate (reference level). Then under direct TRUS guidance, the needle tip is advanced to the level of the seminal vesicles.
- Step 3. The needle is connected to the syringe containing of HA. After aspirating to be certain that we are not in a vessel, we proceed to inject between 6 and 8 cc within the space between the seminal vesicles and the apex of the prostate. This is performed under TRUS guidance to see and verify the new space created by the injection of HA (Fig. 6). The total injected amount allows us to create the new space >2 cm.
- Step 4. The needle is removed and all needles treatment is placed under TRUS Guidance. It can be performed as an outpatient. After the discharge from the theater clinic, the patient continues normal-life activities

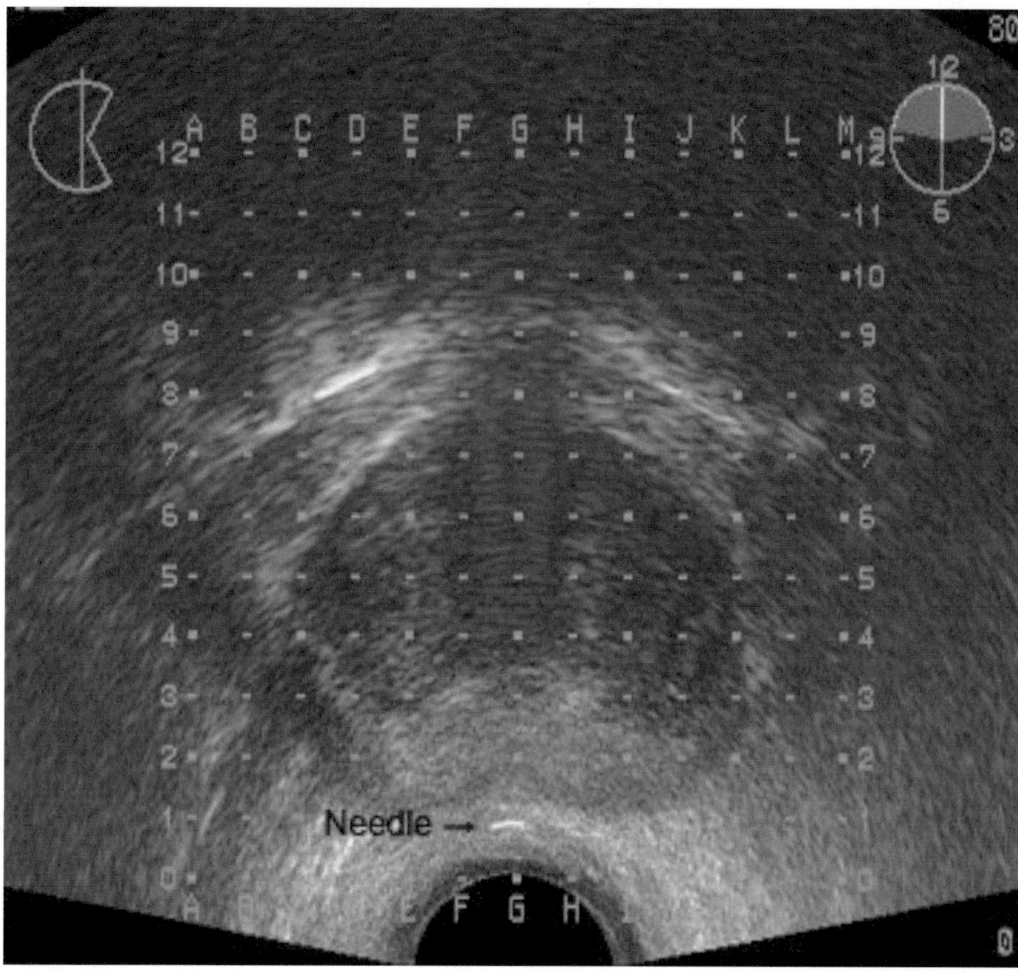

Figure 5. The needle tip is placed in the perirectal fat

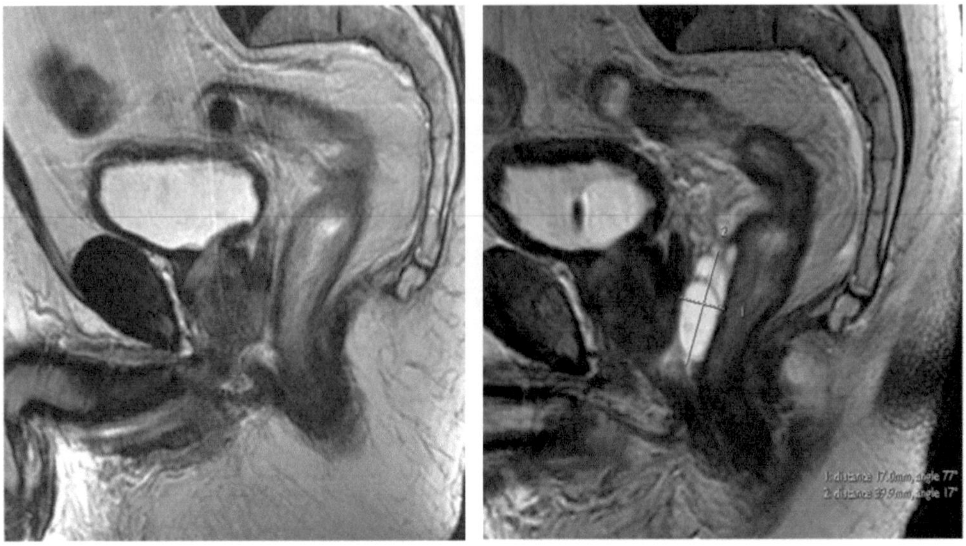

Figure 6. Magnetic resonance image demonstrating the additional perirectal space created by the hyaluronic acid injection

5. Results

In our Centre a total of 70 patients have been treated with this technique and is the first in the medical literature using in patients with favorable risk prostate cancer. Our technique has the great advantage of being practically a one-time procedure which prevents any movement of the needles.

In our series acute and late genitourinary toxicity grade 2 or more was not observed in any patient. The median of flow rate test pretreatment in our study was 12.5 ml/s (3-30 ml/s) but acute urinary retention was seen in only 1 patient, requiring a temporary postimplant bladder catheter during seven days, this results are better than other investigators [13-16].

The lasted follow-up visit the sexual preservation rate was 89% in patients who were potent preoperatively and not receiving hormonal therapy, this result is similar to that other investigators.

The late grade I genitourinary toxicity caused by our treatment was significantly associated with the dose administered to the PTV represented by D90 (p=0.050).

In our study no gastrointestinal toxicity, such as anal pain, rectal bleeding, diarrhea, anal ulcer and/or rectourethral fistula has been observed after treatment. We believe that the increase in distance between rectum and posterior prostatic capsule created by the peri-rectal injection of hyaluronic acid is enough to provide a significant radiation dose reduction from HDR brachytherapy and have significantly smaller incidence of mucosal damage [11, 12].

The actuarial biochemical control in our series was 100% and 88% respectively for low and intermediate risk groups at 32 months, but is too early to draw final conclusion respect to biochemical control.

6. Conclusions

High dose rate brachytherapy as monotherapy in one fraction with a transperineal hyaluronic acid injection into the peri-rectal fat to decrease rectal toxicity for patients with favorable risk prostate cancer is feasible and very well tolerated with advantages compared to LDR and HDR brachytherapy as monotherapy using the fractionation schema of 4 fractions administered 2 times daily during two days.

HDR monotherapy in one fraction resulted in a low genitourinary morbidity and no gastrointestinal toxicity but clinical and biochemical control rates will be reported as longer follow-up.

Author details

Pedro J. Prada

Address all correspondence to: pprada@telecable.es

Department of Radiation Oncology, Hospital Universitario Marques de Valdecilla, Santander, Spain

References

[1] Mettlin CJ, Murphy GP, McDonald CJ, et al. The National cancer data base report on increase use of brachytherapy for the treatment of patients with prostate carcinoma in the USA. Cancer 1999; 86: 1877-1882.

[2] Lee RW, Moughan J, Owen J, et al. The 1999 Patterns of care Study of radiotherapy in localized prostatic carcinoma. A comprehensive survey of prostate brachytherapy in the United States. Cancer 2003; 98 (9): 1987-1994.

[3] Ash D, Flynn A, Battermann J, Reijke T, et al. ESTRO/EAU/EORTC recomendations on permanent seed implantation for localizad prostate cancer. Radiotherapy and Oncology. 2000, 57:315-321.

[4] Battermann JJ, Boon TA, Moerland A et al. Results of permanent prostate brachytherapy, 13 years of experience at a single institution. Radiotherapy and Oncology 2004; 71:23-28.

[5] Fleming I, Cooper JS, Henson DE, et al. AJCC Cancer staging Manual, 5th edn. Philadelphia, Pennsylvania; Lippincitt-Raven, 1997.

[6] Zelefsky MJ, Leibel SA, Gaudin PB, et al. Dose escalation with three-dimensional conformal radiation therapy affects the outcome in prostate cancer. Int J Radiat Oncol Biol Phys 1998; 41:491-500.

[7] Brenner DJ, Martinez AA, Edmundson GK, et al. Direct evidence that prostate tumors show high sensitivity to fractionation (low alpha/beta ratio), similar to late-responding normal tissue. Int J Radiat Oncol Biol Phys 2002;52:6-13.

[8] Duchesne GM, Peters LJ. What is the alpha/beta ratio for prostate cancer? Rationale for hypofractionated high-dose-rate brachytherapy.[editorial]. Int J Radiat Oncol Biol Phys 1999;44:747-748.

[9] Fowler JF. The radiobiology of prostate cancer including new aspects of fractionated radiotherapy. Acta Oncol 2005;44:265-276.

[10] Fowler JF. The linear-quadratic formula and progress in fractionated radiotherapy. Br J Radiol 1989;62:679-694.

[11] Prada PJ, Fernandez J, Martinez A, et al. Transperineal injection of hyaluronic acid in the anterior peri-rectal fat to decease rectal toxicity from radiation delivered with intensity modulated brachytherapy or EBRT for prostate cancer patients. Int J Oncol Biol Phys. 2007; 69 (1):95-102.

[12] Prada PJ, González H, Menéndez C, et al. Transperineal Injection of Hyaluronic Acid in the Anterior Peri-rectal Fat to Decrease Rectal Toxicity from Radiation Delivered with Low Dose Rate Brachytherapy for Prostate Cancer Patients. Brachytherapy. 8(2): 210-217, 2009.

[13] Ghadjar P, Keller T, Rentsch C A, et al. Toxicity and early treatment outcomes in low and intermediate-risk prostate cancer managed by high-dose-rate brachytherapy as a monotherapy. Brachytherapy 2009; 8:45-51.

[14] Martin T, Baltas D, Kurek R, et al. 3-D conformal HDR brachytherapy as monotherapy for localized prostate cancer. A pilot study. Strahlenther Onkol 2004; 180:225-232.

[15] Yoshioka Y, Takayuki N, Yoshida K, et al. High-dose-rate interstitial brachytherapy as a monotherapy for localized próstata cáncer: treatment description and preliminary results of a phase I/II clinical trial.. Int J Oncol Biol Phys 2000; 48(3):675-681.

[16] Konishi K, Yoshioka Y, Isohashi F, et al. Correlation between dosimetric parameters and late rectal and urinary toxicities in patients treated with high-dose-rate brachytherapy used as monotherapy for prostate cancer. Int J Oncol Biol Phys 2009; 75(4): 1003-1007.

Section 4

Prostate Cancer Markers

Chapter 8

Testosterone Measurement and Prostate Cancer

Tine Hajdinjak

Additional information is available at the end of the chapter

http://dx.doi.org/10.5772/52525

1. Introduction

Testosterone is important growth factor for prostate cells. If testosterone availability drops, prostate cells stop thriving. Benign prostate shrinks and the same happens with prostate cancer cells. Larger decrease in testosterone availability means larger reduction in prostate cells mass. Although only reduction in testosterone levels will not, in most occasions, permanently heal prostate cancer, it causes its regression and significantly delays further progression of prostate cancer. Therefore, reduction of body's testosterone level is important prostate cancer treatment modality. When surgical removal of prostate due to cancer is not an opinion (for example because of advanced age, significant comorbidity or because cancer has already spread beyond prostate) or was unsuccessful as noted by rising PSA, which indicates cancer growth, serum testosterone value becomes very important factor in treatment related decisions. If testosterone values are high, reduction of testosterone level will be helpful – it is expected prostate cells will react, shrink, PSA will fall. If testosterone values are already low, their further reduction with different agent may be possible. If testosterone values are already at the lowest reachable levels, other ways of treatment should be sought. After reduction of testosterone levels in the body (castration), prostate cancer cells with time (sometimes months, sometimes years, sometimes decades) develop alternative signaling mechanisms and ways of paracrine androgens supply. It is estimated this happens in a third of all prostate cancer patients [1].

As this chapter focuses primarily on prostate cancer, some topics, like free-testosterone or salivary testosterone measurements are not included, because although they are related to testosterone measurement in general, they are, at least at present (things may change in the future), not used in day-to-day care of prostate cancer patients. All testosterone values mentioned relate to serum testosterone measurements.

2. Some characteristics of testosterone

Testosterone is principal male androgen, sex hormone and anabolic steroid. It is found not only in humans, but also in many other vertebrates. In males, testosterone is secreted by Leydig cells in testicles, in females by theca cells in ovaries. Small amount is produced also in zona reticularis of adrenal cortex in both genders and in placenta. Chemically (figure 1), it is white powder, soluble in methanol, name is17beta-Hydroxyandrost-4-en-3-on or 4-Androsten-17beta-ol-3-on, Chemical Abstracts Service number 58-22-0, ATC code G03BA03. It is a controlled substance, in US by Drug Enforcement Administration (DEA). It's inactive epimer – difference in configuration of OH at C17 - is called epitestosterone. Testosterone's biosynthesis starts from cholesterol. Metabolism: up to one tenth of testosterone is converted by 5-alpha reductase to dihydrotestosterone, less than 0.5% by aromatase to estradiol. Most of testosterone is deactivated and excreted as glucoronides.

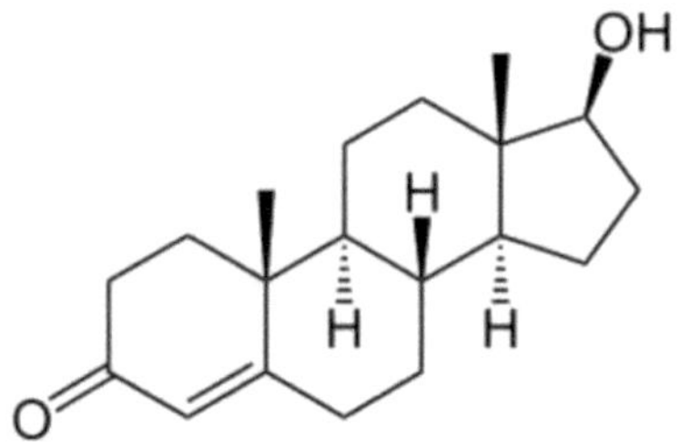

Figure 1. Testosterone structure (Picture in public domain – Wikimedia: NEUROtiker)

3. Reasons for testosterone measurement in prostate cancer

Testosterone measurement in prostate cancer patients has more than 40 years history [2]. Confirmation of castrate testosterone level is necessary before identifying prostate cancer as castration resistant. Castrate states are at present defined as serum testosterone level below 20 ng/dl (=0.69 nmol/l) or below 50 ng/dl (=1.73 nmol/l) [3], but it was not always this way and different testosterone measurement methods have important implications.

Need for controlling quality of chemical castration treatment of prostate cancer steams from reports of up to 15% castration failures [4,5]. This means LHRH treated patients may not reach castration levels of testosterone due to different reasons [6], not only non-compliance, application failures, but also other reasons, for example problems with depot formulation resorption due to granuloma formation on injection site [7] or may simply need more frequent dosages [8].

Further reason for testosterone measurements in prostate cancer patients lies in reports of correlation between success of castration and time to PSA progression: better castration (lower testosterone value) gives longer time to progression [9,10]. Therefore hormonal treatment of prostate cancer should not be followed with PSA measurement only (as indirect indication of treatment success), but also with testosterone measurement [11].

Before any treatment, at diagnosis, serum testosterone value is predictor of disease aggressiveness – lower testosterone values are related to less differentiated cancer and worse prognosis [12]. For all stated reasons, measurement of serum testosterone is important for clinicians who treat prostate cancer patients.

After long term of androgen suppression with LHRH (GnRH) analogues, sometimes testosterone levels do not recover after stopping treatment (which may be due to permanent dysfunction of Lydig cells), therefore application of LHRH drugs may be stopped in selected patients [13]. However, this should be confirmed and followed with testosterone measurement.

But testosterone measurements are not important only for urologists, who, apart from main reason – decisions related to prostate cancer management, use it for example also for aging male symptomatology and evaluation of patients with erectile dysfunction. Also other medical specialties, like endocrinology, pediatrics, gynecology or oncology use testosterone measurements for their conditions, like diagnosing and monitoring hyper- or hypo- androgenic disorders in women, like polycystic ovary syndrome, alopecia, acne, hirsutism or hypoactive sexual desire disorder; androgen secreting neoplasms; congenital syndromes with ambiguous genitalia... Pediatrics and endocrinology were in the past probably most frequent users of testosterone assays, but nowadays most laboratories receive most testosterone requests from urologists.

4. Prostate cancer incidence will increase in future

Prostate cancer is already most frequently diagnosed cancer among men in the developed world. As a cause of death among males, it is second in the USA and third in Europe. Large increase in prostate cancer incidence in recent years is not only due to availability of PSA (biochemical marker, which is useful for screening purposes) and due to better awareness of doctors and population at large, but in large part also due to changes in population pyramid and increased life expectancy. As breast cancer, which is most common in females over 60 years of age, also prostate cancer is cancer of older people. For example, in Slovenia (which may be in health related issues regarded somewhere in-between developed western and less advanced other parts of the world), incidence of prostate cancer increased 50% from 2000 to 2011 [14]. At the same time, population at main risk (males above age 60) increased 28%. Therefore more than half of increase of prostate cancer incidence can not be attributed to, as some people, even health care professionals, claim, "artificial" increase of incidence due to "over-screening", but simply to the fact that population at risk has significantly increased. And among those (males between 55 and 70), screening is most appropriate because life expectancy also increases (at present, for 75 year old man in Slovenia it is on average more than 10 years) and therefore cancer control is worthwhile.

In our country, recently prostate cancer incidence has been higher compared to breast cancer. Cause for this is not better prostate cancer "screening", but simple fact of changes in population pyramid, in numbers of populations at risk: relation between males and females in most important age range for prostate and breast cancer detection has changed – number of males grows significantly faster than number of females. In year 2000, 700 more females reached age of 60 compared to males, in 2011, 500 more males reached age 60 compared to females [15]. Although among oldest old, number of females will remain higher compared to men, present big gap in number of men compared to women in age group 50-70 is getting smaller and smaller and this also contributes to further increase of significance of prostate compared to breast cancer.

According to population pyramid, further increase of burden due to prostate cancer is expected, for example in our country, until year 2050, when overall population in Slovenia will, according to present trends, decrease from current 2 to 1.9 million, but number of males, age 60 or more, will peak at 1.8 times the number in 2011. Similar trend is expected to happen in most countries in the world sooner or later and therefore prostate cancer will remain important health problem in future.

5. Need for hormonal treatment of prostate cancer may not decrease in future

Despite facts about prostate cancer incidence, presented in section 4 and despite undeniable proof that population based PSA prostate cancer screening reduces mortality due to prostate cancer [16], it seems some professional bodies, like U.S. preventive services task force [17,18] recently advised against screening.

Further, among young UK general practitioners, during non-formal conversation, in year 2012, one can easily hear claims like "PSA – oh I thought it is NOT for screening, it is only for follow up purposes, only for patients, who have diagnosis of prostate cancer already" (personal experience).

With this recent trend by policy-makers, it seems hopes of urologists, who treat prostate cancer patients, that we will in the future find only very few patients, who will present with stage of disease, where nothing else but hormonal treatment would be possible or hormonal treatment will become necessary during the course of their disease, are dispelled. As it seems focus of attention is turned away from early detection and managing (watchful waiting, not necessary treating patients with prostate cancer), towards second and third line treatments for advanced disease, testosterone measurement in patients with prostate cancer will become even more important in the future.

6. Different hormonal treatments influence testosterone differently

Different drugs for hormonal treatment of prostate cancer have different effects on serum testosterone. Non-steroidal antiandrogens increase overall serum testosterone levels. Steroidal antiandrogen (cyproterone) reduces testosterone levels, but not to castrate values. Often old patients take two 100 mg tablets daily and testosterone values are than commonly around 7 nmol/l. With proper dosing (3 times 100 mg daily), values nearing castration levels have been reported (mean 2.5 nmol/l, [19]), on the other side, with dose 200 mg daily, relatively small decrease only to low-normal levels has been reported for healthy young to middle-aged men (mean 11.4 nmol/l [20]).

LHRH agonists injections are supposed to universally reduce testosterone levels to castration values, but sometimes this is not the case. LHRH antagonists are gaining popularity very slowly with similar effect on testosterone. They may reduce testosterone levels in a proportion of patients a bit further compared to LHRH agonists [21] and they do not cause microsurges of testosterone, which are often present with every re-dosing of LHRH agonists.

Surgical castration remains a viable opinion in many countries and for many patients. Steroids are available to further reduce serum androgen levels in castrate resistant disease states by blocking adrenal production. 5 alpha reductase inhibitors may, according to some theories, play a role in combination treatment.

In the past, castrate values of testosterone were achieved with estrogens, like stilbestrol. Due to side effects (blood cloths), this is not used any more. Ketoconazole, inhibitor of steroid synthesis, is still available for fast testosterone levels reduction, but in practice is is used mainly in experimental settings after chemotherapy failure in castration resistant states [22].

Typical testosterone responses to some hormonal agents are summarized in Table 1.

Agent	Typical testosterone response
non-steroidal antiandrogen (bicalutamide, flutamide)	increase (may go above 30 nmol/l)
steroidal antiandrogen (cyproterone acetate)	decrease, very dependent on dosage regimen, with 3x100 mg it may approach, but not reach castrate values, in a few days
GnRH (LHRH) agonists (triptorelin, goserelin, leuporolide)	designed to decrease levels below castrate values (below 1.73 nmol/l), may take a month after first application to reach castrate level
GnRH antagonists (degarelix)	designed to decrease levels below castrate values without surges
surgical castration (bilateral orchiectomy)	gold standard, decrease below castration level in few hours, however, adrenal androgens remain
ketoconazole	decrease below castration levels if dose is high enough in 2-4 days, but sometimes variable response, corticosteroids should be supplemented simultaneously
estrogens (stilbestrol – of historical interest only)	decrease below castration levels after approx. 5 days, later surges may appear

Table 1. Typical serum testosterone responses to different hormonal agents. In practice, individual responses may vary significantly, therefore confirmation with individual measurement is important.

7. Methods for serum testosterone measurement

With introduction of indirect RIA techniques (double isotope derivative dilution technique) to measure serum testosterone in 1970ties and later automated chemiluminescent assays, serum testosterone values became widely available to practicing urologists.

Manufacturers mainly use similar principles of assays. As an example of principle, Abbott's chemiluminescent assay is described [23]. It is "delayed one step", competitive heterogeneous assay. First, testosterone in serum sample is displaced from sex binding globulin (SHBG) with low-pH buffer. Sample is mixed with microparticles, coated with mouse monoclonal anti-testosterone antibody. After incubation, addition of labeled testosterone (in this case, conjugated with alkaline phosphatase), follows. Labeled testosterone binds to unoccupied sites on microparticles, coated with the antibodies against testosterone. More testosterone in the sample – less sites are free for labeled testosterone to bind. After another incubation, reaction mixture is transferred to cells, where microparticles fix and bind. Wash step follows – it removes unbound conjugate (labeled testosterone and other substances which may interfere with next step). Then, labeled antigen is visualized and measured. Signal is inversely proportional to amount of testosterone in the sample – as according to principle of competitive assay – stronger signal indicates more added, with marker conjugated testosterone present, therefore less "original" testosterone in the sample. In Abbott's example, 4-methylumbelliferyl phosphate is added and alkaline phosphatase, conjugated to added testosterone, hydrolyzes phosphate from 4-methylumbelliferryl phosphate to 4-methylumbelliferone, which fluorescence is measured [23].

In direct RIA methods, principle is the same, only marking of competing antigen is performed with radioactive substance instead of alkaline phosphatase or other enzymatic, fluorescence-based technique. Large variability was observed for direct RIA methods [24]. In indirect RIA methods, quantification follows organic solvent extraction and purification steps with monitoring of procedural losses. Although correlations between indirect RIA and mass spectrometry methods are good (above 0.9), absolute concentrations were reported to be significantly higher, probably (as in direct assays), due to cross-reaction of immunoreactive material [25].

Indirect assays (extraction and chromatography followed by RIA) are not available any more in our practice. Main method for serum testosterone determination in most present day clinical laboratories around the world (perhaps it is different in parts of US) is still direct automated chemiluminescent assay [26]. This assay mixes antibodies directly with serum and skips extraction step. This holds true for all direct assays, not only chemiluminescent but also radio-immuno (RIA) based.

Mass spectrometry (MS) of steroid compounds, which includes testosterone, has a long history of research and development [27]. It is coupled to liquid chromatography (LC, a separation technique in which the mobile phase is liquid) or gas chromatography (GC, a separation technique where the mobile phase is gas). After first separation and before ionization, in the past, derivatization (conversion of chemical compound into derivative) was often used to improve, for example, ionization efficiency and other characteristics of analyte[28]. With development of more sensitive techniques, today derivatization seem not included any more in a typical setting for testosterone determination with HPLC-tandem mass spectrometry. Sample must be ionized before ions are separated according to mass and charge in the spectrometer. Among methods of ionization are for example atmospheric pressure photoionization (suggested to be most optimal for testosterone analysis) or (less optimal for testosterone) electrospray ionization. Tandem mass spectrometry (MS/MS) means that spectrometry is performed in an arrangement in which ions are subjected to two or more sequential stages of analysis (which may be separated spatially or temporally).

High throughput LC/MS/MS has become gold standard for measurement of testosterone and other well defined steroid substances in biological fluids. GC/MS can also be used to quantify testosterone, but represents today mainly a "discovery tool" which provides "integrated picture of individual's metabolome" [29].

Some characteristics of testosterone assays are summarized in Table 2.

Type	Characteristics
chemiluminescet	uses antibodies, direct, most laboratory platforms (Abbott, Siemens, Roche) have their own antibodies, which all cross react to some extent to other substances and give consistent, but different results, typically higher than reference methods in/near castrate range
RIA – radio -immuo assay	uses antibodies, rarely in use those days, typically good results if indirect – radio- immuno - detection after chromatography step, for direct RIA's, same as for chemiluminescence – problems with antibody selectivity
LC-MS/MS: liquid chromatography – tandem mass spectrometry	uses molecular mass based identification, indirect, uses different liquid chromatography methods to extract testosterone from sample (for example "high turbulent flow") and tandem mass spectrometry to confirm and quantify sample, gold standard
GC-MS: gas chromatography – mass spectrometry	uses molecular mass based identification, indirect, research mainly, useful for profiling different steroids in the sample, reference method, issues with "in-house" development, sample preparation, most labor and resource intensive

Table 2. Most prevalent types of testosterone assays.

8. Units for testosterone measurement

Guidelines [3] state testosterone values in ng/dl only and some countries still use old values (for example US, Germany, Belgium), but in many countries laboratory results only in SI units - International System of Units - (nmol/l) - are available (for example Slovenia). Some articles, to further confusion, use other combinations, like ng/ml or mg/dl. To allow easier reference to practicing physicians, in Table 3, some typical serum testosterone values are presented in different units.

Conversion factors: as molecular formula of testosterone is $C_{19}H_{28}O_{2,}$ molecular mass of testosterone is 288.42 g/mol. Therefore, if value in ng/dl is available, multiply it with 0.0347 nmol/l / ng/dl to get value in nmol/l. If value in nmol/l is available and one needs ng/dl, value in nmol/l should be multiplied by 28.8 ng/dl / nmol/l to get ng/dl. 1 ng/ml (or microg/l) = 100 ng/dl.

Clinical meaning	value
normal morning value for males, above	12 nmol/l (= 346 ng/dl = 3.46 ng/ml)
advised supplementation for healthy males, regardless of symptoms, below	8 nmol/l (= 231 ng/dl = 2.31 ng/ml)
"old" castration value	1.73 nmol/l (= 50 ng/dl = 0.5 ng/ml)
median value for premenopausal females	1.39 nmol/l (= 40 ng/dl = 0.4 ng/ml)
"Morote's" value	1.11 nmol/l (= 32 ng/dl = 0.32 ng/ml)
"new" castration value	0.69 nmol/l (= 20 ng/dl = 0.2 ng/ml)

Table 3. Typical serum testosterone values in different units. "Morote's" value represents level of serum testosterone, determined with direct chemiluminescent immuno assay in prostate cancer patients on hormonal treatment, above which shorter time to progression was observed compared to patients with testosterone values below this level [9]. For curiosity, median value for premenopausal females can also be used as guideline for supplementation in hypoactive sexual desire disorder [30].

9. Daily rhythm of testosterone

Circadian and "ultradian" mean testosterone level fluctuations peak is around 8 AM and through level around 8 PM. Over this, there is a 90 min oscillation in testosterone values as reflection of pulsatile secretory pattern.

Sleeping increases testosterone values [31]. Some even claim sleep, not circadian rhythm to be more important for regulation of testosterone [31]. Pattern of physical activity (physical work or training in the morning versus evening) does not influence testosterone concentrations or testosterone diurnal pattern [32]. Food (mixed meal) decreases testosterone value, if blood is taken 1-2 hours after, by 30% in comparison to overnight fast [33]. Better sleep increases testosterone value [34]. Anxiety may increase testosterone levels, it was even suggested, patient's samples on the day of admission to hospital should not be used because anxiety may be associated with increased testosterone level [35]. On LHRH agonists, diurnal pattern is expected to be abolished [36]. Age reduces circadian fluctuations [37].

Due to stated variations in testosterone levels during the day, morning fasting blood samples are standard.

http://dx.doi.org/10.5772/52525

10. What can one expect from direct chemiluminescent assays –Example

Wide availability of automated testosterone assays should make easy for clinicians to follow prostate cancer patients testosterone levels, as at present almost every clinical laboratory offers testosterone measurement with one of direct chemiluminescent assays methods.

Aim was to evaluate use of such a testosterone measurement tool in every-day clinical practice and consequences that might follow. Claims from some pharmaceutical company representatives on their LHRH agonist formulations to be better than others were also addressed.

10.1. Materials and methods

In a cross-sectional audit study, serum testosterone level was determined in all patients on 3-month LHRH formulations, treated in out-patient clinic in two months period. Blood samples were taken immediately before the next injection. Only patients, who previously received more than one injection and with previous injection exactly 3 months or less before examination were eligible.

Three preparations were found to be used: Diphereline (triptorelin 11.25 mg), Eligard (modern leuprolide formulation, 22.5 mg) and Zoladex (goserelin 10.8 mg).

Further 10 samples were taken from patients with surgical castration performed more than 6 months ago, who appeared on regular follow up out-patient visit during the study period.

Testosterone measurement was performed with direct chemiluminescent microparticle immunoassay Architect from Abbott Laboratories. According to procedural leaflet, functional sensitivity of this assay was 0.49 nmol/l (95% confidence interval 0.38 – 0.59) and analytical sensitivity 0.28 nmol/l.

As SI units (nmol/L) are obligatory in our country, all testosterone measurements were originally reported in SI units and conversion to US units (ng/dl) was performed for the purpose of this report using conversion factor of 0.0347.

For statistical evaluation of differences between groups of patients on different LHRH agonist formulations, analysis of variance between groups was calculated using open source statistical software R [38].

10.2. Results

125 patients aged 50 to 92 (median 74 years, lower quartile 70, upper quartile 78 years) were included.

For the whole group, serum testosterone values ranged from 14 ng/dl (0.5 nmol/l, lowest reportable result) to 107 ng/dl (3.7 nmol/l), median 37 ng/dl (1.3 nmol/l), lower quartile 32 ng/dl (1.1 nmol/l), upper quartile 58 ng/dl (2.0 nmol/l).

According to those results, considering castrate level of 20 ng/dl (=0.694 nmol/l), only 7% of patients on LHRH treatment and 2/10 patients after surgical castration could be classified to castrate state of disease. Considering castrate level of 50 ng/dl (1.735 nmol/l), 66% of patients on chemical castration and 8/10 patients after surgical castration would comply.

Testosterone measurement results, according to LHRH agonist, are presented in Table 4. According to analysis of variance, differences between groups of patients, treated with different LHRH agonists, were not significantly different (F=0.69, p=0.5).

LHRH formulation	N	TST:min-max	TST-median	TST-75%	TST-90%
triptorelin 11.25 mg	53	20-98	37	58	72
goserelin 10.8 mg	41	14-107	37	52	69
leuprolide 22.5 mg	21	14-84	49	63	72

Table 4. Testosterone measurement results with Abbot Architect assay in patients on different 3-month LHRH agonists. Samples were taken immediately before next injection. TST – testosterone. Units: ng/dl (1,73nmol/L=50 ng/dl). Differences between different LHRH formulations were not statistically significant.

11. Problems with direct testosterone immunoassays

Large differences were reported from measurements of the same serum sample with chemiluminescent assays from different manufacturers [39,40]. Direct RIA techniques were not better [41]. In the low range (values of interest for castration control in patients with prostate cancer), which was close to range of female testosterone levels, direct assays gave results more than 20% different from the gold standard [41]. Abbot Architect assay was also reported to give consistently up to 20% higher results compared to standard in this range of values [39].

One of the reasons for variability is in the fact that antibodies are different among manufacturers, with different cross-reactivity profiles. All present direct chemiluminescent assays are matrix dependent, which was extensively studied by the British group [42]. It was confirmed there was significant cross-reactivity for example with dehydroepiandrosteronesulphate (DHEA-S) [43]. The described issue is not only in urology regarding testosterone – also other areas of endocrinology where steroid hormones measurements are important, have reported and discussed similar issues [44,45]. College of American Pathologists proficiency testing revealed in 2008, highest mean compared to lowest mean for testosterone, to differ by factor 2.8 [46]. Differences for mass spectrometry assays were much lower, by factor 1.4.

12. Problems with mass spectrometry testosterone assays

Mass spectrometry (MS) assays are not commercially available in classical sense, but are to much larger extent dependent on each laboratory's own development. As mass spectrometry technology is capable of very high sensitivity and specificity, those assay are accepted as gold standard. But, they are more than direct commercial assays dependent on proper calibration and sample preparation[47]. Research has shown biases as high as 25.3% for testosterone values near castrate ranges [47]. Others reported up to 26% of results outside total error limit of 14% due to improper calibration and between-run calibration [48]. Although MS techniques are becoming standard assays for steroid hormones, this presents several challenges, for example affordability for smaller laboratories, high operating costs of equipment, need for standardization of MS assays and in many occasions, actually setting new reference ranges [49] and relating them to physiological and pathological conditions, as happens with testosterone, where castrate values have been moved from 50 ng/dl to 20 ng/dl.

13. Castrate testosterone values in different prostate cancer studies

Serum testosterone value around 1.735 nmol/l or 50 ng/dl as castrate level for the purpose of hormonal treatment of prostate cancer was used already in 1970'ties [2]. Later, some LHRH formulations were designed to achieve serum testosterone below this value in 95% of treated patients. It was accepted as standard value in guidelines [50]. Guidelines have at present gone even a step further and stated testosterone levels above 50 ng/dl to be in-sufficient and additional hormonal manipulation to be warranted in such patients [3]. It is further generally accepted patients with surgical castration to have lower levels of testosterone – around 15 ng/dl and certainly below 30 ng/dl [51]. As surgical castration provides lower testosterone levels, there were always claims one should aim as low as possible with testosterone levels and should try to reach below 20 ng/dl – for example in a small study of 38 patients, treated with LHRH agonists, Oefelein found 5% did not reach values below 50 ng/dl and 13% did not reach values below 20 ng/dl [52]. This movement, which aims to decrease castrate testosterone level, was further supported by publication which claims patients with castrate testosterone levels below 32 ng/dl (1.1 nmol/l) – Morote's value - to have longer time to biochemical progression [9]. In their study, which also used chemiluminescent antibody testosterone assay, in 25% of patients testosterone levels above 50 ng/dl were identified. Further, with serial measurements, 55% of patients on chemical castration had testosterone values found above 20 ng/dl [8]. Studies which use HPLC/MS/MS for determination of testosterone levels do see lower values [53].

Some studies seem to oversee guidelines and post their own castrate testosterone levels, which are significantly higher and set to a value which offers approximately 95% successful castration. In their article on testosterone escape, group from Norway claims their castration level is 2.8 nmol/l which equals 81 ng/dl [6]. This value was selected as their laboratory's upper normal limit for women. And with this value, they identified 10% of patients who failed to reach this castration level. The present study was similar to this in testing patient's serum for testosterone at the end of 3 month dosing interval, which may also influence results.

Another group from Turkey, which evaluated influence of androgen deprivation therapy on hand function in 2008 article used radioimmunoassay for testosterone measurement and in a castrate group mean value of testosterone was 52 ng/dl +- 35 ng/dl [54]. One can assume for approximately half of their patients testosterone levels were not in castrate area according to guidelines. Surgical castration study, using chemiluminescent assay, found values up to or above 50 ng/dl for surgically castrated patients [55]. Further surgical castration study found patients on LHRH treatment before surgical castration to have values above 50 ng/dl in 28% of patients and after surgical castration in up to 8% [56]. Unfortunately method of testosterone measurement is not stated in this article, but it correlates perfectly with data presented here, where chemiluminescent method was used. Further, recent LHRH agonists report from Canada, which also used "competitive immunoassay using direct chemiluminescent technology" [57], found median testosterone values for different LHRH agonists to be (in nmol/l) 1.2, 1.3, 1.1 and 1.3 and in two of five formulations, upper quartal value was 1.8, indicating 25% of patients on particular formulation to be even above "old" castration value of 1.72 nmol/l (50 ng/dl). Another study from Canada, also using chemiluminescent immunoassays, although claiming they were "newer technology", indicates risk for breakthrough levels of serum testosterone (value measured higher than castrate value) in patients on LHRH agonist injections to be 5.4% and 2.2% (for castration values 1.1 nmol/l and 1.7 nmol/l, respectively) per each LHRH injection [58]! Cancer control was claimed to be inferior in patients with breakthroughs of serum testosterone measured [58].

14. Direct testosterone assays and prostate cancer – The verdict

Probably one of most important reasons for observed discrepancies in testosterone measurements lies in "matrix" issue, in cross-reactivity. Immunolite assay and Abbot Architect both cross-react with DHEA and give consistently higher values for serum testosterone in range of castration male values [39,42]. Therefore results of studies, which use direct chemiluminescent testosterone assays in clinical setting cannot be compared to studies, which use chromatography followed by mass spectrometry techniques, because they do not measure the same things.

Inaccuracy of present day direct testosterone assays is already recognized in the field of female and male testosterone replacement, in pediatrics [59] and should be recognized also in the field of prostate cancer. Until indirect testosterone assays applying mass spectroscopy become widely available, publications should set realistic values of castrate levels and precisely state measurement methods used. They may be universally available in the USA, but in Europe, even western university hospitals are not quick in replacing direct immuno-assays with gas chromatography methods – for example in Ghent they changed only recently, also for reasons like "one can not publish any more anything about testosterone without this method". And even mass spectrometry methods show significant errors and inconsistencies.

On the downside, it becomes clear using direct present day techniques to control castration methods (either chemical or surgical) is not appropriate and invariably leads to disputable results. Above findings also in part explain long term debate about subcapsular or classical simple orchiectomy and part of an occasional finding of non-castrate testosterone level after orchiectomy [56]. Also our own impulse for studying the field come from initial observations that patients after surgical castration have higher testosterone values compared to guideline's requests.

On the upside, direct chemiluminescent assays do measure something. They can unmask occasional testosterone outlier (skipped dose of drug, granuloma formation or an individual in need for more frequent dose of a drug – reduced dose interval, as explained for example in dr. Garnick's editorial comment [8]). They can identify hypogonadal men with prostate cancer before starting androgen deprivation therapy, who have very bad prognosis or may in the future benefit from modified treatments, like incorporating early use of new antiandrogens (for example MDV3100 [60]). They are necessary if one embarks on "on demand" re-dosing of LHRH agonists [61].

It is obvious chemiluminescent direct testosterone measurements do not show only testosterone values and as such can not serve as a tool to decide which LHRH agonist reduces testosterone more compared to other drugs. But results of such assays, as for example Abbot Architect testosterone assay, are consistent [39] and according to published and our results, there are great differences in measured levels of androgens in patients on LHRH agonist therapy (740%, from 0.5 to 3.7 nmol/L, 14 – 107 ng/dL). Perhaps, at present a pure speculation, chemiluminescent assays, which give consistent results, only with some cross-reactivity and therefore systematic overestimation of testosterone values in the low range, like Architect and Immunolite, can give estimation of overall serum androgen levels. Importance of extratesticular androgens is becoming more and more evident [62,63]. This may explain findings from Morote et al, who used same technically problematic direct chemiluminiscent assay and found correlation between assay results and time to biochemical progression [9] or from Perachino et al, who found even correlation between assay results and survival [10]. Also Hashimoto et al [64], although failing to provide details about their testosterone assay and reporting questionably low testosterone values, report usefulness of testosterone measurement for prediction of antiandrogen treatment results – when testosterone levels were low, no additional clinical benefit of antiandrogen treatment was observed, when testosterone was higher, antiandrogens were useful. If future can confirm those propositions, direct testosterone tests, despite their imprecision for their original purpose, may well serve us in selecting patients for antiandrogen addition to castration or for secondary hormonal treatment, especially in perspective of new androgen manipulating drugs, like abiraterone acetate (Zytiga) and MDV3100 [60].

15. Conclusions

Serum testosterone levels provide objectivity for proper prostate cancer disease states characterization. Testosterone level before treatment may add to prognosis. More importantly, testosterone levels during treatment become main issue in individual's prostate cancer treatment decisions, as soon as increasing PSA levels indicate failure of primary local treatment.

Apparent difference between guidelines (which ask for 20ng/dl) and practice in serum testosterone values of hormonally treated prostate cancer patients was investigated and could be explained in methodologies of testosterone determination. Most present day available testosterone assays in hospitals are direct assays, which overestimate testosterone values in the castrate range. Antibodies cross-react with other androgens in serum (which prevail in low testosterone range) and result is overall androgen estimation, not pure testosterone value. Studies should recognize this and find use for this "overall androgen" value, which is, contrary to indirect mass spectroscopy assays, universally available and was found to be related to disease progression and treatment results. Further, it is useful for identification of high risk patients with low testosterone values at diagnosis and identification of patients with poor response to LHRH agonists. Testosteron results are necessary for prolongation of interval between injections, which may be possible in approximately half of patients on LHRH agonists treatment where values are well below castration levels and at the same time, some patients may need injections of LHRH agonists in shorter intervals. In the future, tests which estimate not only pure testosterone, but overall androgen level, may become clinically relevant with awareness of prostate cancer cell's ability to use different androgen molecules and as a consequence patient tailored use of new androgen manipulating drugs.

Acknowledgements

Study was strongly supported by Prim. KarelKisner, Former Head of Department of Urology in UKC Maribor, Slovenia and Mag. MaksimiljanGorenjak, Head of Department of Laboratory Medicine at the same institution.

Author details

Tine Hajdinjak[1,2,3]

Address all correspondence to: tine.hajdinjak@gmail.com

1 Center UROL Maribor, Slovenia

2 Medical Faculty, University of Maribor, Maribor, Slovenia

3 Division of Urology, Department of Surgery, General Hospital Murska Sobota, Slovenia

References

[1] Bianco FJ Jr. Paradigms in androgen/castrate resistant states of prostate cancer in a biomarker era. Urol. Oncol. 2008;26(4):408–14.

[2] Shearer RJ, Hendry WF, Sommerville IF, Fergusson JD. Plasma testosterone: an accurate monitor of hormone treatment in prostatic cancer. Br J Urol. 1973;45(6):668–77.

[3] Mottet N, Bellmunt J, Bolla M, Joniau S, Mason M, Matveev V, idr. EAU guidelines on prostate cancer. Part II: Treatment of advanced, relapsing, and castration-resistant prostate cancer. Eur. Urol. 2011;59(4):572–83.

[4] Peyromaure M, Rebillard X, Ruffion A, Salomon L, Villers A, Soulie M. Time-course of plasma testosterone in patients with prostate cancer treated by endocrine therapy. Prog. Urol. 2008;18(1):2–8.

[5] Morote J, Esquena S, Abascal JM, Trilla E, Cecchini L, Raventós CX, et al. Failure to maintain a suppressed level of serum testosterone during long-acting depot luteinizing hormone-releasing hormone agonist therapy in patients with advanced prostate cancer. Urol. Int. 2006;77(2):135–8.

[6] Yri OE, Bjoro T, Fossa SD. Failure to achieve castration levels in patients using leuprolide acetate in locally advanced prostate cancer. Eur. Urol. 2006;49(1):54–58; discussion 58.

[7] Shiota M, Tokuda N, Kanou T, Yamasaki H. Incidence rate of injection-site granulomas resulting from the administration of luteinizing hormone-releasing hormone analogues for the treatment of prostatic cancer. Yonsei Med. J. 2007;48(3):421–4.

[8] Morote J, Planas J, Salvador C, Raventós CX, Catalán R, Reventós J. Individual variations of serum testosterone in patients with prostate cancer receiving androgen deprivation therapy. BJU Int. 2009;103(3):332–335; discussion 335.

[9] Morote J, Orsola A, Planas J, Trilla E, Raventós CX, Cecchini L, et al. Redefining clinically significant castration levels in patients with prostate cancer receiving continuous androgen deprivation therapy. J. Urol. 2007;178(4 Pt 1):1290–5.

[10] Perachino M, Cavalli V, Bravi F. Testosterone levels in patients with metastatic prostate cancer treated with luteinizing hormone-releasing hormone therapy: prognostic significance? BJU Int. 2010;105(5):648–51.

[11] Schulman CC, Irani J, Morote J, Schalken JA, Montorsi F, Chlosta PL, et al. Testosterone measurement in patients with prostate cancer. Eur. Urol. 2010;58(1):65–74.

[12] Schatzl G, Madersbacher S, Thurridl T, Waldmüller J, Kramer G, Haitel A, et al. High-grade prostate cancer is associated with low serum testosterone levels. Prostate. 2001;47(1):52–8.

[13] Pedraza R, KwartAM. Hormonal therapy for patients with advanced adenocarcinoma of the prostate: is there a role for discontinuing treatment after prolonged androgen suppression? Urology. 2003;61(4):770–3.

[14] Slora: Slovenija in rak (Slovenian cancer registry) [Internet]. [accessed 2012 aug 8]. Available from: http://www.slora.si/

[15] Prebivalstvenapiramida (Statistical office of the Republic of Slovenia) [Internet]. [accessed 2012 aug 8]. Available from: http://www.stat.si/Piramida.asp

[16] Schröder FH, Hugosson J, Roobol MJ, Tammela TLJ, Ciatto S, Nelen V, et. al. Prostate-cancer mortality at 11 years of follow-up. N. Engl. J. Med. 2012 15;366(11):981–90.

[17] Chou R, Croswell JM, Dana T, Bougatsos C, Blazina I, Fu R, et al. Screening for prostate cancer: a review of the evidence for the U.S. Preventive Services Task Force. Ann. Intern. Med. 2011;155(11):762–71.

[18] Prostate Cancer: We Can Do Better: Editorial on Screening for Prostate Cancer from USPSTF Chair Dr. Virginia Moyer [Internet]. [accessed 2012 aug 8]. Available from: http://www.uspreventiveservicestaskforce.org/prostatecancerscreening/prostatecanoped.htm

[19] Appu S, Lawrentschuk N, Grills RJ, Neerhut G. Effectiveness of cyproterone acetate in achieving castration and preventing luteinizing hormone releasing hormone analogue induced testosterone surge in patients with prostate cancer. J. Urol. 2005;174(1):140–2.

[20] Morse HC, Leach DR, Rowley MJ, Heller CG. Effect of cyproterone acetate on sperm concentration, seminal fluid volume, testicular cytology and levels of plasma and urinary ICSH, FSH and testosterone in normal men. J. Reprod. Fertil. 1973;32(3):365–78.

[21] Masson-Lecomte A, Guy L, Pedron P, Bruyere F, Rouprêt M, Nsabimbona B, et al. A switch from GnRH agonist to GnRH antagonist in castration-resistant prostate cancer patients leads to a low response rate on PSA. World journal of urology. 2012. DOI: 10.1007/s00345-012-0841-1.

[22] Heyns W, Drochmans A, van der Schueren E, Verhoeven G. Endocrine effects of high-dose ketoconazole therapy in advanced prostatic cancer. ActaEndocrinol. 1985;110(2):276–83.

[23] Novotny M, Wilson HD. Testosterone testing: an immunoassay with improved accuracy in samples from both males and females. CLI [Internet]. 2005; Accessed 2012 Aug 8. Available from: http://www.cli-online.com/fileadmin/pdf/pdf_general/testosterone-testing-an-immunoassay-with-improved-accuracy-in-samples-from-both-males-and-females.pdf

[24] Stanczyk FZ, Cho MM, Endres DB, Morrison JL, Patel S, Paulson RJ. Limitations of direct estradiol and testosterone immunoassay kits. Steroids. 2003;68(14):1173–8.

[25] Hsing AW, Stanczyk FZ, Bélanger A, Schroeder P, Chang L, Falk RT, idr. Reproducibility of serum sex steroid assays in men by RIA and mass spectrometry. Cancer Epidemiol. Biomarkers Prev. 2007;16(5):1004–8.

[26] Newman JD, Doery JCG. Assessing hypogonadism in men - how helpful are current testosterone assays? AustFam Physician. 2008;37(8):670–1.

[27] Friedland SS, Lane GH, Longman RT, Train KE, O'Neal MJ. Mass Spectra of Steroids. Anal. Chem. 1959;31(2):169–74.

[28] Santa T, Al-Dirbashi OY, Fukushima T. Derivatization reagents in liquid chromatography/electrospray ionization tandem mass spectrometry for biomedical analysis. Drug DiscovTher. 2007;1(2):108–18.

[29] Krone N, Hughes BA, Lavery GG, Stewart PM, Arlt W, Shackleton CHL. Gas chromatography/mass spectrometry (GC/MS) remains a pre-eminent discovery tool in clinical steroid investigations even in the era of fast liquid chromatography tandem mass spectrometry (LC/MS/MS). J Steroid BiochemMol Biol. 2010;121(3-5):496–504.

[30] Palacios S. Hypoactive Sexual Desire Disorder and current pharmacotherapeutic options in women. Womens Health (LondEngl). 2011;7(1):95–107.

[31] Andersen ML, Alvarenga TF, Mazaro-Costa R, Hachul HC, Tufik S. The association of testosterone, sleep, and sexual function in men and women. Brain Res. 2011;1416:80–104.

[32] Sedliak M, Finni T, Cheng S, Kraemer WJ, Häkkinen K. Effect of time-of-day-specific strength training on serum hormone concentrations and isometric strength in men. Chronobiol. Int. 2007;24(6):1159–77.

[33] Lehtihet M, Arver S, Bartuseviciene I, Pousette A. S-testosterone decrease after a mixed meal in healthy men independent of SHBG and gonadotrophin levels. Andrologia. 2012. doi: 10.1111/j.1439-0272.2012.01296.x.

[34] Penev PD. Association between sleep and morning testosterone levels in older men. Sleep. 2007;30(4):427–32.

[35] Robinson MR, Thomas BS. Effect of hormonal therapy on plasma testosterone levels in prostatic carcinoma. Br Med J. 1971;4(5784):391–4.

[36] Grant JB, Ahmed SR, Shalet SM, Costello CB, Howell A, Blacklock NJ. Testosterone and gonadotrophin profiles in patients on daily or monthly LHRH analogue ICI 118630 (Zoladex) compared with orchiectomy. Br J Urol. 1986;58(5):539–44.

[37] Copinschi G, Van Cauter E. Effects of ageing on modulation of hormonal secretions by sleep and circadian rhythmicity. Horm. Res. 1995;43(1-3):20–4.

[38] R Core Team. R: A Language and Environment for Statistical Computing. Vienna, Austria; Available from: www.R-project.org

[39] Taieb J, Mathian B, Millot F, Patricot M-C, Mathieu E, Queyrel N, et al. Testosterone measured by 10 immunoassays and by isotope-dilution gas chromatography-mass spectrometry in sera from 116 men, women, and children. Clin. Chem. 2003;49(8): 1381–95.

[40] Moal V, Mathieu E, Reynier P, Malthièry Y, Gallois Y. Low serum testosterone assayed by liquid chromatography-tandem mass spectrometry. Comparison with five immunoassay techniques. Clin. Chim. Acta. 2007;386(1-2):12–9.

[41] Sacks SS. Are routine testosterone assays good enough? ClinBiochem Rev. 2005;26(1): 43–5.

[42] Middle JG. Dehydroepiandrostenedionesulphate interferes in many direct immunoassays for testosterone. Ann. Clin. Biochem. 2007;44(Pt 2):173–7.

[43] Warner MH, Kane JW, Atkin SL, Kilpatrick ES. Dehydroepiandrosteronesulphate interferes with the Abbott Architect direct immunoassay for testosterone. Ann. Clin. Biochem. 2006;43(Pt 3):196–9.

[44] Pearson Murphy BE. Lack of specificity of urinary free cortisol determinations: why does it continue? J. Clin. Endocrinol. Metab. 1999;84(6):2258–9.

[45] Wartofsky L, Handelsman DJ. Standardization of hormonal assays for the 21st century. J. Clin. Endocrinol. Metab. 2010;95(12):5141–3.

[46] Soldin SJ, Soldin OP. Steroid hormone analysis by tandem mass spectrometry. Clin. Chem. 2009;55(6):1061–6.

[47] Vesper HW, Botelho JC. Standardization of testosterone measurements in humans. J. Steroid Biochem. Mol. Biol. 2010;121(3-5):513–9.

[48] Thienpont LM, Van Uytfanghe K, Blincko S, Ramsay CS, Xie H, Doss RC, et al. State-of-the-art of serum testosterone measurement by isotope dilution-liquid chromatography-tandem mass spectrometry. Clin. Chem. 2008;54(8):1290–7.

[49] Stanczyk FZ, Clarke NJ. Advantages and challenges of mass spectrometry assays for steroid hormones. J. Steroid Biochem. Mol. Biol. 2010;121(3-5):491–5.

[50] Mohler J, Bahnson RR, Boston B, Busby JE, D'Amico A, Eastham JA, et al. NCCN clinical practice guidelines in oncology: prostate cancer. J NatlComprCancNetw. 2010;8(2):162–200.

[51] Oefelein MG, Feng A, Scolieri MJ, Ricchiutti D, Resnick MI. Reassessment of the definition of castrate levels of testosterone: implications for clinical decision making. Urology. 2000;56(6):1021–4.

[52] Oefelein MG, Cornum R. Failure to achieve castrate levels of testosterone during luteinizing hormone releasing hormone agonist therapy: the case for monitoring serum testosterone and a treatment decision algorithm. J. Urol. 2000;164(3 Pt 1):726–9.

[53] Sharifi R, Browneller R. Serum testosterone suppression and potential for agonistic stimulation during chronic treatment with monthly and 3-month depot formulations of leuprolide acetate for advanced prostate cancer. J. Urol. 2002;168(3):1001–4.

[54] Soyupek F, Soyupek S, Perk H, Ozorak A. Androgen deprivation therapy for prostate cancer: effects on hand function. Urol. Oncol. 2008;26(2):141–6.

[55] Vickers MA Jr, Lamontagne DP, Guru KA, Satyanarayana RK, Vickers KE, Menon M. Autologous tunica vaginalis and subcapsular orchiectomy: a hormonal therapy for prostate cancer. J. Androl. 2004;25(3):375–81.

[56] Issa MM, Lendvay TS, Bouet R, Young MR, Petros JA, Marshall FF. Epididymal sparing bilateral simple orchiectomy with epididymoplasty: preservation of esthetics and body image. J. Urol. 2005;174(3):893–7.

[57] Venkateswaran S, Margel D, Yap S, Hersey K, Yip P, Fleshner NE. Comparison of serum testosterone levels in prostate cancer patients receiving LHRH agonist therapy with or without the removal of the prostate. Can UrolAssoc J. 2012;6(3):183–6.

[58] Pickles T, Hamm J, Morris WJ, Schreiber WE, Tyldesley S. Incomplete testosterone suppression with luteinizing hormone-releasing hormone agonists: does it happen and does it matter? BJU international. 2012. doi: 10.1111/j.1464-410X.2012.11190.x.

[59] Tomlinson C, Macintyre H, Dorrian CA, Ahmed SF, Wallace AM. Testosterone measurements in early infancy. Arch Dis Child Fetal Neonatal Ed. 2004;89(6):F558–F559.

[60] Eichholz A, Ferraldeschi R, Attard G, de Bono JS. Putting the brakes on continued androgen receptor signaling in castration-resistant prostate cancer. Molecular and Cellular Endocrinology. 2012;360(1-2):68-75.

[61] Oefelein MG. Words of wisdom. Re: determining dosing intervals for LHRH agonists based on serum testosterone levels: a prospective study. Eur. Urol. 2008;54(1):235–6.

[62] Mostaghel EA, Nelson PS. Intracrine androgen metabolism in prostate cancer progression: mechanisms of castration resistance and therapeutic implications. Best Pract. Res. Clin. Endocrinol. Metab. 2008;22(2):243–58.

[63] Luu-The V, Bélanger A, Labrie F. Androgen biosynthetic pathways in the human prostate. Best Pract. Res. Clin. Endocrinol. Metab. 2008;22(2):207–21.

[64] Hashimoto K, Masumori N, Hashimoto J, Takayanagi A, Fukuta F, Tsukamoto T. Serum testosterone level to predict the efficacy of sequential use of antiandrogens as second-line treatment following androgen deprivation monotherapy in patients with castration-resistant prostate cancer. Jpn. J. Clin. Oncol. 2011;41(3):405–10.

Chapter 9

Describing Prostate Cancer Dynamics: Second Look at PSA-Doubling Time and PSA-Specific Growth Rate

Glenn Tisman

Additional information is available at the end of the chapter

http://dx.doi.org/10.5772/53179

1. Introduction

Physicians responsible for patient care focus on readily available clinical and trending laboratory data to help direct the patient's clinical course and evaluate efficacy of therapy. Most clinicians fail to incorporate newer parameters of tumor response such as tumor growth rate when evaluating patient treatment response. Available now, is a wealth of dynamic growth parameters that shed new light on tumor biology and should be used in clinical decision-making.

What follows is in part a review of former paradigms of prostate tumor growth. Later, focus is directed to newer techniques to assist in evaluating targeted drug effects on the kinetics of prostate and other cancers. The discussion introduces the concept of tumor or marker specific growth rate (SGR) and challenges historical results obtained by use of the classic tumor or marker doubling time (PSA-DT).

As we proceed with this discussion, a mobile device App for hand-held computers including the iPhone, iPad, or iPod is presented. This conveniently facilitates a more sophisticated tumor and marker analysis at the bedside or in the clinic.

2. Historical perspective of tumor growth kinetics, exponential and Gompertzian kinetics

Though there is occasional homage paid to Gompertzian tumor growth, for practical purposes, when we care for patients, tumors are frequently undergoing exponential expansion.

In the absence of tumor mutation or perturbation by therapy the growth rate of exponentially growing tumors is constant. Rarely, there may be periods of interrupted growth.

Gompertzian growth [1, 2, 3] is best described by a sigmoid-shaped curve. At tumor initiation growth is occult, slow and remains subclinical for several years. A second phase is the rapid, clinically apparent exponential phase lasting for a few years followed by the slower terminal growth phase as the tumor approaches 35-40 doublings representing a volume approaching 1000 cc or a tumor diameter of 10 cm Figure 1. The duration of tumor growth from inception is several years and for three quarters of that period the tumor is clinically undetectable. At the time of discovery, the oncologist is attending to the last quarter of tumor growth.

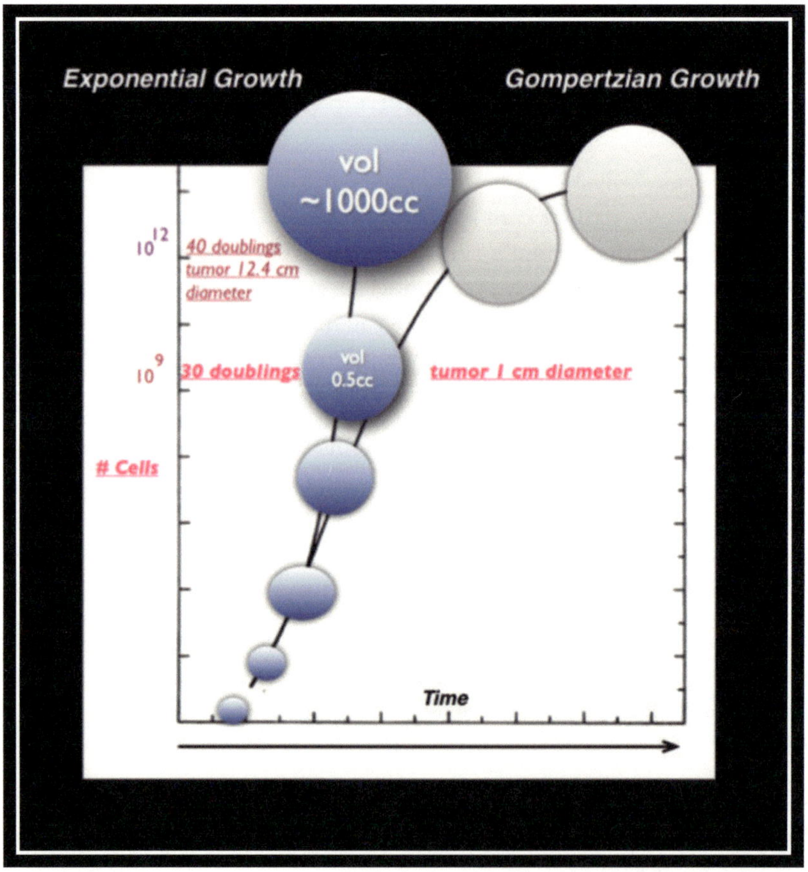

Figure 1. Note the differences between the exponential and Gompertzian growth curves. The lethal burden of tumor is approximately 1000 cc or ~35-40 doublings. In the clinic when tumors reach 0.5-1 cm in diameter (30 doublings or 10^9 cells) they are measurable and follow the exponential growth curve, the steeper the slope the larger the tumor specific growth rate (SGR). Nonetheless, many feel that when looking at the entire lifespan of malignant tumors (over several years) tumor growth may better be described by Gompertzian kinetics [3].

3. Exponential growth

In 1934 Mottram [4, 5] reported work on the rat tar wart. Tar warts are tar-carcinogen induced neoplasms of the skin starting 75-100 days after the continuous painting of the rat's neck with tar. Histologically, some warts appear benign while others are clearly malignant.

Using the tar wart tumor growth model, Mottram was the first to describe tumor expansion as exponential. Exponentially growing tumors graphically produce straight lines by plotting linear time on the x-axis versus the log (at any base) of either tumor area, tumor cell number, tumor volume or tumor diameter on the y-axis see Figure 2.

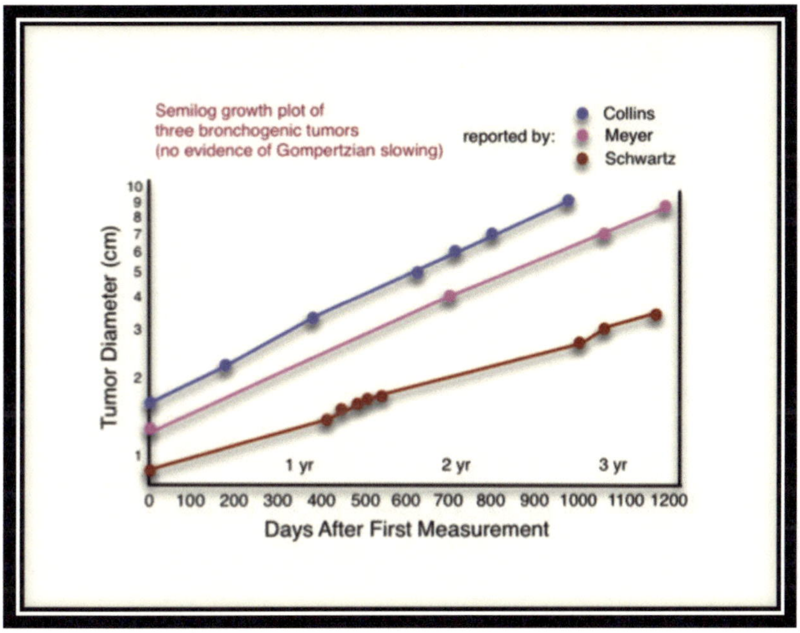

Figure 2. Friberg, Collins, Spratt, Steel, Schwartz affirmed that in the clinic, an exponential growth pattern adequately described tumor growth for most patients. A semi-log plot of tumor diameter vs. time illustrates the linear relationship characteristic of exponential growth.

Twenty years later Laird [6, 7] reported on the growth of transplanted tumors in the rat. Under her specific laboratory conditions, most tumor growth could be described in terms of the Gompertzian model. Her experiments lead her to accept that for her laboratory model; most transplantable, rapidly growing tumors could be described in Gompertzian terms.

Studies of tumor growth in clinic patients have been described in terms of both exponential and Gompertzian models. Nevertheless, several investigators reported data that was inconsistent with the Gompertzian model for the majority of their patients. These authors engaged routine imaging of both metastatic and primary pulmonary lesions in an attempt to resolve whether exponential growth could be confirmed in the clinic. Friberg, Collins, Spratt, Steel, Schwartz [8, 9, 10, 11, 12,13] affirmed that in the clinic, an exponential growth pattern adequately described tumor growth for most patients Figures 2, 3.

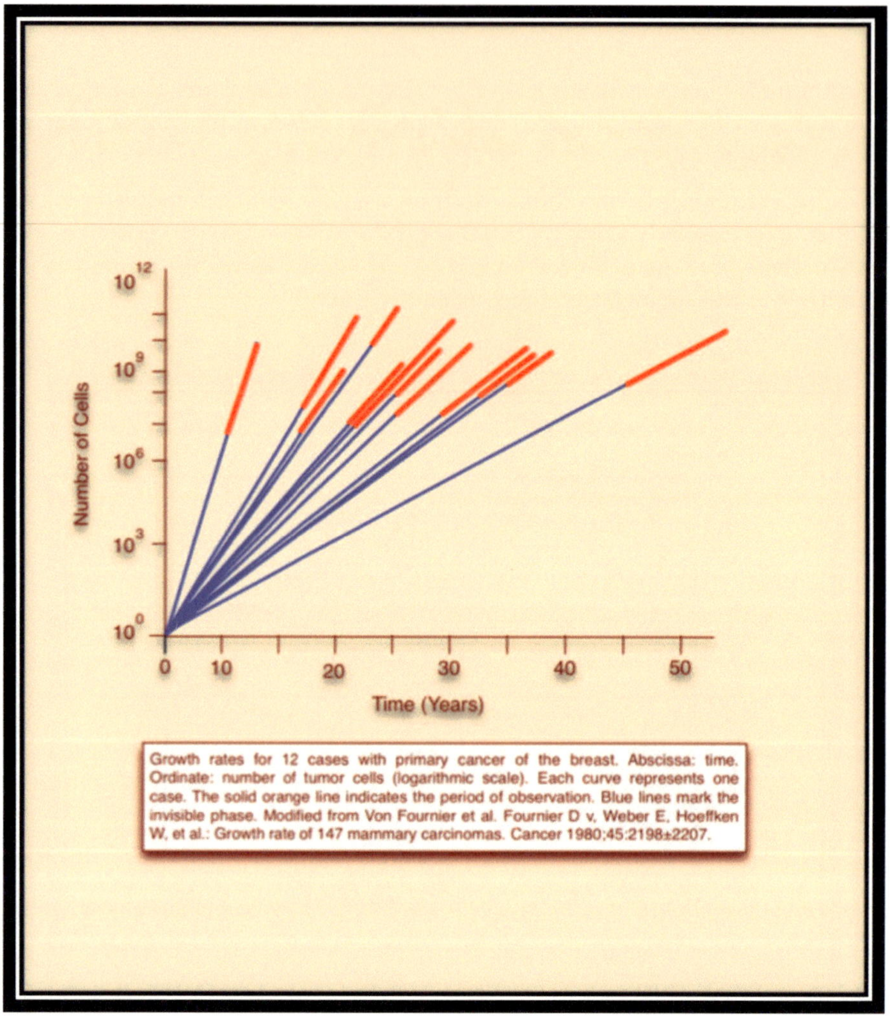

Figure 3. Von Fournier et al. confirm a straight-line (by semi-log plot) relationship for patients with breast tumors supporting the model of exponential growth model.

4. The tumor marker as a surrogate for tumor growth exemplified by PSA and prostate cancer

4.1. PSA Velocity (PSA-V)

PSA-V is the rate of change in serum PSA over time. PSA-V = 1/2 ((PSA_2-PSA_1/t_1 in years) + (PSA_3 – PSA_2/t_2 in years)), where PSA_1 is the first, PSA_2 the second and PSA_3 the third PSA measurement. Time represents the interval (in years) between PSA measurements. It is recommended that three PSA measurements obtained over 24 months yields optimal accuracy. A PSA-V exceeding 0.75 ng/ml/year is highly predictive of prostate cancer. PSA-V is more useful than PSA doubling time (PSA-DT) in the pretreatment setting to help identify those men with life-threatening disease [14].

Studies confirm that the PSA tumor marker reflects prostate tumor growth and PSA dynamic changes are useful for predicting clinical outcome in several situations such as tumor recurrence and overall survival [15].

Klotz [16] reviewed the value of PSA as a tumor marker in patients with prostate cancer. He noted that use of a single serum value of PSA is inadequate for predicting patient survival. However, the PSA-V as ng/ml/yr. was a marker of disease biology. D'Amico [17] included preoperative PSA-V in determining subsequent risk of death from prostate cancer in 1095 men with clinically localized prostate cancer that underwent prostatectomy and radiation therapy [18]. A PSA-V >2 ng/ml/yr the year before prostatectomy, was associated with lymph node metastases, an advanced pathologic stage, and high-grade disease. This threshold level of PSA-V was associated with a significantly shortened time to recurrence, death from prostate cancer, and death from any cause. Strikingly, men with a PSA rise of >2.0 ng/ml had prostate cancer-specific mortality rates nine times those with a PSA-V <2 ng/ml.

4.2. Tumor marker Doubling Time (DT)

Miyamoto [19] studied the growth of hepatic metastases in colorectal cancer patients. He established that a tumor marker could accurately reflect tumor volume and its changes. Using the CEA tumor marker he reported an almost equal and parallel correlation between CEA doubling time and hepatic tumor volume doubling time.

PSA-DT Figure 4 is the time it takes for the serum PSA to double. Evidence indicates PSA-DT closely mirrors prostate tumor volume doubling time. Kato et al. in 2008 [20] undertook an attempt to correlate prostate tumor volume to serum PSA level. Kato's group calculated that for each ng/ml increment of serum PSA, there was a 0.302 cc increase in total tumor volume and a 0.7% increase in relative tumor volume. Total tumor volume in cc was given as V(cc) = 3.476 + 0.302 X PSA (ng/ml) while the percent tumor volume Volume(%) = 11.331 + 0.704 X PSA (ng/ml).

Babaian et. al. [21] reported that multivariate regression analysis of tumor volume as a function of PSA, grade and stage demonstrated that log PSA had the strongest association with tumor volume. Tanaka [22] reported that among significant preoperative and postoperative parameters, calculated cancer volume remained an independent predictive parameter in multivariate analysis (P <0.01). Tumor volume, as calculated by preoperative parameters, was an independent predictor of biochemical recurrence in patients who had undergone radical prostatectomy. Vollmer et al. [23] used a compartmental model and first order kinetics to develop the calculation necessary to relate serum PSA to tumor volume. They found that the resulting model was a good fit to the observed kinetic data of PSA measured after biopsy or prostatectomy. The model also predicted a linear relationship between PSA and the sum of volumes of benign and malignant tissues.

Until evidence to the contrary, it is assumed that similar to colorectal tumors and CEA, there is a reasonable relationship between serum PSA and its kinetics allowing its use as a predictor of changes of prostate tumor volume and growth kinetics.

An important point when using serum PSA in calculations is that an exact interval for testing remains controversial, some investigators stress that the interval between PSA-DT determinations should approach 3-6 months [24] to limit error due to random variation of PSA values. Using a third generation highly sensitive PSA assay, our laboratory changes in PSA are precise to the third decimal point and allow educated decision-making based on monthly determinations.

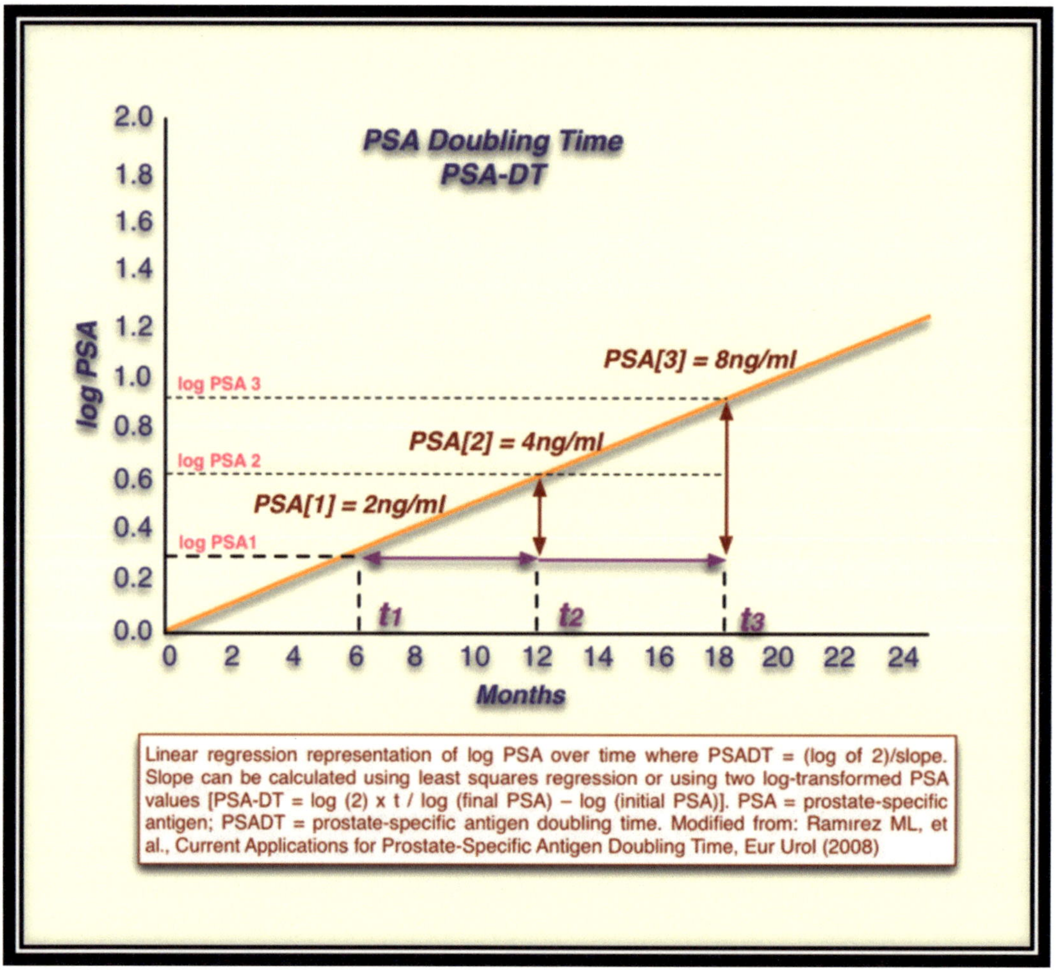

Figure 4. This figure is a semi-log plot of logs PSA (y-axis) vs. time (x-axis) [26]. Note the linear relationship, indicating that the rise of PSA values follows an exponential expansion of PSA.

Historically, PSA kinetics for watchful waiters included PSA-DT. A PSA-DT of >10 yr. can be considered favorable; a PSA-DT of <3-4 yr. suggests a change in biology and consideration should be given to an alternative therapy [25]. PSA kinetics should always be combined with other diagnostics such as endorectal ultrasound; endorectal MRI, digital rectal exam and repeat prostate biopsies approximately every 6-12 months.

4.3. PSA-DT as a surrogate for drug activity

PSA is one of the major androgen receptor-dependent target genes [27], and clinical monitoring is used to detect early stage disease as well as the emergence of recurrent tumor after therapy [28, 29, 30] and changes mirror changes in tumor bulk and indicate response to drugs. The graphic representation of PSA-DT is illustrated and its formula is given in Figure 4 [26].

Kelloff et al. [31], reviewed the use of PSA-DT as a surrogate for tumor response to drugs in patients with prostate cancer. They concluded that protocols that demonstrate significant changes in PSA-DT might be used to support accelerated approval of newer therapies. There is data to suggest PSA-DT in castrate resistant patients is predictive of outcome after chemotherapy [32]. An important caveat is expressed by Newling's review [33] of the subject which concluded that though dynamic changes in the PSA such as PSA-DT are commonly used in clinical trials of new drug therapies, PSA-DT might be affected by other factors including assay variations and false elevations of serum PSA caused by irritation of bladder catheters, prostatitis and cystitis. A substantial incidence of transient elevations of PSA (55%) was reported following combined external beam radiation and brachytherapy for prostate cancer [34]. These complicating issues should always be considered before PSA-DT is used to modify therapy.

Most recently, newer targeted and immunotherapies were found to produce paradoxical effects on PSA kinetics. Newling [33] argues that PSA should therefore be used as a secondary end point while overall survival still remains the gold standard in evaluating therapeutic efficacy for patients with hormone refractory disease.

5. Defining PSA response

Investigators participating in new prostate cancer drug trials commonly define PSA response according to the Bubley guidelines [35] for phase II clinical trials in androgen-independent prostate cancer. The guidelines qualify the following categories of PSA: PSA normalization, PSA $<=0.2$ ng/ml; PSA decrease, PSA decline $\geq 50\%$, confirmed by a second PSA value 4 or more weeks later; PSA progression, PSA $\geq 25\%$ increase over the baseline (and an increase in the absolute value PSA level by at least 5 ng/mL). Though useful for evaluating clinical trials, these PSA changes lack sensitivity when evaluating subtle drug effects vs. prostate tumor growth [36,37, 38].

Therasse [39, 40], in his thesis reports on MRI and PSA as tools in a RECIST evaluation used to define tumor response in prostate cancer patients with measurable soft tissue lesions. When comparing MRI soft tissue responses to serum PSA changes, the correlation of PSA and MRI showed agreement in 14 of the 20 (70%) patients.

6. PSA-DT and Survival of prostate cancer patients

The importance of PSA-DT in predicting survival is illustrated by Freedland et al. [41] Figure 5. This chart presents data for a group of patients experiencing biochemical recurrence of PSA after prostatectomy. Under these circumstances, PSA-DT clearly defined prostate cancer survival into four groups: 1) PSA-DT >=15 months, 2) PSA-DT 9-14 months 3) PSA-DT 3-8.9 months, 4) PSA-DT <3 months. For this study, PSA-DT is clearly a surrogate for prostate cancer-specific survival.

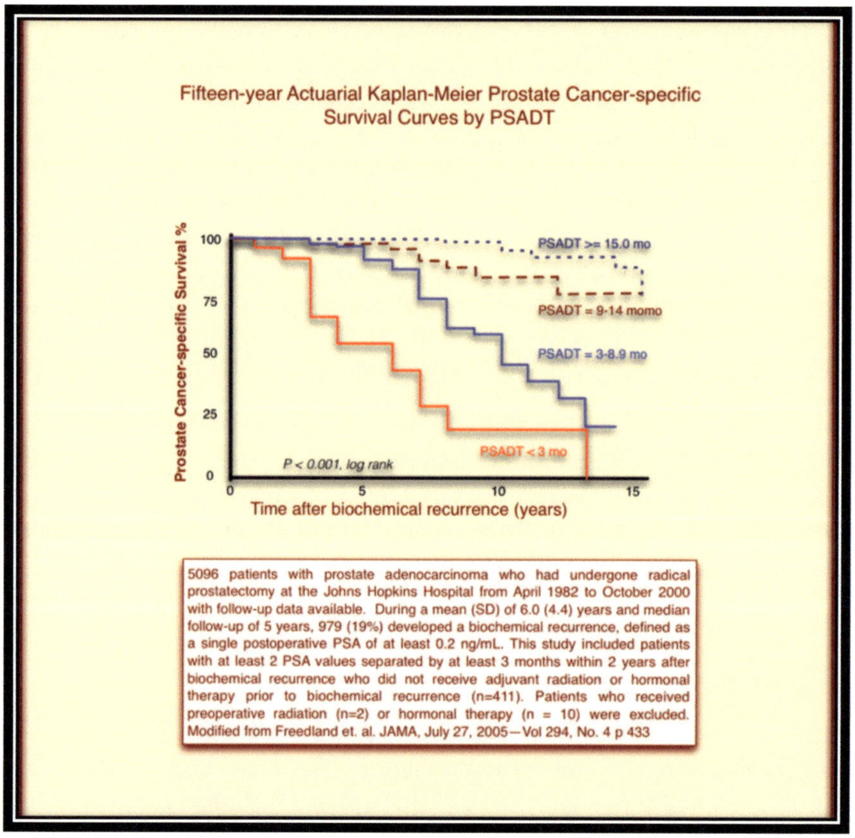

Figure 5.

7. PSA in the era of biologic and targeted therapy

A wealth of data establishes PSA as a marker of tumor aggressiveness, tumor stage, drug response and survival. Controversy and concern persists regarding PSA's role as a marker of disease stabilization and response induced by cytostatic and immunotherapies when compared to cytolytic therapies. An evaluation of the difficulties surrounding PSA interpretation has been addressed [42].

Two vaccine trials, Sipuleucel-T (Provenge) [43, 44, 45] and the TRICOM PROSTVAC [46, 47] demonstrated a significant overall survival benefit without any consistent decline in PSA, raising questions about the value of PSA response for non-hormonal, non-cytotoxic therapies. In addition, wide fluctuations have been observed in PSA values due to a transient effect of some drugs on PSA production seemingly independent of cell proliferation. The independent, non-proliferative effect of drugs on PSA expression should be considered when interpreting PSA response data. These aberrant PSA effects must be considered together with imaging results and clinical evaluation of the patient. Nevertheless, it has been consistent that post therapy a >50% PSA decline in pre-treatment PSA carries a significant overall survival advantage [48, 35].

Kelly [48] reported on 110 assessable patients treated on seven sequential protocols at Memorial Sloan-Kettering Cancer Center for hormone-refractory prostate cancer a statistically significant survival advantage in 110 patients with >50% PSA decline (>25 months survival) versus those without a 50% PSA decline (8.6 months survival). These results suggest that post therapy PSA declines can be used as a surrogate end point to evaluate new agents in hormone-refractory prostate cancer and criteria for response need prospective validation for phase III trials. Smith et al. [49] showed that a PSA decline > 50% for at least 8 weeks resulted in a longer mean survival time of 91 weeks versus 38 weeks for patients showing a smaller PSA reduction. An improved PSA response was associated with prolonged survival in the TAX 327 study (Docetaxel plus Prednisone or Mitoxantrone plus Prednisone for Advanced Prostate Cancer), with a median survival of 33 months when the PSA was normalized (<4 ng/mL) versus 15.8 months for an abnormal PSA [50, 51].

Heidenreich [52], the chair of the European Association of Urology oversaw the EAU 2012 Prostate Cancer Guidelines. He acknowledged that the PSA has been validated to be the most clinically useful tumor marker of treatment failure following local therapy and of tumor response as well as of tumor progression following hormonal treatment.

8. Assessment of molecularly targeted, cytostatic or anti-angiogenic agents

Bellmunt [53] and others expressed concern that PSA response criteria are not established to properly evaluate molecularly targeted cytostatic or anti-angiogenic agents [54]; therefore, certain drug-specific limitations may exist when using PSA or PSA-DT as an indicator of progression or response. One clear example was noted in a study of sorafenib (Nexavar) in castrate resistant prostate cancer, in which two patients with PSA progression were found to have dramatic resolution of bony disease [55]. Therapy-associated PSA "surge" has been described after effective chemotherapy. PSA surge occurs with Samarium^{153} radiotherapy, androgen deprivation and chemotherapy and is generally transient. The surge may be due to rapid lysis of prostate cancer cells thus spilling intracellular contents into the intravascular space [56]. Similarly, 10 of 16 patients who discontinued sorafenib and did not receive other therapy demonstrated post-discontinuation PSA declines of 7–52% [57]. The review by Bellmunt [58, 59] notes that several targeted therapies caused prolongation of the PSA-DT as well as significant suppression of PSA levels. The era of targeted therapy for prostate cancer is just beginning and will require changes in how we interpret PSA kinetics.

9. Considerations in evaluating tumor growth effects of targeted therapies

Newer targeted therapies are often cytostatic or cytolentic (slowing proliferation) [60], resulting in disease stabilization, improved quality of life and extended survival. Examples of such drugs include sorefinib (Nexavar) [61], axitinib (Inlyta) for renal cell carcinoma [62], and mTOR inhibitors (everolimus (Afinitor) [63] and temsirolimus (Torisel)). Dasitinib (Sprycel) and sorefinib (Nexavar) are active in prostate cancer. Dasatinib is active in chronic granulocytic leukemia and GIST, inhibits BCR/ABL tyrosine kinase, KIT, PDGFR and Src tyrosine kinase amongst other targets. The Src tyrosine kinase is instrumental in driving hormone-independent prostate cancers [64]. Dasatinib is active in castrate resistant prostate cancer and may be administered safely with docetaxel [65, 66].

These newer therapies target not only the tumor cell but also modify the supporting stroma and microvasculature. The cytostatic/cytolentic effects may leave the tumor dimensionally intact, stable on imaging studies but with slower or absent growth for extended periods of time. Some imaging techniques such as PET and MRI [67], able to quantify such metabolic effects, may enhance clinical evaluation while CT images appear unchanged.

There is mounting evidence that stabilization of tumor growth significantly prolongs overall survival to a degree similar to patients experiencing an objective response judged by RECIST or RECIST 1.1 criteria (Response Evaluation Criteria in Solid Tumors). This raises concern and new calls for modification of current RECIST categories to include new definitions for targeted responses [68].

Simple reductions in PSA levels as defined by Bubley [35] have not yet been validated as a surrogate end point for use in clinical trials of agents with novel mechanisms of action. As indicated, cytotoxic chemotherapy alone, in combination with molecular-targeted agents, or the sole use of targeted therapies, produces different and at times transient and paradoxical changes in serum PSA and further studies are needed to further define this issue.

As questions have emerged concerning the utility of PSA levels as a surrogate end point, the Prostate Cancer Clinical Trials Working Group reviewed the criteria for outcome measures in clinical trials that evaluate systemic treatment for patients with progressive prostate cancer. Recommendations conclude that PSA responses may be delayed in trials of non-cytotoxic agents, and rising PSA levels in the absence of other signs of progression should not lead to discontinuation of trials. This recommendation might lead to much consternation between the patient and doctor where discussion of the latest PSA value is often the primary subject during follow-up visits.

10. Projected tumor size and projected PSA uncover hidden drug activity

Now that surrogacy of static values of PSA and PSA-DT is being questioned for targeted therapies, new techniques of response evaluation are under study. One attempt to quantitate treatment efficacy redirects attention from PSA-DT to PSA-specific growth rate (PSA-SGR) [69, 70, 71]. Generally ignored, **projected tumor and marker value** play a particularly important role in uncovering and quantifying hidden, cytostatic or cytolentic drug effects. Projected tumor volume or marker value is calculated prior to the initiation of therapy and based on the specific growth rate constant (SGR) before the start of therapy. The projected value is illustrated in Figure 7. This growth projection captures the inherent tumor SGR before therapy and predicts what the outcome (projected tumor or marker volume/value) would be at any future date in the absence of treatment or tumor mutation. Older cytotoxic drugs, when effective, inhibit innate growth by programmed cell death and apoptosis resulting in autophagy and tumor cell lysis [60, 72]. This results in a measurable reduction of tumor size. Interestingly, these drugs are often in part cytostatic or cytolentic and depending on dose may result in stable disease. Keep in mind that prolongation of cytostatic or cytolentic suppression by any drug may eventually induce cytotoxicity and cell lysis [60] Figure 6.

Different combinations of static/lytic drug activity may result in reduced tumor/marker size or complete tumor growth inhibition without clinically detectable change in tumor size. Under these circumstances, use of **projected** growth uncovers hidden suppression of proliferation. A common clinical scenario occurs when during treatment, a tumor increases in size but much less than **projected**. Unless the clinician calculates what the **projected** tumor size should be, the true degree of tumor suppression is not appreciated Figure 7.

10.1. Mathematical relationships of exponentially growing tumors and projected tumor marker or tumor size/volume

The mathematical expression for exponential expansion of growth is: $V_t = V_0 e^{\alpha t}$ where the tumor volume at time V_t is predictable and is the product of the starting tumor volume [V_0] and [e = 2.71828, the base of the natural logarithm raised to the product of the specific growth rate constant α or (SGR) and the duration of growth Δt or (t_1-t_0)].

This is given as $V_t = V_0 e^{SGR * \Delta t}$ and mathematical rearrangement yields $SGR = \frac{\ln(\frac{V2}{V1})}{t2 - t1}$

Inhibitory drug effects slow SGR and are precisely quantifiable by calculating changes of SGR and the tumor size before and after therapy. Tumor size after therapy should be compared to the **projected** tumor size the same time after therapy. The current standard for clinical oncologists is comparison of tumor size before and after therapy while neglecting comparison with the **projected** tumor size. Differences between post therapy tumor size and the post therapy projected tumor size are the clue to hidden responses that are almost never evaluated by the clinical oncologist. These often-subtle differences between projected and post therapy tumor sizes may reveal hidden growth stimulation (mutation or idiosyncratic drug effect) as well as subtle growth inhibition, which may lead to prolonged clinical stability.

The following relationships, extracted from Mehrara's analysis [69,70,71] define projected tumor volume: $\int_{ti}^{t} \Delta\ SGR\,(t) * dt = \ln(\frac{Vn}{Vi}) - \ln(\frac{Vt}{Vi})$ where V_n = **projected** tumor volume, V_t = volume of tumor at the time of response evaluation and V_i is the volume at the initiation of therapy. The tumor response or TR = - $\ln(V_t/V_n)$ where V_t is the volume of treated tumor and V_n is the hypothetical or projected tumor volume, both evaluated at the time of efficacy assessment. These relationships are the model for the growth kinetics of exponentially growing tumors and generally require the use of at least a handheld computer to facilitate evaluation in the clinic. This is further discussed in the appendix.

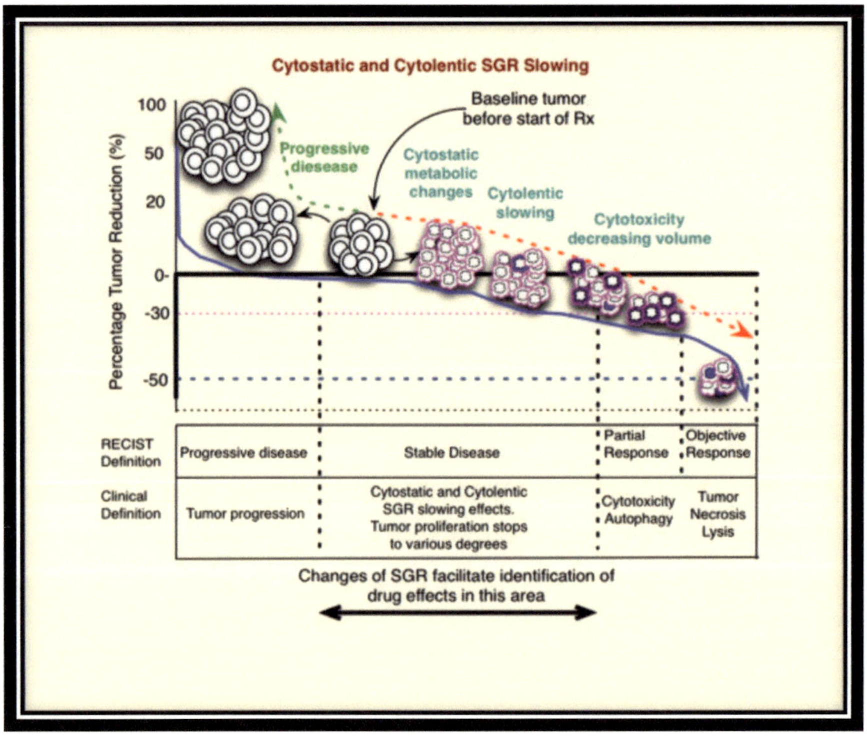

Figure 6. *In vitro and in vivo,* a clear distinction between cytostatic and cytolytic drugs does not exist. Low-dose cytolytic chemotherapy may exert cytostasis or so-called cytolentic slowing of cell proliferation leading to cell lysis, while targeted therapy's prolonged cytostatic metabolic effects (or large doses of targeted therapy) may induce cytolysis and autophagy (autophagocytosis). Regardless of mechanism of cell inhibition, the SGR and the TR (treatment response) calculations clearly and objectively define and quantitate drug efficacy (TR value).

Picture a 4.0 cm diameter (14.1 cc) pulmonary metastasis. At the time of discovery two months before the start of therapy the tumor was 3 cm (33.5 cc). The pre-therapy SGR for this tumor = 1.46%/d (tumor volume was expanding by 1.46%/d). Sixty-one days of therapy was administered and the tumor grew to 4.5 cm (47.7 cc). SGR decreased from 1.46%/d to 1%/d. Clinicians unaware of SGR and the projected tumor volume at this point might declare drug resistance however; **the projected tumor volume was actually 80.6 cc** and the tumor reached only 47.7 cc. Even though the tumor grew, therapy was significantly effective in slowing growth (59% of intrinsic tumor growth was inhibited)! The parameter for treatment efficacy, TR was +0.5. A positive value for TR means that therapy had some inhibitory activity against the tumor, the larger the value the better. A negative value means therapy was associated with growth stimulation. The value of TR is useful as an objective standard comparator to help evaluate efficacy between different treatments.

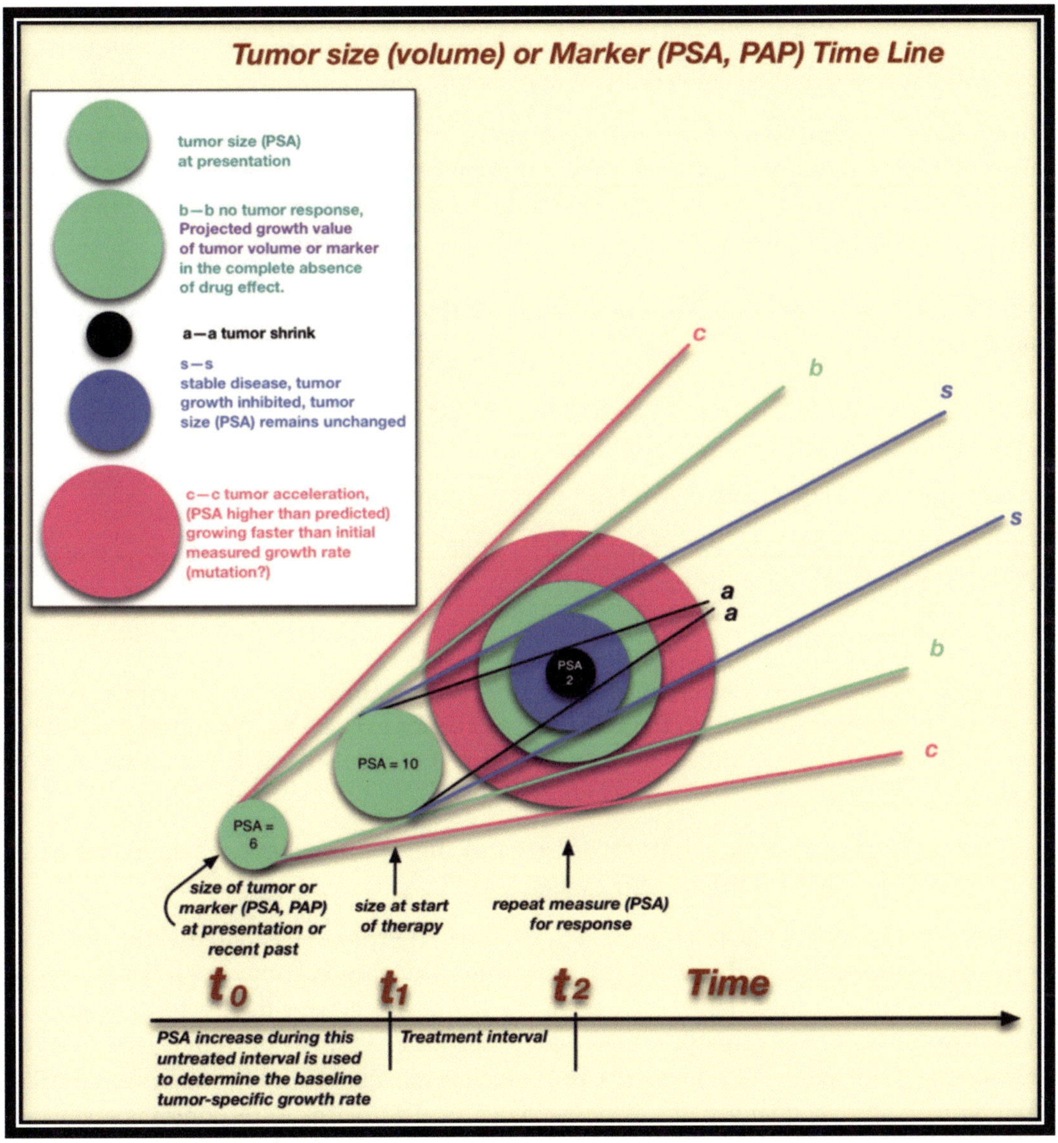

Figure 7. Tumor size (volume) or Marker (PSA, PAP) Time Line

Figure 7 illustrates potential tumor responses to drug treatment. Some of the responses such as positive and negative deviation from the **projected PSA** value or **projected tumor volume** are routinely overlooked in the clinic because **projected sizes** for these parameters must be calculated in advance (projected volume is illustrated by the largest b-b green circle at t_2). SGR is calculated based on tumor or PSA growth between t_0 and t_1. Deviations from **projected values** reveal subtle drug-tumor interactions. In the appendix we discuss straightforward evaluation of all five-treatment outcome scenarios illustrated above by a hand-held computer.

Until now, most attempts to capture drug effects vs. prostate tumors employed changes of PSA-DT. However, Mehrara [70] presented newer assessments of PSA-DT compared to PSA-SGR that cast doubt on the validity of that historic collection of work.

What follows is a general listing of consequences of drug-tumor interaction. These potential tumor or marker responses Figures 6, 7 are important to understand because subtle changes in tumor proliferation may be the only drug-induced tumor response and may go unnoticed when evaluating targeted therapy by RECIST/RECIST 1.1 response criteria.

10.2. Targeted therapies might require SGR calculations to evaluate the full spectrum of tumor response

Figures 6, 7 display tumor responses evaluable in the clinic. RESIST 1.1 criteria follow for comparison.

1. Disease stabilization (complete inhibition of pre-therapy SGR)

The marker or tumor's **inherent growth rate** is inhibited causing it or its surrogate marker value to remain unchanged during therapy.

2. Uninterrupted growth

The tumor or marker continues its calculated pre-therapy growth rate without change during therapy. The growth noted in the surrogate marker or tumor after therapy is predictable and equal to the projected tumor growth based on the calculated SGR before the start of therapy.

3. Tumor "response" of varied degree (note: at the time of response evaluation the tumor may be larger than the pre-therapy value)

Tumor or marker growth is inhibited and at post-therapy response evaluation the tumor or its surrogate marker is **less than the projected value**. This response may be difficult to identify since the tumor or its marker may have reached a size greater than before the start of therapy however, tumor or marker post therapy is **not as large as projected** based on the pre-therapy SGR Figure 7. A computer calculation comparing pre- and post-therapy SGR is required to accurately quantify this response category. TR (treatment response) is easily calculable and offers an objective and continuous value for the degree of response. TR is used as either a "tumor response" or "tumor marker response", to quantitate the effect of therapy. This continuous variable is useful to directly compare treatment efficacy between differing therapies.

Mehrara [71] defined some limitations for the current use of treatment response including: 1) PR and CR as defined in RECIST and other methods are no longer of value for quantifying responses to cytostatic/cytolentic drugs. Combinations of cytolytic and cytostatic/cytolentic therapies add further difficulty to response interpretation. A further problem arises when drugs are used at the extremes of dosing where tumor-killing activity may change from cytostatic/cytolentic to cytolytic and vise versa. 2) Classically, no consideration is given to the persistence of tumor SGR and or its inhibition during the course of therapy. Clinically, this is a trap for the oncologist if response is based solely in terms of whether the tumor marker or size is decreased at the end of therapy 3) The advantage of TR as a continuous variable (as opposed to a discrete variable used to compartmentalize responses such as CR, PR, SD) is that TR is a measurement of inhibitory (+TR) as well as accelerating (-TR) drug effects and is directly comparable between therapies and independent of mechanism of drug action.

A simple statement that the marker or tumor is larger post therapy is no longer adequate to evaluate tumor responses.

4. The size of the tumor or its surrogate marker decreases after therapy.

This may be a partial or complete return to normal, manifest by partial or complete disappearance of tumor/marker abnormality.

5. Tumor acceleration and deceleration

Tumor **acceleration** occurs when the tumor or marker growth rate (SGR) after therapy is greater than the pre-therapy or baseline SGR and SGR = (SGR after Rx − SGR before Rx) / (t2−t1) is a negative value. Tumor growth rate acceleration is positive and may indicate the presence of a tumor-accelerating mutation or an unexpected untoward drug effect.

Tumor **deceleration** occurs when SGR before therapy is greater than SGR after therapy and is expressed as: $SGR \text{ deceleration} = (SGR \text{ after Rx} - SGR \text{ before Rx}) / (t2 - t1)$ this is a negative value.

The rate of change calculations are based on the pre-therapy calculated SGR and its rate of change is calculated at the end of therapy and is expressed as: Acceleration or deceleration of the SGR: $\Delta SGR / \Delta t$. Or EDITOR use $(SGR_2\text{-}SGR_1)/(T_2\text{-}T_1)$.

Note: In the presence of multiple tumor targets the sum of tumor diameters or volumes is used as an approximation. Clonal heterogeneity (a mosaic of tumors growing at different growth rates and or demonstrating a mixed response) may make some tumors inadequate for analysis.

In 1999 an attempt to write a specific dogma evaluating tumor response resulted in the RECIST 1.0 criteria, later updated 2009 as RECIST 1.1 [73]. Note the absence of drug-response based on the concept of projected tumor growth.

RECIST 1.1 criteria

Complete Response (CR): Disappearance of all target lesions. Any pathological lymph nodes (whether target or non-target) must have reduction in short axis to <10 mm.

Partial Response (PR): At least a 30% decrease in the sum of diameters of target lesions, taking as reference the baseline sum of diameters.

Progressive Disease (PD): At least a 20% increase in the sum of diameters of target lesions, taking as reference the smallest sum on study (this includes the baseline sum if that is the smallest on study). In addition to the relative increase of 20%, the sum must also demonstrate an absolute increase of at least 5 mm. (Note: the appearance of one or more new lesions is also considered progression).

Stable Disease (SD): Neither sufficient shrinkage to qualify for PR nor sufficient increase to qualify for PD, taking as reference the smallest sum diameters while on study.

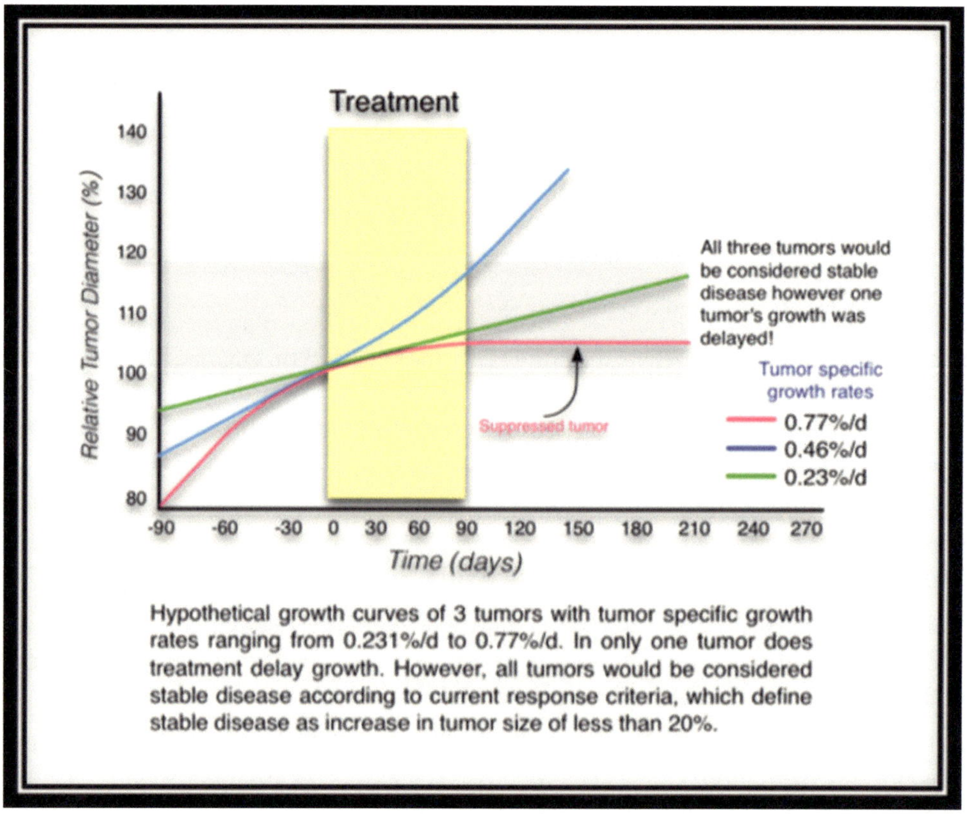

Figure 8. Weber [74] reveals the difficulty of classifying real growth inhibition within the RECIST1.1 criteria of stable disease. Real or suppressed tumor growth is illustrated by the pink growth curve only.

Weber noted that the RECIST 1.1 disease stabilization category does not differentiate between a drug that slows tumor growth and the complete lack of drug effect Figure 8. The RECIST 1.1 definition for disease progression is >5 mm absolute increase in size in addition to >20% increase compared with the nadir. In this figure, though all three tumors do not meet the progressive disease criteria and thus would be termed stable, the growth of the third was slowed by therapy. Though all three are termed stable, note the subtle difference between the two tumors showing a continued and uninterrupted pre-therapy growth rate (SGR), compared to the slowed growth rate of the tumor depicted by the red line. Surely there is a drug effect vs. the red tumor. This active drug could be overlooked in spite of its potential to increase survival if maintained for a sufficient period of time.

In a review of a group of patients treated with targeted therapies, Tourneau [75] revealed clinical evidence where investigators overlooked subtle cytostatic/cytolentic (slowing of SGR) drug activity Figure 6, 8. The group analyzed 50 patient participants in 18 targeted therapy drug trials. Among the 44 patients who withdrew from study because of disease progression according to the investigators' assessment, 18 patients (41%) demonstrated a favorable slowing trend in tumor specific growth rate. Among the 18, 5 had disease progression according to RECIST 1.1 according to retrospective reassessment of on-study imaging and occurrence of no new lesion during study treatment. Their preliminary evaluation concluded that a substantial proportion of patients treated with targeted agents were removed from protocol in spite of possibly benefitting from therapy.

Ferte et al. [76] studied metastatic renal cell carcinoma patients treated with sorafenib (Nexavar) and everolimus (Afinitor). Analysis of tumor SGR clearly revealed drug effects that would have been missed had RECIST response criteria been applied. Tumor response was assessed before, during, at the time of tumor progression and after drug discontinuation. Tumor growth rate was computed by dividing tumor shrinkage by the time between two related evaluations (% RECIST x 100 /day).

In two different patient populations (IGR and TARGET) tumor growth rate significantly decreased following sorafenib (-23.6 vs. 20 (IGR) and -19 vs. 22 (TARGET)) and everolimus (-5.2 vs. 30 (IGR)). The great majority of patients (IGR) had a decrease in the tumor growth rate during vs. before therapy, regardless of the RECIST evaluation, both with sorafenib (28/29) or everolimus (36/37). Growth rate after sorafenib or everolimus interruption was significantly higher than at the time of progression in both settings (IGR) (14.6 vs. 31 and 17.9 vs. 32.1 respectively). No significant difference was observed between growth rate before or after therapy for either sorafenib or everolimus (IGR). They concluded that SGR evaluation revealed: 1) better evaluation of tumor response, regardless of RECIST criteria, 2) had independent prognostic value, 3) the possibility that continuation of sorafenib or everolimus after disease progression might be beneficial to patients by sustaining a continued suppression of tumor growth.

The following section presents a model of tumor growth rate expressed as an executable algorithm in the form of an Apple App that quantitates subtle changes of tumor specific growth rate (SGR).

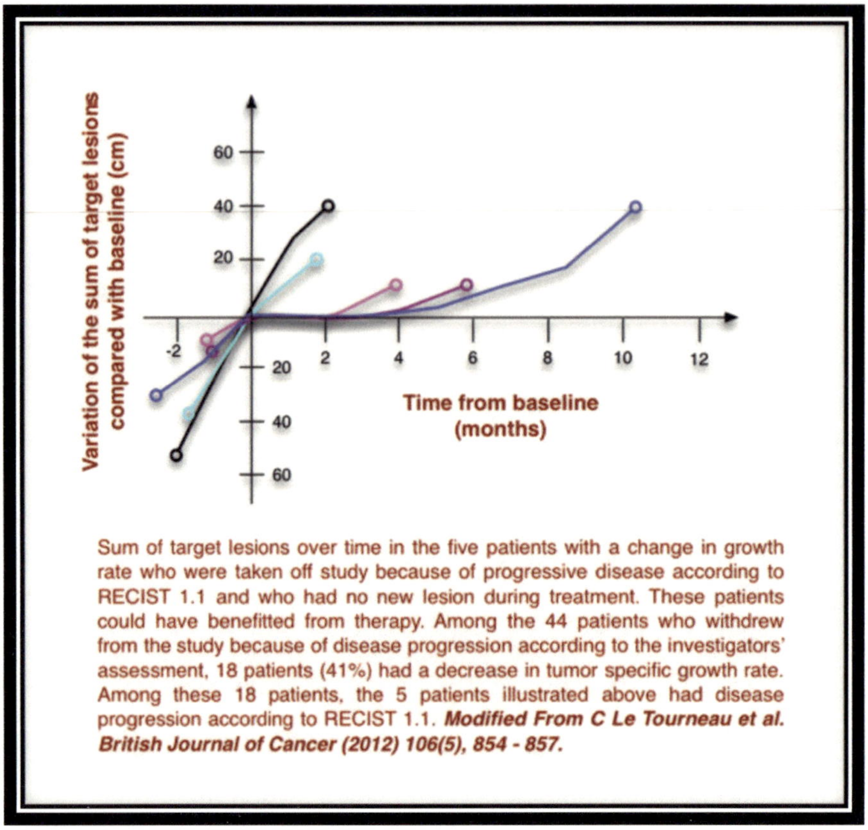

Figure 9. Following a patient's tumor size often reveals subtle changes in the slope of the tumor measurement or marker growth curve as revealed above. These subtle changes in growth rate are not associated with a significant decrease of tumor size or marker value. As Le Tourneau et al. and Ferte et al. demonstrate, subtle changes in tumor growth rate are not evaluated as a response when applying RECIST 1.1 criteria nevertheless, they do represent a true cytostatic effect of targeted therapies that may translate into a meaningful prolonged survival.

11. SGR is a useful tool to identify subtle drug-associated tumor or marker kinetic changes of tumors

Mehrara, as part of his PhD thesis at the Department of Radiation Physics, University of Gothenburg, Goteborg, Sweden presented an analysis of tumor growth kinetics based on the tumor specific growth rate constant (SGR). The analysis assumes that for most practical purposes clinically observable tumor growth follows exponential growth. Additionally, this is true for the surrogate PSA tumor marker. SGR is rapidly calculable by hand-held mobile devices and facilitates the rapid identification of tumor responses easily overlooked in the clinic, many of which are not readily apparent without computer analysis. Occasionally, changes of SGR uncover subtle tumor stimulation.

Construction of the exponential growth curve, similar in shape to the mid portion of the Gompertzian curve Figure 1, requires just two different measurements of tumor volume (or diameter, area, cell number) or a surrogate marker at two different times to satisfy the exponential growth equation: $Vt = V0\,e^{at}$. Here "α" is the exponential growth constant, and V_t and V_0 are the tumor volume at times t and t_0, respectively. This model implies that tumor volume can increase indefinitely and the growth rate of a tumor is proportional to its volume and dV/dt =aV .

SGR is the relative change in tumor volume per unit time calculable as percent increase or decrease of tumor volume per unit time. Excluding mutations, for exponentially growing tumors, SGR is constant, *i.e.*, SGR or α is independent of tumor volume or age. Faster growing tumors have higher SGR values, SGR=0 represents non-growing tumors; a negative SGR represents tumor regression. In 1956 Collins et al. [9] graphically introduced the concept of tumor doubling time. The DT formulation was proposed in 1961 [10]: $DT = (t_2\text{-}t_1) * \ln(2) / [\ln(V_2/V_1)]$. Other relationships of importance include the specific growth rate, $SGR = \ln(V_2/V_1)/(t_2\text{-}t_1)$ and $DT = \ln(2)/SGR$. These equations are descendants of the primary exponential growth equation, $V_t = V_0e^{at}$

Mehrara expresses concerns based on his mathematical treatment of SGR and DT suggesting that for clinical studies, SGR is the best indicator of tumor growth. Tumor growth rate, especially but not limited to urology circles, is usually quantified as DT i.e. PSA-DT. Because of the subtle mathematical relationship between SGR and DT, use of DT alone to evaluate therapeutic effects may give erroneous results.

Mehrara's studies revealed that DT has several drawbacks when used to describe tumor or tumor marker growth rates. The shortfalls include 1) for brief measurement time intervals, or high volume and very small measurement uncertainties the mean DT can either overestimate or underestimate the average growth rate; 2) DT approaches infinity for very slow growing tumors and is mathematically limited while SGR is a continuous variable no mater the speed and 3) the non normal frequency distribution of DT values restricts use of parametric statistics thus reducing use of more discriminatory statistics especially when studying small samples [77]. Unlike DT, SGR is definable for all tumor volume changes no matter how small, and it is Gaussian (normally) distributed allowing use of parametric statistics. SGR is more accurate to use when considering growth fraction, cell loss rate, and tumor growth rate heterogeneity. For these reasons, Mehrara opines that SGR be used instead of DT, to quantify tumor growth rate.

Accuracy and clinical outcome analysis comparing SGR and DT would be a valuable area of research in light of the cytostatic changes leading to subtle changes of growth rate characteristic of targeted therapies. Later, an in depth illustration of the differences between DT and SGR will help illuminate this issue.

Collins and Schwartz [9, 10] both analyzed several tumors in patients as they defined the use of tumor volume doubling time. Note that for bronchogenic lung cancers a semi-logarithmic plot of tumor diameter (y-axis) versus a linear time period (x-axis) produces a near straight line Figure 2.

12. Measuring tumor growth

It is imperative to depend on sensitive and precise marker assays. Guess [38] tried to address this problem by use of splines or line segments to average all PSA-DT values in an attempt to better detect therapy-induced changes of PSA-DT. Unfortunately, this computerized technique is cumbrous for most to apply.

The accurate and reproducible measurement of tumor diameters from imaging studies is critical. Keep in mind that occasionally plain radiographs of larger lesions are preferred because CT imaging may slice through a lesion at variable levels producing aberrant results for elliptical lesions.

A closer look at differences between DT and SGR.

The mathematical relationship between DT and SGR as revealed by the exponential growth model is important because as displayed in Figure 10, sole use of tumor volume doubling time (TV-DT) or tumor marker doubling time (PSA-DT) rather than tumor or marker specific growth rate as a measure of treatment outcome may be destined for failure depending on the magnitude of differences in the clinical study. Applying the exponential model of tumor growth to published studies reporting only DT as displayed here Table 1,2 and Figures 11,12 reveals discordant conclusions from those using SGR. Note that the DT is mathematically logarithmically related to the inverse of the exponential growth constant (SGR): SGR = ln(2)/DT.

The opposite results using SGR compared to those obtained with DT are critical since prostate cancer research is steeped in the use of the PSA-DT to predict survival, tumor dissemination, relapse, and tumor response to drugs and hormones and to radiation efficacy. In the prostate cancer literature use of DT as a parameter of response is established canon.

Mehrara reveals that DT is not normally symmetrically distributed (non-Gaussian distribution) and its use as an indicator of treatment response could yield inaccurate conclusions. Changes in DT over-predict drug effects in slow growing tumors while they under-predict in rapidly growing tumors and DT is essentially of no value for tumor volumes (or markers) that show no change in value (stable disease) where DT approaches infinity see Figure 10.

Work by others confirms the importance of the tumor or marker-specific growth rate. Stein et al. [46] studied a combination of equations that simultaneously modeled both tumor/ PSA regression and tumor/PSA exponential growth. They found that only the exponential growth equation with its specific growth rate constant (PSA-SGR) predicted a statistically significant high mortality hazard ratio of 5.14 (95% confidence interval, 3.10 - 8.52) in his study group of patients with prostate cancer. The disease regression formula was unable to predict patient mortality.

http://dx.doi.org/10.5772/53179

13. Why PSA-SGR is more useful than PSA-DT

As noted in Figure 10, when SGR is fast and increases 1% from 4 to 5%/day, the doubling time changes 1.3-fold from 4 to 3 days (a slight change). However, when the SGR is slower and increases 1% from 1 ▪ 2%/d, doubling time changes four-fold from 69 to 17 days (a large change). A DT of 1-day does not represent the same growth rate when the tumor is slowing as when the tumor is rapidly growing. As the absolute value of SGR approaches zero, DT approaches infinity and is of no practical use other than to say the tumor or marker is stable. Because of the DT-SGR relationship at the extremes of tumor or marker growth, therapy-induced changes in doubling times at the extremes of SGR do not accurately represent the magnitude of the impact of therapy.

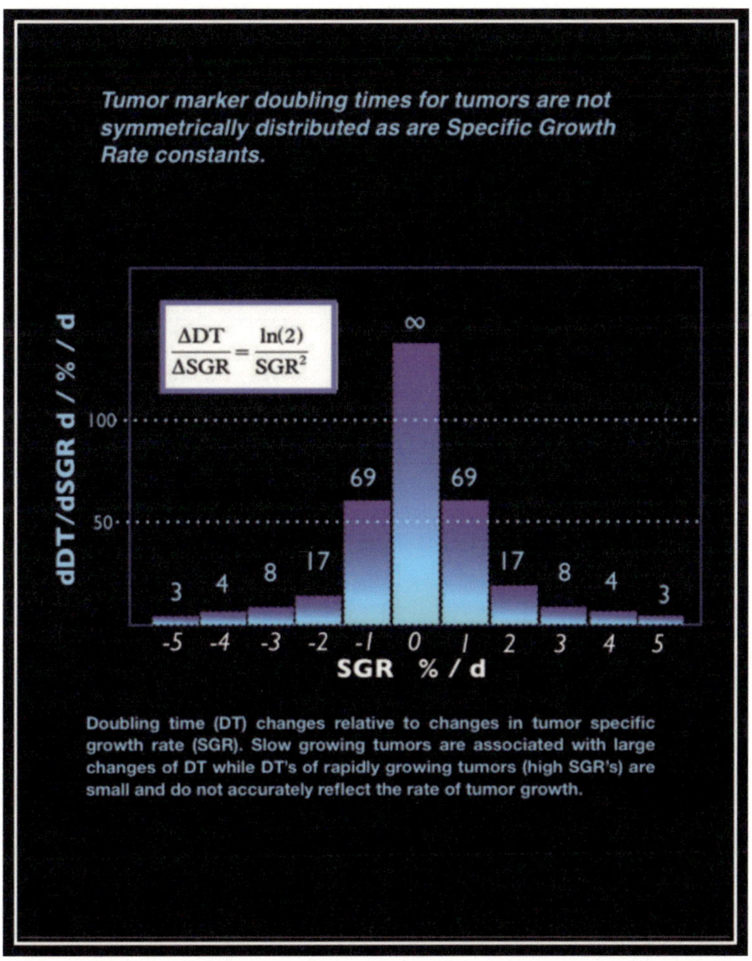

Figure 10. This figure, modified from Mehrara [70], displays the variation of tumor volume doubling time or tumor marker doubling time (DT) per unit change of tumor specific growth rate (SGR) based on:.

14. Clinical application of DT and SGR: Discordant results

Mehrara retrieved data from two previously published clinical studies [70]. The first by Guess et al. [38] Table 1 who studied the effect of modified citrus pectin (MCP) on PSA-DT of 12 prostate cancer patients. Mehrara extracted data and analyzed for both PSA-DT and PSA-SGR before and after therapy. The difference between PSA-DT before and after treatment was not found to be statistically significant by the paired t-test (p = 0.27). Nevertheless, when transforming PSA-DT to PSA-SGR the difference before and after MCP treatment is statistically significant by the paired t-test (p = 0.003) and nonparametric Wilcoxon matched pairs signed rank test: p = 0.002. Thus, a therapy initially deemed ineffective by PSA-DT analysis, when analyzed for a group of patients based on PSA-SGR proved to be highly significant Table 1.

Effect of modified citrus pectin (MCP) on PSA-DT and PSA-SGR

Patient	Before Rx PSA-DT (mo)	After Rx PSA-DT (mo)	Before Rx PSA-SGR (%/mo)	After Rx PSA-SGR (%/mo)
A	3.97	13.34	17.46	5.16
B	5.67	10.11	12.22	6.86
C	1.14	2.91	60.80	23.82
D	3.37	7.71	20.57	8.99
E	1.58	16.49	43.87	4.20
F	10.5	7.97	6.60	8.70
G	2.66	11.95	26.06	5.80
H	3.64	3.27	19.04	21.20
I	2.04	4.96	33.98	13.97
J	2.33	3.24	29.75	21.39
K	6.29	-155.49	11.02	-0.45
L	5.12	-645.51	13.54	-0.11
	Nonparametric Wilcoxon matched pairs signed rank: p = 0.42 Parametric Paired t-test p = 0.2704		Nonparametric Wilcoxon matched pairs signed rank: p = 0.002 Parametric Paired t-test p = 0.0027	

Table 1. Guess et al. [38] studied the effect of modified citrus pectin (MCP) on PSA-DT of 12 prostate cancer patients. Mehrara extracted that data and analyzed both PSA-DT and PSA-SGR before and after therapy. The difference between PSA-DT before and after treatment was not statistically significant by the paired t-test (p = 0.27). Nevertheless, when transforming PSA-DT to PSA-SGR the difference before and after MCP treatment is statistically significant by the paired t-test (p = 0.003) and nonparametric Wilcoxon matched pairs signed rank test: p = 0.002.

A second analysis of original data by Nishida et al. (1999) [78] was based on a study of the correlation of tumor volume and the CA19-9 tumor marker of pancreatic cancer patients Table 2. The correlation between CA19-9-DT and tumor volume-DT was statistically significant (p<0.0001). However, after converting tumor-volume-DT to TV-SGR and CA19-9-DT to CA19-9-SGR, correlation between CA19-9-SGR and TV-SGR was no longer statistically significant (p>0.3). Since SGR is the preferred parameter, the initial analysis of Nishida may benefit from a second look.

Relationship between CA19-9-DT and TV-DT vs. CA19-9-SGR and TV-SGR				
Patient	**CA19-9 DT (Days)**	**Tumor-DT (Days)**	**CA19-9-SGR %/day**	**Tumor-SGR %/day**
A	8.3	34.8	8.4	2
B	39.7	44.6	1.7	1.6
C	46.3	34.5	1.5	2
D	36.5	21.2	1.9	3.3
E	30.4	47.7	2.3	1.5
F	67.1	112.8	1	0.6
G	44.7	70.6	1.6	1
H	24.7	18.4	2.8	3.8
I	42.7	50.6	1.6	1.4
J	137.5	231.6	0.5	0.3
K	42.3	39.3	1.6	1.8
	Linear regression: $r^2 = 0.89$ $p < 0.0001$		Linear regression: $r^2 = 0.09$ $p = 0.37$	

Table 2. This table displays the extracted data from Nishida's study [78] of the correlation of tumor volume and the CA19-9 tumor marker of pancreatic cancer patients. The correlation between CA19-9-DT and tumor volume-DT was statistically significant (p<0.0001). However, after converting tumor-volume-DT to TV-SGR and CA19-9-DT to CA19-9-SGR, correlation between CA19-9-SGR and TV-SGR was no longer statistically significant (p>0.3).

Most prostate cancer studies employ changes in the PSA-DT. PSA-DT values are not normally distributed and thus not readily subject to more sensitive parametric statistical analysis. However, PSA-specific growth rate is normally distributed and parametric statistics can be applied. Nonparametric statistical methods lose discriminatory power especially for clinical studies of smaller groups of patients [77].

During a cursory review of the literature we found two additional studies, one dealing with the effects of celecoxib on PSA-DT Figure 11 and the other investigating the effects of a combination of calcitriol and naproxin on PSA-DT of prostate cancer patients Figure 12.

Smith et al. [79] Figure 11 studied the biologic activity of celecoxib, a selective cyclooxygenase-2 inhibitor, in men with recurrent prostate cancer using change in PSA-DT as the primary outcome variable. We carefully extracted the data from his graphic report. We applied the Wilcoxon matched-pairs signed rank test [two tailed] (for nonparametric distribution of

PSA-DT) to the data. PSA-DT before versus after celecoxib was highly significant: $p = 0.0006$. After transformation of PSA-DT to PSA-SGR, the Paired t-test [two tailed] for parametric distribution of PSA-SGR suggests that the celecoxib effect lacked statistical significance $p = 0.213$!

A second study by Srinivas [80] Figure 12 evaluated naproxen in combination with calcitriol in patients with early recurrent prostate cancer. All patients received 45 μg of calcitriol (DN101, Novacea, South San Francisco, CA, USA) orally once a week with naproxen 375 mg twice a day and were evaluated for a biochemical PSA response and a change in PSA doubling time (PSA-DT). Testing the efficacy of the combination therapy using changes of PSA-DT by the non-parametric Wilcoxon matched-pairs signed rank test [two tailed] $p = 0.037$ a significant difference. However, after transforming PSA-DT to PSA-SGR ($SGR_{PSA} = \ln(2)/DT_{PSA}$), analysis with the parametric Paired t-test [2-tailed] indicate naproxen plus calcitriol was not effective in slowing tumor growth, $p = 0.213$.

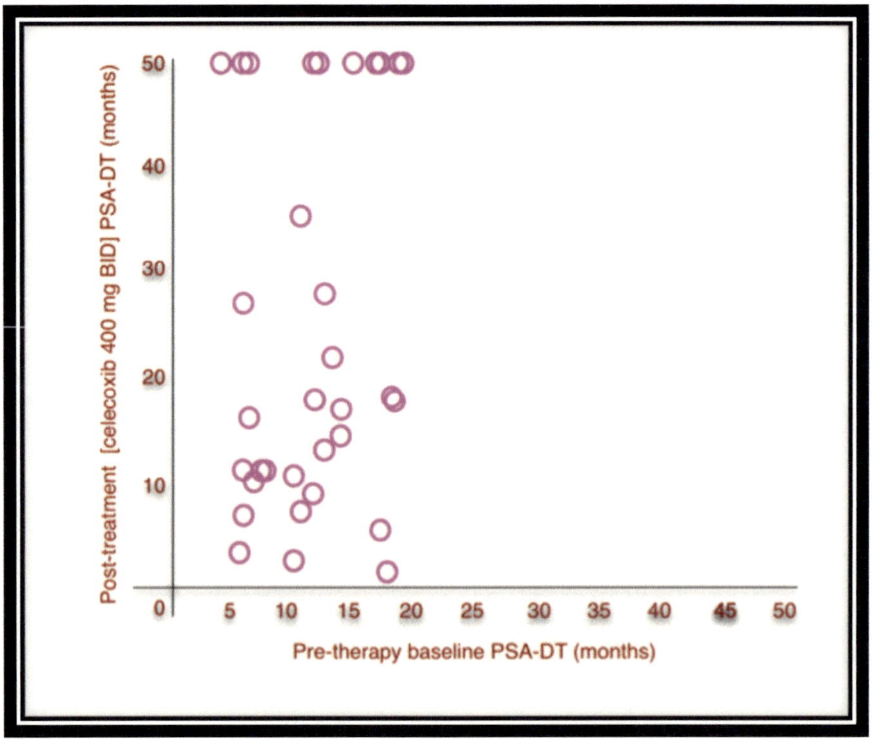

Figure 11. Smith et al. [79] studied the biologic activity of celecoxib, a selective cyclooxygenase-2 inhibitor, in men with recurrent prostate cancer using change in PSA-DT as the primary outcome variable. We retrieved their graphic data for our own analysis. A histogram of the PSA-DT paired differences for before and after celecoxib appears normally distributed. Applying the parametric Paired t-test statistic for significance of the difference yields $p = 0.0002$. Next, we transformed the same (before-after celecoxib PSA-DT data with to PSA-SGR before and after pairs and applied the paired t-test. Contrary to the statistical analysis for celecoxib induced change of PSA-DT, changes of PSA-SGR revealed that the celecoxib difference was no longer significant, $p = 0.213$!

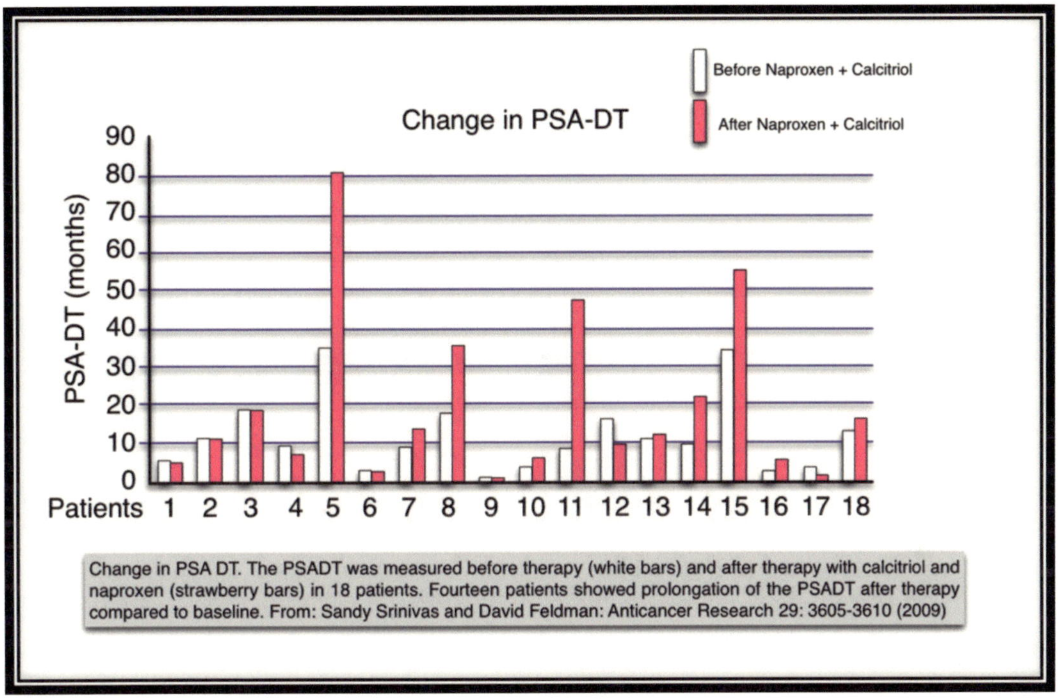

Figure 12. Sinivras and Feldman [80] evaluated naproxen in combination with calcitriol in patients with early recurrent prostate cancer. All patients received 45 µg of calcitriol (DN101, Novacea, South San Francisco, CA, USA) orally once a week with naproxen 375 mg twice a day and were evaluated for a biochemical PSA response and a change in PSA doubling time (PSA-DT). Applying the paired t-test for statistical significance (before PSA-DT and after PSA-DT) resulted in p = 0.034. Nevertheless, after transforming PSA-DT to PSA-SGR (PSA-SGR = ln(2)/PSA-DT), analysis with the paired t-test [2-tailed] suggested naproxen plus calcitriol was not effective in slowing tumor growth, p = 0.213.

The non-linear relationship between the SGR and DT may be responsible for erroneous interpretations of treatment effects reported in prior prostate cancer trials that published results solely in terms of changes in PSA-DT Figure 10.

15. Evaluation of tumor and surrogate marker drug responses, rate of change of response: *SGR* acceleration = (*SGR* after Rx − *SGR* before Rx) / ($t2-t1$) ; A positive number

The dynamic of PSA change was used as an early predictor of overall survival after a short exposure to docetaxel therapy (4 doses). Knowledge that a drug may extend survival after just a short exposure would minimize toxicity from ineffective drugs. Hannenin's work [81] found that a rapid rate of PSA decline expressed as PSA half-life <70 days was associated with a longer overall-survival Figure 13. This result was independent of other known markers of survival and allowed for a greater survival differentiation than PSA suppression alone. Response-time evaluations may play a new role in determining drug efficacy earlier than usual. I would propose study of an alternate expression for tumor acceleration or deceleration in terms of SGR as: SGR (accel…decal) = SGR2-SGR1/(t_2-t_1). The value of this expression may be positive for acceleration or negative for deceleration.

De Crevoisier [82] found that a PSA decline 6 weeks after the start of EBRT when used as monotherapy and 3 months after the start of androgen deprivation therapy (ADT) in patients treated with combined ADT and external beam radiation is predictive of progression and specific survival.

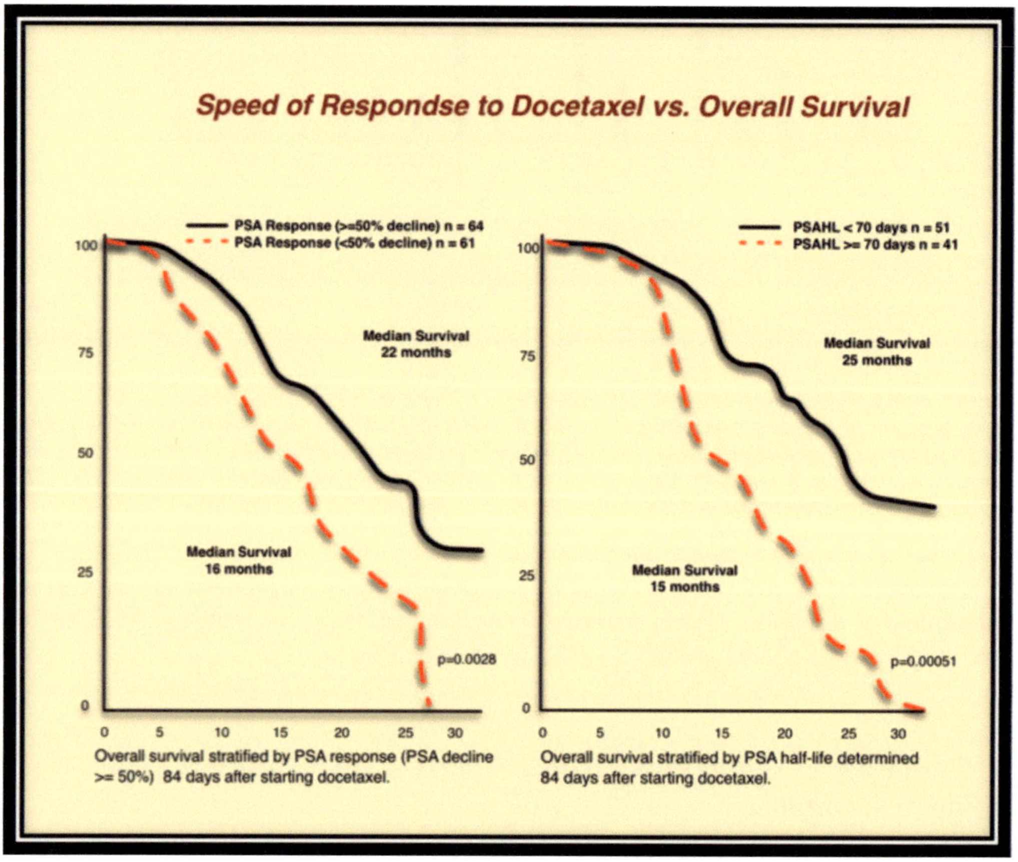

Figure 13. Treatment-associated tumor/marker deceleration in response to docetaxel. The magnitude of rate of change (acceleration-deceleration) of SGR resulting from therapy is an early predictor of prostate-specific survival.

Figure 14 illustrates a computer analysis of a prostate cancer patient treated with docetaxel. A pelvic node is noted to grow over 4.5 months from 1.3 to 1.6 cm in greatest dimension. This establishes the pre-therapy SGR of 0.46%/d and the tumor volume (assuming a sphere) before starting therapy is 2.1 cc. Fifty-one days of therapy induces a decrease of tumor diameter to 0.9 cc and a decrease of tumor volume to 0.38 cc. Had the tumor grown uninterrupted the project-

http://dx.doi.org/10.5772/53179

ed tumor volume would have been 2.7 cc. In this case, the value for deceleration of SGR for the tumor: is given as $(SGR2 \text{ after Rx} - SGR1 \text{ before Rx}) / (t2 - t1) = -0.021\% / d / d$.

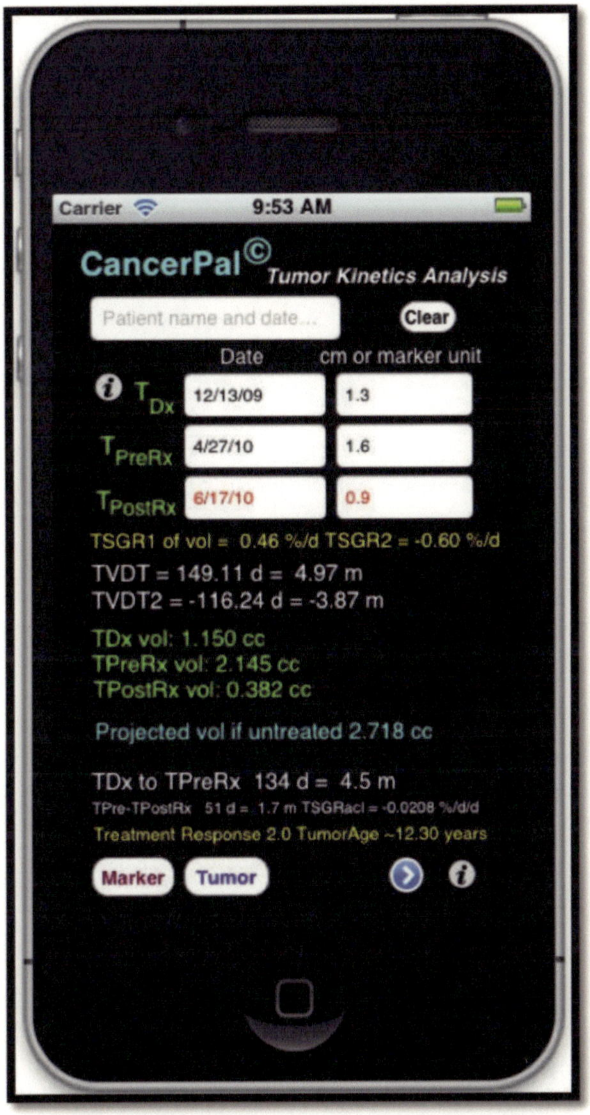

Figure 14. This calculation displays results for a patient treated with docetaxel (see text).

This is an objective measure of the rate of change of SGR. The treatment response is displayed as = + 2.0. This assigns a calculated continuous variable as a measure of the degree of response and is used to objectively compare docetaxel efficacy to any other administered drug. Positive TR values represent tumor reduction compared to the **projected** tumor size while a negative TR represents tumor growth relative to the **projected** size. Estimated age of tumor, here approximated ~ 12.3 years, is a calculated value based on the initial SGR of 0.46%/d in the absence of therapy. This assumes constant, continuous exponential growth over many years. Tumor age calculations are gross approximations and notoriously subject to large error.

Figure 15 illustrates the evaluation for a 68 year-old man undergoing watchful waiting for a Gleason score 3+3 = 6, T1c prostate cancer. Three PSA values are displayed for three sequential dates. When the patient was asked if he had changed medication between 3/2/11 and 5/1/11 he noted he was ingesting a new Chinese herbal mixture sold to enhance energy and libido.

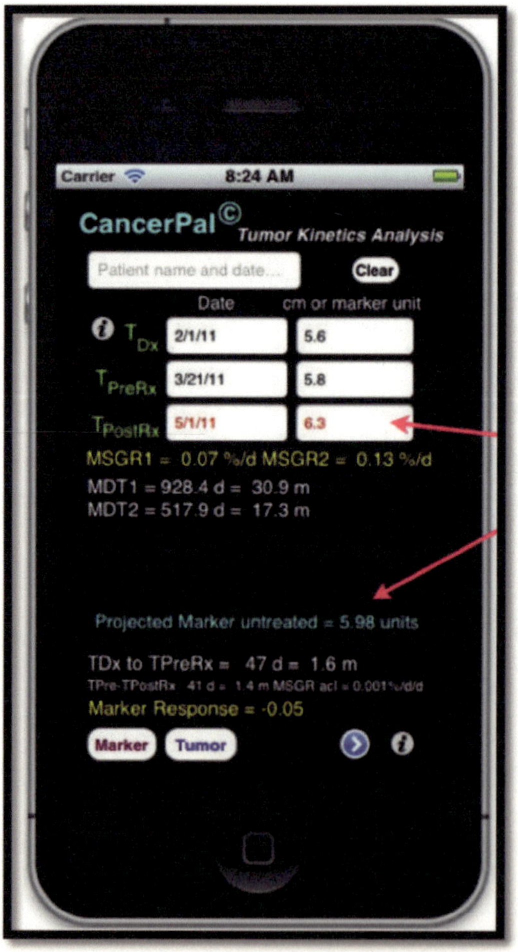

Figure 15. Evaluation of a 68 year-old man undergoing watchful waiting for a Gleason score 3+3 = 6, T1c prostate cancer. The patient was ingesting a stimulatory Chinese herb.

Subtle acceleration of the tumor marker value was uncovered by inspection of the projected PSA value for 5/1/11 as compared to the actual measured value for that date. Notice the confirmative quantitative measures given by the calculation Figure 14 of the marker specific growth rate $MSGR_2$ = 0.13%/d compared to $MSGR_1$ = 0.07 %/d; marker doubling time MDT2 = 17.3 months compared to the initial MDT_1 = 30.9 months; by both the positive value for MSGR acceleration = +0.001%/d/d and by the negative value for marker response MR = -0.05. Based on the marker-specific growth rate (MSGR) for the first interval TDx thru TPRx (the date at initiation of therapy) of 0.07%/d, the App calculated the expected PSA on 5/1/11 to be 5.98 ng/ml. However, the measured value was higher = 6.3 ng/ml. The negative value for MR of -0.05 indicates a negative marker response thus PSA expansion (marker acceleration confirmed this = +0.001%/d/d). We suspected that the Chinese herb might have caused subtle acceleration of PSA production and or tumor growth. Other explanations for acceleration of the PSA value include decreased clearance of PSA or the subtle appearance of a mutated, faster growing clone of PSA-producing tumor cells. Note that in the absence of knowledge of the inherent initial PSA-SGR between 2/1/11 and 3/2/11 and calculation of the expected **projected** value of PSA for 5/1/11, the subtle PSA acceleration would have been missed.

16. Predicting approximate tumor size or marker value for any arbitrary date in the future

Assuming untreated clinical cancers and their markers expand at a relatively constant exponential rate, it is possible to predict values for tumor diameter, volume and marker for any arbitrary future date. Figure 16 displays a PSA projection made for a patient with newly diagnosed prostate cancer who asked if a preplanned three-month holiday before initiation of therapy could jeopardize his chance for a curative procedure. The prediction, assuming constant exponential expansion of serum PSA, is that the PSA value upon returning from sabbatical would increase from 9.4 to 16.28 ng/ml. This alarmed the patient and he cancelled the trip to initiate therapy.

17. Unique treatment paradigms may be suggested by analysis of tumor growth rate

Figure 17 illustrates results for a patient with pancreatic cancer post Whipple procedure who was found on 6/4/10 to have an enlarged peri-aortic mass = 1.8 cm (3.1 cc). Repeat CT on 8/27/10 noted increased size to 2.9 cm (12.8 cc). Therapy with gemcitabine was initiated on 8/27/10. Post therapy reevaluation of the mass on 12/24/10 revealed growth to 3.1 cm (15.6 cc). The patient was discouraged and frightened and thought he had wasted precious

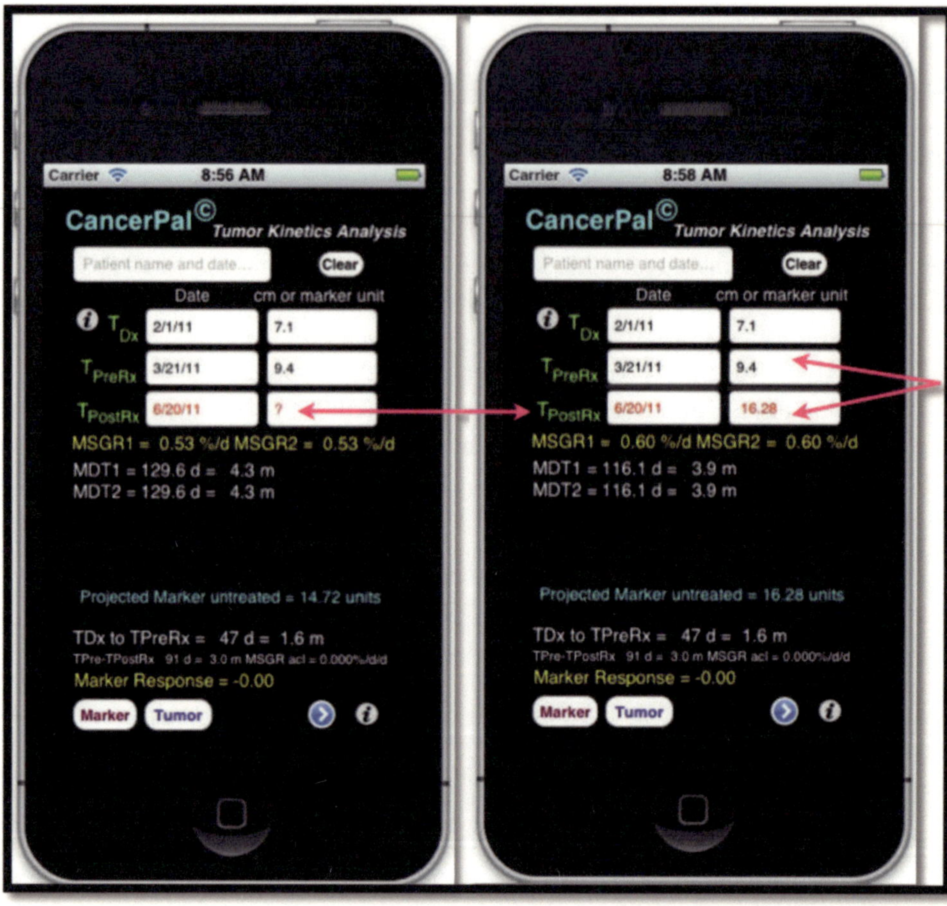

Figure 16. PSA projection made for a patient with newly diagnosed prostate cancer

time and subjected himself to undo toxicity for no gain. However, evaluation revealed that had the tumor never been treated with gemcitabine it would have reached the **projected volume** of 96.9 cc by 12/24/10. Thus, based on the initial exponential growth rate from 6/4/10 thru 8/27/10, the tumor volume was actually 84% **less than what it would have been** had no drug been given (15.6 cc vs. 96.9 cc).

This patient experienced substantial tumor suppression by gemcitabine in spite of its growth. Under these circumstances, when there are poor second choices for effective therapy, instead of discarding gemcitabine, perhaps addition of another compound with differing toxicity might be a reasonable option.

http://dx.doi.org/10.5772/53179

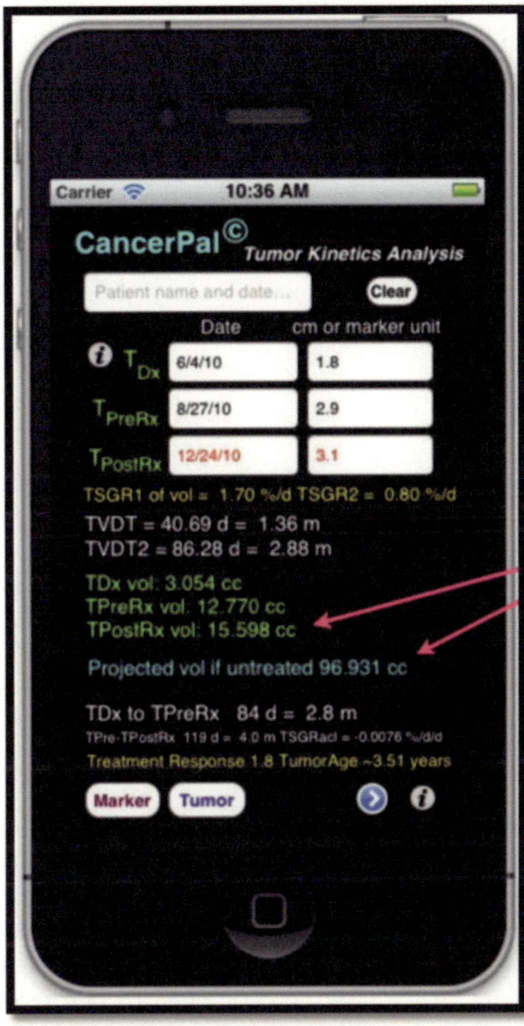

Figure 17. The tool we developed to facilitate calculation of tumor kinetics is named CancerPal©. The software App is available from Apple Corporation's App store. The App analyzes kinetic changes of tumor markers and or tumor diameter/volume/area and is run on the iPhone, iPad, or iPod. Clinical use is facilitated by the small size and portability of the new hand-held devices. The App is routinely used in our clinic for objectively measuring subtle drug effects on tumor and the dynamics of surrogate tumor markers. A video tutorial of the App is available at www.healthsciencereports.com.

18. Conclusion

Several principles of prostate cancer management rely on the absolute and dynamic values of various formulations of PSA i.e. PSA-V, PSA-DT and PSA-SGR. This review introduces SGR, a parameter that is underused and closely reflects the true growth rate of tumors undergoing exponential expansion. Several instances are presented where results of studies employing PSA-DT yield statistically divergent results after converting PSA-DT to PSA-SGR. It is recommended that for some studies results be reevaluated in terms of PSA specific growth rate, PSA-SGR.

Newly introduced targeted therapies require innovative techniques to evaluate drug efficacy. Tumor or tumor marker specific growth rate and the concept of **projected** tumor or marker value are tools capable of quantitatively evaluating subtle effects of targeted drugs. Calculation of the **projected** tumor size and tumor marker values is critical to properly evaluate subtle drug-tumor proliferative outcomes.

Appendix

CancerPal©

It is important to realize that CancerPal© remains an experimental tool used strictly for analysis of clinical and laboratory data by cancer researchers, pharmacists or clinical research radiation and medical oncologists. The methods used in designing this tool have been discussed primarily in the references listed below with special attention given to the work of Mehrara et al. PNA, A Limited Liability Corporation, cannot be held responsible for any treatment modifications or recommendations made based on this research tool.

What CancerPal© does

CancerPal© evaluates whether a chemotherapy or targeted therapy should be continued alone, possibly dropped or added to by revealing concealed drug activity causing suppression of the tumor specific growth rate. The app uncovers occult efficacy of drugs by comparing the measured drug-induced tumor size vs. the projected tumor size or projected tumor-marker value that would occur in the absence of any therapy. Sudden changes in tumor growth rate suggesting drug related tumor stimulation or a detrimental, growth-promoting mutation is rapidly identified. CancerPal© may uncover hidden tumor acceleration unexpectedly caused by drugs, immunosuppression or alternative therapies thought to be harmless

CancerPal© uses a tumor's specific growth rate (TSGR) defined as percentage increase in volume per day or percentage increase in the specific tumor marker per day thus avoiding errors inherent in the doubling time calculation which consistently overestimates the growth rate of slowly growing tumors and underestimates the growth rate of rapidly growing tumors.

This app predicts the tumor diameter or tumor marker value at any time in the future assuming constant exponential tumor or tumor marker growth over the period of observation. This, when compared to the actual measured tumor diameter or marker value, identifies tumor response, stability or acceleration. The app predicts a tumor marker or diameter at any time point in the future based on patient-specific tumor kinetics. CancerPal© may quickly alert the clinician of emergence of a mutant, more aggressive, rapidly dividing clone of tumor cells suggesting a review of therapy. Analysis based on continual exponential growth for the relatively short time (several months) in the multi-year history of tumor growth has been found to be more useful for kinetic calculations in spite of some tumors demonstrating Gompertzian growth over the long haul (several years)

Continuous variables for Tumor Response (TR) and Marker Response (MR) allow for quantitation of drug/biological response modulator effects. Negative values of TR and MR indicate tumor acceleration, values close to or equal to zero indicate lack of response while positive values confirm beneficial tumor response. Responses are numerically quantitated and elusive disease stability may now numerically be defined by a continuous variable. Drugs previously thought to be of no value may be found to induce useful and profound disease stability

The software is helpful for those patients followed by watchful waiting/active surveillance for prostate or any other cancer. Prostate tumors changing biological behavior are immediately identified in a quantitative and objective manner by rapidly uncovering changes in PSA kinetics without the errors inherent in the PSA doubling time (PSA-DT) parameter. The software can help determine whether metastectomy is a reasonable treatment modality for some patients with pulmonary metastasis [83].

CancerPal© uses the exponential growth constant as described by John Spratt to extrapolate backwards to approximate the time of tumor initiation in years based on the rate of growth

Patient data required for analysis

Three dates and three associated measurements of a tumor marker or tumor diameter

- TDx (date at diagnosis + marker value or tumor diameter in cm)
- TPreRx (date of initiation of Rx + marker value or tumor diameter in cm)
- TPostRx (date of measurement of drug effect + tumor marker value or diameter in cm).

CancerPal© information output:

- Tumor Specific Volume Growth Rates for two intervals ($TSGR_1$ and $TSGR_2$)
- Tumor Marker Specific Growth Rates for two intervals ($MSGR_1$ and $MSGR_2$)
- Tumor Specific Growth Rate acceleration and deceleration
- Tumor Volume Doubling Times for two intervals (TVDT)
- Tumor Marker Doubling Time for two intervals (MDT)
- Projected TSGR and MSGR at any user designated time in the future
- Treatment Response as both Tumor Response and Tumor Marker Response, both as continuous numerical values used to quantitate the effect of therapy. Negative numbers reveal growth acceleration; values of zero reveal no effect and positive values indicate varying degrees of therapeutic efficacy.

- Tumor volumes in cc are calculated for TDx, TPreRx and TPostRx.
- Extrapolates back to the time of tumor initiation thus calculating how long it took for the tumor to reach the initial tumor diameter.
- Calculates approximate time to death in the absence of therapy, assuming constant tumor growth rate.

Acknowledgements

Peter Jahn, Whittier, CA for manuscript review and discussion, mathematical suggestions and statistical considerations.

Author details

Glenn Tisman

Whittier Cancer Research Building, Whittier, CA, USA

References

[1] Bassukas ID. Comparative gompertzian analysis of alterations of tumor growth patterns. Cancer Res 1994, Aug 15; 54(16): 4385-92.

[2] Demicheli R, Foroni R, Ingrosso A, Pratesi G, Soranzo C, Tortoreto M. An exponential-gompertzian description of lovo cell tumor growth from in vivo and in *vitro data*. Cancer Res 1989, Dec 1; 49(23): 6543-6.

[3] Norton L. A gompertzian model of human breast cancer growth. Cancer Res 1988, Dec 15;48(24 Pt 1):7067-71.

[4] Mottram JC. On the correlation between malignancy and the rate of growth of tar warts in mice. Cancer Res 1934, Dec; 22(4): 801-30.

[5] Mottram JC. A further consideration of the growth rates of tar warts in mice and of their autografts. The American Journal of Cancer 1936; 28(1): 115-20.

[6] Laird AK. Dynamics of normal growth. Annual Report 1964; 6971:52.

[7] Laird AK. Dynamics of tumour growth: Comparison of growth rates and extrapolation of growth curve to one cell. Br J Cancer 1965; 19(2): 278.

[8] Friberg S, Mattson S. On the growth rates of human malignant tumors: Implications for medical decision-making. J Surg Oncol 1997, Aug; 65(4): 284-97.

[9] Collins VP, Loeffler RK, Tivey H. Observations on growth rates of human tumors. Am J Roentgenol Radium Ther Nucl Med 1956, Nov; 76(5): 988-1000.

[10] Schwartz M. A biomathematical approach to clinical tumor growth. Cancer 1961; 14:1272-94.

[11] Spratt JS, Spjut HJ, Roper CL. The frequency distribution of the rates of growth and the estimated duration of primary pulmonary carcinomas. Cancer 1963, Jun; 16:687-93.

[12] Spratt Jr JS, Spratt TL. Rates of growth of pulmonary metastases and host survival. Ann Surg 1964; 159(2): 161.

[13] Steel GG, Lamerton LF. The growth rate of human tumours. Br J Cancer 1966, Mar; 20(1): 74-86.

[14] Loeb S, Kettermann A, Ferrucci L, Landis P, Metter EJ, Carter HB. PSA doubling time versus PSA velocity to predict high-risk prostate cancer: Data from the Baltimore longitudinal study of aging. Eur Urol 2008, Nov; 54(5): 1073-80.

[15] Tosoian J, Loeb S. PSA and beyond: The past, present, and future of investigative biomarkers for prostate cancer. ScientificWorldJournal 2010; 10:1919-31.

[16] Klotz L, Teahan S. Current role of PSA kinetics in the management of patients with prostate cancer. European Urology Supplements 2006, Apr; 5(6): 472-8.

[17] D'Amico AV, Chen MH, Roehl KA, Catalona WJ. Preoperative PSA velocity and the risk of death from prostate cancer after radical prostatectomy. N Engl J Med 2004, Jul 8; 351(2): 125-35.

[18] D'Amico AV, Chen MH, de Castro M, Loffredo M, Lamb DS, Steigler A, et al. Surrogate endpoints for prostate cancer-specific mortality after radiotherapy and androgen suppression therapy in men with localised or locally advanced prostate cancer: An analysis of two randomised trials. Lancet Oncol 2012, Feb; 13(2): 189-95.

[19] Miyamoto S. A chronological study of hepatic metastasis from colorectal cancer. Jpn J Gastroenterol Sur 1991;24:1990-6.

[20] Kato RB, Srougi V, Salvadori FA, Ayres PP, Leite KM, Srougi M. Pretreatment tumor volume estimation based on total serum psa in patients with localized prostate cancer. Clinics (Sao Paulo) 2008, Dec; 63(6): 759-62.

[21] Babaian RJ, Troncoso P, Steelhammer LC, Lloreta-Trull J, Ramirez EI. Tumor volume and prostate specific antigen: Implications for early detection and defining a window of curability. J Urol 1995, Nov; 154(5): 1808-12.

[22] Tanaka N, Fujimoto K, Hirayama A, Nakai Y, Chihara Y, Anai S, et al. Calculated tumor volume is an independent predictor of biochemical recurrence in patients who underwent retropubic radical prostatectomy. Adv Urol 2012; 2012:204215.

[23] Vollmer RT, Humphrey PA. Tumor volume in prostate cancer and serum prostate-specific antigen. Analysis from a kinetic viewpoint. Am J Clin Pathol 2003, Jan; 119(1): 80-9.

[24] Carter HB, Pearson JD, Waclawiw Z, Metter EJ, Chan DW, Guess HA, Walsh PC. Prostate-specific antigen variability in men without prostate cancer: Effect of sampling interval on prostate-specific antigen velocity. Urology 1995, Apr; 45(4): 591-6.

[25] Van den Bergh RC, Roemeling S, Roobol MJ, Wolters T, Schröder FH, Bangma CH. Prostate-specific antigen kinetics in clinical decision-making during active surveillance for early prostate cancer--a review. Eur Urol 2008, Sep; 54(3): 505-16.

[26] Ramírez ML, Nelson EC, Devere White RW, Lara PN, Evans CP. Current applications for prostate-specific antigen doubling time. Eur Urol 2008, Aug; 54(2): 291-300.

[27] Lonergan PE, Tindall DJ. Androgen receptor signaling in prostate cancer development and progression. J Carcinog 2011; 10:20.

[28] Bidart JM, Thuillier F, Augereau C, Chalas J, Daver A, Jacob N, et al. Kinetics of serum tumor marker concentrations and usefulness in clinical monitoring. Clin Chem 1999, Oct; 45(10): 1695-707.

[29] Nash AF, Melezinek I. The role of prostate specific antigen measurement in the detection and management of prostate cancer. Endocr Relat Cancer 2000, Mar; 7(1): 37-51.

[30] Ryan CJ, Smith A, Lal P, Satagopan J, Reuter V, Scardino P, et al. Persistent prostate-specific antigen expression after neoadjuvant androgen depletion: An early predictor of relapse or incomplete androgen suppression. Urology 2006;68(4):834-9.

[31] Kelloff GJ, Coffey DS, Chabner BA, Dicker AP, Guyton KZ, Nisen PD, et al. Prostate-specific antigen doubling time as a surrogate marker for evaluation of oncologic drugs to treat prostate cancer. Clin Cancer Res 2004, Jun 1; 10(11): 3927-33.

[32] Oudard S, Banu E, Scotte F, Banu A, Medioni J, Beuzeboc P, et al. Prostate-specific antigen doubling time before onset of chemotherapy as a predictor of survival for hormone-refractory prostate cancer patients. Ann Oncol 2007, Nov; 18(11): 1828-33.

[33] Newling DW. Issues with the use of prostate-specific antigen as a surrogate end point in hormone-resistant prostate cancer. European Urology Supplements 2009, Jan;8(1): 13-9.

[34] Singh AK, Guion P, Susil RC, Citrin DE, Ning H, Miller RW, et al. Early observed transient prostate-specific antigen elevations on a pilot study of external beam radiation therapy and fractionated MRI guided high dose rate brachytherapy boost. Radiat Oncol 2006; 1:28.

[35] Bubley GJ, Carducci M, Dahut W, Dawson N, Daliani D, Eisenberger M, et al. Eligibility and response guidelines for phase II clinical trials in androgen-independent

prostate cancer: Recommendations from the prostate-specific antigen working group. J Clin Oncol 1999, Nov; 17(11): 3461-7.

[36] WOO TCS, Richard Choo MD, Mary Jamieson RN, Chander BSNDS. Vitamin D3 (cholecalciferol) in the treatment of biochemically-relapsed prostate cancer. .

[37] Guess BW, Scholz MC, Strum SB, Lam RY, Johnson HJ, Jennrich RI. Modified citrus pectin (MCP) increases the prostate-specific antigen doubling time in men with prostate cancer: A phase II pilot study. Prostate Cancer Prostatic Dis 2003;6(4):301-4.

[38] Guess B, Jennrich R, Johnson H, Redheffer R, Scholz M. Using splines to detect changes in PSA doubling times. Prostate 2003, Feb 1; 54(2): 88-94.

[39] Therasse P, Arbuck SG, Eisenhauer EA, Wanders J, Kaplan RS, Rubinstein L, et al. New guidelines to evaluate the response to treatment in solid tumors. European organization for research and treatment of cancer, national cancer institute of the United States, national cancer institute of canada. J Natl Cancer Inst 2000, Feb 2; 92(3): 205-16.

[40] Therasse, P. Response assessment in cancer clinical trials. Doctorate thesis; Erasmus University, Rotterdam, 2006.

[41] Freedland SJ, Humphreys EB, Mangold LA, Eisenberger M, Dorey FJ, Walsh PC, Partin AW. Risk of prostate cancer-specific mortality following biochemical recurrence after radical prostatectomy. JAMA 2005, Jul 27; 294(4): 433-9.

[42] Armstrong AJ, Eisenberger MA, Halabi S, Oudard S, Nanus DM, Petrylak DP, et al. Biomarkers in the management and treatment of men with metastatic castration-resistant prostate cancer. Eur Urol 2012, Mar; 61(3): 549-59.

[43] Gupta S, Carballido E, Fishman M. Sipuleucel-T for therapy of asymptomatic or minimally symptomatic, castrate-refractory prostate cancer: An update and perspective among other treatments. Onco Targets Ther 2011; 4:79-96.

[44] Garcia JA. Sipuleucel-T in patients with metastatic castration-resistant prostate cancer: An insight for oncologists. Ther Adv Med Oncol 2011, Mar; 3(2): 101-8.

[45] Bitting RL, Armstrong AJ, George DJ. Management options in advanced prostate cancer: What is the role for sipuleucel-t? Clinical Medicine Insights: Oncology; 5:325-32.

[46] Stein WD, Gulley JL, Schlom J, Madan RA, Dahut W, Figg WD, et al. Tumor regression and growth rates determined in five intramural NCI prostate cancer trials: The growth rate constant as an indicator of therapeutic efficacy. Clin Cancer Res 2011, Feb 15; 17(4): 907-17.

[47] Madan RA, Bilusic M, Heery C, Schlom J, Gulley JL. Clinical evaluation of TRICOM vector therapeutic cancer vaccines. Semin Oncol 2012, Jun; 39(3): 296-304.

[48] Kelly WK, Scher HI, Mazumdar M, Vlamis V, Schwartz M, Fossa SD. Prostate-specific antigen as a measure of disease outcome in metastatic hormone-refractory prostate cancer. J Clin Oncol 1993, Apr; 11(4): 607-15.

[49] Smith DC, Dunn RL, Strawderman MS, Pienta KJ. Change in serum prostate-specific antigen as a marker of response to cytotoxic therapy for hormone-refractory prostate cancer. Journal of Clinical Oncology 1998; 16(5): 1835-43.

[50] Berthold DR, Pond GR, Soban F, de Wit R, Eisenberger M, Tannock IF. Docetaxel plus prednisone or mitoxantrone plus prednisone for advanced prostate cancer: Updated survival in the TAX 327 study. J Clin Oncol 2008, Jan 10; 26(2): 242-5.

[51] Berthold DR, Pond GR, de Wit R, Eisenberger M, Tannock IF, TAX 327 Investigators. Survival and PSA response of patients in the TAX 327 study who crossed over to receive docetaxel after mitoxantrone or vice versa. Ann Oncol 2008, Oct; 19(10): 1749-53.

[52] Heidenreich A, Bolla M, Joniau S, Van Der Kwast TH, Matveev V, Mason MD, et al. Guidelines on prostate cancer. Eur Urol 2008; 53(1): 68-80.

[53] Bellmunt J, Rosenberg JE, Choueiri TK. Recent progress and pitfalls in testing novel agents in castration-resistant prostate cancer. Eur Urol 2009; 56(4): 606.

[54] Loriot Y, Massard C, Fizazi K. Recent developments in treatments targeting castration-resistant prostate cancer bone metastases. Ann Oncol 2012, May; 23(5): 1085-94.

[55] Dahut WL, Scripture C, Posadas E, Jain L, Gulley JL, Arlen PM, et al. A phase II clinical trial of sorafenib in androgen-independent prostate cancer. Clin Cancer Res 2008, Jan 1; 14(1): 209-14.

[56] Thuret R, Massard C, Gross-Goupil M, Escudier B, Di Palma M, Bossi A, et al. The postchemotherapy PSA surge syndrome. Ann Oncol 2008, Jul; 19(7): 1308-11.

[57] Chi KN, Ellard SL, Hotte SJ, Czaykowski P, Moore M, Ruether JD, et al. A phase II study of sorafenib in patients with chemo-naive castration-resistant prostate cancer. Ann Oncol 2008, Apr; 19(4): 746-51.

[58] Bellmunt J, Rosenberg JE, Choueiri TK. Recent progress and pitfalls in testing novel agents in castration-resistant prostate cancer. Eur Urol 2009; 56(4): 606.

[59] Bellmunt J, Oh WK. Castration-resistant prostate cancer: New science and therapeutic prospects. Ther Adv Med Oncol 2010, May; 2(3): 189-207.

[60] Rixe O, Fojo T. Is cell death a critical end point for anticancer therapies or is cytostasis sufficient? Clin Cancer Res 2007, Dec 15; 13(24): 7280-7.

[61] Nabhan C, Tolzien K, Lestingi T, Kelby SK, Galvez AG, Bitran JD. Activity of sorafenib (SOR) in chemotherapy-failure castration-resistant prostate cancer (CRPC). ASCO/GU Proceedings 2010; 122.

[62] Carmichael C, Lau C, Josephson DY, Pal SK. Comprehensive overview of axitinib development in solid malignancies: Focus on metastatic renal cell carcinoma. Clin Adv Hematol Oncol 2012 May; 10(5): 307-14.

[63] Baselga J, Campone M, Piccart M, Burris HA, Rugo HS, Sahmoud T, et al. Everolimus in postmenopausal hormone-receptor-positive advanced breast cancer. N Engl J Med 2012, Feb 9; 366(6): 520-9.

[64] Kung HJ. Targeting tyrosine kinases and autophagy in prostate cancer. Horm Cancer 2011, Feb; 2(1): 38-46.

[65] Adamo V, Noto L, Franchina T, Chiofalo G, Picciotto M, Toscano G, Caristi N. Emerging targeted therapies for castration-resistant prostate cancer. Front Endocrinol (Lausanne) 2012; 3:73.

[66] Agarwal N, Sonpavde G, Sternberg CN. Novel molecular targets for the therapy of castration-resistant prostate cancer. Eur Urol 2012, May; 61(5): 950-60.

[67] Brindle K. Watching tumours gasp and die with MRI: The promise of hyperpolarised 13C MR spectroscopic imaging. Br J Radiol 2012, Jun; 85(1014): 697-708.

[68] Rosen MA. Use of modified RECIST criteria to improve response assessment in targeted therapies: Challenges and opportunities. Cancer Biol Ther 2010, Jan; 9(1): 20-2.

[69] Mehrara E, Forssell-Aronsson E, Ahlman H, Bernhardt P. Specific growth rate versus doubling time for quantitative characterization of tumor growth rate. Cancer Res 2007, Apr 15; 67(8): 3970-5.

[70] Mehrara E, Forssell-Aronsson E, Ahlman H, Bernhardt P. Quantitative analysis of tumor growth rate and changes in tumor marker level: Specific growth rate versus doubling time. Acta Oncol 2009; 48(4): 591-7.

[71] Mehrara E, Forssell-Aronsson E, Bernhardt P. Objective assessment of tumour response to therapy based on tumour growth kinetics. Br J Cancer 2011, Aug 23; 105(5): 682-6.

[72] Elmore S. Apoptosis: A review of programmed cell death. Toxicol Pathol 2007, Jun; 35(4): 495-516.

[73] Eisenhauer EA, Therasse P, Bogaerts J, Schwartz LH, Sargent D, Ford R, et al. New response evaluation criteria in solid tumours: Revised RECIST guideline (version 1.1). Eur J Cancer 2009, Jan; 45(2): 228-47.

[74] Weber WA. Assessing tumor response to therapy. J Nucl Med 2009, May; 50 Suppl 1:1S-10S.

[75] Le Tourneau C, Servois V, Diéras V, Ollivier L, Tresca P, Paoletti X. Tumour growth kinetics assessment: Added value to RECIST in cancer patients treated with molecularly targeted agents. Br J Cancer 2012, Feb 28; 106(5): 854-7.

[76] Ferte C, Albiges L, Soria JC, Loriot Y, Fizazi K, Escudier BJ. The use of tumor growth rate (TGR) in evaluating sorafenib and everolimus treatment in mrcc patients: An in-

tegrated analysis of the TARGET and RECORD phase III trials data. J Clin Oncol 30, 2012 (suppl; Abstr 4540).

[77] Motulsky H. Intuitive statistics a nonmathematical guide to statistical thinking. Second Ed. New York: Oxford University Press; 2010k.

[78] Nishida K, Kaneko T, Yoneda M, Nakagawa S, Ishikawa T, Yamane E, et al. Doubling time of serum CA 19-9 in the clinical course of patients with pancreatic cancer and its significant association with prognosis. J Surg Oncol 1999, Jul; 71(3): 140-6.

[79] Smith MR, Manola J, Kaufman DS, Oh WK, Bubley GJ, Kantoff PW. Celecoxib versus placebo for men with prostate cancer and a rising serum prostate-specific antigen after radical prostatectomy and/or radiation therapy. J Clin Oncol 2006, Jun 20; 24(18): 2723-8.

[80] Srinivas S, Feldman D. A phase II trial of calcitriol and naproxen in recurrent prostate cancer. Anticancer Res 2009, Sep; 29(9) : 3605-10.

[81] Hanninen M, Venner P, North S. A rapid PSA half-life following docetaxel chemotherapy is associated with improved survival in hormone refractory prostate cancer. Can Urol Assoc J 2009, Oct; 3(5): 369-74.

[82] De Crevoisier R, Slimane K, Messai T, Wibault P, Eschwege F, Bossi A, et al. Early PSA decrease is an independent predictive factor of clinical failure and specific survival in patients with localized prostate cancer treated by radiotherapy with or without androgen deprivation therapy. Ann Oncol 2010, Apr; 21(4): 808-14.

[83] Lee JH, Gulec SA, Kyshtoobayeva A, Sim MS, Morton DL. Biological factors, tumor growth kinetics, and survival after metastasectomy for pulmonary melanoma. Ann Surg Oncol 2009, Oct; 16(10): 2834-9.

Section 5

Medical Treatment

Chapter 10

Rational Categorization of the Pipeline of New Treatments for Advanced Cancer – Prostate Cancer as an Example

Sarah M. Rudman, Peter G. Harper and Christopher J. Sweeney

Additional information is available at the end of the chapter

http://dx.doi.org/10.5772/53092

1. Introduction

1.1. The problem

Whilst improvements in patient survival have been realized for a number of haematological and solid malignancies in the last 30 years, new efficacious systemic anti-cancer treatments are still needed. The current, widely used drug development paradigm is often associated with a poor conversion rate from experimental to licensed drug. This process involves a significant investment of resources from sponsors, investigators and patients and to date has only lead to a limited chance of success. At present there are in excess of 800 anti-cancer agents in development and less than 10 new FDA approvals each year [1]. In order to address this problem there has been considerable debate concerning the best trial methodology to rationalize this process, with discussion of the timing, sequence and design of appropriate trials [2]. At present in many tumour types including breast, lung, renal cell and prostate cancer, the pipeline of new agents is crowded. In order therefore to use the available financial and patient resource wisely, it is crucial to identify the key important pathways in oncogenesis that in turn may help and prioritize the drugs with the most promise.

1.2. A promising future

In recent years advances in molecular biology have aided our understanding of the pathogenesis of cancer. This has occurred concurrently with technological advances allowing rational drug design and development (such as tyrosine kinase inhibitors, monoclonal antibodies and anti-sense oligonucleotides). Combining these two advances has been very beneficial in the drug development process such that we now have a wealth of opportunities. The challenge now is how to rationally categorize and prioritize the many strategies that can be deployed. In the discussion below, we propose a rational process to evaluate the merits of different strategies and use prostate cancer as an example. The different strategies include focusing on cytotoxic agents, synthetic lethality strategies, angiogenesis, oncogene addiction pathways and activated survival pathways such as those driven by systems of inflammation and/or metabolism.

2. Building on past successes – Cytotoxics and agents targeting key biological pathways

2.1. Cytotoxic agents

Cytotoxic chemotherapy has had an established role for many cancer types for many decades with the ability to eradicate some cancers, prevent relapse from micrometastatic disease in others and offer life prolonging or palliative benefit in other cancers. With respect to prostate cancer, a role for cytotoxic chemotherapy in the treatment of metastatic castrate refractory prostate cancer (CRPC) was first established using mitoxantrone in 1996, when it was shown to provide effective palliation of pain symptoms compared to prednisolone alone without prolongation of overall survival [3]. This was not associated with a survival benefit and to date the only class of cytotoxic agents to improve survival in metastatic prostate cancer are the taxanes [4]. Docetaxel was licensed in metastatic CRPC patients in 2004 following a phase III study of docetaxel plus prednisone versus mitoxantrone plus prednisone. The taxanes block cells in the G2/M phase of the cell cycle by stabilizing microtubules in the mitotic spindle thereby rendering them unable to separate during mitosis. Cancer cells sensitivity to taxanes is often short lived and resistance develops. The mechanism of this is poorly understood, although over expression of P-glycoprotein and mutations in the tubulin gene have been described [5]. Whilst the non-specific targeting of cycling cells by cytotoxic agents is not classed as targeted therapy, ongoing efforts do exist to introduce new cytotoxic agents to the prostate cancer arena. The aim of improving efficacy and delivery whilst minimizing toxicity underlies this development. In this era of personalized medicine, cytotoxic agents may continue to have a role especially where tumours do not harbour an obvious upregulated or mutated pathway to target. This approach has already led to the development and approval of the synthetic taxane - cabazitaxel for use in the second line metastatic CRPC setting. In the international multicentre phase III TROPIC trial, patients who had progressed on docetaxel were randomized to receive cabazitaxel plus prednisone or mitoxantrone plus prednisone. An improvement in overall survival of 2.4 months was seen (15.1 months versus 12.7 months $HR=0.7$ $p<0.001$) [6].

In addition to new members of existing cytotoxic drug classes, new mechanisms of drug delivery continue to be developed. Nanoparticle albumin bound (nab) paclitaxel and docetaxel use albumin as a vehicle to improve drug delivery to the tumour. This approach has proven to be successful using nab-paclitaxel (Abraxane®) in metastatic breast cancer where it delivered a 49% higher dose of drug to patients than a conventional solvent based approach. In addition, higher response rates were seen with an overall response rate of 33% (versus 19% for standard paclitaxel) and increased time to progression from 16.9 to 22 weeks [7]. Both agents are also in development in prostate cancer, where phase II trials are currently evaluating nab-paclitaxel and nab-docetaxel in the CRPC population. Other novel drug delivery strategies include water soluble biodegradable polyglutamate polymer with linked chemotherapeutic molecules (e.g. paclitaxel poligumex, Opaxio®) [8,9] and a nanoparticle bound docetaxel agent (BIND014) has also recently entered phase I clinical trials [10] (Table 1)

Drug	Class	Study Design	Results	Current phase of clinical development	Reference
Androgen receptor blockers					
Abiraterone	CYP 17 lyase inhibitor	Randomised placebo controlled phase III trial in post-docetaxel and chemo naïve CRPC pts.	Overall survival adv 3.9 months in post chemo population Chemo naïve study stopped early. Median OS not yet reached for Abiraterone	Licensed in post-docetaxel pts Awaiting license in chemo naïve pts	[26, 28, 29]
Enzalutamide /MDV3100	Androgen receptor antagonist	Phase III randomized placebo controlled AFFIRM study	Overall survival adv 4.8 months. Favourable toxicity profile. 0.6% seizure rate	Phase III trials in chemo-naïve setting completed accrual	[33, 34]
Orteronel/ TAK700	17,20 lyase inhibitor	Phase I-II dose escalation study in metastatic CRPC pts accrued.	RPIID is 400mg BID, no DLTs	Phase II trial accruing in asymp CRPC pts, pts without mets but rising PSA & in combination with docetaxel in met CRPC pts.	[30, 31]
TOK-001	AR antagonist, CYP 17 lyase inhibitor, ↓AR levels			Phase I-II in CRPC pts (ARMOR1) currently accruing	[113]
Histone deacetylase (HDAC) inhibitors					
Panobinostat	HDAC inhibitor	Phase I completed in combination with docetaxel/pred and phase II completed as single agent in CRPC pts	Safe as single agent and in combination. IV formulation going forward	Phase I-II with Bicalutamide in CRPC pts accruing	[37]

Vorinostat	HDAC 6 inhibitor	Phase I with safety study with docetaxel q21 days and vorinostat q1-14 days Phase II in post chemo CRPC pts receiving 400mg vorinostat orally	12 pts enrolled but 5 DLTs reported. Trials suspended due to excess toxicity 27 pts but terminated due to excess toxicity. Significant toxicity seen. 44% G3 AE's	Phase I in combination with temsirolimus planned	[38, 39]
SB939	HDAC inhibitor (multiple classes)	Phase I dose escalation trial in solid malignancies	MTD 80mg, RPIID 60mg, DLTs were fatigue, troponin elevation & QTc prolongation	Phase II single agent study in recurrent/met prostate cancer accruing	[114]
Romidepsin	Depsipeptide HDAC inhibitor	Phase II in chemo naïve met CRPC pts. 13 mg/m2 q1,8,15 every 28 days	35 pts enrolled. 2 pts had PR "/>6months. 11 pts stopped due to toxicity. N&V, fatigue & anorexia	Combination studies with cytotoxic agents planned	[115]
HSP90 inhibitors					
IPI-504 (Retaspmycin)	17-AAG analogue HSP90 inhibitor	Phase II study in CRPC patients stratified by prior chemotherapy at 400mg/m^2	No PSA or RECIST responses seen. G5 ketoacidosis and hepatic failure observed	Clinical development ongoing in NSCLC	[43]
STA9090	2nd gen HSP90 inhibitor	Phase I dose escalation studies with IV wkly and twice wkly admin	Wkly admin - MTD 216mg/m^2 DLTs due to amylase elevation, diarrhoea & fatigue Twice weekly – MTD as yet not reached	Phase II prostate trials planned	[44]
17AAG (Tanespimycin)	1st gen HSP90 inh	Phase II in metastatic CRPC pts. 300mg/m^2 weekly for ¾ weeks	Trial stopped after 1st phase due to lack of PSA response. G3 fatigue	No further prostate trials	[41, 42]
siRNA against AR	Nanoparticle technology	In pre-clinical development			[10]

Table 1. The Androgen Receptor pathway

New classes of cytotoxic agents are also in development in prostate cancer. These are members of the epothilone family and the halichondrin B analogue - eribulin. The epothilones are macrolide antibiotics that also act by stabilizing microtubules. They are water soluble and as such do not have to be administered in a lipophilic solution, therefore reducing the allergic reaction rate compared to taxanes. To date the epothilone - ixabepilone is licensed for use in metastatic chemo-refractory breast cancer, although it has also shown activity and acceptable toxicity in a phase II study in a mixed chemo naïve and post chemotherapy CRPC population [11]. Clinical development of several members of this family in prostate cancer continues. Patupilone or naturally occurring Epothilone B and sagopilone (a fully synthetic compound) have also shown activity in post docetaxel and chemo naïve CRPC patients respectively [12, 13].

Eribulin mesylate (or Halaven, Eisai Co.) is a synthetic analogue of the marine sponge natural product Halichondrin B that is a potent naturally occurring mitotic inhibitor. Eribulin binds predominantly with high affinity to the ends of microtubules leading to mitotic arrest and ultimately apoptosis. Eribulin is also licensed for use in metastatic chemotherapy refractory breast cancer patients although a phase II study in both chemotherapy naive and pretreated prostate cancer patients has been performed. Most activity was demonstrated in the chemotherapy naïve cohort with a 22.4% PSA response rate and 8.8% overall response rate [14].

Another successful cytotoxic strategy for targeting prostate cancer metastases with radiation has been the studies using the alpha-emitter Radium 223. This radiopharmaceutical that acts as a calcium mimic can selectively target bone lesions from prostate cancer whilst its low penetrance alpha-emissions are cytotoxic to cancer cells. Its half life of 11.4 days also favours its use as a cancer treatment. Having proven its safety in phase I and II trials [15], the phase III ALSYMPCA trial was stopped early after a pre-planned efficacy interim analysis following recommendations from the independent data monitoring committee on the basis of a significant improvement in overall survival and favourable toxicity profile. In this large study of 922 patients, Radium-223 significantly improved overall survival in patients by 2.8 months (HR 0.695 95% CI 0.552-0.875) in addition to delaying the time to first skeletal-related event by 5.2 months (HR 0.610 95% CI 0.461-0.807) [16].

2.2. Targeting key biological pathways

A leading premise for the treatment for advanced prostate cancer is to target the androgen receptor (AR) axis or to identify cases where a single pathway mutation is thought to drive carcinogenesis. It is proposed that triaging the current pipeline of agents can be directed by building on prior successes. In light of recent advances in our knowledge of AR pathway signaling, further exploration of this pathway is warranted. Moreover, since molecular interrogation of distinct clones driving individual prostate cancers is now possible, treatment of these tumours with agents targeting these mutations would also be desirable. In the past the prostate cancer treatment paradigm has been to expose the patient to an established sequence of agents in a 'one size fits all' approach – which may have missed identifying a drug with major activity in a few patients. A strategy that is being increasingly more recognized is the need to characterize a patient's cancer and select the most appropriate treatment for that cancer phenotype. It is also important to ensure that critical appraisal of pre-clinical and clinical research continues to help guide these endeavors to identify oncogene addiction pathways.

3. Extinguishing the AR axis

The androgen dependence of prostate cancer on testosterone was first observed as early as 1941 when the effect of castration on androgen levels in prostate cancer was studied [17]. This lead to the introduction of androgen deprivation therapy and the generation of the castrate state where serum levels of testosterone are reduced to <50ng/dl or 1.7nmol/l. This treatment is initially effective in 80-90% of patients and results in PSA or radiological responses and clinical improvement in the patient's symptoms. Eventually, the patient's cancer progresses despite serum testosterone levels continuing to be low. The current term used to describe this state is 'castrate resistant prostate cancer' which has replaced the misleading term 'hormone-refractory prostate cancer'. CRPC more accurately describes the ongoing dependence of the cancer on AR signaling despite low measureable testosterone levels.

Ligand independent AR signaling is thought to occur in the majority of CRPC tumours via activation of oncogenes such as ERBB2 or H-*ras* and through MAP kinase signaling [18, 19]. A small proportion of CRPC tumours will also harbour amplifications or point mutations in the ligand-binding domain of the androgen receptor gene leading to altered responsiveness to ligands [20]. A third mechanism of action bypasses androgen receptor in favour of an alternative signaling pathway [21].

The evidence for ongoing androgen sensitivity is also strengthened by the observation of up regulation of AR protein levels in hormone resistant versus hormone sensitive paired xenografts [21] as well as in patient tumour samples [22, 23]. Maintained intra-tumoural levels of testosterone and dihydrotestosterone are also observed despite castrate serum androgen levels [24].

In addition to testicular androgen production, extragonadal sites of androgen synthesis also contribute to testosterone levels. These *de novo* adrenal and intra-tumoural pathways utilize the 17α-hydroxylase and C17, 20-lyase activity of the CYP17A1 enzyme involved in the steroid biosynthesis pathway. The importance of this pathway was initially clinically exploited with the use of ketoconazole, a weak reversible inhibitor of CYP17. Anti-tumour activity was demonstrated with a PSA response rate of 20-62% in phase II trials and a median duration of response of 3-7 months [25]. However its use was associated with significant toxicity and up to 20% of patients discontinued treatment. This toxicity profile has not been observed with the more potent CYP17 inhibitor abiraterone acetate. This agent has successfully reawakened interest in further manipulation of the AR axis in CRPC patients. After successful phase I and II clinical trial development [26, 27] randomized double blind placebo controlled phase III trials of abiraterone plus prednisolone versus placebo plus prednisolone in chemotherapy naïve and post docetaxel patients were conducted. Results in post docetaxel patients revealed a statistically significant increase in median overall survival of 3.9 months in favour of abiraterone as well as improvements in time to PSA progression, radiological PFS and PSA response rate [28]. More recent results from the interim analysis of chemotherapy naïve patients have also shown significant activity in favour of abiraterone with the interim data monitoring committee recommending unblinding and crossover for patients receiving prednisone alone [29]. Abiraterone was also well tolerated with the predominant toxicities being hypertension, hypokalaemia and fluid retention. These are the expected consequences of the mineralocorticoid excess resulting from the accumulation of precursors upstream of CYP17. These have subsequently been managed with the concomitant use of steroids or the mineralocorticoid antagonist eplerenone.

Orteronel (or TAK 700, Takeda Pharmaceuticals) is another 17,20 lyase inhibitor which has also advanced to phase III CRPC trials after successful phase I and II development [30, 31]. This inhibitor is now in phase III trials as a single agent in asymptomatic CRPC patients and in patients with a rising PSA but no detectable metastatic disease as well as in phase I/II trials in a number of prostate cancer settings including in combination with docetaxel in metastatic CRPC patients.

In addition to steroid biosynthesis inhibitors, further manipulation of the AR axis in castrate patients has been demonstrated using MDV3100 or enzalutamide. First generation anti-androgens such as bicalutamide, flutamide and nilutamide competitively inhibit the AR ligand binding domain. This response is often transient as castration resistance develops which may in part be a consequence of the partial agonist activity of this class [21]. These observations led to the rational design of enzalutamide, an orally available anti-androgen with superior AR binding compared to bicalutamide, and no AR agonist activity in bicalutamide-resistant and AR-over expressing cell lines [32]. A phase I/II study of enzalutamide in 140 post-chemotherapy metastatic CRPC patients demonstrated a PSA response rate of 56% (78/140 patients), soft tissue responses in 22% (13/59 patients), and a median time to progression of 47 weeks. enzalutamide was well tolerated with the most common grade 3 or 4 adverse events being fatigue that resolved with a dose reduction [33]. This activity was confirmed in the multicentre double blind placebo controlled phase III AFFIRM trial comparing enzalutamide against placebo. This trial of 1199 docetaxel pre-treated patients was also stopped early due to a 4.8 months overall survival benefit for enzalutamide compared to placebo with all subgroups benefiting [34].

Other agents in development that manipulate the androgen receptor axis are shown in table 1. In addition to agents intrinsic to the androgen receptor pathway, inhibitors of chaperone proteins may also be important targets. Histone deacetylases (HDAC) are enzymes which remove acetyl groups from proteins and in so doing modulate the protein-protein interactions of co-activators associated with AR binding. HDAC enzymes are over expressed in certain solid tumours including prostate cancer, where high expression levels are associated with poor outcome [35]. HDAC over expression in prostate cancers is also often co-existent with genetic rearrangements in the ETS (E-twenty six) gene family. These genetic alterations have been found in up to 70% of prostate cancers and may interact with HDAC's already known to be upstream regulators and downstream transducers of the ETS transcription factors family [36]. The preclinical rationale for HDAC inhibition in prostate cancer has led to early phase clinical development of several HDAC inhibitors. Phase I/II studies of panobinostat both as a single agent and in combination with docetaxel confirmed the safety of this approach [37]. In the single arm study, all patients developed progressive disease despite evidence of acetylated histones in peripheral blood mononuclear cells, however 5 out of 8 (63%) patients in the combination study had a ≥ 50% reduction in PSA value. At present a study in combination with bicalutamide in CRPC patients is recruiting. However trials involving single agent vorinostat (an HDAC6 inhibitor known to acetylate tubulin and stabilize microtubules) have been terminated early due to excess toxicity with no significant activity [38, 39].

The other major group of agents that are involved in post-translational modification of the AR axis are heat shock proteins. These are proteins that ensure the maintenance of oncogenic protein homeostasis in the presence of stress factors such as hypoxia or acidotic conditions. Heat shock protein 90 (HSP 90) is an ATP-dependent multi-chaperone complex implicated in the function of the AR. The AR is stabilized by the interaction with HSP 90 that allows it to interact with androgens [40]. Pre-clinical models have shown HSP 90 inhibition leads to decreased AR expression and function and a phase I trial of 17-AAG both as a single agent and in combination with cytotoxic chemotherapy demonstrated drug safety [41]. The subsequent phase II study however failed to reach its primary endpoint and was terminated [42]. Significant toxicity was observed with the 17-AAG analogue retaspmycin (or IPI-504) [43] although clinical development of the second generation HSP90 inhibitor STA9090 has confirmed safety in phase I trials and is proceeding [44]. Studies are planned to determine whether the newer HSP90 agents can hit target and decrease activity with a suitable toxicity profile or whether the therapeutic window is too narrow for safe use of these agents.

In addition, small interfering RNA's (siRNA's) are a class of double stranded RNA molecules that are now known to exist as important gene regulatory factors in both plant and animal systems. Selective targeting of the androgen receptor by siRNA molecules may further silence the AR signaling pathway in prostate cancer. This may be made viable by nanoparticle technology being able to facilitate use of otherwise undeliverable agents. The development of these agents is currently hampered by the need for safe systemic delivery of these agents without the off target and immune stimulation problems encountered with other nucleic acid medicines such as plasmid DNA and anti-sense oligonucleotide [45].

4. An advanced understanding of cancer biology comes of age

4.1. Specific targeting of DNA repair mechanisms

In recent years one successful targeted approach has been to exploit the vulnerability of tumors with an impaired DNA damage repair mechanism by inhibiting a second DNA repair pathway and as such commit the cancer cell to die. This concept of synthetic lethality has been most successfully demonstrated in patients bearing tumors with *BRCA-1/-2* mutations where homologous recombination (HR) mechanisms are already known to be inadequate. This hypothesis has reactivated the development of poly (ADP-ribose) polymerase (PARP) inhibitors. PARP is an enzyme that is crucial in the base excision repair pathway. When this repair mechanism is inhibited in the presence of pre-existing impaired HR then efficient

DNA repair is prevented and apoptosis occurs. Following pre-clinical and more recently proof of concept clinical trials in patients with *BRCA* mutated breast and ovarian carcinoma, the PARP inhibitor olaparib has demonstrated significant activity [46]. Whilst it is hoped that the application of these agents may broaden to include sporadic tumours in which mutations in DNA pathways may also be found, there has also been considerable interest in other tumours types where these mutations may be found. The inherited *BRCA-2* mutation is associated with a 20% lifetime risk of developing prostate cancer that often occurs before 65 years of age. The subsequent tumors are often of high Gleason score, more advanced stage at diagnosis and patients have a shorter survival than patients with sporadic prostate cancers [47]. One of three prostate cancer patients with germ-line BRCA variant had a prolonged response to olaparib in a phase 1 trial [48]. In addition to BRCA mutated cancers, pre-clinical evidence has also demonstrated a sensitivity of tumours with phosphatase and tensin homolog (PTEN) deficiency to PARP inhibition [49]. This is one of the most commonly mutated genes in human cancers where it has a role in genome stability. PTEN deficiency is associated with an HR defect that sensitizes tumours cells to PARP inhibition using the same mechanism as BRCA mutated cancers.

At present, the clinical development of olaparib has been focused on breast and ovarian cancer. Studies in prostate cancer are underway with the PARP inhibitor veliparib (or ABT888) in combination with temozolamide in a phase I study recruiting patients with metastatic prostate cancer. In addition a phase I study using the Merck PARP inhibitor - MK4827 is currently recruiting to a prostate cancer enriched second stage following encouraging phase I study data in advanced solid malignancies [50].

4.2. Oncogene addiction pathways

The development of drugs targeting tumours driven by so-called 'oncogene addictions' has lead to some success. Examples include imatinib targeting the *bcr-abl* translocation in CML and mutated *c-kit* in GIST, trastuzumab and laptinib in HER-2 positive breast cancers BRAF inhibitors in melanomas with BRAF mutations. Molecular studies in prostate cancer have to date identified mutations of this type in less than 20% of all sporadically occurring prostate cancers. Analysis of a cohort of 206 prostate cancer cases found the common BRAF mutation V600E in 10.2% (or 21/206 cases) [51], whilst PI3 kinase mutations were found in only 3% of a separate cohort [52]. Drugs inhibiting BRAF as well as PI3 kinase mutations may lead to meaningful responses in patients with tumors been driven by these mutations. It is hoped that further "oncogene addiction" pathways will be uncovered and be able to be drugged.

4.3. Ligand and transcription factor driven survival pathways

Whilst it is often hoped that mutations in a single molecular pathway will be uncovered as the crucial oncogenic event in tumour development and its abrogation lead to meaningful anticancer activity, to date this has been rarely found to be the case for sporadic tumours. Another approach is to consider the factors that cause and/or are associated with the development as well as the survival of cancer. The role of androgens and androgen receptor is clear for prostate cancer. Other biological approaches associated with cancer development and survival include the metabolism and inflammatory systems. In both cases, there is epidemiological, preclinical and pathological data implicating these systems in the development of prostate cancer. In comparison to the "oncogene addiction" phenomenon, these cancers are driven by altered expression of ligands and control mechanisms (such as transcription factors). Knowledge of these pathways has provided valuable clues for the treatment of cancer.

5. Targeting the metabolism system

Incidence and disease specific mortality in prostate cancer exhibit marked global variation with the highest levels seen in Western Europe, North America and the lowest in Asia [53]. It is assumed that whilst this is accounted for by a significant genetic component, that diet and lifestyle factors may also contribute. Epidemiological studies also support an association between dietary fat intake, poor prognosis and risk of relapse [54]. In order to identify new pathways that are important in prostate cancer pathogenesis, evaluating a role for the metabolism system and its key components is crucial.

Cancer cells are already known to differ from normal cells in some of the fundamental metabolic pathways they employ. Most cancer cells generate energy by primarily metabolizing glucose by glycolysis followed by lactate production. This occurs in contrast to normal cells in which glucose is catabolised by oxidative phosphorylation, a primarily aerobic process. Proliferating cancer cells also exhibit increased glucose uptake compared to normal cells. This results in tumour cells with glycolytic rates over 200 times higher than those of normal tissues and allows efficient generation of macromolecules needed for new cancer cell production. This so-called Warburg hypothesis was initially thought to be the fundamental cause of cancer, however it is now thought to explain how tumours may flourish in low oxygen environments [55]. These observations suggest that differences in metabolism between normal tissues and cancer cells may be important in oncogenesis.

Insulin and insulin-like growth factors (IGF-1) are extracellular hormones and growth factors that regulate important metabolic pathways such as fatty acid and sterol synthesis as well as growth factor signaling via the PI3 kinase and MAP kinase pathways. Their activation may stimulate tumourigenesis by activating one or both of these mitogenic pathways and disrupting fat metabolism.

IGF-I and IGF-II bind to the IGF-1 receptor, a tyrosine kinase receptor that is known to be upregulated following castration in animal models [56]. It has been implicated in the development of the castrate resistant state with evidence that inhibition of the IGF-1 receptor may enhance the effect of castration in xenograft models [57]. Targeting the IGF-1 receptor is therefore an attractive therapeutic target in CRPC. Several IGF-1 receptor inhibitors are currently being evaluated in clinical trials and candidates include both monoclonal antibodies and small molecule tyrosine kinase inhibitors. Cixutumumab (or IMC-A12) is a fully human IgG1 subclass monoclonal antibody that has reached phase II of clinical development. A single agent study of chemotherapy naïve asymptomatic patients noted that the drug was well tolerated with grade 3 fatigue and hyperglycaemia the worst toxicity seen and 29% of patients had stable disease [58]. Future trials with this agent are planned or ongoing including in the first line metastatic setting with androgen deprivation therapy (SWOG S0925) based on supporting preclinical data [57].

Drug	Class	Study Design	Results	Current phase of clinical development	Reference
Insulin-like growth factor receptor inhibitors					
Cixitumumab /IMC-A12	IGF-1 R inh	Phase II study in chemo naïve CRPC Asx pts 10mg/kg q2 wkly or 20mg/kg q3 wkly	29% disease stab >6 mths. Worst toxicity G3 fatigue & ↑glycaemia	Phase II Neoadj +ADT in high risk pts + Temsiro in met CRPC + 1st line met+ADT	[58]
Figitumumab /CP-751871	IGF-1 R inh	Phase Ib in adv solid tumours in comb with docetaxel 75mg/m2	46 pts - MTD not reached. 4PR and 12 pts with disease stab >6months. G3/4 febrile neutropenia, fatigue 10/18 CRPC pts had >5 CTC with 60% response	Phase III studies recruiting in NSCLC (ADVIGO 1016). Phase II in breast, prostate, colorectal & Ewings sarcoma	[59, 60]
Ganitumab/ AMG 479	IGF-1 R inh	Phase I dose escalation study in adv solid malign of IV q2 wkly	53 pts - 1DLT – G3 ↓plts & transminitis. MTD not reached – maxdose 20mg/kg. ↑ in serum IGF-1	Phase II studies recruiting in Ex Stage small cell with platinum, +Everolimus in colorectal, in carcinoid & pNETs	[61]
Lisitinib/ OSI-906	Dual kinase inhibitor of Insulin & IGF-1 R	Phase I continuous dose escalation study in adv solid tumours using BID & QD dosing Phase I intermittent dosing in adv solid tumours	57 pts – MTD reached 400mg QD, 150mg BID. DLTs were ↑ QTc & G3 hyperglycaemia SD >12 weeks seen in 18/43 pts MTD 600 mg	Phase III recruiting in Adrenocortical Ca Phase II + Erlotinib in Breast	[62, 116]
AMP Kinase activators					
AICAR (Aminoimidazole-4-caboxamide-1-b-riboside	AMP mimetic	Preclinical studies show inhibition of prostate cancer cell proliferation	Inhibition of tumour growth in prostate cancer xenograft models		[78, 117]

A-769662	AMP K subunit act.	Delay tumour development & decrease tumour incidence in PTEN def mice			[79]
Metformin	Indirect	44% reduction in prostate cancer cases compared to Caucasian controls		Phase II recruiting in loc adv or met CRPC and in loc disease as prevention against MS with ADT	[80]
Resveratrol	Indirect	Phase I single dose safety study in colon ca pts with hepatic metastases	Results are awaited	Phase I/II currently recruiting as neoadj in colon carcinoma pts	[82]
mTOR inhibitors					
Temsirolimus	mTOR inhibitor	Phase II study in CRPC patients post first line docetaxol chemotherapy. Pts receive maintenance temsirolimus 25mg/m2 weekly	Currently recruiting	Phase II recruiting in chemo naïve CRPC pts, in comb with cixutumumab in met CRPC, in CRPC after no response to chemo with bevacizumab & PI/II with docetaxel	[118]
Everolimus	mTOR inhibitor via mTORC1	Phase II study in castrate resistant prostate cancer of bicalutamide and everolimus compared to bicalutamide alone	*In vivo* evidence of synergy between mTOR and AR pathways. Study ongoing but 8 pts enrolled. 6/8 responses in PSA. Well tolerated with no unexpected toxicity	Phase I/II in met CRPC with docetaxel & bevacizumab, in post chemo pts with carbo/pred, in neoadj setting in int/high risk localized disease & in first line met/ locally adv setting	[72, 73, 74]
PI3 kinase inhibitors					
XL-147	Class I PI3K isoform inhibitor	Phase I dose escalation study in adv solid malig of continuous daily dosing or d1-21 of 28 day cycle	68pts – DLT G3 rash. Inhibition of PI3K & ERK demonstrated. Prolonged stable disease observed	Recruiting to Phase I study in solid tumours and Phase I/II in breast & endometrial carcinoma	[65]

GDC-0941	Pan PI3K inhibitor	Phase I dose escalation study. GDC-0941 given QD for 21 out of 28 day cycle. BID cohorts also recruited	36 pts enrolled, dose escalation ongoing. QD dosing safe up to 254mg, BID dosing safe up to 180mg. 3 DLTs – headache, pl eff and red TLCO	Phase I study recruiting in NSCLC & Met breast cancer in comb. With paclitaxel or carbo +/- bevacizumab	[66]
BKM120 BEZ235	Pan class I PI3K inhibitor	Phase I dose escalation study. BKM120 PO QD	30 pts enrolled from 12.5-150mg. MTD 100mg. PD data suggests active drug at 100mg. 8/10 PR on FDG-PET	Phase I/II currently accruing in HER2+ Met breast ca. Also recruiting in combination with GSK 1120212	[67]
Akt inhibitors					
GSK 2141795 GSK 2110183	Akt inhibitor			First-in-human phase I study of GSK 2141795 in advanced solid malig, also recruiting in combination with GSK 1120212	
Perifosine	Oral Akt inhibitor	CRPC pts with rising PSA but no detectable mets. 900mg loading dose then 100mg daily	20% pts had a PSA reduction but did not meet PSA response criteria. DLTs included hypoNa, arthritis, photophobia, hyperuricaemia	Recruiting phase III in multiple myeloma with bortezomib +/- dex , phase I in recurrent paediatric solid tumours	[70]
MK2206	Highly selective non ADP comp Akt inhibitor	Phase I dose escalation study 30-90mg QOD in 28 day cycles in tx-refractory solid tumours	MTD established at 60mg QOD. PD efficacy confirmed with dec pAKT levels. SD seen in 6/19 pts	Phase II bicalutamide +/- MK2206 in pts after local therapy + rising PSA, Phase I in com with docetaxel is recruiting	[71]

Table 2. The Metabolic Syndrome

A second IGF-1 receptor antibody is the human IgG2 subclass antibody figitumumab. This was evaluated in a phase I dose escalation trial during which the maximum feasible dose was established as 20mg/kg intravenously every 21 days [59]. A phase Ib dose escalation study in combination with docetaxel then enrolled 46 predominantly metastatic CRPC patients. This combination was well tolerated with no MTD reached and the toxicity profile included nausea, febrile neutropenia, anorexia, fatigue and hyperglycaemia. A 22% response rate was observed with a disease stabilization rate of 44% for ≥ 6 months [60]. A phase II study of this combination has completed accrual and results are awaited. A third monoclonal antibody ganitumumab (or AMG478, Amgen) is also in clinical development and whilst safe in phase I dose escalation studies, its focus for ongoing development is in lung and colorectal carcinoma [61]. OSI-906 or linsitinib is a first in class inhibitor of both the insulin and IGF-1 receptors. It has been evaluated in phase I dose escalation safety studies where MTDs of 400mg QD and 150 mg BID were reached. The dose limiting toxicities were the known class effects hyperglycaemia and prolongation of the QTc interval. Whilst further development of this compound continues in adrenocortical and breast carcinomas [62], a phase II study of linsitinib in asymptomatic or mildly symptomatic CRPC patients has completed accrual and results are awaited.

An important downstream intracellular signaling pathway that has been implicated in prostate cancer pathogenesis, progression and the development of castration resistance is the PI3K/Akt/mTOR pathway. Phosphatidylinositol-3 kinase (PI3K) activation results in the phosphorylation of phosphatidylinositol 4,5-bisphosphate (PIP2) to generate the second messenger phosphatidylinositol 3-5triphosphate (PIP3) that activates the Akt signal transduction cascade. Reports suggest that PI3K signaling may play a critical role in castration resistance allowing prostate cancers to maintain continued proliferation in low androgen environments [63]. In addition, the PI3K isoforms p85 and p110b appear to have a role in regulating AR-DNA interactions and the assembly of the AR based transcriptional complex [64]. There are numerous PI3K inhibitors in clinical development, XL147 (Exelixis) is a class I isoform inhibitor whilst SF1126 (Semafore), GDC0941 (Genentech) and BEZ234 (Novartis) are pan PI3K inhibitors. All agents have successfully completed phase I dose escalation studies and preliminary results suggest that these agents are well tolerated and have favourable pharmacokinetic-pharmacodynamic profiles [65 - 67]. Further tumour specific phase I/II studies are ongoing, although at present no prostate specific studies are in progress.

The Akt's are a family of three serine/threonine kinases – AKT-1, AKT-2, & AKT-3. Phosphorylation of AKT modulates multiple downstream cellular functions including apoptosis, metabolism and proliferation. Enhanced pAKT correlates with more aggressive histological and pathological prostate cancer stage, and a worse prognosis underlining its importance as a druggable target and possible role as a prognostic biomarker [68, 69]. There are several classes of Akt inhibitors currently in clinical development including those inhibiting the catalytic and the pleckstrin homology (PH) domains. Perifosine, an alkylphospholipid inhibiting the PH domain has reached phase II in CRPC patients. Unfortunately although well tolerated this agent did not exhibit significant activity [70]. The pan-AKT inhibitors GSK2141795 and MK2206 with simultaneous targeting of both AKT-1 and AKT-2 are considered potentially superior to single isoform inhibitors. MK2206 was well tolerated in a phase II dose escalation study with an observed MTD of 60mg. Pharmacodynamic endpoints were met with a measurable reduction in pAKT levels. In addition, 6 of 19 patients achieved stable disease [71]. Further development continues in a number of tumour types

http://dx.doi.org/10.5772/53092

both as single agent and in combination with chemotherapy. Of note a phase I study in combination with docetaxel is currently recruiting, as is a randomized phase II study of bicalutamide +/- MK2206 in prostate cancer patients with a rising PSA after definitive local therapy. GSK2141795 and GSK 2110183 also entered phase I development with results of first in human safety studies pending.

Mammalian target of rapamycin (mTOR) is also a serine/threonine kinase downstream of PI3K which interacts with the mTOR complexes mTORC1 and mTORC2 to regulate cell proliferation and inhibit apoptosis. Proof of principle that the PI3K pathway can be successfully targeted for clinical use in cancer has been demonstrated by the development of the rapamycin analogs - temsirolimus and everolimus that inhibit the mTORC1 kinase. Temsirolimus is an intravenous formulation which was the first compound in this class to be approved by the FDA for first line treatment in poor risk patients with advanced renal cell cancer. Everolimus an oral formulation is also approved for use in advanced renal cell cancer but in the second line setting. Single agent studies of these agents in the prostate cancer setting have been performed but were considered disappointing with a short time to progression (2.5 months) and no radiographic or PSA responses [72]. Everolimus has also been evaluated in combination with docetaxel in CRPC patients. The recommended phase II dose was 10mg everolimus and 70mg/m2 docetaxel, 3 patients had a PSA response and the combination was well tolerated with fatigue and haematological toxicities the most common [73]. Further studies with both agents in prostate cancer continue with a similar study involving temsirolimus in combination with docetaxel, as well as studies with cixitumumab and bevacizumab. A randomized study in hormone responsive patients of bicalutamide +/- everolimus is currently recruiting with early results suggesting the combination was well tolerated with PSA responses observed in six of eight patients [74]. Studies in the neoadjuvant and localized disease setting are also ongoing.

Finally, AMP kinase is a serine/threonine kinase that is activated by metabolic stressors that deplete ATP and increase AMP levels. Its activity is also under the control of hormones such as adiponectin and leptin as well as cytokines [75]. The activation of AMP kinase reduces insulin levels, as well as increasing ATP producing activities (glucose uptake, fatty acid oxidation) and suppressing ATP-consumption (synthesis of fatty acids, sterols, glycogen and proteins). AMP kinase therefore acts as a metabolic switch controlling glucose and lipid metabolism. Decreased AMP kinase activity is thought to contribute to the metabolic abnormalities involved in the metabolic syndrome [76]. In addition polymorphisms in a gene locus encoding one of the AMPK subunits correlates with prostate cancer risk [77].

Activators of AMP kinase activity may be direct or indirect. Several direct AMP kinase activators act either by allosteric binding to AMP kinase subunits or as an AMP mimetic. These agents aminoimidazole-4-caboxamide-1-b-riboside (AICAR), A-769662 and PT1 are at an early stage of clinical development. AICAR has been shown to inhibit prostate cancer cell proliferation and tumour growth in xenograft models [78]. However its further development may be limited by its poor specificity for AMPK and low oral bioavailability. To date no interventional oncology studies have been undertaken. The recent publication of the crystal structure of AMP kinase subunits has allowed rational drug design of A-769662 and

PT1. A769662 has been shown to delay tumour development and decrease tumour incidence in PTEN deficient mice [79].

The indirect activator metformin is a well established treatment for type II diabetes mellitus. Its use is associated with a 44% risk reduction in prostate cancer cases compared with controls in Caucasian men [80]. The mechanism of metformin's antitumour effect is not completely understood, although it is hypothesized that metformin may decrease circulating glucose, insulin and IGF-1 levels by inhibiting hepatic gluconeogenesis resulting in increased signaling through the insulin/IGF-1 pathway [81]. Its action in prostate cancer is currently under evaluation in a number of clinical trials, these include as a preventative treatment for metabolic syndrome in men on androgen deprivation therapy and as first line therapy in locally advanced or metastatic prostate cancer patients. Finally, resveratrol is a phytoalexin produced by plants when under attack by pathogens. It is found in the skin of grapes, grape products, red wine and mulberries and is thought to have anticancer properties. These were first identified when it was shown to inhibit tumourigenesis in a mouse skin cancer model [82]. Its indirect action on AMP kinase remains to be elucidated although its anticancer action has been explored in a number of tumour types. Clinical trials using resveratrol have explored potential roles in preventing and treating diabetes, Alzheimers disease and weight loss. In addition safety studies of its use in colorectal carcinoma patients with liver metastases have been conducted and the results are awaited. As yet no studies in prostate cancer are planned.

6. Inflammation

Numerous studies have implicated inflammation in the development of prostate cancer and its metastases. Pathologists have recognized focal areas of epithelial atrophy in the periphery of the prostate (proliferative inflammatory atrophy - PIA), where prostate cancers typically arise and these areas are associated with acute or chronic inflammation and can show morphological transitions in continuity with high grade PIN [83]. This could indicate a role of PIA as a cancer precursor [84]. Putative causes of these lesions are infection or dietary oxidants. To date, the identification of an infectious agent directly involved in prostate carcinogenesis has been elusive. However, it is possible that one or more infectious agents may be indirectly involved in prostate carcinogenesis by being initiators of the inflammatory lesion (PIA). Interesting data includes serologic evidence of *T. vaginalis* infection being associated with a higher prostate cancer risk overall, and an almost two-fold risk for poorly differentiated disease [85] as well as greater prostate cancer specific mortality (HR: 1.5; 95% CI: 1.0, 2.2) [86]. It is also of note that hereditary susceptibility genes which encode proteins with infectious response function: RNASEL and MSR1 (macrophage scavenger receptor 1) have been associated with prostate cancer [83]. Single nucleotide polymorphism's of anti-oxidant genes have also been associated with prostate cancer and include OGG1 (repair from oxidized DNA), MnSOD [88]. Also the incidence of prostate cancer has been decreased with anti-oxidants such as lycopene and NSAIDs [87].

One possible mediator of the inflammation that leads to cancer and is instigated by oxidative stress from a diverse arrays of causes is NFκB activation. Specifically, it has been shown that a vicious cycle of oxidative stress causing DNA damage and consequent influx of inflammatory cytokines into the microenvironment results in further production of proteases, angiogenic factors, growth factors and immunosuppressive cytokines. Examples of NFκB controlled proteins found in prostate cancer include COX-2, XIAP, CXCR4, macrophage inhibitory cytokine-1 (MIC-1), IL-6, IL-8, IL-1, CXCL12, and the CXCR4 [89].

NFκB is a protein complex that controls DNA transcription and is activated by numerous factors including cytokines, free radicals, receptor activator of nuclear factor kappa-B (RANK), and microbial pathogens [90]. Upon activation, the NFκB dimers translocate to the nucleus with activation of numerous genes controlling cell growth, differentiation, inflammatory responses and apoptosis. Aberrant regulation of NFkB has previously been linked to inflammatory states and cancer. Moreover, NFκB controls many of the hallmarks of cancer including: invasion (IL-6); angiogenesis (IL-8, VEGF); propagation through the cell cycle (cyclin D1); and evasion of apoptosis (cIAP-1, TRAF-2, Bcl-X_L) [91 - 95]. As such, NFκB activation has clear-cut biological plausibility as a driver of cancer progression and CRPC. In tumor cells, NFκB is constitutively active either due to mutations in genes encoding the NFκB transcription factors themselves or in genes that control NFκB activity (such as IκB genes) or due to tumor cells secreting activation factors (e.g. IL-1). Constitutive NFκB activation in prostate cancer is found in both tumor and its associated stroma and occurs early in the disease process [96 - 100]. It is of note that preclinical work has mechanistically connected NFκB activation to development of prostate cancer with a metastatic phenotype [97]. Specifically, loss of the Ras GTPase-activating protein (RasGAP) gene DAB2IP lead to increased EZH2 and in turn induced NFκB activation which in turn resulted in metastatic prostate cancer in an orthotopic mouse tumor model.

Drugs targeting the inflammatory system are in preclinical and clinical development. The agents can be classified as upstream or direct inhibitors of nuclear factor kappa B or inhibitors of products of NFκB activation Table 3. This is a very new area but one which may lead to significant improvements.

Drug	Class	Study Design	Results	Current phase of clinical development	Reference
Upstream agents					
EZH2inhibitor (Enhancer of Zeste protein)	Polycomb grp protein	Pre-clinical studies only Ectopic expression of miRNAs impt in EZH2 action inhibit cell growth & tumourigenesis			[119]

Custirsen OGX-011	Clusterin Inhibitor (antisense oligo)	Randomised phase II in mCRPC with PD on or within 6m docetaxel (D) D/Pred/C or Mito/ Pred/C	42 pts – 3/23pts with PR in D/P/C OS 15.8 mths M/P/C OS 11.5 mths Toxicity similar in both arms	Phase III Docetaxel +/- Custirsen in mCRPC as 1st & 2nd line recruiting	[120]
Bortezomib	Proteosome inhibitor	Phase II study of bortezomib with addition of MAB on progression. Bortezomib given d1,4,8,11 for 3 cycles	No activity in addition to docetaxel or paclitaxel (phase I) and high rates of PN observed. When given as single agent or MAB – 11/15 CR with TTP 5.5 months	Results awaited for phase I study with mitoxanthrone	[121, 122, 123]
Carfilzomib	Selective proteosome inhibitor	Phase I trial in relapsed or refractory haem malig, d1-5 IV 1.2-20mg/m2	MTD 15mg/m2 – DLT of feb neutropenia & G4 thrombocytopenia. 2/29 responses	No prostate specific trials recruiting	[124]
Denosumab (bone)	Anti-RANKL antibody	Randomised phase III trial denosumab vs zoledronic acid in mCRPC with bone mets	Median time to first SRE 20.7m denosumab vs 17.1m zoledronic acid HR 0.82 p=0.00002	Phase III study investigating lens opacification in men on demosumab and ADT	[125]
Direct agents					
Silibinin (derived from Milk Thistle)	Via down regulation of epithelial-mesenchymal transition regulators	Phase II single arm study in PC pts with localized disease prior to prostatectomy. Pts given 13g/day	Transient high blood concentration observed but low tissue concentration. Response results awaited		[126]
Flavopiridol (Alvocidib)	Cyclin dependent kinase inhibitor	Phase II single agent study in met CRPC pts. 72 hour IV infusion at 40-60 mg/m2/day	36 pts enrolled. No objective responses. 14% pts met 6 month PFS endpoint.	Further development in germ cell tumours & gastric/GOJ ca	[127]
Thalidomide	IκB kinase inhibitor	Phase II studies docetaxel (75mg/m2) and docetaxel/ bevacizumab (15mg/m2) +/- thalidomide (200mg/m2)	60 pts enrolled. 90% PSA decline of >50%. Median TTP 18.3 months, median OS 28.2 months. Manageable toxicity but all pts had G3/4 neutropenia	Phase III placebo controlled trial in recurrent hormone sensitive non metastatic PC	[128, 129]

Lenolidamide		Phase II trial after biochemical relapse with LHRH agonists & phase I/II trial as single agent 5mg or 25 mg	159 pts enrolled. Med TTP PSA 15 vs 9.6 mths. Thalidomide well tolerated, 47% DR. 60 pts enrolled, 25mg ass with greater change in PSA slope but higher toxicity	Phase III in met CRPC pts, docetaxel/ prednisone +/- lenolidamide	[130, 131]
Parthenolide analogue (derived from *Tanacetum parthenium*)	NFκB inhibitor	Dimethylamino-partehnolide (DAMPT) with superior solubility & bioavailability	DAMPT inhibited NFkB DNA binding & expression of NFkB regulated anti-apoptotic proteins	Phase I dose escalation trial currently recruiting in pts with haem malig	[132]
Downstream agents					
Siltuximab	αIL-6 Ab	Phase II study in met CRPC pts post docetaxel. 6mg/kg IV q14d for 12 cycles	53 pts enrolled. PSA response rate 3.8%, RECIST SD rate 23%. High baseline IL-6 levels ass with poor prognosis	Phase I study in combination with docetaxel in met CRPC pts	[133]
Celecoxib	NSAID				
CNTO888	α-chemokine ligand 2 Ab	Preclinical studies of CNTO888 2mg/kg twice weekly ip in vivo prostate cancer model	Reduced tumour burden by 96% at 5 weeks also synergistic with docetaxel	Phase II in met CRPC pts post docetaxel results awaited	[134]
Plerixafor BKT140	αCXCR4			Focus of clinical dvpt in AML, phase I/II studies recruiting	

Table 3. The Inflammatory System

7. Other key pathways

With time, it is anticipated that more pathways and targets key to prostate cancer growth will be identified. Angiogenesis inhibition has been successful in other cancers but minimal activity was seen in trials with Sunitinib [101] and Bevacizumab [102]. Similarly, targeting the HGF-MET axis is supported by preclinical work [103] and some activity has been seen with MET inhibition. However, Cabozantinib – a tyrosine kinase inhibitor that inhibits multiple receptor tyrosine kinases (RTKs) with growth-promoting and angiogenic properties (MET (IC_{50} in enzymatic assays= 1.8nM), VEGFR2 (0.035nM), RET (3.8nM), and KIT (4.6nM) has significant and intriguing clinical activity in bony disease and some activity in soft tissue disease. This suggests the effect may be due to concurrent inhibition of two relevant pathways.

Cabozantinib has been studied in multiple solid tumors and has shown a broad spectrum of activity with tumour regression in patients with a variety of diseases. It's activity in medullary thyroid cancer is based on RET inhibition [104]. Of particular relevance to prostate cancer, a phase II discontinuation study of 168 men with progressive metastatic CRPC received Cabozantinib initially for 12 weeks [105]. Patients with PR continued open-label cabozantinib, patients with stable disease were randomized to cabozantinib or placebo, whilst patients with progression were discontinued. Trial accrual was halted after enrollment of 168 patients due to the significant activity observed. 78% patients had bone metastasis and significantly 86% of these had a complete or partial response on bone scan as early as week 6. 64% patients had improved pain and 46% patients reported lower narcotic analgesia use. To date the median PFS has not been reached. Most common related Grade 3/4 AEs were fatigue (11%), HTN (7%), and hand-foot syndrome (5%). Osteoclast and osteoblast effects were observed: 55% had declines of ≥50% in plasma C-Telopeptide; 56% of patients with elevated tALP had declines of ≥50%.

Interestingly numerous lines of preclinical and clinical evidence implicate MET and VEGFR activation in bone metastases as well as prostate cancer, especially castration resistant disease. Specifically, androgen deprivation increases MET expression in prostate cancer cells [106, 107] and c-met has been shown to be upregulated in CRPC and may be a factor that supports CRPC cells in the castrate state [106, 108]. Androgen deprivation also increases expression of c-met's ligand, Hepatocyte Growth Factor (HGF) in the stroma. Increased expression of MET and HGF may contribute to disease progression following androgen deprivation therapy. This may be a compensatory mechanism as HGF/cMET activity enhances Leydig cell steroidogenetic activity [109]. It is also of note that increased expression of MET and/or HGF correlate with prostate cancer metastasis and disease recurrence [110, 111]. In addition, VEGF has been shown to activate MET signaling via neuropilin-1. Osteoblasts and osteoclasts also express MET and VEGFRs and osteoclasts secrete HGF. This supports the notion that MET signaling not only supports the tumor, but also bone turnover which provides a fertile microenvironment for prostate cancer growth [112]. These observations provide a strong rationale for dual inhibition of VEGFR2 and MET as a therapeutic strategy in men with CRPC and bone metastases. As such, cabozantinib may not only have single agent activity but also enhance abiraterone activity by simultaneously blocking a putative resistance/survival mechanism to hormonal therapy and abrogating bone turnover and making the microenvironment less hospitable for cancer growth. Given these many reasons, it is logical to hypothesize that combining these two active agents against CRPC will result in even more substantial clinical benefit.

8. Conclusion & future directions

It is clear from the foregoing discussion that increased biological knowledge and drug development technologies has resulted in a vast number of agents for clinical trial testing. However, it is paramount that judicious trial designs are employed and match the drug to the tumor by ensuring that the target is present. It is also quite certain that no single drug will work given the inherent multiple redundant survival pathways. This is probably more apparent for castration resistant disease. Therefore, one can argue that waiting for metastatic disease or castrate resistant disease to assess a new drug is a defeatist approach, and that an assessment earlier in the disease spectrum to prevent the emergence of resistance is a more proactive and promising approach to improve outcomes in prostate cancer. The conduct of a study in patients with a biochemical relapse after definitive localized therapy provides a major opportunity for drug development. This approach allows the analysis of a drug in isolation and as well as an assessment and effective triage of the numerous new agents that are now available for testing. Also the primary pathology can be interrogated to look for activation of the pathway and provides an opportunity to biologically direct the evaluation of drugs relevant to a given a pathway in an individual's cancer. Ultimately, key combinations simultaneously targeting the essential and multiply redundant pathways driving cancer survival and resistance mechanisms can be developed. This has been a successful strategy for treatment of HIV and AIDS where the early use of Highly Active Anti-retroviral Therapy (HAART) has made major advances. With time and judicious clinical development, it is possible to develop a similar strategy such as Highly Effective Early Prostate Cancer Therapy (HEEPT) for patients with rapidly progressive PSA rises after definitive local therapy and have a long life expectancy. Early use of a highly effective combination therapy will hopefully eradicate the disease and prevent patients from dying from recurrent disease that may otherwise have been lethal and more difficult to treat if waited until later in the disease

Author details

Sarah M. Rudman[1], Peter G. Harper[1] and Christopher J. Sweeney[2]

1 Dept of Oncology, Guys & St Thomas' NHS Foundation Trust, Great Maze Pond, London, SE1 9RT, UK

2 Lank Center for Genitourinary Oncology, Dana Farber Cancer Institute, 450 Brookline Ave, Boston, MA, USA

References

[1] Sridhara R, Johnson J R, Justice R et al: Review of oncology and haematology drug product approvals at the US Food and drug administration between July 2005 and December 2007. J Natl Cancer Inst 2010 102(8) 578-9

[2] Lo Russo P M, Anderson A B, Boerner S A et al. Making the investigational oncology pipeline more efficient and effective: are we headed in the right direction? Clin Cancer Res 2010 16(24) 5956-62

[3] Tannock IF, Osoba D, Stockler MR et al: Chemotherapy with mitoxantrone plus prednisone or prednisone alone for symptomatic hormone resistant prostate cancer: a

Canadian randomized trial with palliative end-points. J Clin Oncol 1996 14(6) 1756-64

[4] Tannock I F, de Wit R, Berry WR et al: Docetaxel plus prednisone or mitoxantrone plus prednisone for advanced prostate cancer. N Engl J Med 2004 351 1502-12 2004

[5] Morris PG & Fornier MN: Microtubule active agents: beyond the taxane frontier. Clin Cancer Res 2008 14 7167-7172

[6] De Bono J S, Oudard S, Ozguroglu M et al: Prednisone plus cabazitaxel or mitoxantrone for metastatic castrate resistant prostate cancer progressing after docetaxel treatment: a randomized open label trial. Lancet 2010 376 (9747) 1147-54

[7] Gradishar WJ, Tjulandin S, Davidson N et al: Phase III trial of nanoparticle bound paclitaxel with polyethylated castor oil based paclitaxel in women with breast cancer. J Clin Oncol 2005 23(31) 7794-803

[8] Mita M, Mita A, Sarantopoulos J et al: Phase I study of paclitaxel poliglumex administered weekly for patients with advanced solid malignancies. Cancer Chemother Pharmacol 2009 64(2) 287-295

[9] Beer TM, Ryan C, Alumkal J et al: A phase II study of paclitaxel poliglumex in combination with transdermal oestradiol for the treatment of metastatic castrate resistant prostate cancer after docetaxel chemotherapy. Anticancer drugs 2010 21(4) 433-438

[10] Farokhzad OC, Cheng J, Teply BA et al: Targeted nanoparticle aptamer bioconjugates for cancer chemotherapy in vivo. Proc Natl Acad Sci USA 2006 103(16) 6315-6320

[11] Liu G, Chen YH, Dipaola R et al: Phase II trial of weekly ixabepilone in men with metastatic castrate-resistant prostate cancer (E3803): a trial of the eastern co-operative oncology group. Clin Genitourin Cancer 2012 10(2) 99-105

[12] Chi KN, Beardsley E, Eigl BJ et al: A phase II study of patupilone in patients with metastatic castrate-resistant prostate cancer previously treated with docetaxel: Canadian Urologic Oncology group study P07a. Ann Oncol 2012 23(1) 53-58

[13] Beer TM, Smith DC, Hussain A et al: Phase II study of sagopilone plus prednisone in patients with castrate-resistant prostate cancer: a phase II study of the Department of Defense Prostate Cancer Clinical Trials Consortium. Br J Cancer 2012 doi 10.1038/bjc.2012.339

[14] De Bono J S, Molife R, Sonpavde G et al: Phase II study of eribulin mesylate (E7389) in patients with metastatic castration-resistant prostate cancer stratified by prior taxane therapy. Ann Oncol 2012 23(5) 1241-1249

[15] Nilsson S, Parker C, Haugen I et al: Alpharadin, a novel, highly targeted alpha pharmaceutical with a good safety profile for patients with CRPC and bone metastases: Combined analyses of phase I and II clinical trials. 2010 Genitourinary cancer symposium abstract 106

http://dx.doi.org/10.5772/53092

[16] Sartor AO, Heinrich D, O'Sullivan JM et al: Radium-223 chloride (Ra-223) impact on skeletal-related events (SREs) and ECOG performance status (PS) in patients with castration-resistant prostate cancer (CRPC) with bone metastases: Interim results of a phase III trial (ALSYMPCA). J Clin Oncol 2012 30 suppl abstrc 4551

[17] Huggins C & Hodges CV. Studies on prostate cancer, I: the effect of castration of estrogen and of androgen injection on serum phosphatases in metastatic carcinoma of the prostate. Cancer Res 1941 1 293-297

[18] Craft, N, Shostak Y, Carey M et al: A mechanism for hormone-independent prostate cancer through modulation of androgen receptor signaling by the HER-2/neu tyrosine kinase. Nat. Med. 1999 5 280–285

[19] Gioeli, D, Ficarro SB, Kwiek JJ et al: Androgen receptor phosphorylation. Regulation and identification of the phosphorylation sites. J Biol Chem. 2003 277 29304–29314

[20] Veldscholte, J Ris-Stalpers C, Kuiper GG et al: A mutation in the ligand binding domain of the androgen receptor of human LNCaP cells affects steroid binding characteristics and response to anti-androgens. Biochem. Biophys. Res. Commun. 1990 173 534–540

[21] Chen CD, Welsbie DS, Tran C et al: Molecular determinants of resistance to anti-androgen therapy. Nature Medicine 2004 10 (1) 33-39

[22] Mitsiades N, Schultz B, Taylor S et al: Increased expression of androgen receptor and enzymes involved in androgen synthesis in metastatic prostate cancer: targets for novel personalized therapies. J Clin Oncol 2009 27: (15 suppl) abstr 5002

[23] Koivisto PA & Hellin H J: Androgen receptor gene amplification increases tissue PSA protein expression in hormone-refractory prostate carcinoma. Am J Pathol 1999 189(2) 219-223

[24] Mohler JL, Gregory CW, Ford OH. The androgen axis in recurrent prostate cancer. Clin Cancer Res 2004 10 440-448

[25] Figg WD, Liu Y, Arlen P et al. A randomized phase II trial of ketoconazole plus alendronate versus ketoconazole alone in patients with androgen independent prostate cancer and bone metastases. J Urol 2005 173 790-796

[26] Attard G, Reid A H M, A'Hern R et al: Selective inhibition with Cyp 17 with abiraterone acetate is highly active in the treatment of castrate-resistant prostate cancer. J Clin Oncol 2010 27 (23) 3742-3748

[27] Reid AH, Attard G, Danila DC et al. Significant and sustained anti-tumour activity in post docetaxel castration resistant prostate cancer with the CYP17 inhibitor abiraterone acetate. J Clin Oncol 2010 28 1489-1495

[28] De Bono JS, Logothetis CJ, Molina A et al: Abiraterone and increased survival in metastatic prostate cancer. N Engl J Med 2011 364(21) 1995-2005

[29] Ryan CJ, Smith MR, De Bono JS et al: Interim analysis (IA) results of COU-AA-302, a randomized, phase III study of abiraterone acetate (AA) in chemotherapy-naive patients (pts) with metastatic castration-resistant prostate cancer (mCRPC). J Clin Oncol 2012 suppl. Abstrc LBA 4518

[30] Petrylak DP, Gandhi JG, Clark WR et al: Phase I results from a phase I/II study of orteronel, an oral, investigational, nonsteroidal 17,20-lyase inhibitor, with docetaxel and prednisone (DP) in metastatic castration-resistant prostate cancer (mCRPC). J Clin Oncol 2012 30 suppl abstrc 4656

[31] Dreicer R, Agus DB, Bellmunt J et al: A phase III, randomized, double-blind, multicenter trial comparing the investigational agent orteronel (TAK-700) plus prednisone (P) with placebo plus P in patients with metastatic castration-resistant prostate cancer (mCRPC) that has progressed during or following docetaxel-based therapy. J Clin Oncol 2012 20 suppl abstrc TPS4963

[32] Chen Y, Clegg NJ, Scher HI. Anti-androgens and androgen-depleting therapies in prostate cancer: new agents for an established target. Lancet Oncol 2009 10 981-991

[33] Scher HI, Beer TM, Higano CS et al: Antitumour activity of MDV3100 in castration-resistant prostate cancer: a phase 1-2 study. Lancet 2010 375 (9724) 1437-1446

[34] De Bono JS, Fizazi K, Saad F et al: Primary, secondary, and quality-of-life endpoint results from the phase III AFFIRM study of MDV3100, an androgen receptor signaling inhibitor. J Clin Oncol 2012 30 suppl abstrc 4519

[35] Bolden JE, Peaert MJ, Johnstone RW. Anticancer activities of histone deacetylase inhibitors. Nat Rev Drug Discov 2006 5 769-784

[36] Welsbie DS, Xu J, Chen H et al: Histone deacetylases are required for androgen receptor function in hormone-sensitive and castrate – resistant prostate cancer. Cancer Res 2009 69 958-966

[37] Rathkopf D, Wong BY, Ross RW et al: A phase I study or oral panobinostat alone and in combination with docetaxel in patients with castration-resistant prostate cancer. Cancer Chemother Pharmacol 2010 66 (1) 181-9

[38] Bradley D, Rathkopf D, Dunn R et al: Vorinostat in advanced prostate cancer patients progressing on prior chemotherapy (National Cancer Institute Trial 6862): trial results and interleukin-6 analysis: a study by the Department of Defense Prostate Cancer Clinical Trial Consortium and University of Chicago Phase 2 Consortium. Cancer 2009 115 (23) 5541-9

[39] Schneider BJ, Kalemkerian GP, Bradley D et al. Phase I study of vorinostat in combination with docetaxel in patients with advanced and relapsed solid malignancies. Invest New Drugs 2012 30(1) 249-257

[40] Powers MV, Workman P: Targeting of multiple signaling pathways by heat shock protein 90 molecular chaperone inhibitors. Endocr Relat Cancer 2006 13 (Suppl 1): S125-S135

[41] Solit DB, Egorin M, Valentin G et al: Phase I pharmacokinetic and pharmacodynamic trial of docetaxel and 17-AAG (17-allylamino-17-demethoxygeldanamycin). J Clin Oncol 2004 22 (14 Suppl) Abstr 3032

[42] Heath EI, Hillman DW, Vaishampayam U et al: A phase II trial of 17-allylamino-17-demethoxygeldanamycin in patients with hormone-refractory metastatic prostate cancer. Clin Cancer Res 2008 14 (23) 7940-7946

[43] Oh W, Stadler WM. Srinivas S et al: A single arm phase II trial of IPI-504 in patients with castration resistant prostate cancer (CRPC). Presented at ASCO Genitourinary symposium 2009 Abstract 219

[44] Goldman JW, Raju RN, Gordon GA et al: A Phase 1 dose-escalation study of the Hsp90 inhibitor STA-9090 administered once weekly in patients with solid tumors. J Clin Oncol 2010 28:15s (suppl; abstr 2529)

[45] Oh Y K & Park T G. siRNA delivery systems for cancer treatment. Adv Drug Deliv Rev 2009 61(10) 850-862

[46] Tutt A, Robson M, Garber J E et al. Oral poly(ADP-ribose) polymerase inhibitor olaparib in patients with BRCA1 or BRCA2 mutations and advanced breast cancer: a proof of concept trial. Lancet 2010 376 235-244

[47] Gallagher DJ, Gaudet MM, Pal P et al: Germline BRCA mutations denote a clinicopathologic subset of prostate cancer. Clin Cancer Res 2010 16 (7) 2115-21

[48] Fong PC, Boss DS, Yap TA et al: Inhibition of poly(ADP-ribose) polymerase in tumours from BRCA mutations carriers. N Engl J Med 2009 361 123-134

[49] Mendes-Pereira AM, Martin SA, Brough R et al: Synthetic lethal targeting of PTEN mutant cells with PARP inhibitors. EMBO Mol Med 2009 1 (6-7) 315-22

[50] Sandhu SK, Wenham RM, Wilding G et al: First-in-human trial of a poly(ADP-ribose) polymerase (PARP) inhibitor MK-4827 in advanced cancer patients (pts) with antitumor activity in BRCA-deficient and sporadic ovarian cancers. J Clin Oncol 28:15s 2010 (suppl abstr 3001)

[51] Cho N Y, Choi M, Kim B H et al: Braf and Kras mutations in prostatic adenocarcinoma. Int J Cancer 2006 119(8) 1858-62

[52] Sun X, Huang J, Homma T et al: Genetic alterations in the PI3K pathway in prostate cancer. Anticancer Res 2009 29(5) 1739-43

[53] Hsing A W & Devesa S S: Trends and patterns of prostate cancer: what do they suggest? Epidemiol Rev 2001 23 3-13

[54] Strom S S, Yamamura Y, Forman MR et al: Saturated fat intake predicts biochemical failure after prostatectomy. Int J Cancer 2008 122 2581-5

[55] Warburg O. On the origin of cancer cells. Science 1956 123 309-314

[56] Nickerson T, Pollak M Huynh H: Castration-induced apoptosis in the rat ventral prostate is associated with increased expression of genes encoding insulin-like growth factor binding proteins 2,3,4 and 5. Endocrinology 1998 139(2) 807-810

[57] Plymate S R, Haugk K, Coleman I et al: An antibody targeting the type I insulin-like growth factors receptor enhances the castration induced response in androgen-dependent prostate cancer. Clin Can Res 2007 13(21) 6429-39

[58] Higano CS, Alumkal JJ, Ryan CJ et al: A phase II study of cixutumumab (IMC-A12), a monoclonal antibody (MAb) against the insulin-like growth factor 1 receptor (IGF-IR), monotherapy in metastatic castration-resistant prostate cancer (mCRPC): Feasibility of every 3-week dosing and updated results. Presented at the ASCO Genitourinary Symposium 2010 Abstract 189

[59] Haluska P, Shaw H M, Batzel G N et al: Phase I dose escalation study of the anti insulin-like growth factor-I receptor monoclonal antibody CP-751,871 in patients with refractory solid tumours. Clin Cancer Res 2007 13 5834-55840

[60] Molife LR, Fong PC, Pacagnella L et al: The insulin-like growth factor-I receptor inhibitor figitumumab (CP-751, 871) in combination with docetaxel in patients with advanced solid tumours: results of a phase Ib dose-escalation, open-label study. Br J Cancer 2010 103 (3) 332-9

[61] Tolcher AW, Sarantopoulos J, Patnaik A et al: Phase I, pharmacokinetic, and pharmacodynamic study of AMG 479, a fully human monoclonal antibody to insulin-like growth factor receptor 1. J Clin Oncol 2009 27 (34) 5800-7

[62] Carden CP, Lim ES, Jones RL et al: Phase I study of intermittent dosing of OSI-906, a dual tyrosine kinase inhibitor of insulin-like growth factor-1 receptor (IGF- 1R) and insulin receptor (IR) in patients with advanced solid tumors. J Clin Oncol 2010 28:15s (suppl; abstr 2530)

[63] Mulholland DJ, Dedhar S, Wu H et al: PTEN & GSK3beta: key regulators of progression to androgen-independent prostate cancer. Oncogene 2006 25(3) 329-337

[64] Jia S, Liu Z, Zhang S et al: Essential roles of PI(3)K-p110b ▪ in cell growth, metabolism and tumourigenesis. Nature 2008 454 776-9

[65] Edelmann G, Bedell C, Shapiro G et al: A phase I dose escalation study of XL147 (SAR205408), a PI3K inhibitor administered orally to patients with advanced malignancies. J Clin Oncol 2010 28 15s (suppl;abstrc 3004)

[66] Von Hoff DD, LoRusso P, Tibes R et al: A first in human phase I study to evaluate the pan-PI3K inhibitor GDC-0941 administered QD or BID in patients with advanced solid tumours. J Clin Oncol 2010 28:15s (suppl;abstr 2541)

[67] Baselga J, De Jonge MJ, Rodon J et al: A first-in-human phase I study of BKM120, an oral pan-class I PI3K inhibitor, in patients (pts) with advanced solid tumours. J Clin Oncol 28:15s 2010 (suppl;abstr 3003)

[68] Kreisberg J I, Malik S N, Prihoda T J et al: Phosphorylation of Akt (ser473) is an excellent predictor of poor clinical outcome in prostate cancer. Cancer Res 2004 64 5232-5236

[69] Ayala G, Thompson t, Yang G et al: High levels of phosphorylated form of Akt-1 in prostate cancer and non-neoplastic prostate tissues are strong predictors of biochemical recurrence. Clin Cancer Res 2004 10 6572-6578

[70] Chee K G, Longmate J, Quinn D I et al: The AKT inhibitor perifosine in biochemically recurrent prostate cancer: a phase II California/Pittsburgh cancer consortium trial. Clin Genitourin Cancer 2007 5(7) 433-7

[71] Tolcher AW, Yap TA, Fearen I et al: A phase I study of MK-2206, an oral potent allosteric Akt inhibitor in patients with advanced solid tumours. J Clin Oncol 2009 27 15s (suppl;abstrc 3503)

[72] George D J, Armstrong A J, Creel P: A phase II study of RAD001 in men with hormone-refractory metastatic prostate cancer (HRPC). ASCO Genitourinary Cancers Symposium 2008: abstract 181

[73] Ross R W, Manola J, Oh W K et al: Phase I trial of RAD001 and docetaxel in castration resistant prostate cancer with FDG-PET assessment of RAD001 activity. J Clin Oncol 2008 26 abstrc 5069

[74] Pan C, Ghosh P, Lara P et al: Encouraging activity of bicalutamide and everolimus in castration-resistant prostate cancer (CRPC): Early results from a phase II clinical trial. J Clin Oncol 2011 suppl. 11 abstrc 157

[75] Hardie D G. AMP-activated/SNF-1 protein kinases: conserved guardians of cellular energy. Nat Rev Mol Cell Biol 2007 8 774-785

[76] Luo Z, Saha AK, Xiang X et al: AMPK, the metabolic syndrome and cancer. Trends Pharmacol Sci 2005 26 69-76

[77] Matsui H, Suzuki K, Ohtake N et al: Genome wide linkage analysis of familial prostate cancer in the Japanese population. J Hum Genet 2004 49 9-15

[78] Xiang X, Saha A K, Wen R et al: AMP-activated protein kinase activators can inhibit the growth of prostate cancer cells by multiple mechanisms. Biochem Biophys Res Commun 2004 321 161-7

[79] Huang X, Wullschleger S, Shapiro N et al: Important role of the LKB1-AMPK pathways in suppressing tumourigenesis in PTEN-deficient mice. Biochem J 2008 412 212-21

[80] Wright J L & Stanford J L: Metformin use and prostate cancer in Caucasian men: results from a population-based case-control study. Cancer Causes Control 2009 20 1617-22

[81] Pollak M: Insulin and insulin-like growth factor signaling in neoplasia. Nat Rev Cancer 2008 8 915-28

[82] Jang M, Cai L, Udeani G O et al: Cancer chemopreventive activity of resveratrol, a natural product derived from grapes. Science 1997 275 218-220

[83] De Marzo AM, De Weese TM, Platz EA et al: Pathological and molecular mechanisms of prostate carcinogenesis: implications for diagnosis, detection, prevention and treatment. J Cell Biochem 2004 91 459-477

[84] De Marzo AM, Marchi VL, Epstein JI & Nelson WG: Proliferative inflammatory atrophy of the prostate: implications for prostate carcinogenesis. Am J Pathol. 1999 59 (22) 1985-1992

[85] Sutcliffe S, Giovanucci E, Alderete JF et al: Plasma antibodies against Trichomonas vaginalis and subsequent risk of prostate cancer. Cancer Epidemiol Biomarkers Prev 2006 15(11) 939-945

[86] Stark JR, Judson G, Alderete JF et al: Prospective study of Trichomonas vaginaslis infection and prostate cancer incidence and mortality: Physicians health study. J Natl Cancer Inst 2009 101 (20) 1406-1411

[87] Nelson WG, De Marzo AM, Isaacs WB et al: Mechanisms of disease: prostate cancer. N Engl J Med 2003 349 366-381

[88] Li H, Kantoff PW, Giovanucci E et al: Manganese superoxide dismutase polymorphism, prediagnostic antioxidant status and risk of clinically significant prostate cancer. Cancer Res 2005 65(6) 2498-2504

[89] Dobrovolskaia MA & Kozlov SV: Inflammation & Cancer:when NFκB amalgamates the perilous partnership. Curr Cancer Drug Targets 2005 5(5) 325-344

[90] Ghosh S, Bhattacharya S, Sirkar M et al: Leishmania donovani suppresses activated protein1 and NF-κB activation in host macrophages via ceramide generation: involovement of extracellular signal-regulated kinase Infect Immun 2002 70(12) 6828-6838

[91] Helbig G, Christopherson KW, Bhat-Nakshatri P et al: NK-κB promotes breast cancer cell migration and metastasis by inducing the expression of the chemokine receptor CXCR4. J Biol Chem 2003 278(24) 21631-21638

[92] Zong WX, Edelstein LC, Chen C et al: The prosurvival Bcl-2 homolog Bfl-1/A1 is a direct transcriptional target of NF-κB that blocks TNF alpha induced apoptosis. Genes Dev 1999 13 (4) 382-387

[93] Dolcet X, Llobet D, Pallares J et al: NF-kB in development and progression of human cancer.Virchows Archiv 2005 446 (5) 475-482

[94] Wang CY, Mayo MW, Baldwin AS: TNF and cancer therapy-induced apoptosis: potentation by inhibition of NF-κB. Science 1996 274: 784-787

[95] Karashima T, Sweeney P, Kamat A et al: Nuclear factor κB mediates angiogenesis and metastasis of human bladder cancer through the regulation of interleukin-8. Clin Cancer Res 2003 9(7) 2786-2797

[96] Ammirante M, Luo JL, Grivennikov S et al: B-cell derived lymphotoxin promotes castration resistant prostate cancer. Nature 2010 464 302-5

[97] Min J, Zaslavsky A, Fedele G et al: An oncogene-tumor suppressor cascade drives metastatic prostate cancer by coordinately activating Ras and nuclear factor-κB. Nat Med 2010 16(3) 286-294

[98] Sweeney C, Li L, Shanmugam R et al: Nuclear factor-kappaB is constitutively activated in prostate cancer in vitro and is overexpressed in prostatic intraepithelial neoplasia and adenocarcinoma of the prostate. Clin Cancer Res 2004 10(16) 5501-5507

[99] Lessard L, Begin LR, Gleave ME et al: Nuclear localization of nuclear factor-κB transcription factors in prostate cancer: an immunohistochemical study 2005 93(9) 1019-1023

[100] Lessard L, Mes-Masson AM, Lamarre L et al. NF κB nuclear localization and its prognostic significant in prostate cancer BJU Int. 2003 91(4) 417-420

[101] Michaelson MD, Oudard S, Ou Y et al: Randomized, placebo-controlled, phase III trial of sunitinib in combination with prednisone (SU+P) versus prednisone (P) alone in men with progressive metastatic castration-resistant prostate cancer (mCRPC). J Clin Oncol 2011 29 suppl abstrc 4515

[102] Heidenreich A, Pfister DJ, Thüer D et al: Docetaxel versus docetaxel plus bevacizumab in progressive castration-resistant prostate cancer following first-line docetaxel. J Clin Oncol 2010 28 suppl abstrc e15006

[103] Varkaris A, Corn PG, Gaur S et al: The role of HGF/c-met signaling in prostate cancer progression and c-met inhibitors in clinical trials. Exp Opin Investig Drugs 2011 20 (12) 1677-84

[104] Kurzrock R, Sherman SI, Ball DW et al: Activity of XL-184 (Cabozantinib), an oral tyrosine kinase inhibitor, in patients with medullary thyroid cancer. J Clin Oncol 2011 29 2660-2666

[105] Hussain M, Sweeney C, Corn PG et al: Cabozantanib (XL184) in metastatic castration-resistant prostate cancer (mCRPC): Results from a phase II randomized discontinuation trial. J Clin Oncol 2011 29 (Suppl) abstrc 4516

[106] Humphrey PA, Zhu X, Zarnegar R et al: Hepatocyte growth factor and its receptor (c-MET) in prostatic carcinoma. Am J Pathol. 1995 147 (2) 386-396

[107] Verras M, Lee J, Xue H et al: the androgen receptor negatively regulates the expression of c-Met: implications for a novel mechanism of prostate cancer progression. Cancer Res 2007 67 (3) 967-975

[108] Tu WH, Zhu C, Clark C et al: Efficacy of c-Met inhibitor fpr advanced prostate cancer. BMC Cancer 2010 10 556

[109] Del Bravo J, Catizone A, Ricci G et al: Hepatocyte growth factor-modulated rat Leydig cell functions. J Androl. 2007 28(6) 866-874

[110] Knudsen BS, Gmyrek GA, Inra J et al: High expression of the Met receptor in prostate cancer metastasis to bone. Urology 2002 60(6) 1113-1117

[111] Humphrey PA, Halabi S, Picus J et al: Prognostic significance of plasma scatter/hepatocyte growth factor levels in patients with metastatic hormone refractory prostate cancer: results from Cancer & Leukaemia group B 150005/9480. Clin Genitourin Cancer 2006 4(4) 269-274

[112] Grano M, Galimi F, Zambonin G et al: Hepatocyte growth factor is a coupling factor for osteoclasts and osteoblasts in vitro. Proceedings of the National Academy of Sciences of the United States of America. 1996 93(15) 7644-7648

[113] Bruno RD, Vasaitis TS, Gediya LK et al: Synthesis and biological evaluations of putative metabolic stable analogs of TOK-001: head to head anti-tumour efficacy evaluation of TOK-001 and Abiraterone in LAPC-4 human prostate cancer xenograft model. Steroids 2011 76(12) 1268-1279

[114] Yong W, Goh B, Toh H et al: Phase I study of SB939 three times weekly for 3 weeks every 4 weeks in patients with advanced solid malignancies. J Clin Oncol 27:15s, 2009 (suppl; abstr 2560)

[115] Molife LR, Attard G, Fong PC et al: Phase II, two-stage, single arm trial of the histone deacetylase inhibitor (HDAC) romidepsin in metastatic castration-resistant prostate cancer (CRPC). Ann Oncol 2010 21: 109-113

[116] Evans T, Lindsay CR, Chan E et al: Phase I dose-escalation study of continuous oral dosing of OSI-906, a dual tyrosine kinase inhibitor of insulin-like growth factor-1 receptor (IGF-1R) and insulin receptor (IR), in patients with advanced solid tumors. J Clin Oncol 28:15s, 2010 (suppl; abstr 2531).

[117] Ben Sahra I, Laurent K, Loubat A et al: The antidiabetic drug metformin exerts an anti-tumoural effect in vitro and in vivo through a decrease in cyclin D1 level. Oncogene 2008 27 2576-3586

[118] Emmenegger U, Berry SR, Booth C et al: Phase II study of maintenance therapy with temsirolimus (TEM) after response to first-line docetaxel (TAX) chemotherapy in castration-resistant prostate cancer (CRPC). J Clin Oncol 2011 29 Suppl 7 Abstrc 160

[119] Lu J, Me ML, Wang L et al: MiR-26a inhibits cell growth and tumorigenesis of nasopharyngeal carcinoma through repression of EZH2.Cancer Res 2011 71(1) 225-233

[120] Saad F, Hotte S, North S et al: Randomized Phase 2 Trial of Custirsen (OGX-011) with Docetaxel or Mitoxantrone in Patients with Metastatic Castrate-Resistant Prostate Cancer: CUOG Trial P06c. Clin Cancer Res 2011 Epub ahead of print.

[121] Hainsworth JD, Meluch AA, Spigel DR et al; Weekly docetaxel and bortezomib as first-line treatment for patients with hormone-refractory prostate cancer: a Minnie Pearl Cancer Research Network phase II trial. Clin Genitorurin Cancer 2007 5(4) 278-283

[122] Cresta S Cessa C, Catapano CV et al: Phase I study of bortezomib with weekly paclitaxel in patients with advanced solid tumours. Eur J Cancer 2008 44 (13) 1829-1834

[123] Kraft AS, Garrett-Mayer E, Wahlquist AE et al: Combination therapy of recurrent prostate cancer with the proteosome inhibitor Bortezomib plus hormone blockade. Cancer Biol Ther 2011 12(2) 119-124

[124] O'Connor OA, Stewart AK, Vallone M et al: A phase I dose escalation study of the safety and pharmacokinetics of the novel proteosome inhibitor carfilzomib in patients with haematological malignancies. Clin Cancer Res 15 (22) 7085-91

[125] Fizazi K, Carducci M, Smith M et al: Denosumab versus zoledronic acid for treatment of bone metastases in men with castrate-resistant prostate cancer: a randomized double blind study. Lancet 2011 377 813-822

[126] Flaig TW, Glode M, Gustafson D et al: A study of high-dose oral silybin-phytosome followed by prostatectomy in patients with localized prostate cancer. Prostate 2010 70(8) 848-855

[127] Liu G, Gandara DR, Lara PN et al: A phase II trial of flavopiridol in patients with previously untreated metastatic androgen-independent prostate cancer. Clin Cancer Res 2004 10(3) 924-928

[128] Ning Y-M, Gulley JL, Arlen PM et al: Phase II trial of bevacizumab, thalidomide, docetaxel and prednisone in patients with metastatic castration resistant prostate cancer. J Clin Oncol 2010 28(12) 2070-2076

[129] Dahut WL, Gulley JL, Arlen PM et al: Randomised phase II trial of docetaxel plus thalidominde in androgen-independent prostate cancer. J Clin Oncol 2004 22 2532-2539

[130] Figg WD, Huassain MH, Gulley JL et al: A double blind randomized crossover study of oral thalidomide versus placebo for androgen dependent prostate cancer treated with intermittent androgen ablation. J Urol 2009 181(3) 1104-1113

[131] Keizman D, Zahurak M, Sinibaldi V et al: Lenolidamide in non-metastatic biochemically relapsed prostate cancer: results of a phase I/II double-blinded randomized study. Clin Cancer Res 2010 16(21) 5269-5276

[132] Shanmugam R, Kusumanchi P, Cheng L et al: A water soluble parthenolide analogue suppresses in vivo prostate cancer growth by targeting NFkB & generating reactive oxygen species. Prostate 2010 70(10) 1074-1086

[133] Dorff TB, Goldman B, Pinski JB et al: Clinical and correlative results of SWOG S0354: a phase II trial of CNTO 328 (Siltuximab), a monoclonal antibody against interleukin-6, in chemotherapy pre-treated patients with castration resistant prostate cancer. Clin Cancer Res 2010 16(11) 3028-3034

[134] Loberg RD, Ying C, Craig M et al: Targeting CCL-2 with systemic delivery of neutralizing antibodies induced prostate cancer tumour regression in vivo. Cancer Res 2007 67(19) 9417-9424

Chapter 11

Novel Therapeutic Settings in the Treatment of Castration-Resistant Prostate Cancer

Miguel Álvarez Múgica, Jesús M. Fernández Gómez,
Antonio Jalón Monzón,
Erasmo Miguelez García and
Francisco Valle González

Additional information is available at the end of the chapter

http://dx.doi.org/10.5772/52288

1. Introduction

Prostate cancer is the most common non-dermatological malignant disease in men in western countries. According to the American Cancer Society in 2010, the incidence of prostate cancer was 217,730 cases with 32,050 deaths from the disease [1]. Overall, the actuarial 10 and 15 years survival are 93% and 77% respectively [1]. The rise in incidence and improved survival of prostate cancer over the past decades have often been attributed to prostate cancer screening and early detection. Definite evidence supporting this relationship is, however, still pending. There are also alternative explanations such as improved treatment at advanced stages that could lower prostate cancer mortality. Because of earlier detection, up to 90% of new cases in the post prostate-specific antigen (PSA) era present with clinically localized disease, the majority of which do well regardless of treatment regimen undertaken. Overall, those with advanced prostate cancer at time of diagnosis remains essentially incurable, and do poorly after androgen withdrawal therapy developing progressive disease that is resistant to further hormone manipulation. For these patients with castration-resistent prostate cancer (CRPC), and particularly patients with metastatic disease, options till few years ago have been limited. However, as newer agents become available, higher rate of biochemical and clinical response are being achieved, providing a new hope for the management of these patients [2].

CRPC is defined as patients with serum castration levels of testosterone (< 50 ng/dL or < 1.7 nmol/L), PSA and/or clinical progression to castration, and progression despite anti-androgen withdrawal for at least 4-6 weeks. PSA progression is defined as three consecutive rises of PSA, 1 week apart, resulting in two 25% increases over the nadir, with a PSA level > 2 ng/dL above the nadir. Clinical progression includes progression of bone lesions (two or more lesions on bone scan) or soft tissue progression using Respond Evaluation Criteria In Solid Tumors (RECIST) criteria [3].

Although patients with CRPC have, by definition, castrate levels of circulating testosterone, most tumors continue to remain dependent on androgen and on signaling from the androgen receptor (AR). This may occur through constitutive activation of the AR (gene amplification, alternative splicing, AR-activating gene mutations), intratumoral production of androgen, promiscuity of the AR (and binding of other hormones), activation of downstream targets by dysregulation of transcription factors (eg, binding of the frequently rearranged and overexpressed ETS oncogenic factors to androgen-regulated promoters), and alternative yet unidentified mechanisms [1, 2].

CRPC status includes patient cohorts with significantly different median survival times and different sensitivity to second hormonal manipulations. However, the vast majority of patients eventually develop progressive disease that is resistant to further hormone manipulation. We now know that although this group of patients progress to androgen deprivation, they might still be hormone-sensitive. Until 2004, cytotoxic chemotherapy was considered to be relatively ineffective in men with CRPC. In 2004, 2 landmark trials, TAX 327 and Southwest Oncology Group (SWOG) 99-16, showed for the first time a survival benefit in men with metastatic HRPC. Specifically, docetaxel-based chemotherapy demonstrated a median improvement in survival of 2.5 months as compared with mitoxantrone and prednisone in metastatic HRPC [4, 5]. Regimens that include docetaxel, have demonstrated higher rates of objective and biochemical PSA response, as well as longer survival durations. In contrast, metastatic CRPC has become a more complicated disease to be properly treated. Since then, newer treatments in this stage of the disease have been approved optimizing survival and quality of life.

2. Mechanisms involved in the development and progression of the disease

To understand prostatic growth in diseased states, it is important to understand the hormonal influences at play in normal prostate development and function. Testosterone is the primary circulating androgen in men. Within the prostate, testosterone is converted to a more potent androgen dihydrotestosterone (DHT) by the action of intracellular 5α-reductase enzymes [6]. Circulating DHT levels are low (1 : 10) when compared with testosterone, whereas in the prostate, this ratio is reversed, making DHT the primary prostatic androgen [7].

Dihydrotestosterone is essential for the development of the prostate gland. Inside the prostate, both testosterone and DHT bind to the androgen receptor (AR), stimulating the AR signalling axis that promotes cell-cycle regulation, cell survival and lipogenesis [8]. Although both the androgens are capable of binding AR, DHT has a stronger affinity than testosterone and a slower dissociation rate [9, 10]. DHT is also more potent at stimulating prostatic growth than testosterone [9]. These combined effects of DHT enhance the androgen signalling pathway in tissues where 5α-reductase enzymes are highly expressed [10].

Depending on the developmental stage of the individual, DHT signalling could promote the differentiation of the male external genitalia (gestation) or the maturation of the prostate gland (puberty) [7]. Throughout adulthood, DHT androgen signalling acts as a regulator of homoeostasis, maintaining the prostate epithelium by balancing cell proliferation and cell death [8]. Unlike testosterone, DHT does not exhibit an age-related decline in serum concentration. Some studies have shown a steady decline of testosterone every decade in healthy men [11, 12], whereas the levels of DHT either decline slightly or remain unchanged [13, 14]. It has been suggested that DHT levels remain constant in ageing individuals because the pathway of conversion from testosterone is saturated at low levels of testosterone. Morgentaler and Traish present a critical revision of the traditional view of T and PC [15]. They use a saturation model that is consistent with regression of cancer when T is reduced to castrate levels but lacks observed growth when serum T is increased. The saturation model starts from the observation that PCa growth is sensitive to variation in serum T concentrations at or below the castrate range and is insensitive to T variation above this concentration. Considering the actual interest in using T replacement therapies in men, a new definition of the relationship between T and PCa is of considerable importance. Evidence supports the hypothesis that T administration in hypogonadal men without PCa does not increase the risk for PCa growth if T levels are normalised [16-18].

Compelling evidence that implicates DHT as the primary prostatic androgen comes from the discovery of the Dominican pseudohermaphrodites or Guevedoce. This population has a deficiency in 5α-reductase and therefore their DHT levels are markedly lower, whereas their testosterone levels remain normal [19]. The prostate of these affected men is non-palpable and the prostate volume is one-tenth that of normal age-matched controls. Administration of DHT in these individuals results in prostate enlargement, strongly implicating DHT as a necessary component of prostate growth and development [20].

Androgen receptor signaling remains active even with castrate levels of serum testosterone, contrary to the previous notion that disease progression after gonadal ablation necessarily implied androgen-independent escape mechanisms. This is supproted by studies, which report high intratumoral androgens, continued AR signaling [21], and overexpression of enzymes key to androgen síntesis, which suggests that CRPC may synthesize androgens de novo [22, 23]. Until recently, available strategies that target the AR, such as antiandrogens, ketoconazole, estrogens or glucocorticoids, result in modest beneficit. New drugs such as abiraterone, or MDV 3100 have shown a much more supression activity of the AR by different pathways.

The key components of DHT production are the 5α reductase enzymes. There are two well-characterised isoforms, type 1 and type 2 [24, 25]. Type 1 is present throughout all stages of life and is primarily localised in extraprostatic tissues including the non-genital skin, liver and certain brain regions. Although type 1 expression was originally thought to be absent from the prostate gland, certain studies have found type 1 within the prostatic tissue predominantly localised to the secretory luminal epithelium [26]. The type 2 5α-reductase isoform is prevalent in the prostatic tissue as well as the genital skin, seminal vesicle and epididymis. Although this isoform is present through all stages of prostate development, it has a single wave of expression in the skin and scalp that begins at birth and ends at ages 2–3 years [26]. Type 2 5α-reductase is deficient in the Guevedoce and therefore these individuals do not generate enough DHT to promote normal development of the prostate gland and the man's external genitalia [20].

3. Natural history of prostate cancer

Although the natural history of prostate cancer (PCa) has not been fully elucidated, it is thought to arise from damaged prostate epithelium and progressively develop over many decades [27]. Prostate disease is heterogeneous and multifocal, further complicating the understanding of its progression. Based on autopsy studies, about one-third of men over the age of 50 years display histological evidence of PCa. However, a majority of these cases remain clinically insignificant, underscoring the variability in PCa and the protracted nature of this disease [3, 28].

The likelihood of disease progression of PCa is difficult to predict. Detection of cancer from a biopsy can result in a localised diagnosis; however, upon a prostatectomy, it may be revealed that the disease had grown outside the margins of the gland or even had metastasised. Conversely, certain men diagnosed with PCa may live out their natural lives without suffering any morbidity or mortality from the disease.Therefore, it becomes imperative to determine whether or not a particular lesion will stay localised or spread beyond the confines of the gland [3]. The usually slow progression of prostate cancer allows delaying or avoiding definitive treatment (active surveillance) in selected patients if some prerequisites are fulfilled. The younger a candidate is for active surveillance, the more strict the tumour-related criteria that should be used [29].

Research has revealed insights into the likely progression of prostate tumours. It has been shown that certain high-grade tumours proceed on a more aggressive course than low-grade, well-differentiated tumours and therefore should be managed accordingly [30]. The Gleason score is one of the most powerful prognostic factors in prostate cancer [31]. In elderly patients with clinically localised, conservatively managed prostate cancer, the probability to survive the disease for at least 10 years ranges from 77% to 98% when the Gleason score is 7 or less, whereas this rate is only 33–75% in patients with a Gleason score of 8–10 [32]. The prolonged nature of PCa progression highlights the opportunities for clinical therapeutic interventions that could reduce the risk of disease development and slow it or treat the existing disease. Through the Cancer and Leukimia Group B (CALGB) cooperative study group, Halabi and colleagues performed a polled analysis combining data from 6 trials and more than 1100 patients with CRPC accured from 1991 to 2001 [33], and created a prognostic model for risk stratification of metastatic CRPC patients. The observed median survival durations (in months) were 7.5 (95% confidence interval [CI] 6.2–10.9], 13.4 (95% CI 9.7–26.3],

18.9 (95% CI 16.2–26.3], and 27.2 (95% CI 21.9–42.8] for the first, second, third, and fourth risk groups, respectively. The factors involved in this model can be broadly divided into clinical variables that reflect the condition of the host (eg, performance status, anemia, fatigue), the tumor burden (eg, sites of metastatic disease, PSA level, alkaline phosphatase level), or the biologic aggressiveness of the cancer itself (eg, lactate dehydrogenase [LDH] levels, Gleason sum).

The clinical course of metastatic castration-resistant prostate cancer has changed considerably, primarily because of factors such as earlier diagnosis, stage migration and changes in clinical practice patterns. Earlier initiation of androgen-deprivation therapy and the increased use of diagnostic imaging have contributed to earlier detection of metastatic disease in androgen-deprived patients. Furthermore, new treatments have further extended the time to the terminal phase of the disease, extimating the duration of the course of metastatic castration-resistant prostate cancer measured from the first documented metastasis (in the castrate state) until death may now extend beyond 5 years.

4. Mechanisms and targets in CRPC

The key for the development of new drugs and to optimize androgenic suppression in advanced stages of CRPC is the identification and characterization of molecular targets and mechanisms that lead to tumor growth. Disease progression involves the development of cellular adaptive pathways of survival in an androgen-depleted environment [34]. Experimental evidence assigns an important role to the continuous activation of the androgenic receptors (ARs) in tumor growth, as well as alternative independent routes [35]. In general, resistance mechanisms can be divided into 6 groups.

- *Increased Expression of Enzymes Involved in Steroidogenesis.* Studies have suggested that, in CRPC patients, even castrate serum levels of androgen are still sufficient for AR activation and able to maintain cancer cells survival. Indeed, the intratumoral levels of testosterone in CRPC patients are equal of those found in noncastrate patients [36]. The source of these androgens is thought to be derived from the synthesis of androgens directly in prostate cancer cells due to an upregulation of the enzymes and activation of the routes necessary for the synthesis of androgens such as testosterone and dihydrotestosterone [34, 37, 38]. Also bone metastases contain intact enzyme pathways for conversion of adrenal androgens to testosterone and dihydrotestosterone [36]. Montgomery and colleagues showed that there was marked reversal of the DHT : testosterone ratio in the metastatic tumor. These tumor cells express significantly lower levels of SRD5A2, which catalyses the conversion of testosterone to DHT, and higher levels of UGT2B15 and UGT2B17, which mediate the irreversible glucuronidation of DHT metabolites. Marked up regulation of CYP19A1, which mediates the aromatization of testosterone to estradiol, was also observed in the metastases samples [34, 36-38].
- *Increased Expression of AR.* The overexpression of AR have been involved in the progression of prostate cancer [34]. The activated AR pathways observed in these CRPC patients

has been postulated as a result of genetic phenomena that promotes increased sensitivity of AR. DNA amplifications are responsible for AR overexpression and for its activation in presence of low levels of ligand (androgens) [34, 38].

- *AR Gene Mutations and Altered Ligand Specificity.* While the androgens are the main factors of tumor growth and AR signaling, the presence of AR mutations leads to its activation by nonandrogenic steroid molecules and antiandrogens [34]. The majority AR mutations are point mutations in the AR ligand-binding domain, and initially this was considered relevant to explain why 10–30% of patients receiving antiandrogens treatment experience paradoxical PSA drop on cessation of treatment [35]. However the AR mutations could occur in other regions such as the amino terminus or the DNA binding domain that confer oncogenic properties to the AR [37]. At the present, the role of AR mutations in the anti-androgen withdrawal phenomena is called into questioned and a new explanation is offered since the discovery of alternative splicing of the AR. In fact, in recent reports [39, 40], it was shown that splice variants of AR with deletion of exons 5, 6, and 7 could result in AR capable to translocate to the nucleus without ligand binding.

- *Downstream Signaling Receptor for Androgens.* One of the most important mechanisms in the development of castration resistance is the activation of different signal transduction pathways in CRPC cells. They could enhance the activity of the AR or its coactivators in the presence of low levels or even in the absence of androgen. These include other receptors such as epithelial growth factors, insulin growth factors, and tyrosine-kinase receptor [40].

- *Bypass Pathways.* The induction of bypass pathways independent of AR, is an important mechanism of castration resistance, that can overcame apoptosis induced by androgen-deprivation therapy. One such example of this is the up-regulation of antiapoptotic proteins, including the protein Bcl-2 gene [34, 40].

- *Stem Cells.* Prostatic cancer stem cells are rare and undifferentiated cells that do not express AR on their surface, being independent of androgens to survive [34]. Currently it is thought that these cells can be responsible for maintaining tumor growth and development, because they are able to survive under androgen-deprivation therapy. The identification of these cells is possible based on the expression of surface protein ($\alpha 1 \beta 1$ integrin and CD133), which could allow new targets therapies [34].

5. New therapeutics settings in the treatment of castration resistant prostate cancer

Being able to predict which patients will develop metastasis and death with rising PSA levels after treatment with androgen ablation is essential for deciding therpeutic interventions and gauging prognosis. The major biologic processes under therpeutic investigation in prostate cancer involve growth and survival, chemotherapy and hormone therapy resistance, extragonadal androgen production, modulation of the androgen receptor, angiogenesis, the bone interface, immune surveillance and escape, epigenetic regulation and stem cell renewal. A better understanding of this mechanisms responsible for prostate cancer growth and metastatic spread has allowed for the development of a wide array of new therapies.

The growth of prostate cancer is originally androgen dependent and metastatic tumors are generally treated with androgen ablation therapy, with or without antiandrogen supplementation [41, 42, 43]. However, resistance to hormonal therapy occurs within 12–18 months (remissions last on average 2-3 years, progression occurs even under castration [37, 44, 45], referred to as hormone-refractory or CRPC [41]. Resistance to hormones (in patients with metastatic disease) is probably shorter than 2-3 years, using PSA. Until recently, patients with castration-resistant prostate cancer had limited treatment options after docetaxel chemotherapy. However, in 2010, new options emerged [46]. The three nonhormonal systemic approaches that have been found to prolong survival are docetaxel as first line [4] chemotherapy, cabazitaxel as second-line cytotoxic chemotherapy [46, 47] and a vaccine named sipuleucel-T [48]. A new hormonal manipulation with abiraterone acetate [45] also showed to prolong survival in CRPC.

The current palliative treatment options for patients with CRPC can be divided in different groups such as secondary hormonal therapies, chemotherapy agents, vaccine-based immune therapy, bisphosphonates, radiotherapy and novel targets.

5.1. Antiandrogen therapies

Drugs that reduce circulating levels of androgens or that competitively inhibit the action of androgens remain central to the treatment of prostate cancer. The surgical or medical castration with orchiectomy or gonadotropin-releasing hormone (GnRH) agonists, respectively, suppresses testicular testosterone generation. However, the duration of response to castration is short [12–33 months) and, in almost all patients, is followed by the emergence of a castration-resistant phenotype [34]. The combination with antiandrogens to achieve the maximum androgen blockade (MAB) did not prove to prolong survival and 30% of the patients have a drop in PSA after discontinuing antiandrogens [3, 43]. For patients whose disease progresses after a MAB, antiandrogen can be discontinued [49], or can be switched to an alternative antiandrogen as showed in several reports [3, 43]. High-dose [150 mg daily) bicalutamide as second-line hormonal therapy resulted in ≥50% PSA reduction in 20%–45% of patients [12, 34].

- **Oral Glucocorticoids** (10 mg/day) can result in temporary PSA responses for 25% of the patients, presumably due to adrenal androgen suppression [34, 50].
- **Diethylstilboestrol** (DES), a synthetic estrogen, as well as the other estrogens, suppresses the hypothalamic-pituitary-gonadal axis and it reduces ≥50% the total PSA in 26% to 66% of patients with CRPC. However, the important thromboembolic toxicity limited is use [50,51].
- **Ketoconazol** is an antifungal agent that can be given to CRPC patients after antiandrogen withdrawal because it inhibits cytochrome P-450 enzyme-mediated steroidogenesis in testes and adrenal glands and when given at high-dose (1200 mg/day) or low dose (600

mg/day) it resulted in ≥50% PSA reduction in 27% to 63% and 27 to 46%, of patients, respectively [49]. However, the narrow therapeutic window of ketoconazole + hydrocortisone versus hydrocortisone alone must be kept in mind due to secondary effects of ketoconazole.

- **Abiraterone acetate**, a prodrug of abiraterone, is a potent and highly selective inhibitor of androgen biosynthesis that blocks cytochrome P450 c17 (CYP17] a critical enzyme in androgen synthesis in the testes, adrenals and in the tumor itself [52]. This enzyme catalyzes two sequential reactions: the conversion of pregnenolone and progesterone to their 17-α-hydroxy derivates and the subsequent formation of dehydroepiandrosterone (DHEA) and androstenedione, respectively. These two androgens are precursors of testosterone. As a result, plasma testosterone levels are significantly lower than those achieved with conventional hormone therapies; in addition, a reduction in intratumoral levels of androgens is obtained. The COU-AA-301, a phase III trial in post-docetaxel refractory CRPC, resulted in a significant improvement in overall survival in the abiraterone group [53]. Furthermore there is a second randomized phase III trial (COU-AA-302) targeting men with docetaxel and ketoconazole-naïve CRPC showing positive results in the interim analysis in the Abiraterone group, achieving a delay in disease progression and fairly long expected survival. For this reason the study was recently unblinded before completion at the recommendation of the Independent Data Monitoring Committee.

- **MDV3100** (Enzalutamide) is an androgen-receptor antagonist that blocks androgens from binding to the androgen receptor and prevents nuclear translocation and co-activator recruitment of the ligand-receptor complex. It also induces tumour cell apoptosis, and has no agonist activity. MDV 3100 was found clinically active for metastatic castration-resistant prostate cancer patients in ongoing phase I and II trials. The AFFIRM trial (a phase III trial) compared MDV3100 versus placebo in patients with docetaxel-refractory CRPC [34, 54]. The trial will determine the effectiveness of enzalutamide in patients who have previously failed chemotherapy treatment with docetaxel. In November 2011, this trial was halted after an interim analysis revealed that patients given the drug lived for approximately 5 months longer than those taking placebo, estimating a median survival of 18.4 months for men treated with MDV3100, compared with 13.6 months for men treated with placebo. This translates into a 37% reduction in the risk for death with MDV3100 (hazard ratio, 0.631]. As a result, the trial's Independent Data Monitoring Committee recommended that AFFIRM should be stopped earlier and that men who were receiving placebo should be offered MDV3100. The recommendation was based on the fact that the study's prespecified interim efficacy stopping criteria were successfully met. The committee also examined the safety profile to date and determined that MDV3100 demonstrated a risk/benefit ratio that was favorable enough to stop the study. It is expected to file for FDA approval sometime in 2012. There is another phase III trial, known as PREVAIL, that is investigating the effectiveness of enzalutamide with patients who have not yet received chemotherapy [55].

- **Orteronel** (TAK-700]. Is an androgen synthesis inhibitor. It selectively inhibits the enzyme CYP17A1 which is expressed in testicular, adrenal, and prostatic tumor tissues. It is a very promising drug, but we still have to wait for results of two phase III clinical trials currently recruiting participants in CRPC patients and high risk patients [56].

5.2. Chemotherapy

Cabazitaxel is a new tubulin-binding taxane that has shown to be as potent as docetaxel in cell lines, and is the first chemotherapy shown to improve survival in patients with docetaxel-refractory metastatic castration resistant prostatic cancer. Moreover, it has demonstrated antitumor activity in models resistant to docetaxel due to its poor affinity for the ATP-dependent drug efflux pump, a member of the multidrug resistance protein family [57]. The TROPIC trial, a phase III trial in post-docetaxel refractory CRPC, compared cabazitaxel plus prednisone versus mitoxantrone plus prednisolone, in patients with docetaxel-refractory prostate cancer concluding in a significant improvement in overall survival in the cabazitaxel group.

Epothilones, namely, ixabepilone and patupilone, have shown significant activity in men with CRPC [58, 59]. These molecules were evaluated in second-line chemotherapy in two phase II trials after progression with prior taxane [60, 61]. Phase III trials with ixabepilone are in development and two phase II trial of patupilone are completed [59].

Eribulin mesylate (E7389] is a synthetic analog of the marine macrolide halichondrin B, which acts as a novel microtubule modulator with a distinct mechanism of action (different from taxanes) [60]. An open-label, multicenter, single-arm, phase II study was conducted in patients with CRPC stratified by prior taxane therapy [62]. Primary efficacy endpoint was PSA response rate defined as two consecutive ≥50% decreases in PSA levels from baseline. The secondary endpoints were duration of PSA response rate and objective response rate by RECIST criteria. One hundred and eight patients were available for analyses. Of these 50 were taxane pretreated. Eribulin showed activity in patients with metastatic CRPR, especially in those with taxane naïve disease. Side effects, mainly hematological toxicity (grade 3 and 4 leucopenia and neutropenia), fatigue, and peripheral neuropathy were manageable [62].

Satraplatin (JM-216] is an oral third-generation platinum compound evaluated in the SPARC trial, a phase III trial, in combination with prednisone in second-line therapy after docetaxel [34, 51]. In this trial, satraplatin plus prednisone resulted in significant improvement in PFS (11.1 weeks versus 9.7 weeks) but there were no improvement in median overall survival compared with prednisone alone (61.3 weeks versus 61.4 weeks).

Other chemotherapy treatments, studied in CRPC are Mitoxantrone with two pivotal studies in the late 90´s that could not demonstrate to be superior to palliative corticosteroid therapy. Encourarging results with alternative treatments, including Vinorelbine, a semi-synthetic vinca alkaloid, and oral cyclophosphamide, have being obtained in prospective clinical phase II trials. However the lack of representative randomized phase III trials and unknown long-term efficacy are the major problems associatied with all these studies [63, 64, 65].

5.3. Vaccines-based immunotherapy

Sipuleucel-T is an active cellular immunotherapy consisting of autologous peripheral-blood mononuclear cells, including antigen-presenting cells (APCs), which have been activated ex vivo with a recombinant fusion protein known as PA2024, composed of prostatic acid phosphatase (PAP) linked to granulocyte-macrophage colony-stimulating factor (GM-CSF). In the first two randomized trials, sipuleucel-T, the primary endpoint was not accomplished since these studies did not show a significant effect on the time to disease progression comparing with placebo. Despite this, the hazard ratios were in favor of sipuleucel-T [66, 67]. The IMPACT trial, a phase III trial in CPRC asyntomatic patients, resulted in a longer median survival time in the Sipuleucel-T group, with limited toxicity. Approved by the Food and Drugs Administration (FDA), currently Sipuleucel-T is not approved to been used in Europe [68].

GVAX (CGI940/CG8711] is a cellular vaccine composed of two allogeneic prostate cancer cell lines (LNCaP and PC-3] that is genetically modified to secrete GM-CSF [69]. This vaccine showed clinical benefit with limited toxicity in phase I and II trials [70, 71]. However, the two phase III trials (VITAL-1 and VITAL-2] evaluated GVAX against docetaxel plus prednisone in naïve CRPC and both were closed prematurely [70]. The VITAL-1 study was closed when the unplanned futility analysis revealed a <30% chance of meeting its predefined primary endpoint of OS improvement and the VITAL-2 terminated when an interim analysis revealed more deaths in the GVAX arm than in the control [71].

PROSTVAC-VF is a cancer vaccine consisting of a recombinant vaccinia vector as a priming immunization with subsequent multiple booster vaccinations, using a recombinant fowlpox vector. This agent presented in the context of 3 costimulatory molecules (ICAM-1, BLA-7, and LFA-3] which, when taken together, demonstrate an increase in strength of the target immunologic response [48]. This vaccine was evaluated in phase I and II trials. The phase I trial showed PSA stabilization in 40% of patients and limited toxicity and, in the phase II study, patients in the PROSTVAC-VF arm achieved an 8.5-month improvement in median OS [25.1 months versus 16.6 months) and a 44% reduction in the death rate (Hazard ratio 0.56], [72]. Phase III trial are being planned and other vaccines are under current development [73].

5.4. Bone-targeted treatments

Zoledronic Acid. Metastatic prostate cancer has an affinity to spread to the bone. Bone metastases occur in up to 90% of patients with HRPC. These metastases can lead to significant morbidity, including severe pain, fractures, and spinal cord compression tumors in the bone may cause pain, compression, or pathologic fratures, known as skeletal related events (SRE´s). Because of the frequent involvement of vertebrae by metastatic prostate cancer, the incidene of cord compression is of particular concern. Zoledronic acid has been shown to prevent or delay skeletal complications in men with bone metastases, as well as to palliate bone pain [74, 75]. At an average followup of 24 months, there was a significant reduction in the frequency of skeletal related events (SREs) in men receiving zoledronic acid compared to placebo [38 versus 49 percent), and the median time to develop an SRE was significantly longer with zoledronic acid [488 versus 321 days) [76]. Biphosphonates may also have a role in preventing osteopenia that frequently accompanies the use of androgen-deprivation therapy [77, 78]

Denosumab. Is a human monoclonal antibody directed against RANKL that inhibits osteoclast-mediated bone destruction. In a phase III study [79]. Denosumab showed to be better than zoledronic acid for the prevention of skeletal-related events. Although is not yet available in Europe, it is expected to be approved soon.

5.5. External beam radiotherapy and radioisotope drugs

Focal external beam radiation therapy (RT) is a palliative treatment possibility that should be considered for men with CRPC and bone pain that is limited to one or a few sites. Several clinical trials as well as a systematic review of the literature suggest that single treatments with fractionation schedules provide palliation with cost effectiveness and patient convenience [80].

Hemibody RT could also be considered in selected patients with symptomatic disease limited to one side of the diaphragm, in order to rapid pain relief, when multiple bone metastases are present [81]. However, this technique has frequently been replaced by the administration of radioisotope pharmaceuticals which may be associated with less toxicity and are more appropriated for patients with multiple painful lesions [82]. In order for these patients to be treated with radioisotopes the presence of uptake on bone scan due to metastatic disease at sites that correlate with pain is necessary. These radioisotopes are used in men with advanced prostate cancer with osteoblastic bone metastasis. These patients are often characterized by a high ratio of bone to soft tissue metastases. Multiple radioisotopes have been used but the most extensive data are with 89-strontium (89Sr), Radium-223 and 153-samarium [153Sm). Several clinical trials provide the rational for the use of this approach in carefully selected patients [83, 84, 85].

Lexidronam (Samarium 153]. Is a complex of a radioisotope of the lanthanide element samarium with the chelator EDTMP. Particularly useful in patients with CRPC and multiple painful bone metastases, who have relapsed following initial course of hormonal or cytotoxic chemotherapy, and in patients with progressive or recurrent symptoms at the treated sites. The goal in this stage of the disease is to maintain quality of life while managing the symptoms of the progressing cancer. Extensive data support the use of Samarium SM 153 in this group of patients [8, 9].

Alpharadin (Radium-223]. Alpharadin uses alpha radiation from radium-223 decay to kill cancer cells. Radium-223 naturally self-targets to bone metastases by virtue of its properties as a calcium-mimic. Alpha radiation has a very short range of 2-10 cells (when compared to current radiation therapy which is based on beta or gamma radiation), and therefore causes less damage to surrounding healthy tissues (particularly bone marrow). Radium-223 has a half life of 11.4 days, making it ideal for targeted cancer treatment. Furthermore, any Alpharadin that is not taken up by the bone metastases is rapidly cleared to the gut and excreted. In the phase III ALSYMPCA trial [86], Alpharadin succesfully met the primary endpoint of overall survival. When compared with placebo, Radium-223 was associated with improved overall survival (median 14.0 versus 11.2 months; HR, 0.69. A recent phase III trial envolving Alpharadin, showed a significant improvement in the median overall survival in chemo-naïve patients as well as in those treated previously with docetaxel.

5.6. Antiangiogenic strategies

Bevacizumab. Tumor angiogenesis is likely to be an important biologic component of prostate cancer growth and progression. An elevated levels of the potent angiogenic molecule vascular endothelial growth factor (VEGF) have been shown to correlate with advanced clinical stage and survival. Microvessel density in clinically localized prostate cancer is an independent prognostic for progression and survival [87, 88]. Antiangiogenic agents using monoclonal antibodies to VEGF, such as bevacizumab (Avastin®) have been studied in prostate cancer. Although single-agent studies have failed to demonstrate significant results, a phase II trial conducted by the CALGB added bevacizumab to docetaxel and estramustine in men with HRPC; 79% of patients had a greater than 50% decline in PSA level, median time to progression of 9.7 months, and overall median survival of 21 months [89]. On the basis of these promising results, a randomized, double-blind, placebo-controlled, phase III trial has been designed comparing docetaxel 75 mg/m^2 every 3 weeks with prednisone 10 mg orally daily with either bevacizumab 15 mg/kg IV or placebo every 3 weeks (CALGB 90401]. The primary endpoint for this trial is overall survival, and secondary endpoints include progression-free survival, PSA reduction, and grade 3 toxicities. This trial opened in April 2005 and is actively accruing.

Thalidomide. Is a synthetic glutamic acid derivative. Thalidomide was noted to have anti-inflammatory, immunomodulatory and antiangiogenic effects. alone or in combination with docetaxel were studied in phase II trials with promising results. Microvessel density (MVD) has been reported to be higher in prostate cancer tissue than in adjacent hyperplastic or benign tissue [90]. Preclinical evidence also suggests that angiogenesis may play a key role in the development of aggressive prostate cancer lesion [91]. Clinical studies have observed a correlation between increased angiogenesis in primary tumor specimens and the future development of metastatic disease. The apparent importance of angiogenesis in the evolution of prostate cancer provides a rationale for the investigation of antiangiogenesis agents in CRPC. A phase II trial of thalidomide resulted in a > 40% fall in PSA levels in 27% of patients and improvement in clinical symptoms in all responding patients. PSA declines often resulted in striking reductions in measurable disease on positron emission tomographic scan. Thalidomide plus docetaxel versus docetaxel monotherapy, in a phase II trial in patients with metastatic CRPC, showed a ≥50% PSA decrease (53% versus 37%) and improvement in median overall survival (28.9 months versus 14.7 months) for patients in the thalidomide group [92, 93].

The combination of docetaxel, thalidomide, bevacizumab, and prednisolone was also evaluated in a phase II trial with a ≥50% PSA reduction in 89.6% of patients. The median time to progression was 18.3 months and the median overall survival was 28.2 months [93]. More studies are needed before prescribing angiogenesis inhibitors outside clinical trials.

5.7. Other targets

Dasatinib. Is a small molecular kinase inhibitor of Src family kinases (SFK), being studied for prostate cancer because Src signaling is involved in androgen-induced proliferation. In a phase II trial in chemotherapy-naïve patients with metastatic CRPC, dasatinib [100 mg orally

http://dx.doi.org/10.5772/52288

twice daily) showed lack of progression in 43% of patients at week 12 and in 19% in patients at week 24. It also revealed a decrease in the markers of bone metabolism (N-telopeptide and bone alkaline phosphatase) A randomized phase III trial with dasatinib plus docetaxel is ongoing [94].

Ipilimumab. Blockade of the T-cell inhibitory receptor CTL-associated antigen-4 (CTLA-4] augments and prolongs T-cell responses and is a strategy to elicit antitumor immunity [95]. Ipilimumab, an anti-CTLA-4 antibody, was tested in order to potentiate endogenous antitumor immunity to prostate cancer through combination immunotherapy with CTLA-4 blockade and GM-CSF [96]. The results showed that this combination immunotherapy can induce the expansion not only of activated effector CD8 T cells *in vivo* but also of T cells that are specific for known tumor-associated antigens from endogenous immune repertoire.

In a pilot trial of CTLA-4 blockade with ipilimumab patients with CRPC were given a single dose of 3 mg/kg [95]. Results showed that this approach was safe and did not result in significant clinical autoimmunity. PSA modulating effects presented need further investigation in order to be fully understood. Two phase III trials are now recruiting patients in order to compare ipilimumab with placebo [96]. One trial [97] will evaluate this approach in patients with metastatic disease, with at least one bone metastasis, prior treatment with docetaxel, and castrate levels of serum testosterone. The other trial [98] will include patients with metastatic castration-resistant prostate cancer who are asymptomatic or minimally symptomatic and who have not received prior chemotherapy or immunotherapy.

Atrasentan. The Endothelins (ETs) constitute a family of three 21-amino-acid peptides (ET-1, ET-2, and ET-3] that are synthesized as propeptides and are transformed to their active forms by sequential endopeptidase and ET-converting enzyme-mediated cleavage [99]. ETs are regulators of cell proliferation, vasomotor tone, and angiogenesis. The ETs bind to two receptors, endothelin-A (ET-A) and endothelin-B (ET-B), and play an important role in angiogenesis, proliferation, escape from apoptosis, invasion, tumor growth, new bone formation, and bone metastasis [73, 74]. ET and their receptors have emerged as a potential targets in CRPC [99]. Efficacy and safety of ET-A receptor blockade—atrasentan (ABT-627]—have been evaluated in a double-blind, randomized, placebo-controlled, phase II trial [99], Two hundred and eighty-eight asymptomatic patients were randomized to one of three study groups: placebo, 2.5 mg atrasentan, 10 mg atrasentan. Primary endpoint was time to progression. Secondary end points were time to PSA progression, bone scan changes, and changes in bone and tumor markers. Target therapy with atrasentan was well tolerated and results showed a potential to delay progression of CRPC.

Based on these results other phase III studies also evaluated atrasentan. In one of these studies [100], atrasentan did not reduce the risk of disease progression relative to placebo. However exploratory analyses showed that alkaline phosphatase and PSA levels were significantly lower in the treatment arm [90]. Another phase III study (SWOG S0421] tested atrasentan combined with docetaxel/prednisone in metastatic CRPC as a first-line therapy [100]. SWOG trial S0421 closed earlier based on interim finding that atrasentan added to docetaxel and prednisone did not confer additional survival benefit to patients with hormone-refractory prostate cancer. The Data and Safety Monitoring Committee has determined that patients in phase III S0421 receiving atrasentan in addition to a standard chemotherapy regimen for advanced prostate cancer did not have longer survival or longer progression-free survival.

Zibotentan (ZD 4054]. Is another ET-A receptor antagonist, which showed evidence of activity in a randomized phase II trial in men with castrate-resistant prostate cancer and bone metastases [101]. Following these results two phase III trials [102, 103] were conducted. ENTHUSE M0 was discontinued following the results of an early efficacy review by the Independent Data Monitoring Committee. The company has concluded that zibotentan was unlikely to meet its primary efficacy endpoints progression free survival and overall survival. Results from ENTHUSE M1C are still awaited.

Tyrosine kinase inhibitors (TKIs) are important new class of target therapy that interfere with specific cell signaling pathways and thus allow target specific therapy for selected malignancies. Sorafenib and sunitinib have been tested in prostate cancer in phase I and II trials.

Sorafenib. In the first stage of a phase II trial with sorafenib [104] 22 metastatic CRPC were enrolled. Most of the patients [59%) had received prior therapy with docetaxel or mitoxantrone. Sorafenib therapy failed to show >50% PSA reduction [51]. A second stage of the trial was conducted with 24 more patients [105]. Of the 24 patients, 21 had previous chemotherapy with docetaxel. All patients had bone metastases, either alone (in 11] or with soft-tissue disease (in 13]. At a median potential followup of 27.2 months, the median progression-free survival was 3.7 months and the median overall survival was 18.0 months. For the whole trial of 46 patients the median survival was 18.3 months. The authors concluded that sorafenib has moderate activity as a second-line treatment for metastatic castration-resistant prostate cancer in this trial population [106].

Another phase II study [98] included 57 chemotherapy naïve CRPC patients. Fifty-five patients were evaluable. Two of these patients had >50% PSA reduction and 15 patients had stable disease. Analysis of the results from a third phase II trial suggests that sorafenib therapy could affect PSA production or secretion regardless of its antitumor activity [107].

Sunitinib. A phase I/II trial of sunitinib in combination with docetaxel and prednisone showed a PSA response in 56% of patients, a median time to PSA progression of 42.1 weeks, and a partial response of measurable disease in 39% patients [108]. Sunitinib was also tested in CRPC naïve and docetaxel refractory patients in other phase II trials [106, 107]. A phase III trial comparing sunitinib plus prednisone versus prednisone alone, in patients with docetaxel refractory metastatic CRPC, is ongoing. Overall survival is the primary endpoint of this study [109].

Cabozantinib. Is an inhibitor of MET and VEGFR2 [90]. Both the MET and VEGF-type 2 receptor signaling pathways appear to play important roles in the function of osteoblasts and osteoclasts. MET signaling promotes tumor growth, invasion, and metastasis. Results from cabozantinib trial were presented at ASCO Meeting, 2011. The authors concluded that cabozantinib showed clinical activity regardless of prior docetaxel in metastatic CRPC patients, particularly in patients with bone disease, in addition to improvements in hemoglobin and tumor regression.

There are also other potential targets, such as IGF-1R signaling, vitamin D receptor, PTEN, and phosphoinositide 3-kinase signaling; those are quite promising and could lead us to new treatment options [3, 34]. New mechanisms, drugs, and clinically relevant molecular targets show survival advantage and are new options available for patients after traditional chemotherapy. As ongoing studies using all the mentioned agents continue to evolve, our understanding of how and where these agents fit into the treatment paradigm for patients with CRPC will become clearer. Improvements in progression-free survival and OS rates, observed with novel agents, in metastatic prostate cancer have led to a shift in treatment paradigm. The challenge will be to position the current established and expected novel treatments in the new landscape of metastatic prostate cancer and to determine at what point and time in the disease course they can best be administered. It is clear, however, that our knowledge of the biologic mechanisms involved iin teh progression of metastaic castration-resistant prostate cancer has reached a level at which the discovery of more effective targeted approaches will probably futher improve outcomes.

Author details

Miguel Álvarez Múgica[1], Jesús M. Fernández Gómez[2,3], Antonio Jalón Monzón[2], Erasmo Miguelez García[1] and Francisco Valle González[1]

1 Urology Department, Hospital Valle Nalón, Spain

2 Urology Department, HUCA, Spain

3 University of Oviedo, Spain

References

[1] American Cancer Society. http://www.cancer.org (accessed September 2010).

[2] Dolfsson J, Oksanen H, Salo JO, Steineck G. Localized prostate cancer and 30 years of follow-up in a population-based setting. Prostate Cancer Prostatic Dis2000; 3: 37-42.

[3] Scardino PT. The Gordon Wilson Lecture. Natural history and treatment of early stage prostate cancer. Trans Am Clin Climatol Assoc 2000; 111: 201–41.

[4] Tannock IA, de Wit R, Berry WR, Horti J, Pluzanska A, Chi KN, Oudard S, Théodore C, James N, Turesson I, Rosenthal MA, Eisenberger MA. Docetaxel plus Prednisone or Mitoxantrone plus Prednisone for Advanced Prostate Cancer. N Engl J Med 2004; 351: 1502-12.

[5] Petrylak DP, Tangen CM, Hussain MHA, et al. Docetaxel and estramustine compared with mitoxantrone and prednisone for advanced refractory prostate cancer. N Engl J Med 2004; 351: 1513–20.

[6] Zhu YS, Sun GH. 5α-reductase isozymes in the prostate. J Med Sci 2005; 25: 1–12.

[7] Marks LS. 5α-reductase: history and clinical importance. Rev Urol 2004; 6(suppl 9): 11–21.

[8] Dutt SS, Gao AC. Molecular mechanisms of castration-resistant prostate cancer progression. Fut Oncol 2009; 5: 1403-13.

[9] Pereira de Jésus-Tran K, Côté PL, Cantin L, Blanchet J, Labrie F, Breton R. Comparison of crystal structures of human androgen receptor ligand-binding domain complexed with various agonists reveals molecular determinants responsible for binding affinity. Protein Sci 2006; 15: 987–99.

[10] Askew EB, Gampe RT Jr, Stanley TB, Faggart JL, Wilson EM. Modulation of androgen receptor activation function 2 by testosterone and dihydrotestosterone. J Biol Chem 2007; 282: 25801–16.

[11] Morley JE, Kaiser FE, Perry HM III et al. Longitudinal changes in testosterone, luteinizing hormone, and follicle-stimulating hormone in healthy older men. Metabolism 1997; 46: 410–3.

[12] Harman SM, Metter EJ, Tobin JD, Pearson J, Blackman MR. Longitudinal effects of aging on serum total and free testosterone levels in healthy men. Baltimore Longitudinal Study of Aging. J Clin Endocrinol Metab 2001; 86: 724–31.

[13] Gray A, Feldman HA, McKinlay JB, Longcope C. Age, disease, and changing sex hormone levels in middle-aged men: results of the Massachusetts Male Aging Study. J Clin Endocrinol Metab 1991; 73: 1016–25.

[14] Pirke KM, Doerr P. Age related changes in free plasma testosterone, dihydrotestosterone and oestradiol. Acta Endocrinol (Copenh) 1975; 80: 171–8.

[15] Morgentaler A, Traish AM. Shifting the paradigm of testosterone and prostate cancer: the saturation model and the limits of androgen-dependent growth. Eur Urol 2009; 55: 310–21.

[16] Morgentaler A, Rhoden EL. Prevalence of prostate cancer among hypogonadal men with prostate-specific antigen levels of 4.0 ng/ml or less. Urology 2006; 68: 1263–7.

[17] Lane BR, Stephenson AJ, Magi-Galluzzi C, Lakin MM, Klein EA. Low testosterone and risk of biochemical recurrence and poorly differentiated prostate cancer at radical prostatectomy. Urology 2008; 72: 1240–5.

[18] Sofikerim M, Eskicorapci S, Oruc O, Ozen H. Hormonal predictors of prostate cancer. Urol Int 2007; 79: 13–8.

[19] Imperato-McGinley J, Guerrero L, Gautier T, Peterson RE. Steroid 5α-reductase deficiency in man: an inherited form of male pseudohermaphroditism. Science 1974; 186: 1213–5.

[20] Imperato-McGinley J, Zhu YS. Androgens and male physiology the syndrome of 5α-reductase-2 deficiency. Mol Cell Endocrinol 2002; 198: 51–9.

[21] Titus MA, Schell MJ, Lih FB, et al. Testosterone and dihydrotestosterone tissue levels in recurrent prostate cancer. Clin Cancer Res 2005; 11: 4653-7.

[22] Stanbrough M, Bubley GJ, Ross K, et al. Increased expresión of genes converting adrenal androgens to testosterone in androgen-independent prostate cancer. Cancer Res 206; 66: 2815-25.

[23] Holzbeierlein J, Lal P, La Tulippe E, et al. Gene expresión analysis of human prostate carcinoma Turing hormonal therapty identifies androgen-responsive genes and mechanisms of therapy resistance. Am J Pathol 204; 164: 217-27.

[24] Andersson S, Russell DW. Structural and biochemical properties of cloned and expressed human and rat steroid 5α-reductases. Proc Natl Acad Sci USA 1990; 87: 3640–4.

[25] Jenkins EP, Andersson S, Imperato-McGinley J, Wilson JD, Russell DW. Genetic and pharmacological evidence for more than one human steroid 5α-reductase. J Clin Invest 1992; 89: 293–300.

[26] Wright AS, Thomas LN, Douglas RC, Lazier CB, Rittmaster RS. Relative potency of testosterone and dihydrotestosterone in preventing atrophy and apoptosis in the prostate of the castrated rat. J Clin Invest 1996; 98: 2558–63.

[27] Rittmaster RS. 5α-reductase inhibitors in benign prostatic hyperplasia and prostate cancer risk reduction. Best Pract Res Clin Endocrinol Metab 2008; 22: 389–402.

[28] Gudmundsson J, Sulem P, Steinthorsdottir V et al. Two variants on chromosome 17 confer prostate cancer risk, and the one in TCF2 protects against type 2 diabetes. Nat Genet 2007; 39: 977–83.

[29] Klotz L. Active surveillance for prostate cancer: a review. Curr Urol Rep 2010; 11: 165–71.

[30] Chodak GW, Thisted RA, Gerber GS et al. Results of conservative management of clinically localized prostate cancer. N Engl J Med 1994; 330: 242–8.

[31] Epstein JI. An update of the Gleason grading system. J Urol 2010; 183: 433–40.

[32] Lu-Yao GL, Albertson PC, Moore DF et al. Outcomes of localized prostate cancer following conservative management. JAMA 2009; 302: 1202–9.

[33] Halabi S, Small E, Kantoff P, et al. Prognostic model for predicting survival in men with hormone-refractory metastatic prostate cancer. J Clin Oncol 2003; 21: 1232-7.

[34] Attard G, Sarker D, Reid A, Molife R, Parker C, De Bono JS. Improving the outcome of patients with castration-resistant prostate cancer through rational drug development. Br J Cancer 206; 95 (7): 767-74.

[35] Cooperberg MR, Lubeck DP, Meng MV, Mehta SS, Carroll PR. The changing face of low-risk prostate cancer: trenes in clinical presentation and primary management. J Clin Oncol 2004; 22: 2141-9.

[36] Harris WP, Mostaghel EA, P. S. Nelson, and B. Montgomery, "Androgen deprivation therapy: progress in understanding mechanisms of resistance and optimizing androgen depletion," Nature Clinical Practice Urology 2009; 6 (2): 76–85.

[37] Attar RM, Takimoto CH, Gottardis MM. Castration-resistant prostate cancer: locking up the molecular escape routes Clinical Cancer Research 2009: 15 (10); 3251–5.

[38] Serafini AN, Houston SJ, Resche I, et al. Palliation of pain associated with metastático bone cancer using samarium-153 lexidronam: a double-blind placebo-controlled clinical trial. J Clin Oncol 1998; 16: 1574-81.

[39] Sun S, Sprenger CT, Vessella RL. Castration resistance in human prostate cancer is conferred by a frequently occurring androgen receptor splice variant. J Clin Invest 2010; 120: 2715-30.

[40] Watson PA, Chen YF, Balbas M. Constitutively active androgen receptor splice variants expressed in castration-resistant prostate cancer require full-length androgen receptor. Proceedings of the National Academy of Sciences of the United States of America 2010; 107: 16759–65.

[41] Marques RB, Dits NF, Erkens-Schulze S, Weerden WM, Jenster G. Bypass mechanisms of the androgen receptor pathway in therapy-resistant prostate cancer cell models. PLoS ONE 2010; 5: 13500-5.

[42] Crawford ED, Eisenberger MA, McLeod DG. A controlled trial of leuprolide with and without flutamide in prostatic carcinoma. N Eng J Med 1989; 321: 419-24.

[43] Eisenberger MA, Blumenstein BA, Crawford ED. Bilateral orchiectomy with or without flutamide for metastatic prostate cancer. N Eng J Med 1998; 339: 1036-42.

[44] Harris WP, Mostaghel EA, Nelson PA, Montgomery B. Androgen deprivation therapy: progress in understanding mechanisms of resistance and optimizing androgen depletion. Nature Clin Prac Urol 2009; 6: 76-85.

[45] Ang JA, Olmos D, De Bono JS. CYP17 blockade by abiraterone: further evidence for frequent continued hormone-dependence in castration-resistant prostate cancer. Br J Cancer 2009; 100: 671-5.

[46] Paller CJ, Antonarakis ES. Cabazitaxel: a novel second-line treatment for metastatic castration-resistant prostate cancer. Drug Design, Develop Ther 2011; 5: 117-24.

[47] Pal SK, Twardowski P, Sartor O. Critical appraisal of cabazitaxel in the management of advanced prostate cancer. Clin Interv Aging 2010; 5: 395-402.

[48] Sonpave G, Slawin KM, Spencer DM, Levitt JM. Emerging vaccine therapy approaches for prostate cancer. Rew Urol 2010; 12: 25-34.

[49] Small EJ, Halabi S, Dawson NA. Antiandrogen withdrawal alone or in combination with ketoconazole in androgen-independent prostate cancer patients: a phase III trial (CALGB 9583). J Clin Oncol 2004; 22 (6): 1025-33.

[50] Berthold DR, Sternberg CN, TannockIF. Management of advanced prostate cancer after first-line chemotherapy. J Clin Oncol 2005; 23: 8247-52.

[51] Kim SJ, Kim SM. Current treatment strategies for castration-resistant prostate cancer. Korean J Urol 2011; 52: 157-65.

[52] O'Donell A, Judson I, Dowsett M, et al. Hormonal impact of the 17 alpha-hydrosylase/C(17,20)-lyase inhibitor abiraterone acetate (CB7630) in patients with prostate cancer. Br J Cancer 2004; 90: 2317-25.

[53] de Bono JS, Logothetis CJ, Molina A, et al. Abiraterone and increased survival in metastatic prostate cancer. New Engl J Med 2011; 364: 1995-2005.

[54] Safety and Efficacy Study of MDV3100 in Patients With Castration-Resistant Prostate Cancer Who Have Been Previously Treated With Docetaxel-based Chemotherapy (AFFIRM).

[55] ClinicalTrials.gov, United States National Institutes of Health. Retrieved 2011-11-06. "A Safety and Efficacy Study of Oral MDV3100 in Chemotherapy-Naive Patients With Progressive Metastatic Prostate Cancer (PREVAIL)". "NCT01212991".

[56] Kaku T, Hitaka T, Ojida A, Matsunaga N, Adachi M, Tanaka T, Hara T, Yamaoka M, Kusaka M, Okuda T, Asahi S, Furuya S, Tasaka A. Discovery of orteronel (TAK-700), a naphthylmethylimidazole derivative, as a highly selective 17,20-lyase inhibitor with potential utility in the treatment of prostate cancer. Bioorg Med Chem. 2011; 19(21): 6383-99.

[57] Pouessel D, Oudard S, Gravis G, Priou F, Shen L, Culine S. Cabazitaxel for metastatic castration-resistant prostate cancer progressing after docetaxel treatment: the TROPIC study in France. Bull Cancer 2012; 99: 731-741.

[58] Galsky MD, Small EJ, Oh WK. Multi-institutional randomized phase II trial of the epothilone B analog ixabepilone (BMS-247550) with or without estramustine phosphate in patients with progressive castrate metastatic prostate cancer. J Clin Oncol 2005; 23 (7): 1439-46.

[59] Chi KN, Beardsley EK, Venner PM. A phase II study of patupilone in patients with metastatic hormone refractory prostate cancer (HRPC) who have progressed after docetaxel. J Clin Oncol 2008; 26 (15): 5166-71.

[60] Beardsley EK, Saad F, Eigl B. A phase II study of patupilone in patients (patients) with metastatic castration-resistant prostate cancer (CRPC) who have progressed after docetaxel. J Clin Oncol 2009; 27: 5319.

[61] Rosenberg JE, Weinberg VK, Kelly WK. Activity of second-line chemotherapy in docetaxel-refractory hormone-refractory prostate cancer patients: randomized phase 2 study of ixabepilone or mitoxantrone and prednisone. Cancer 2007; 110: 556–63.

[62] Bono JS, Maroto P, Calvo E. Phase II study of eribulin mesylate (E7389) in patients (pts) with metastatic castration-resistant prostate cancer (CRPC) stratified by prior taxane therapy. Ann Oncol 2011; 1: 380-5.

[63] De Bono JS, Oudard S, Ozguroglu M. Prednisone plus cabazitaxel or mitoxantrone for metastatic castration-resistant prostate cancer progressing after docetaxel treatment: a randomised open-label trial. Lancet 2010; 376: 1147-54.

[64] Park SI, Liao J, Berry JE, Li X, Koh AJ, Michalski ME, Eber MR, Soki FN, Sadler D, Sud S, Tisdelle S, Daignault SD, Nemeth JA, Snyder LA, Wronski TJ, Pienta KJ, McCauley LK. Cyclophosphamide creates a receptive microenvironment for prostate cancer skeletal metastasis. Cancer Res 2012; 72(10): 2522-32.

[65] Grenader T, Goldberg A. Reinduction of hormone sensitivity to goserelin following chemotherapy with vinorelbine in castration-resistant prostate cancer. Scientific World Journal 2010; 10: 1814-7.

[66] Small EJ, Schellhammer PF, Higano CS. Placebo-controlled phase III trial of immunologic therapy with Sipuleucel-T (APC8015) in patients with metastatic, asymptomatic hormone refractory prostate cancer. J Clin Oncol 2006; 24: 3089-94.

[67] Higano CS, Schellhammer PF, Small EJ. Integrated data from 2 randomized, double-blind, placebo-controlled, phase 3 trials of active cellular immunotherapy with sipuleucel-T in advanced prostate cancer. Cancer 2009; 115: 3670-9.

[68] Kantoff PW, Higano CS, Shore ND. Sipuleucel-T immunotherapy for castration-resistant prostate cancer. New Eng J Med 2010: 363: 411–2.

[69] Small EJ, Sacks N, Nemunaitis J. Granulocyte macrophage colony-stimulating factor-secreting allogeneic cellular immunotherapy for hormone-refractory prostate cancer. Clin Canc Res 2007; 13: 3883-91.

[70] Hussain M, Smith MR, Sweeney C. Cabozantinib (XL184) in metastatic castration-resistant prostate cancer (mCRPC): results from a phase II randomized discontinuation trial. J Clin Oncol 2011; 29: 4516-9. 71. Cha E, Fong L. Therapeutic vaccines for prostate cancer. Current Opinion Mol Ther 2010; 12 (1): 77-85.

[71] Cha E, Fong L. Therapuetic vaccines for prostate cancer. Current Opinion Mol Ther 2010; 12 (1): 77-85.

[72] Kantoff PW, Schuetz TJ, Blumenstein BA. Overall survival analysis of a phase II randomized controlled trial of a Poxviral-based PSA-targeted immunotherapy in metastatic castration-resistant prostate cancer. J Clin Oncol 2010; 28 (7): 1099-105.

[73] Carducci MA, Jimeno A. Targeting bone metastasis in prostate cancer with endothelin receptor antagonists. Clin Canc Res 2006; 12: 6296-300.

[74] Saad F, Gleason DM, Murray R. A randomized, placebo-controlled trial of zoledronic acid in patients with hormone-refractory metastatic prostate carcinoma. J Nat Canc Inst 2002; 94: 1458-68.

[75] Weinfurt KP, Anstrom KJ, Castel LD, Schulman KA, Saad F. Effect of zoledronic acid on pain associated with bone metastasis in patients with prostate cancer. Ann Oncol 2006; 17 (6): 986-9.

[76] Saad F, Gleason DM, Murray R. Long-term efficacy of zoledronic acid for the prevention of skeletal complications in patients with metastatic hormone-refractory prostate cancer. J Nat Canc Inst 2004; 96: 879-82.

[77] Diamond TH, Winters J, Smith A. The antiosteoporotic efficacy of intravenous pamidronate in men with prostate carcinoma receiving combined androgen blockade: a double blind, randomized, placebo-controlled crossover study. Cancer 2001; 92 (6): 1444-50.

[78] Smith MR, Eastham J, Gleason DM, Shasha D, Tchekmedyian S, Zinner N. Randomized controlled trial of zoledronic acid to prevent bone loss in men receiving androgen deprivation therapy for nonmetastatic prostate cancer. J Urol 2003; 169 (6): 2008-12.

[79] Cavalli L, Brandi ML. Targeted approaches in the treatment of osteoporosis: differential mechanism of action of denosumab and clinical utility. Ther Clin Risk Manag 2012; 8: 253-6.

[80] Chow E, Harris K, Fan G, Tsao M, Sze WM. Palliative radiotherapy trials for bone metastases: a systematic review. J Clin Oncol 2007; 25 (11): 1423-36.

[81] Salazar OM, Sandhu T, Da Motta NW. Fractionated half-body irradiation (HBI) for the rapid palliation of widespread, symptomatic, metastatic bone disease: a randomized Phase III trial of the International Atomic Energy Agency (IAEA). Int J Rad Oncol Biol Physic 2001; 50 (3): 765-75.

[82] Dearnaley DP, Bayly RJ, A'Hern RP, Gadd J, Zivanovic MM, Lewington VJ. Palliation of bone metastases in prostate cancer. Hemibody irradiation or strontium-89?. Clin Oncol 1992; 4 (2): 101-7.

[83] Lewington VJ, McEwan AJ, Ackery DM. A prospective, randomised double-blind crossover study to examine the efficacy of strontium-89 in pain palliation in patients with advanced prostate cancer metastatic to bone. Eur J Canc 1991; 27 (8): 954-8.

[84] Buchali K, Correns HJ, Schuerer M, Schnorr D, Lips H, Sydow K. Results of a double blind study of 89-strontium therapy of skeletal metastases of prostatic carcinoma. Eur J Nuc Med 1988; 14 (7): 349-51.

[85] Sartor O, Reid RH, Hoskin PJ. Samarium-153-lexidronam complex for treatment of painful bone metastases in hormone-refractory prostate cancer. Urology 2004; 63 (5): 940-5.

[86] Cheetham PJ, Petrylak DP. Alpha particles as radiopharmaceuticals in the treatment of bone metastases: mechanism of action of radium-223 chloride (Alpharadin) and radiation protection. Oncology 2012; 26(4): 330-7.

[87] Kelly WK, Halabi S, Carducci M, George D, Mahoney JF, Stadler WM, Morris M, Kantoff P, Monk JP, Kaplan E, Vogelzang NJ, Small EJ. Randomized, double-blind, placebo-controlled phase III trial comparing docetaxel and prednisone with or without bevacizumab in men with metastatic castration-resistant prostate cancer: CALGB 90401. J Clin Oncol. 2012; 30(13): 1534-40.

[88] Redding MB, Surati M. Emerging treatments for castrate-resistant prostate cancer. J Pharm Pract. 2011; 24(4): 366-73.

[89] Weisshardt P, Trarbach T, Dürig J, Paul A, Reis H, Tilki D, Miroschnik I, Ergün S, Klein D. Tumor vessel stabilization and remodeling by anti-angiogenic therapy with bevacizumab. Histochem Cell Biol. 2012; 137(3): 391-401.

[90] Meng LJ, Wang J, Fan WF, Pu XL, Liu FY, Yang M. Evaluation of oral chemotherapy with capecitabine and cyclophosphamide plus thalidomide and prednisone in prostate cancer patients. J Cancer Res Clin Oncol 2012; 138 (2): 333-9.

[91] Emerging novel therapies for advanced prostate cancer. Osanto S, Van Poppel H. Ther Adv Urol 2012; 4 (1): 3-12.

[92] Dahut WL, Gulley JL, Arlen PM. Randomized phase II trial of docetaxel plus thalidomide in androgen-independent prostate cancer. J Clin Oncol 2004; 22 (13): 2532-9.

[93] Ning YM, Gulley JL, Arlen PM. Phase II trial of bevacizumab, thalidomide, docetaxel, and prednisone in patients with metastatic castration-resistant prostate cancer. J Clin Oncol 2010; 28 (12): 2070-6.

[94] National Institutes of Health Clinical Trials database, http://clinicaltrials.gov/.

[95] Small EJ, Tchekmedyian NS, Rini BI, Fong L, Lowy I, Allison JP. A pilot trial of CTLA-4 blockade with human anti-CTLA-4 in patients with hormone-refractory prostate cancer. Clin Canc Res 2007; 13 (6): 1810-5.

[96] Fong L, Kwek SS, O'Brien S. Potentiating endogenous antitumor immunity to prostate cancer through combination immunotherapy with CTLA4 blockade and GM-CSF. Cancer Res 2009; 69 (2): 609-15.

[97] NCT00861614 A Randomized, Double-Blind, Phase 3 Trial Comparing Ipilumumab vs. Placebo Following Radiotherapy in Subjects With Castration Resistant Prostate Cancer That Have Received Prior Treatment With Docetaxel.

[98] NCT01057810 Randomized, Double-Blind, Phase 3 Trial to Compare the Efficacy of Ipilumumab vs Placebo in Asymptomatic or Minimally Symptomatic Patients With Metastatic Chemotherapy-Naïve Castration Resistant Prostate Cancer.

[99] Carducci MA, Padley RJ, Breul J. Effect of endothelin-A receptor blockade with atrasentan on tumor progression in men with hormone-refractory prostate cancer: a randomized, phase II, placebo-controlled trial. J Clin Oncol 2003; 21 (4): 679-89.

[100] Phase III Study of Docetaxel and Atrasentan Versus Docetaxel and Placebo for Patients With Advanced Hormone Refractory Prostate Cancer National Institutes of Health. Clinical Trials 2011, http://clinicaltrials.gov/.

[101] James ND, Caty A, Payne H. Final safety and efficacy analysis of the specific endothelin A receptor antagonist zibotentan (ZD4054) in patients with metastatic castration-resistant prostate cancer and bone metastases who were pain-free or mildly symptomatic for pain: a double-blind, placebo-controlled, randomized Phase II trial. Br J Urol Int 2010; 106 (7): 966-73.

[102] A Phase III Trial of ZD4054 (Zibotentan) (Endothelin A Antagonist) in Non-metastatic Hormone Resistant Prostate Cancer (ENTHUSE M0) NCT00626548.

[103] A Phase III Trial of ZD4054 (Zibotentan) (Endothelin A Antagonist) and Docetaxel in Metastatic Hormone Resistant Prostate Cancer (ENTHUSE M1C) NCT00617669.

[104] Dahut WL, Scripture C, Posadas E. A phase II clinical trial of sorafenib in androgen-independent prostate cancer. Clin Canc Res 2008; 14 (1): 209-14.

[105] Aragon-Ching JB, Jain L, Gulley JL. Final analysis of a phase II trial using sorafenib for metastaticcastration-resistant prostate cancer. Br J Urol Int 2009; 103: 1636-40.

[106] Steinbild S, Mross K, Frost A. A clinical phase II study with sorafenib in patients with progressive hormone-refractory prostate cancer: a study of the CESAR Central European Society for Anticancer Drug Research-EWIV. Br J Cancer 2007; 97 (11): 1480-5.

[107] Chi KN, Ellard SL, Hotte SJ. A phase II study of sorafenib in patients with chemo-naive castration-resistant prostate cancer. Ann Oncol 2008; 19 (4): 746-51.

[108] Zurita AJ, Liu G, Hutson T. Sunitinib in combination with docetaxel and prdnisone in patients (pts) with metastatic hormone-refrectory prostate cancer (mHRPC). J Clin Oncol 2009; 27 (15): 5166-71.

[109] Sonpavde G, Periman PO, Bernold D. Sunitinib malate for metastatic castration-resistant prostate cancer following docetaxel-based chemotherapy. Ann Oncol 2010; 21 (2): 319-24.

Chapter 12

Steroidal CYP17 Inhibitors for Prostate Cancer Treatment: From Concept to Clinic

Jorge A. R. Salvador, Vânia M. Moreira and Samuel M. Silvestre

Additional information is available at the end of the chapter

http://dx.doi.org/10.5772/45948

1. Introduction

The successful application of therapeutic strategies to block the known growth stimulation property of estrogen in breast cancer, namely the aromatase (CYP19) inhibitors formestane (4-OH) and exemestane (Aromasin) [1], has paved the way for the investigation of inhibitors of other P450 enzymes that might impart the growth of hormone-dependent cancers [2]. Cytochrome P450 17α-hydroxylase,$C_{17,20}$-lyase (CYP17) is at the crossroads of androgen and corticoid biosynthesis and has become a valuable target in prostate cancer (PC) treatment [3-8]. Androgens, which are produced in steroidogenic tissues, bind to the androgen receptor (AR) and initiate transcription which in turn results in the synthesis of prostate-specific proteins, as well as in cell proliferation. Systemic ablation of androgen by castration, either surgical or chemical, is highly effective in treating PC when the disease is hormone-dependent [3]. However, within 18-24 months following the onset of primary hormonal therapies, the disease becomes androgen-refractory by mechanisms in which AR-mediated signaling and gene expression is still active despite castrate androgen levels [9]. The FDA approved the combination of docetaxel (Taxotere) *1* and prednisone for the treatment of castrate-resistant PC (CRPC) which improves survival time in about 18 months [10, 11], and cabazitaxel (Jevtana) *2* [12], a novel taxane derivative, for metastatic CRPC (mCRPC) which has progressed following docetaxel therapy (Fig. 1). The immunotherapy Sipuleucel-T (Provenge) is also approved for the treatment of asymptomatic or minimally symptomatic mCPRC. In April 2011, abiraterone acetate (Zytiga) *3* became the first steroidal CYP17 inhibitor to be approved by the FDA for the treatment of docetaxel-resistant mCRPC (Fig. 1) [13, 14]. Following abirateroneacetate *3*, galeterone (TOK-001) *4* (Fig. 1), another steroidal CYP17 inhibitor, with AR antagonistic and ablative activities, is currently undergoing Phase I/II clinical trials for the treatment of chemotherapy-naive CRPC [15, 16].

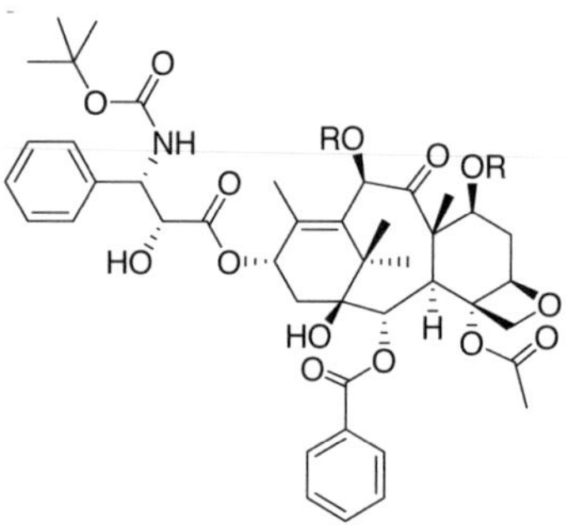

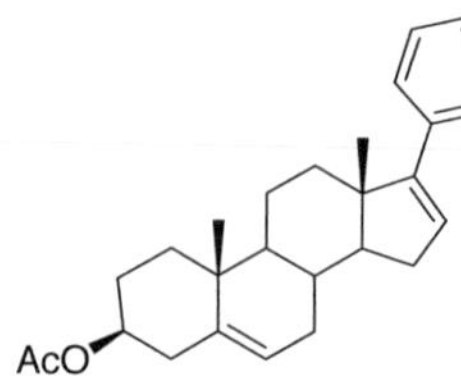

3 Abiraterone acetate (Zytiga®)

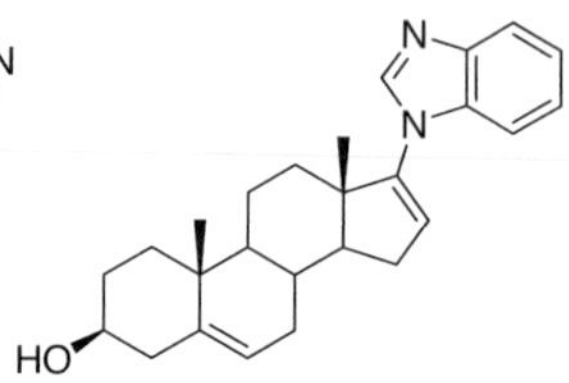

4 Galeterone
TOK-001

1 R = H **Docetaxel (Taxotere®)**
2 R = CH_3 **Cabazitaxel (Jevtana®)**

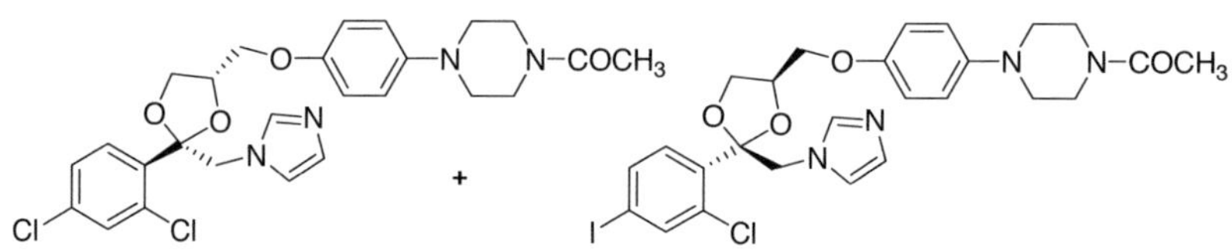

5 Ketoconazole
cis-isomer (1 : 1)

Figure 1. Compounds used in the clinical practice for PC treatment, and galeterone4, currently undergoing clinical trials for the treatment of chemotherapy-naive CRPC.

The first reports on steroidal CYP17 inhibitors date back to about 40 years ago [3, 8, 17-20]. Many different chemistries have been exploited in their development which has been complicated by the fact that no 3D structure of the enzyme is available. Nonetheless, structure-activity analysis has revealed the general features of a good inhibitor and recent docking and modeling studies have further shed some light on the way these molecules interact with the enzyme's active site [21, 22]. Moreover, additional effects of these compounds on other PC-related targets have been studied and disclosed. This chapter will tell the success story of the development of steroidal CYP17 inhibitors from their early discovery days to their very recent introduction into the clinics for the treatment of advanced PC.

2. The CYP17 enzyme: One active site, two activities

The eukaryotic class II cytochrome P450 enzyme CYP17 is an endoplasmic reticulum membrane bound multifunctional protein with 17α-hydroxylase and $C_{17,20}$-lyase activities, both engaged on a single active site (Fig. 2) [23-28].

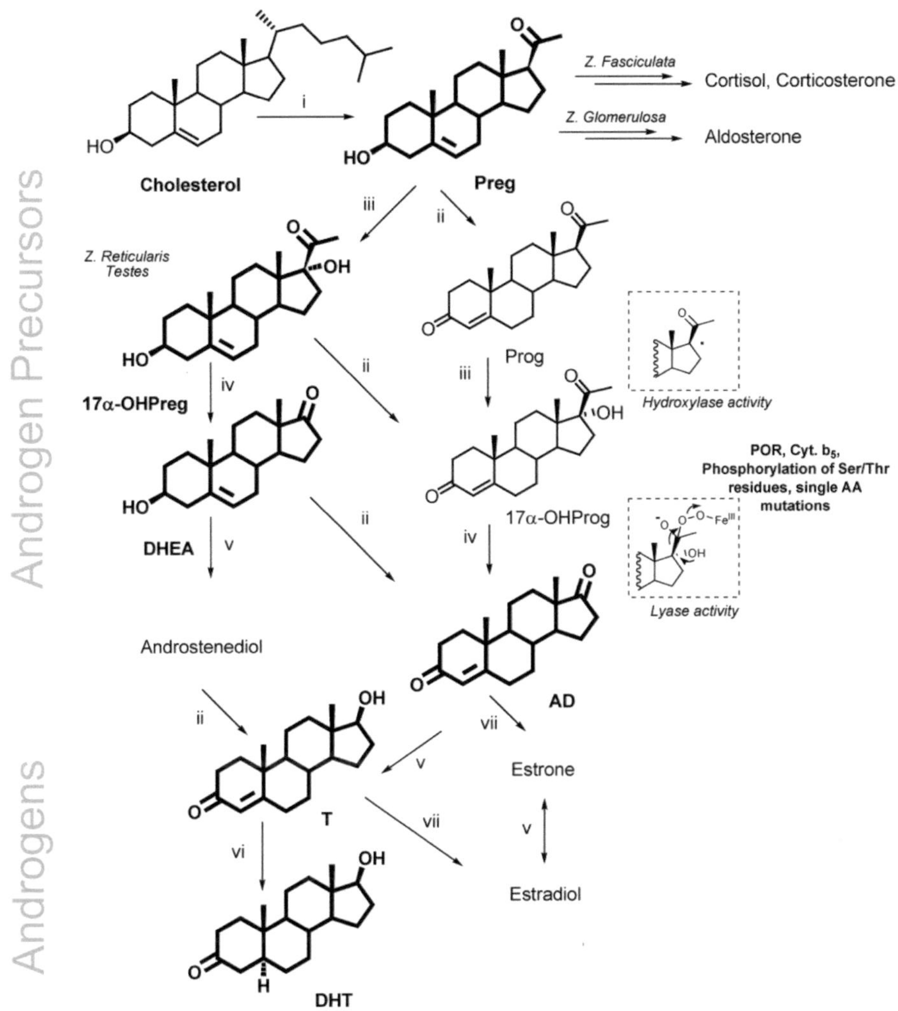

Figure 2. CYP17 and androgen physiology. i. P450 cholesterol side-chain cleavage ($P450_{scc}$); ii. 3β-Hydroxysteroid dehydrogenase, $\Delta^{4,5}$-isomerase; iii. CYP17 (OHase); iv. CYP17 (lyase); v. 17β-Hydroxysteroid dehydrogenase; vi. 5α-Reductase; vii. Aromatase (CYP19).

Alike other cytochrome P450 enzymes, this cysteinato-heme enzyme functions as a monooxygenase by activating and cleaving molecular dioxygen so that one of the atoms is inserted into its substrate while the other gives rise to a water molecule [29, 30]. P450 reductase transfer of electrons in the presence of nicotinamide adenine dinucleotide phosphate (NADPH) is a requisite for both catalytic activities [29, 30]. Its natural substrates are pregnenolone (Preg) and progesterone (Prog) which are first hydroxylated at the 17 position and then their side chain is cleaved to afford 17-keto derivatives (dehydroepiandrosterone, DHEA and androstenedione, AD respectively), which are androgen precursors. The androgens (testosterone, T and dihydrotestosterone, DHT) that result from further metabolization of both DHEA and AD, bind to the AR and initiate transcription, triggering the synthesis of specific proteins and also cell proliferation [31, 32]. Apart from male physiology, androgens are involved in PC development and progression, as at least 80% of human PCs respond favorably to androgen ablation therapy [33-35]. This dependence of PC on androgen signalling has been known for about 70 years [36, 37] and the use of strategies that effectively lower the levels of circulating androgens in PC patients has been the mainstay of PC therapy for several decades.

CYP17 is localized to the adrenals, testes, placenta and ovaries and plays a fundamental role in the synthesis of not only sex steroids but also corticosteroids. The testes are responsible for about 90-95% of the circulating androgens and the adrenals for the remaining 5-10% [38]. Human CYP17 is expressed from a single gene mapped to a specific sub-band of chromosome 10 at q24.3, in steroidogenic tissue [39-41]. This bifunctionality of the product of a single gene has been explained by modulation of the enzyme's $C_{17,20}$-lyase activity by several factors such as the presence of the electron carrier P450 oxidoreductase (POR) [42, 43], cytochrome b5 (cyt. b5) [44-48], the phosphorylation of serine/threonine residues [44, 49-51], and single amino acid mutations [52-55]. The effective ratio of $C_{17,20}$-lyase to 17α-hydroxylase activities is under tight control during development in the human adrenal cortex, and becomes greatly elevated in adrenarche, where a rise in DHEA body concentrations is observed without concomitant increase in glucocorticoid or mineralocorticoid production [56]. Thus, production of the mineralocorticoid aldosterone occurs in the adrenal *zona glomerulosa* where CYP17 is absent. In the *zona reticularis* and in the gonads, the presence of both activities drives the production of sex steroids, whereas overexpression of 17α-hydroxylase activity is fundamental for the production of glucorticoids in the *zona fasciculata*.

The crystal structure of CYP17 remains yet to be determined since purification from its membrane environment and subsequent reconstitution of activity *in vitro* has proved to be a difficult task [26, 29, 30]. However, the availability of some cytochrome P450 crystal structures, such as the ones from prokaryotic P450cam [57, 58], P450BM3 [59-61], and P450 CYPeryF [62], as well as the eukaryotic CYP3A4 [63] and AYP2C9 [64] among others [65], has been a valuable tool in building homology models. In addition, the high-resolution crystal structures of mammalian P450s that are significantly homologous to CYP17 and complexed to a variety of ligands [66] have now been uploaded onto the Protein Data Bank (PDB). A very recent model has been developed based on these crystal structures from closely related mammalian cytochrome P450s [21]. In another approach, a truncated, His-tagged version of human CYP17 was generated from a synthetic complimentary DNA and expressed in *E. coli* [22]. These models were used to dock known CYP17 inhibitors to the active site.

3. Steroidal CYP17 inhibitors

Clinical practice outcomes with ketoconazole *5* (Fig. 1), an orally administered non-steroidal imidazole antifungal agent that was first reported to cause gynecomastia in male patients [67-69], have further evidenced the value of inhibition of the steroid synthesis pathway as a therapeutic strategy for advanced PC. This compound is used clinically as the racemate of the *cis*-isomer [17, 70], and is offered as secondary hormonal therapy to patients with CRPC, despite some significant gastrointestinal and hepatic side-effects when administered in high doses [71-73]. Following ketoconazole *5*, several non-steroidal compounds have been synthesized which displayed better inhibitory properties. In addition, modification of the original core of the enzyme's natural substrates has also afforded very potent steroidal inhibitors [3, 8, 17-20]. Based on the knowledge that was generated by this approach which was recently validated by computational studies, common features were established for optimal interaction between enzyme and substrate. Thus, a good inhibitor should possess a sufficiently large hydrophobic core, comparable to a steroid molecule, and bear electronegative groups at its external positions [74]. The presence of a heteroatom-containing group capable of coordination to the heme iron of CYP17, ofa planar α-face to pack against the I helix; and in addition of hydrogen bonding groups such as the 3β-hydroxylto interact with conserved polar residues in a hydrogen binding network, has proved invaluable for optimal inhibition, as is the case of both abiraterone acetate *3* and galeterone *4* [22].

3.1. Androstanes

The first reports on CYP17 steroidal inhibitors date back to 1971 when Arth et al. synthesized and evaluated testosterone derivatives against rat testicular CYP17, following the observation that testosterone acetate *6* (Fig. 3, Table 1, entry 1) was a potent inhibitor of the enzyme [75]. Almost total abrogation of the enzyme's activity was observed after treatment with 1.5 μM of compounds *7*, *8*, and *10* (Table 1, entries 2-3, and 5), with the acetamide derivative *9* being less potent (Table 1, entry 4). Competitive inhibition of pig CYP17 was reported for the anabolic steroids mestanolone *11*, stanozolol*12*, and furazobol *13* (Fig. 3) [76]. Week inhibition in the high μM range was found with compounds *11* and *13* against the $C_{17,20}$-lyase activity whereas stanozolol *12* inhibited both enzyme activities with IC_{50} values of 2.9 μM and 0.74 μM, for the 17α-hydroxylase and $C_{17,20}$-lyase activities, respectively.

The irreversible inhibition of CYP17 by compound *14* (Fig. 3, Table 1, entry 6) was reported to occur due to the presence of a cyclopropylamino moiety capable of being activated by the enzyme by one-electron oxidation of the nitrogen atom, which causes ring opening to afford a β-iminium radical that covalently binds to the enzyme, while the compound is still bound in the active site [77]. Other related irreversible inhibitors reported include compounds *15-18* (Fig. 3, Table 1, entries 7-10) [78-81]. Compounds *15-17* were potent inhibitors of the human CYP17 at 0.8 and 1 μM, after preincubation with the enzyme (Table 1, entries 7-9). The ki values of the 4-amino derivatives *16-17* and of the sulfoxide derivatives *19-20* were determined using cynomolgous monkey and porcine testicular CYP17, respectively (Table 1, entries 8-9 and 11-12) [82]. Compound *18* also potently inhibited the activity of the monkey cynomolgous CYP17 at 0.1 μM, after preincubation with the enzyme (Table 1, entry 10) [80].

The introduction of heterocyclic moieties into molecules is a commonly used strategy in drug discovery and the design of potent steroidal CYP17 inhibitors based on this feature is an example of success. Thus, several androstane derivatives have been synthesized bearing a heterocycle ring at C17 either connected to it by a carbon (Fig. 4, Compounds *21-50*) or a nitrogen (Fig. 5, Compounds *53-60*) atom. In 1995, Jarman et al. reported the synthesis of abiraterone *21* (Fig. 4), a 17-(3-pyridyl)androstane derivative and a potent irreversible inhibitor of human testicular CYP17 (Table 2, entry 1), about 16- and 9-fold more potent than ketoconazole *5* for the inhibition of the hydroxylase and lyase activities, respectively, with IC_{50} values in the low nM range [86]. Its 3β-acetoxy derivative and prodrug, abiraterone acetate *3* (Table 2, entry 2) has helped to further evidence and establish the utility of specific CYP17 inhibition in metastatic PC (mPC) patients. In 2001, Hartmann et al. reported that the introduction of a pyrimidyl substituent at C17 originated compounds such as *22* and *23* (Fig. 4, Table 2, entries 3-4) which were more potent inhibitors of the human enzyme than both ketoconazole *5* and abiraterone *21*, under the same assay conditions, and that compound *23* effectively lowered T plasma concentrations to castrate levels after administration to mice [87, 88]. The thiazole and furan derivatives *24* and *25* were also synthesized and tested on the monkey cynomolgous enzyme (Fig. 4, Table 1, entries 13-14) [83, 85].

<table>
<tr><th>Entry</th><th>Compound</th><th>Inhibitor concentration (μM)</th><th>% Inhibition[a]</th><th>Ki (nM)</th><th>IC50 (μM)</th><th>Ref.</th></tr>
<tr><td>1</td><td>6</td><td>1.5</td><td>65</td><td>—</td><td>—</td><td rowspan="5">[75]</td></tr>
<tr><td>2</td><td>7</td><td>1.5</td><td>95</td><td>—</td><td>—</td></tr>
<tr><td>3</td><td>8</td><td>1.5</td><td>100</td><td>—</td><td>—</td></tr>
<tr><td>4</td><td>9</td><td>1.5</td><td>85</td><td>—</td><td>—</td></tr>
<tr><td>5</td><td>10</td><td>1.5</td><td>90</td><td>—</td><td>—</td></tr>
<tr><td>6</td><td>14</td><td>—</td><td>—</td><td>90[b]</td><td>4.6[c]</td><td>[77]</td></tr>
<tr><td>7</td><td>15</td><td>0.8</td><td>64</td><td>—</td><td>—</td><td>[78,79]</td></tr>
<tr><td>8</td><td>16</td><td>1</td><td>84</td><td>339[b]</td><td>—</td><td rowspan="2">[80,81]</td></tr>
<tr><td>9</td><td>17</td><td>1</td><td>86</td><td>286[b]</td><td>—</td></tr>
<tr><td>10</td><td>18</td><td>0.1</td><td>79[b]</td><td>—</td><td>—</td><td>[80]</td></tr>
<tr><td>11</td><td>19</td><td>—</td><td>—</td><td>380[c, d]</td><td>1.9[c]</td><td rowspan="2">[82]</td></tr>
<tr><td>12</td><td>20</td><td>—</td><td>—</td><td>380[c, d]</td><td>1.9[c]</td></tr>
<tr><td>13</td><td>24</td><td>0.1</td><td>58[b]</td><td>—</td><td>0.063[b]</td><td rowspan="2">[83-85]</td></tr>
<tr><td>14</td><td>25</td><td>0.1</td><td>53[b]</td><td>—</td><td>—</td></tr>
</table>

Table 1. Inhibition of CYP17 by androstane derivatives. [a]Human CYP17; [b]Determined on cynomolgous monkey testis enzyme; [c]Porcine testicular CYP17; [d]ki for compound 14 under the same assay conditions was 3620 nM.

A series of interesting effects on PC cells other than just CYP17 inhibition was reported by Brodie et al. for the imidazolyl, pyrazolyl, and isoxazolylandrostane derivatives *26-32* (Fig. 4, Table 2, entries 5-11). The isoxazolyl compound *32* was not only a non-competitive inhibitor of human CYP17 but also a competitive inhibitor of 5α-reductase, with potency similar to finasteride, while in addition bearing antiandrogenic activity [89-93]. Its effects were confirmed using PC xenograftmodels, however, its short half-life and relatively low bioavailability were reasoned to limit its efficacy *in vivo* [93-95]. Less successful attempts of CYP17 inhibitors design include the 5′-methyl-2′-thiazolyl androstane *33* (Fig. 4) which was a weak inhibitor of human CYP17 expressed in *E. coli* when compared to ketoconazole *5* [3]. In 2006, Wolfling et al. reported the synthesis of a series of dihydrooxazine derivatives *34-45* (Fig. 4) which low inhibitory activity of CYP17 is most likely due to the bulkiness of the C17 moieties and the absence of a double bond at C16 [96]. The same group later reported the synthesis of the oxazolidone derivative *46* (Fig. 4, Table 2, entry 12) which inhibited the activity of rat testicular $C_{17,20}$-lyase with an IC_{50} value of 3 μM [97]. Similar inhibition of the enzyme was observed with the halogenated oxazoline derivatives *47* and *48* [98], and with the D-ring fused arylpyrazoline *51* (Fig. 4, Table 2, entries 13-14, and 17) [99]. The *N*-phenylpyrazolyl derivatives *49* and *50* were however much less active, with IC_{50} values in the high μM range [100], as was the steroidal D-ring fused oxazolidine *52* (Fig. 4, Table 2, entries 15-16, and 18) [99].

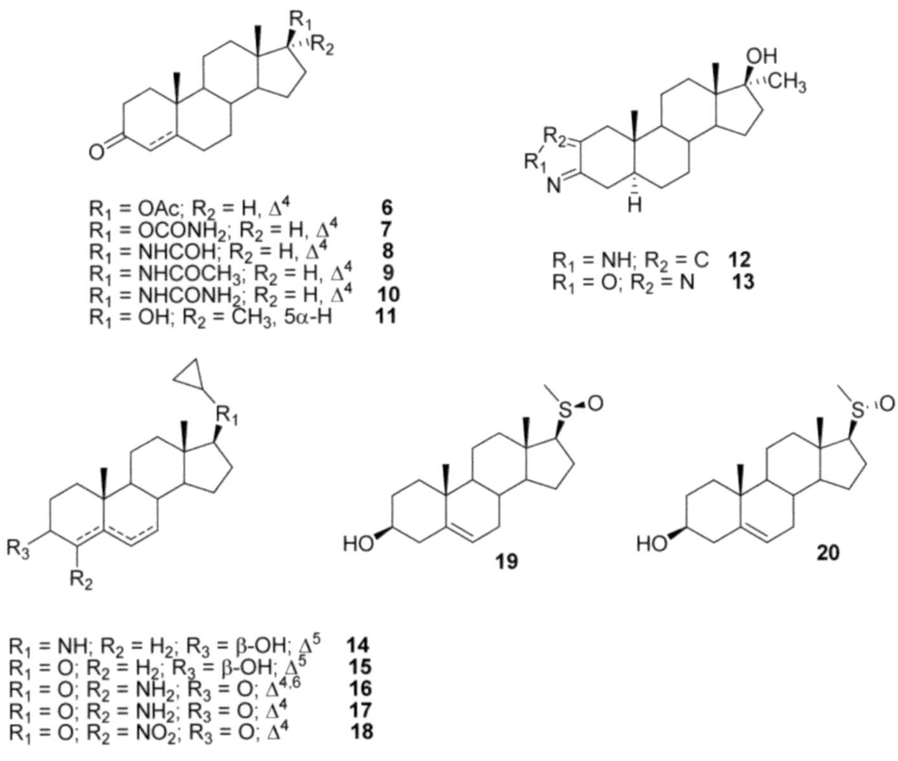

Figure 3. Androstane based CYP17 inhibitors.

In 1996, Njar et al. reported the first steroidal inhibitors of CYP17 bearing a heterocyclic moiety bound to C17 by a nitrogen atom [101], which included compounds *53-55* (Fig. 5, Table 2, entries 19-21), among which the imidazolyl derivative *53* was found to be the most promising [101-104]. Later, in 2005, the same group reported the synthesis of galeterone *4* and its Δ^4-3-keto derivative *56* (Fig. 5, Table 2, entries 22-23) [104-106].

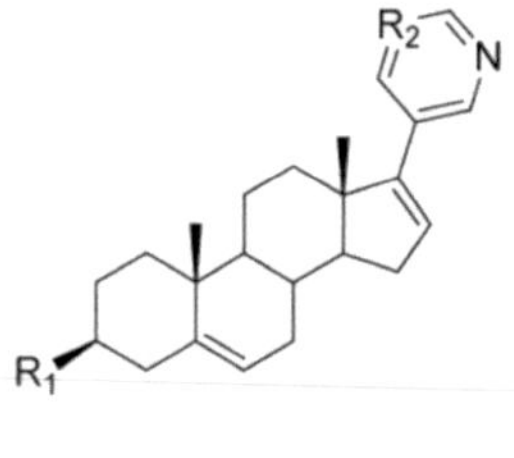

R_1 = OH; R_2 = CH **21**
R_1 = OH; R_2 = N **22**
R_1 = OAc; R_2 = N **23**

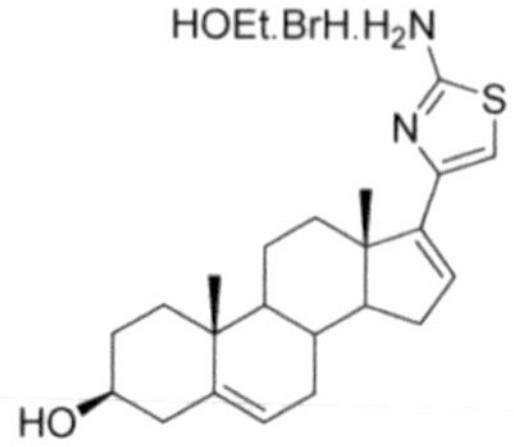

24

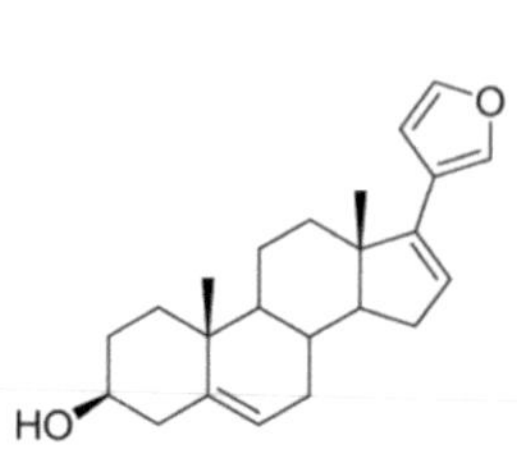

25

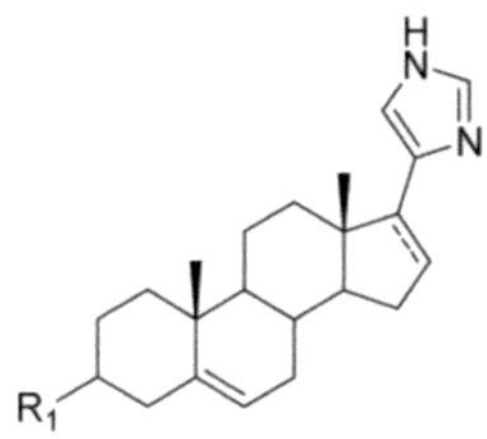

R_1 = β-OH; Δ^5 **26**
R_1 = β-OH; $\Delta^{5,16}$ **27**
R_1 = O; Δ^4 **28**

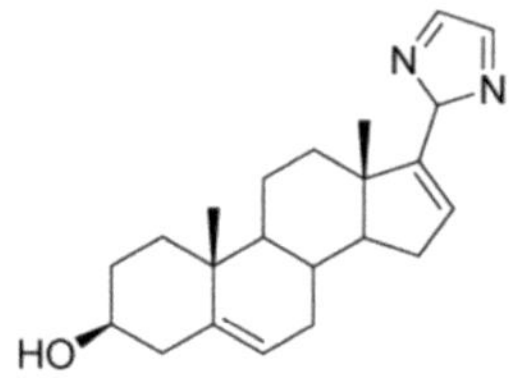

29

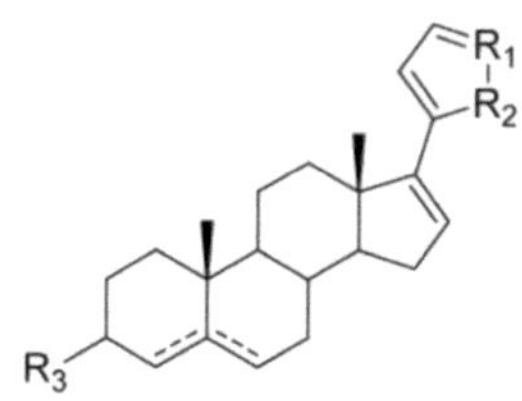

R_1 = N; R_2 = NH; R_3 = OAc **30**
R_1 = N; R_2 = NH; R_3 = O; Δ^4 **31**
R_1 = N; R_2 = O; R_3 = O; Δ^4 **32**

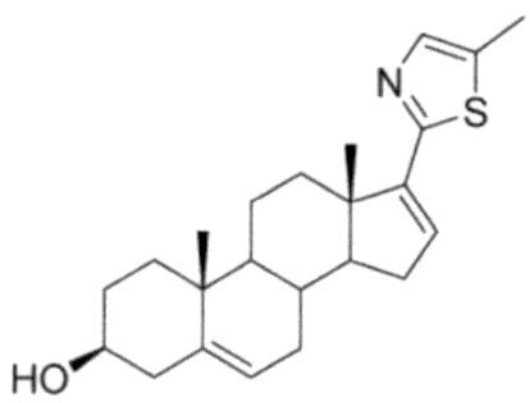

33

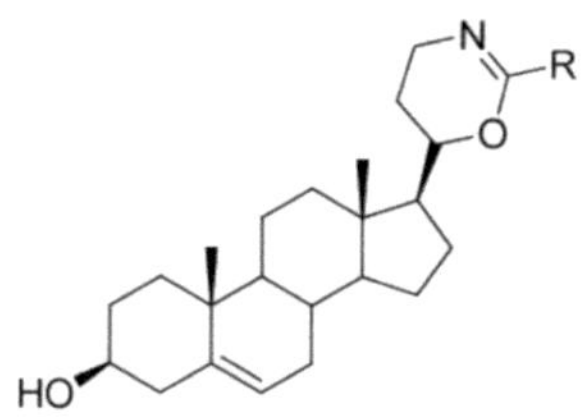

R = Ph **34**
R = 4-chlorophenyl **35**
R = 4-bromophenyl **36**
R = 4-nitrophenyl **37**
R = 4-methoxyphenyl **38**
R = 3,4,5-trimethoxyphenyl **39**

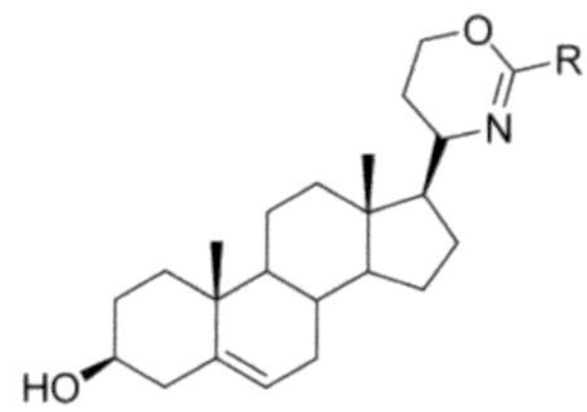

R = Ph **40**
R = 4-chlorophenyl **41**
R = 4-bromophenyl **42**
R = 4-nitrophenyl **43**
R = 4-methoxyphenyl **44**
R = 3,4,5-trimethoxyphenyl **45**

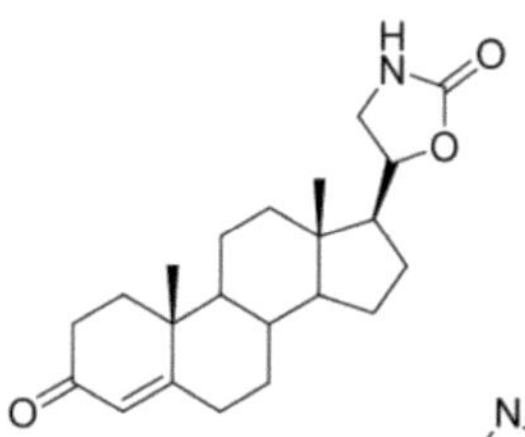

46

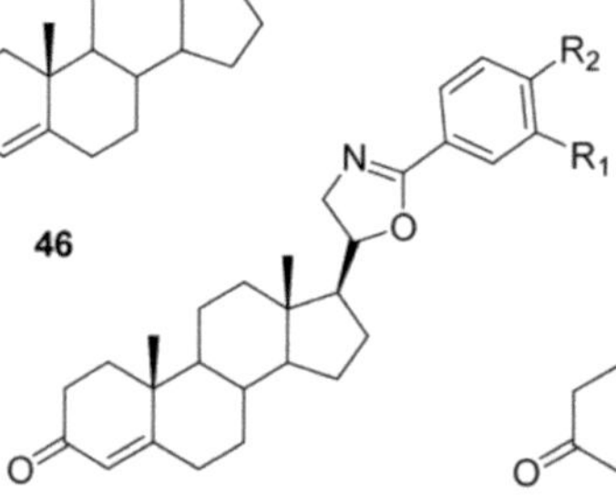

R_1 = Cl, R_2 =H **47**
R_1 = H; R_2 = Br **48**

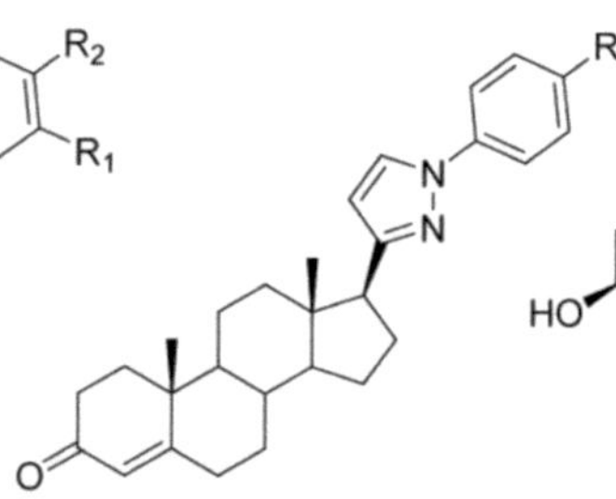

R = CN **49**
R = OCH_3 **50**

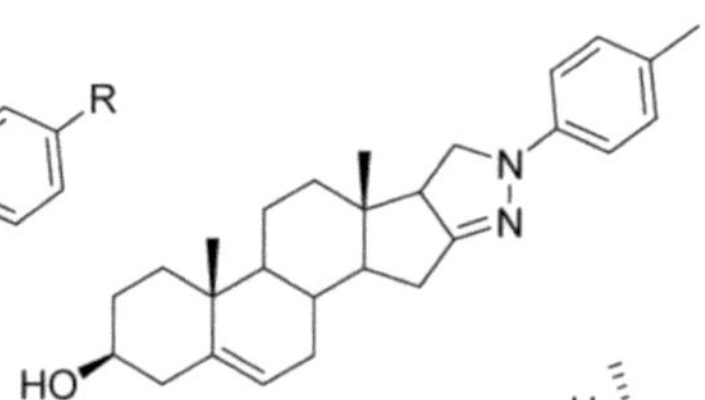

51

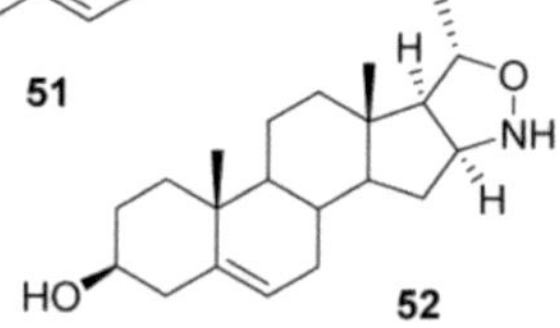

52

Figure 4. Androstane based CYP17 inhibitors.

Entry	Compound	CYP17 inhibition (nM)	Ref.
1	21	Human (OHase): 4 Human (lyase): 2.9	[86,107]
2	3	Human (OHase): 18 Human (lyase): 17	
3	22	Rat: 220 Human: 24 *E.coli* [a]: 30	[87, 88]
4	23	Rat: 1460 Human: 38 *E.coli* [a]: 2500	
5	26	Rat: 91 Human: 66	[89, 90]
6	27	Rat: 49 Human: 24	
7	28	Rat: 79 Human: 58	
8	29	ND[b] Human: 21	
9	30	Rat: 28 Human: 42	
10	31	Rat: 76 Human: 59	
11	32	Rat: 32 Human: 39	
12	46	Rat: 3000	[97]
13	47	Rat: 4800	[98]
14	48	Rat: 5000	
15	49	Rat: 22000	[100]
16	50	Rat: 59000	
17	51	Rat: 5800	[99]
18	52	Rat: 26000	
19	53	Rat: 9 Human: 8 LNCaP-CYP17 cells[c]: 1.25	[102, 103]
20	54	Rat: 8 Human: 7 LNCaP-CYP17 cells[c]: 2.96	
21	55	Rat: 10 Human: 13	

Entry	Compound	CYP17 inhibition (nM)	Ref.
		LNCaP-CYP17 cells[c]: 7.97	
22	4	*E.coli*[a]: 300	[105, 106]
23	56	*E.coli*[a]: 915	
24	61	LNCaP-CYP17 cells[c]: 11500	[4]
25	62	LNCaP-CYP17 cells[c]: 17100	

Table 2. IC_{50} values for androstane CYP17 inhibitors. [a]Recombinant human CYP17 expressed in *E.coli*; [b]ND = Not Determined; [c]Recombinant human CYP17 expressed in LNCaP cells.

Thus, *in vitro* results with compounds *53-55* revealed a high inhibitory potential of the human enzyme expressed in LNCaP cells. In addition, compounds *53* and *55* completely suppressed T and DHT stimulated growth of LNCaP cells below 5 μM, and displayed antiandrogenic activity [102, 108]. *In vivo* experiments confirmed these results and showed that the compounds were however less effective than castration [109]. The C17-benzimidazole derivative *4* became the first example of a CYP17 inhibitor and antiandrogen that could effectively suppress androgen-dependent tumor growth better than castration [105]. In 2007, our group reported the synthesis of the 1*H*- and 2*H*-indazole androstanes *57-60* which despite being poor inhibitors of human CYP17 displayed selective inhibition of PC-3 cells suggesting that mechanisms other than interference with the AR could be involved in their cytotoxicity [5]. We also synthesized a series of steroidal carbamates out of which compounds *61* and *62* (Fig. 5, Table 2, entries 24-25) were inhibitors of human CYP17 with IC_{50} values of 11.5 and 17.1 μM, respectively [4].

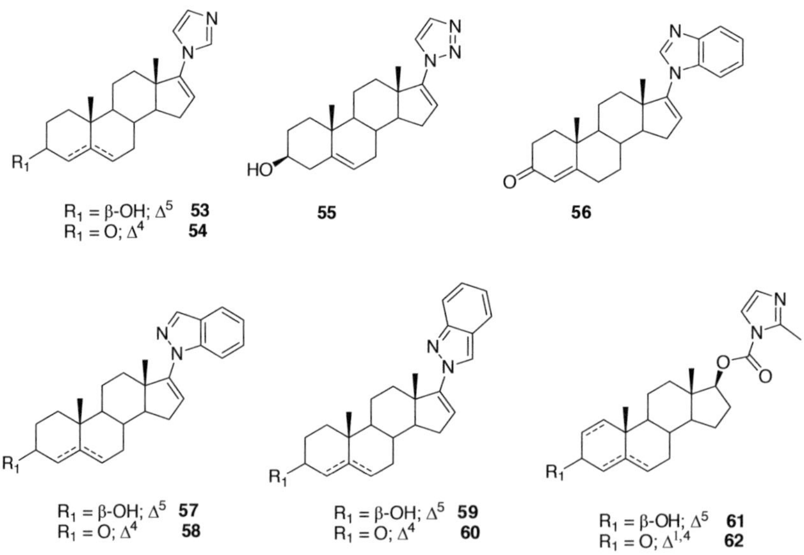

Figure 5. Androstane based CYP17 inhibitors.

3.2. Pregnanes

Among the pregnane CYP17 inhibitors, compounds *63-65* (Fig. 6, Table 3, entries 1-3) bearing 20-substituents with moderate to strong dipole properties were more active than ketoconazole in inhibiting human CYP17, displaying IC_{50} values of 16 to 230 nM and 16 to 190 nM for the hydroxylase and lyase activities, respectively [90, 110, 111]. In 2000, Hartman et al. tested several pregneneoximes *66-76* among which some were potent inhibitors of both rat and human CYP17 (Fig. 6, Table 3, entries 4-11) [112]. Compound *66* was effective *in vivo* and suppressed plasma T concentrations more potently than ketoconazole. The hydroxamic acid derivative *77* (Fig. 6) was not a CYP17 inhibitor [113].

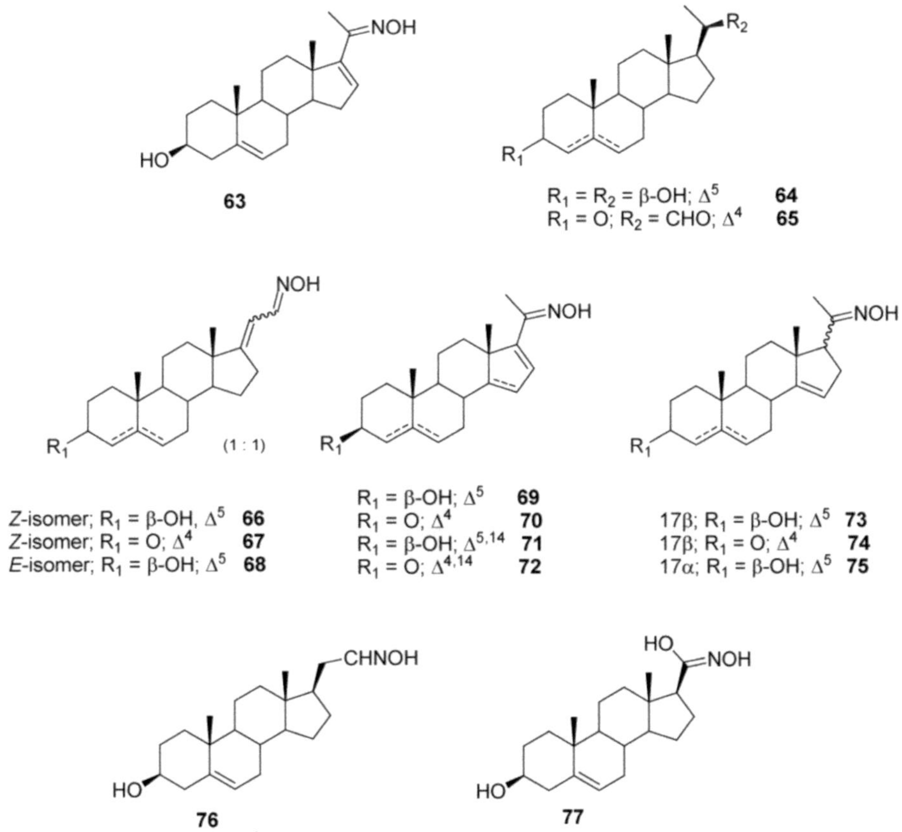

Figure 6. Pregnane based CYP17 inhibitors.

Entry	Compound	CYP17 inhibition (nM)	Ref.
1	63	Human (OHase): 16 Human (lyase): 16	[90, 110, 111]
2	64	Human (OHase): 180 Human (lyase): 190	
3	65	Human (OHase): 230 Human (lyase): 160	[90, 110, 111, 114]
4	66	Rat: 520 Human: 77 *E. coli* [b]: 230	[112]
5	67	Rat: 140 Human: 180	
6	69	Rat: [a] Human: 170 *E. coli* [b]: 520	
7	70	Rat: [a] Human: 100	
8	71	Rat: [a] Human: 200 *E. coli* [b]: 420	
9	72	Rat: [a] Human: 200	
10	74	Rat: 300 Human: 300	
11	76	Rat: 2760 Human: 270	
12	78	Rat: 210 Human: 540	[115, 116]
13	79	Rat: 34000 Human: 1520	
14	80	Rat: 1200	[115]
15	81	Rat: 36000	
16	82	Rat: 9670 Human: 970	[116]
17	83	Rat: 430 Human: 290	
18	84	Rat: 530 Human: 400	

Entry	Compound	CYP17 inhibition (nM)	Ref.
19	85	Rat (OHase): 75.8 Rat (lyase): 55.8	[117]
20	86	Rat: 600	[118]

Table 3. IC_{50} values for pregnane CYP17 inhibitors. [a]≥ 125 μM; [b]*E. Coli* cells coexpressing human CYP17 and NADPH reductase

A difference in the inhibitory potential of rat CYP17 of the aziridinylpregnanes *78-81* was observed between the *S*- and *R*-isomers, the *S*-isomers *78* and *80* being 162 and 30-fold more potent than the *R*-isomers, respectively (Fig. 7, Table 3, entries 12-15) [115]. However, this finding was not corroborated by later studies that used the human enzyme [116]. The activity of compounds *82-85* (Fig. 7, Table 2, entries 16-19) was also reported [116, 117]. Several fluorinated pregnanes *86–91*and *93* were synthesized in search of greater metabolic stability (Fig. 7, Table 3, entry 20, Table 4). Inhibition of the cynomolgous monkey enzyme at 1 μM, following preincubation with the enzyme with compounds *87-93*, is depicted on Table 4[118-122].

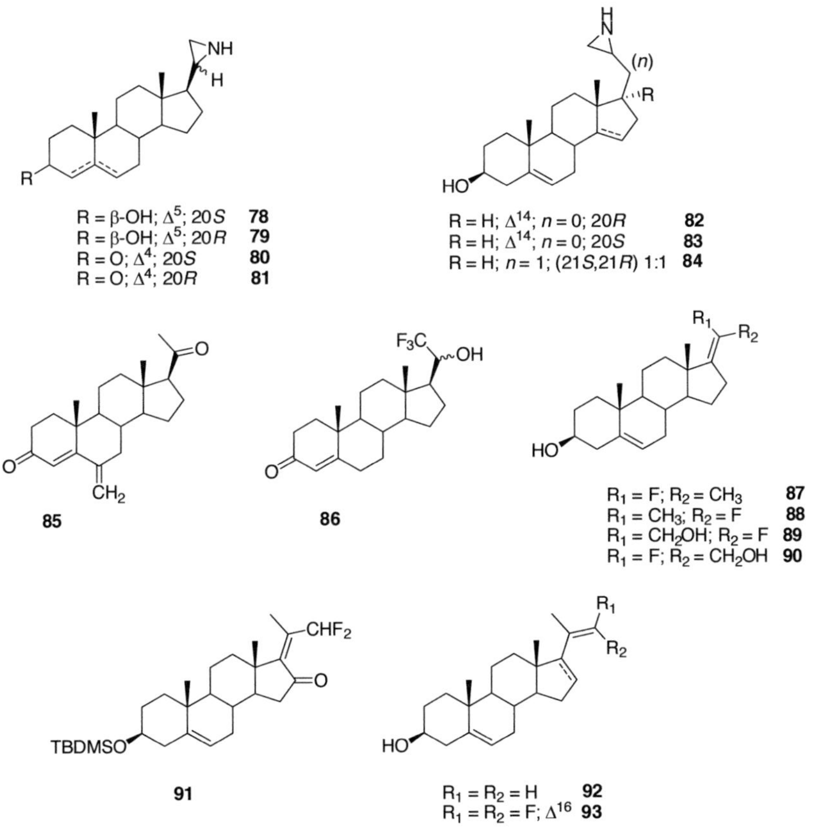

Figure 7. Pregnane based CYP17 inhibitors.

Entry	Compound	% Inhibition	Ref.
1	87	61	[119-121]
2	88	60	
3	89	61	
4	90	94	
5	91	85	[122]
6	92	60	
7	93	62	

Table 4. Inhibition of cynomolgous monkey testicular CYP17 by pregnane derivatives, at 1 μM, following preincubation with enzyme.

3.3. Other steroidal inhibitors

Other reported steroidal inhibitors of CYP17 are depicted on figure 8. The 17-aza derivative *94* inhibited human CYP17 with an IC_{50} value of 4.9 μM [123]. Compound *95* inhibited both 5α-reductase and CYP17 with k_i values of 27 and 14 nM, respectively [124]. The oxime *96* was also a dual inhibitor with the ability to reduce serum and prostatic T and DHT concentrations *in vivo* [125].

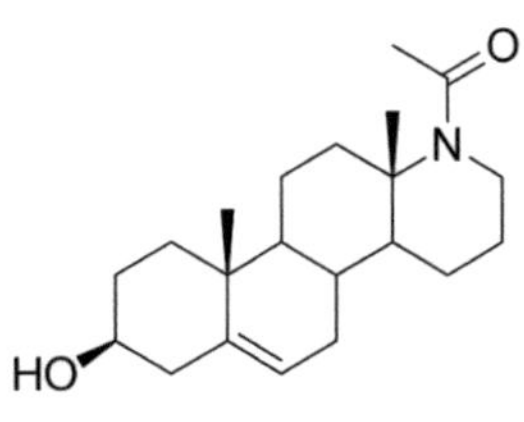

94

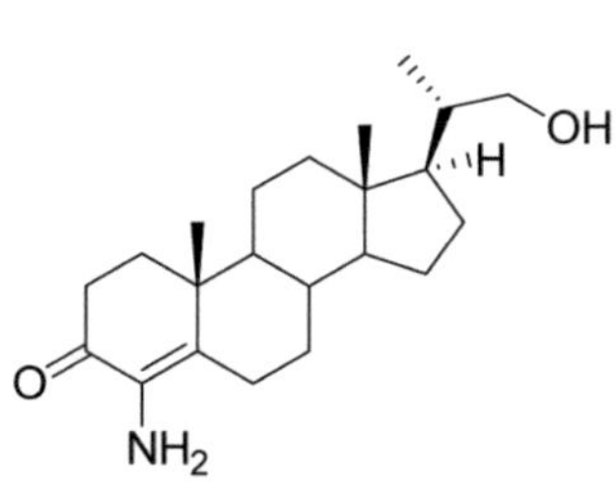

95

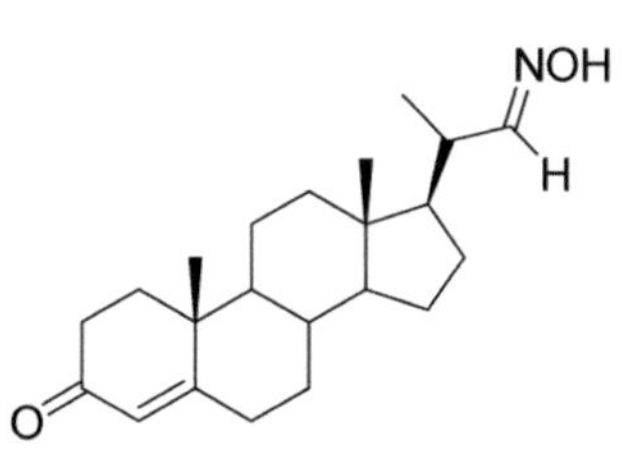

96

Figure 8. Other steroidal inhibitors of CYP17.

4. Abiraterone and galeterone

As previously mentioned, abiraterone acetate *3* (Fig. 1) constitutes the first and still the only steroidal CYP17 inhibitor approved by the FDA in 2011, being indicated for the treatment of mCRPC after chemotherapy [14].

This drug was developed at the Institute of Cancer Research (UK) considering the known efficacy and limitations of ketoconazole in this field and following the observation that non-steroidal 3-pyridyl esters had improved selectivity for the inhibition of CYP17. This led to the preparation of abiraterone *21* (Fig. 4), a $\Delta^{5,16}$-steroid with a 3-pyridyl group bound to C17, which revealed to be a potent and selective irreversible inhibitor of both 17α-hydroxylase and $C_{17,20}$-lyase activities of CYP17 [86, 126, 127]. In fact, it was observed that abiraterone *21* is not only a more potent CYP17 inhibitor than ketoconazole but also is a less effective inhibitor of other CYP450 enzymes, responsible for the significant side effects and potential pharmacological interactions of ketoconazole in PC therapy [14, 128]. Accordingly, preclinical studies in mice demonstrated that abiraterone *21* reduced serumT to castrate levels, in spite of a compensatory significant increase in luteinizing hormone (LH) [126]. However, when abiraterone acetate *3*was tested in human PC patients for the first time as a substitute to gonadotropin-releasing hormone (GnRH) analogues, sustained suppression of T production was not observed due to an increase in LH levels [129]. For this reason, abiraterone *21*was developed to be concomitantly used with GnRH analogues in mCRPC [130]. Studies in xenograft models devoid of testicular and adrenal androgens further evidenced that abiraterone *21* inhibited CRPC growth and thus also seem to suppress androgen production in PC tumors [128].

Several Phase I clinical studies [131, 132] revealed that abiraterone acetate *3* is safe and effective on lowering serum androgen levels in both ketoconazole naïve and exposed patients. In addition, its antitumor activity was nearly equivalent in both groups. However, a significant increase in adrenocorticotrophic hormone (ACTH) was developed leading to hypokalemia and hypertension as the predominant toxicities. In order to reduce these side effects eplerenone, a mineralocorticoid antagonist, was introduced. As the highest studied dosage of abiraterone acetate *3* (1000mg) did not lead to limiting toxicities, the useof 1000mg daily was chosen in additional trials [8, 131, 133 135].

The concomitant use of the corticosteroids dexamethasone or prednisone in the efficacy of abiraterone acetate *3*in several conditions was studied in Phase II trials [133-135]. A significant decrease in hyperaldosteronism-related symptoms was observed and therefore prednisone 5mg b.i.d. was included in all subsequent studies, as well as in the FDA label indication. Other Phase II studies evaluated the efficacy of abiraterone in docetaxel-treated CRPC patients, and continued to evidence the importance of this steroidal drug in this stage of the pathology [135].

A Phase III study compared the use of abiraterone acetate *3*and prednisone versus prednisone alone in 1195 ketoconazole-naïve men with mCRPCshowing disease progression during or after therapy withdocetaxel. The primary endpoint was overall survival and the secondary endpoints were PSA decline, time to PSA progression and progression-free survival. In this study an increased median overall survival in the abiraterone acetate *3*+ predisone group was observed when compared to that of patients treated with prednisone alone (14.8 vs 10.9 months; hazard ratio of 0.65). In addition, all the other endpoints were met and as expected the toxicities caused by CYP17 blockage occurred mostly in the abiraterone acetate *3*+ prednisone group. Another Phase III study set to be completed in 2014 is evaluating the use of abiraterone acetate *3* and prednisone versus prednisone alone in CRPC prior to chemotherapy [136].

Due to all these beneficial results and after the first Phase III studies, in April 2011, abiraterone acetate *3*was approved by the FDA for the treatment of mCRPC after chemotherapy [14].

Abiraterone *3* is being used in the form of its 3β-acetyl prodrug in order to increase its oral bioavailability, and is quickly deacetylated to the active drug once absorbed. In spite of the fact that high-fat meals increase its oral absorption, it is recommended that this drug should be taken on an empty stomach. Other pharmacokinetic studies revealed that this drug is highly bound to plasma proteins and has a plasma half-life of 10-14h [131, 132]. At present, several other clinical trials are ongoing, mainly for the study of the combination of abiraterone acetate *3* with other relevant drugs in PC treatment [137].

Galeterone *4* (Fig. 1) is structurally similar to abiraterone *21* and was rationally designed as an androgen biosynthesis inhibitor via CYP17 inhibition [8]. In fact, as previously mentioned, several research works evidenced that modification of the C17 substituent of Δ^{16}-steroids, particularly by attachment of nitrogen heterocycles, was a relevant strategy to produce potent inhibitors of the enzyme. Following these considerations, Handratta et al. designed and prepared several Δ^{16}-steroidal C17 benzoazoles and pyrazines and evaluated their CYP17 and 5α-reductase inhibitory activities, binding to and transactivation of the AR, as well as their antiproliferative effects against two human PC cell lines (LNCaP and LAPC4). Some of the compounds including *4* and its Δ^4-3-ketone derivative *56* (Fig. 5) were potent CYP17 inhibitors and antagonists of both wild type and mutant AR. These compounds were the first reported examplesbearing such a dual activity. In addition, these steroids inhibited the growth of DHT-stimulated LNCaP and LACP4 PC cells with IC_{50} values in the low micromolar range. Galeterone *4* and compound *56* were further studied for pharmacokinetic properties and antitumor activities against androgen-dependent LAPC4 human prostate tumor xenografts in severe combined immunodeficient (SCID) mice. Galeterone *4* was more effective than castration in its *in vivo* antitumor activity [104]. Taking this into account, Vasaitis et al. demonstrated by *in vitro* and *in vivo* studies that unlike bicalutamide and castration, galeterone *4* also caused down-regulation of AR protein expression, which appears to contribute to its antitumor efficacy. The authors also evidenced that this compound caused a significant regression of LAPC4 tumors in xenograft models, being more potent than castration, and that treatment with galeterone *4* was also very effective in preventing the formation of LAPC4 tumors [138].

An *in vitro* study using high-passage LNCaP cells demonstrated that galeterone *4* inhibited the proliferation of these cells that were no longer sensitive to bicalutamide and had increased AR expression. In addition, the combination of galeterone *4*with inhibitors of signal transduction pathways such as gefitinib and everolimus, was proven to be synergistic when compared to either agent alone and superior to their combination with bicalutamide [139]. Later, *in vivo* studies with LNCaP and high-passage LNCaP tumor xenografts in SCID mice indicated that dual inhibition of AR and mammalian target of rapamycin (mTOR) in castration-resistant models can restore the sensitivity of tumours to anti-androgen therapy. The results observed in this study also indicated that the CYP17 and AR inhibitor galeterone *4* combined with the mTOR inhibitor everolimus may be effective in resistant PC [140].

A very recent *in vitro* study with LNCaP and LAPC4 cells demonstrated that both galeterone *4* and abiraterone *21* directly down-regulated the expression and activation of the AR via multiple mechanisms, in addition to their CYP17 inhibitory activities [141].

Due to the impressive biological activities observed, galeterone *4* is currently being evaluated in a phase I/II open label clinical trial (ARMOR1 study) as a potential drug for the treatment of castration resistant prostate cancer. This study began in 2009 and has as primary outcomes the incidence of adverse effects (phase I) and the proportion of patients with 50% or greater decrease in PSA from baseline (phase II) [137].

Recently, in a continuing study of the clinical candidate *4* and analogues as potential agents for PC treatment, putative metabolites of *4* and metabolically stable derivatives were prepared. Putative metabolites included compounds with no double bonds at C16, C5, or both as well as their corresponding 3-oxo derivatives. Metabolically stable analogues of *4*, developed to optimize its potency and to increase its stability and oral bioavailability, included their 3α-azido, 3ξ-fluoro, 3β-mesylate and 3β-O-sulfamoyl derivatives. Several *in vitro* studies, including CYP17 inhibitory activity, binding to and transactivation of AR, as well as antiproliferative effects against LNCaP and LAPC4 cell lines, demonstrated that none of the compounds were superior to *4* in the observed effects. The 3ξ-fluoro analogue was, however, nearly 2-fold more efficacious *vs* LAPC4 xenografts than *4*. Nonetheless, the toxicity observed with this halogenated compound was of concern [142].

5. Conclusion

PC is one of the most prevalent causes of death in Europe and USA. In spite of important advances in the treatment of localized disease, advanced PC is still incurable. One of the most relevant PC therapeutic strategies involves the inhibition of androgen biosynthesis by

CYP17 inhibition. In fact, starting from the structure of the natural substrates of this enzyme, several steroids, mainly with a heterocyclic ring bound to C17, have been developed over the years as CYP17 inhibitors. All these studies successfully led to the approval of abiraterone acetate *3* by the FDA in 2011 for the treatment of mCRPC after chemotherapy. In addition, other clinical trials involving this drug are being performed in order to expand its clinical usefulness, namely in CRPC prior to chemotherapy and in combination with other drugs. Another steroid that is in Phase I/II clinical trials for CRPC is galeterone *4*, which is structurally similar to abiraterone *21*. However, in addition to bearing a potent and selective CYP17 inhibitory activity, this compound also modulates AR activity. As it is now clear that function of the AR axis remains crucial to a majority of patients with CRPC, its mechanism of action can be of great advantage in PC therapy, either alone or in combination with other AR-modulating agents.In the future it is expected that the invaluable knowledge provided by the use of CYP17 inhibitors in PC treatment will shed more light on the most significant biological pathways involved in this disease. The establishment of a possible role for combination regimens including CYP17 inhibitors in earlier stages of PC as a means to prevent surgery and classical chemotherapy drugs would undoubtedly contribute to improving the quality of life of PC patients.

Acknowledgments

Jorge A. R. Salvador thanks Universidade de Coimbra and Centro de Neurociências e Biologia Celular for financial support. Vânia M. Moreira acknowledges Fundação para a Ciência e a Tecnologia for financial support (SFRH/BPD/45037/2008).

Author details

Jorge A. R. Salvador[1,2], Vânia M. Moreira[3] and Samuel M. Silvestre[4]

*Address all correspondence to: salvador@ci.uc.pt

1 Laboratório de Química Farmacêutica, Faculdade de Farmácia, Universidade de Coimbra,Pólo das Ciências da Saúde, Azinhaga de Santa Comba, Coimbra, Portugal

2 Centro de Neurociências e Biologia Celular, Universidade de Coimbra, Coimbra, Portugal

3 Division of Pharmaceutical Chemistry, Faculty of Pharmacy, Viikinkaari, University of Helsinki, Helsinki, Finland

4 Health Sciences Research Centre, Faculdade de Ciências da Saúde,Universidade da Beira Interior,Covilhã, Portugal

References

[1] Jordan V C and Brodie A M H. Development and evolution of therapies targeted to the estrogen receptor for the treatment and prevention of breast cancer. Steroids 2007;72(1): 7-25.

[2] Brodie A, Njar V, Macedo L F, Vasaitis T S and Sabnis G. The Coffey Lecture: Steroidogenic enzyme inhibitors and hormone dependent cancer. Urologic Oncology: Seminars and Original Investigations 2009;27(1): 53-63.

[3] Moreira V M, Salvador J A R, Vasaitis T S and Njar V C. CYP17 Inhibitors for Prostate Cancer Treatment - An Update. Current Medicinal Chemistry 2008;15(9): 868-899.

[4] Moreira V M A, Vasaitis T S, Guo Z, Njar V C O and Salvador J A R. Synthesis of Novel C17 Steroidal Carbamates. Studies on CYP17 Action, Androgen Receptor Binding and Function, and Prostate Cancer Cell Growth. Steroids 2008;73(12): 1217-1227.

[5] Moreira V M A, Vasaitis T S, Njar V C O, and Salvador J A R. Synthesis and evaluation of novel 17-indazole androstene derivatives designed as CYP17 inhibitors. Steroids 2007;72(14): 939-948.

[6] Owen C P. 17α-Hydroxylase/17,20-Lyase ($P450_{17\alpha}$) Inhibitors in the Treatment of Prostate Cancer: A Review. Anti-Cancer Agents in Medicinal Chemistry 2009;9(6): 613-626.

[7] Pezaro C J, Mukherji D and De Bono J S. Abiraterone acetate: redefining hormone treatment for advanced prostate cancer. Drug Discovery Today 2012;17(5-6): 221-226.

[8] Vasaitis T S, Bruno R D and Njar V C O. CYP17 inhibitors for prostate cancer therapy. Journal of Steroid Biochemistry and Molecular Biology 2011;125(1-2): 23-31.

[9] Ang J E, Olmos D and Bono J S. CYP17 blockade by abiraterone: further evidence for frequent continued hormone-dependence in castration-resistant prostate cancer. British Journal of Cancer 2009;100(5): 671-675.

[10] Mancuso A, Oudard S and Sternberg C N. Effective chemotherapy for hormone-refractory prostate cancer (HRPC): Present status and perspectives with taxane-based treatments. Critical Reviews in Oncology/Hematology 2007;61(2): 176-185.

[11] Harzstark A L and Small E J. Castrate-resistant prostate cancer: therapeutic strategies. Expert Opinion on Pharmacotherapy 2010;11(6): 937-945.

[12] Sartor A O. Progression of metastatic castrate-resistant prostate cancer: impact of therapeutic intervention in the post-docetaxel space. Journal of Hematology & Oncology 2011;4: 18.

[13] Logothetis C J, Efstathiou E, Manuguid F and Kirkpatrick P. Abiraterone acetate. Nature Reviews Drug Discovery 2011;10: 573-574.

[14] Bryce A and Ryan C J. Development and Clinical Utility of Abiraterone Acetate as an Androgen Synthesis Inhibitor. Clinical Pharmacology & Therapeutics 2012;91(1): 101-108.

[15] Vasaitis T S and Njar V C O. Novel, potent anti-androgens of therapeutic potential: recent advances and promising developments. Future Medicinal Chemistry 2010;2(4): 667-680.

[16] Molina A and Belldegrun A. Novel Therapeutic Strategies for Castration Resistant Prostate Cancer: Inhibition of Persistent Androgen Production and Androgen Receptor Mediated Signaling. Journal of Urology 2011;185(3): 787-794.

[17] Jarman M, Smith H J, Nicholls P J and Simons C. Inhibitors of Enzymes of Androgen Biosynthesis: Cytochrome $P450_{17\alpha}$ and 5α-Steroid Reductase. Natural Product Reports 1998;15(5): 495-512.

[18] Baston E and Leroux F. Inhibitors of Steroidal Cytochrome P450 Enzymes as Targets For Drug Development. Recent Patents on Anti-cancer Drug Discovery 2007;2(1): 31-58.

[19] Hartmann R W, Ehmer P B, Haidar S, Hector M, Jose J, Klein C D, Seidel S B, Sergejew T F, Wachall B G, Wächter G A, and Zhuang Y. Inhibition of CYP 17, a New Strategy for the Treatment of Prostate Cancer. Archiv der Pharmazie (Weinheim) 2002;335(4): 119-128.

[20] Schneider G and Wolfling J. Synthetic Cardenolides and Related Compounds. Current Organic Chemistry 2004;8(14): 1381-1403.

[21] Haider S M, Patel J S, Poojari C S, and Neidle S. Molecular Modeling on Inhibitor Complexes and Active-Site Dynamics of Cytochrome P450 C17, a Target for Prostate Cancer Therapy. Journal of Molecular Biology 2010;400(5): 1078-1098.

[22] DeVore N M and Scott E E. Structures of cytochrome P450 17A1 with prostate cancer drugs abiraterone and TOK-001. Nature 2012;482: 116-119.

[23] Nakajin S, Hall P F and Onoda M. Testicular Microsomal Cytochrome P-450 for C_{21} Steroid Side Chain Cleavage. Spectral and Binding Studies. Journal of Biological Chemistry 1981;256(12): 6134-6139.

[24] Nakajin S and Hall P F. Microsomal Cytochrome P-450 from Neonatal Pig Testis. Purification and Properties of a C_{21} Steroid Side-chain Cleavage System (17α-hydroxylase-$C_{17,20}$ lyase). Journal of Biological Chemistry 1981;256(8): 3871-3876.

[25] Nakajin S, Shively J E, Yuan P M and Hall P F. Microsomal Cytochrome P-450 from Neonatal Pig Testis: Two Enzymatic Activities (17α-Hydroxylase and $C_{17,20}$-Lyase) Associated with One Protein. Biochemistry 1981;20(14): 4037-4042.

[26] Zuber M X, Simpson E R and Waterman M R. Expression of Bovine 17α-Hydroxylase Cytochrome P-450 cDNA in Nonsteroidogenic (COS 1) Cells. Science 1986;234(4781): 1258-1261.

[27] Onoda M, Haniu M, Yanagibashi K, Sweet F, Shively J E and Hall P F. Affinity Alkylation of the Active Site of C_{21} Steroid Side-chain Cleavage Cytochrome P-450 from Neonatal Porcine Testis: a Unique Cysteine Residue Alkylated by 17-(Bromoacetoxy)progesterone. Biochemistry 1987;26(2): 657-662.

[28] Hall P F. Cytochrome P-450 C_{21scc}: One Enzyme with Two Actions: Hydroxylase and Lyase. Journal of Steroid Biochemistry and Molecular Biology 1991;40(4-6): 527-532.

[29] Meunier B, Visser S P and Shaik S. Mechanism of Oxidation Reactions Catalyzed by Cytochrome P450 Enzymes. Chemical Reviews 2004;104(9): 3947-3980.

[30] Denisov I G, Makris T M, Sligar S G and Schlichting I. Structure and Chemistry of Cytochrome P450. Chemical Reviews 2005;105(6): 2253-2277.

[31] Gao W, Bohl C E and Dalton J T. Chemistry and Structural Biology of Androgen Receptor. Chemical Reviews 2005;105(9): 3352-3370.

[32] Guyton A C and Hall J E. Textbook of Medical Physiology. Philadelphia: WB Saunders Company; 2000.

[33] Koivisto P, Kolmer M, Visakorpi T and Kallioniemi O P. Androgen Receptor Gene and Hormonal Therapy Failure of Prostate Cancer. American Journal of Pathology 1998;152(1): 1-9.

[34] Isaacs J T and Isaacs W B. Androgen Receptor Outwits Prostate Cancer Drugs. Nature Medicine 2004;10(1): 26-27.

[35] Chatterjee B. The Role of the Androgen Receptor in the Development of Prostatic Hyperplasia and Prostate Cancer. Molecular and Cellular Biochemistry 2003;253(1-2): 89-101.

[36] Huggins C and Hodges C V. Studies on Prostatic Cancer. I. The Effect of Castration, of Estrogen and of Androgen Injection on Serum Phosphatases in Metastatic Carcinoma of the Prostate. Cancer Research 1941;1: 293-297.

[37] Huggins C, Stevens R E and Hodges C V. Studies on Prostatic Cancer. II. The Effect of Castration on Clinical Patients with Carcinoma of the Prostate. Archives of Surgery 1941;43: 209-223.

[38] Denis L J and Griffiths K. Endocrine Treatment in Prostate Cancer. Seminars in Surgical Oncology 2000;18(1): 52-74.

[39] Chung B C, Picado-Leonard J, Haniu M, Bienkowski M, Hall P F, Shively J E and Miller W L. Cytochrome P450c17 (Steroid 17α-Hydroxylase/17,20 Lyase): Cloning of Human Adrenal and Testis cDNAs Indicates the Same Gene is Expressed in Both Tissues. Proceedings of the National Academy of Sciences of the United States of America 1987;84(2): 407-411.

[40] Sparkes R S, Klisak I and Miller W L. Regional Mapping of Genes Encoding Human Steroidogenic Enzymes: $P450_{scc}$ to 15q23-q24, Adrenodoxin to 11q22; Adrenodoxin

Reductase to 17q24-q25; and P450c17 to 10q24-q25.DNA and Cell Biology 1991;10(5): 359-365.

[41] Fan Y S, Sasi R, Lee C, Winter J S, Waterman M R and Lin C C. Localization of the Human CYP17 gene (cytochrome $P450_{17\alpha}$) to 10q24.3 by Fluorescence *in situ* Hybridization and Simultaneous Chromosome Banding. Genomics 1992;14(4): 1110-1111.

[42] Yanagibashi K and Hall P F. Role of Electron Transport in the Regulation of the Lyase Activity of C21 Side-chain Cleavage P-450 From Porcine Adrenal and Testicular Microsomes. Journal of Biological Chemistry 1986;261(18): 8429-8433.

[43] Lin D, Black S M, Nagahama Y and Miller W L. Steroid 17α-Hydroxylase and 17,20-Lyase Activities of P450c17: Contributions of Serine106 and P450 Reductase. Endocrinology 1993;132(6): 2498-2506.

[44] Pandey A V and Miller W L. Regulation of 17,20-Lyase Activity by Cytochrome b_5 and by Serine Phosphorylation of P450c17. Journal of Biological Chemistry 2005;280(14): 13265-13271.

[45] Dharia S, Slane A, Jian M, Conner M, Conley A J and Parker C R. Colocalization of P450c17 and Cytochrome b_5 in Androgen-synthesizing Tissues of the Human. Biology of the Reproduction 2004;71(1): 83-88.

[46] Akhtar M K, Kelly S L, and Kaderbhai M A. Cytochrome b_5 Modulation of 17α-Hydroxylase and 17,20-lyase (CYP17) Activities in Steroidogenesis. Journal of Endocrinology 2005;187(2): 267-274.

[47] Naffin-Olivos J L and Auchus R J. Human Cytochrome b_5 Requires Residues E48 and E49 to Stimulate the 17,20-Lyase Activity of Cytochrome P450c17. Biochemistry 2006;45(3): 755-762.

[48] Akhtar M, Wright J N and Lee-Robichaud P. A review of mechanistic studies on aromatase (CYP19) and 17α-hydroxylase-17,20-lyase (CYP17). Journal of Steroid Biochemistry and Molecular Biology 2011;125(1-2): 2-12.

[49] Zhang L H, Rodriguez H, Ohno S and Miller W L. Serine Phosphorylation of Human P450c17 Increases 17,20-Lyase Activity: Implications for Adrenarche and the Polycystic Ovary Syndrome. Proceedings of the National Academy of Sciences of the United States of America 1995;92(23): 10619-10623.

[50] Pandey A V, Mellon S H and Miller W L. Protein Phosphatase 2A and Phosphoprotein SET Regulate Androgen Production by P450c17. Journal of Biological Chemistry 2003;278(5): 2837-2844.

[51] Souter I, Munir I, Mallick P, Weitsman S R, Geller D H and Magoffin D A. Mutagenesis of Putative Serine-threonine Phosphorylation Sites Proximal to Arg255 of Human Cytochrome P450c17 Does Not Selectively Promote Its 17,20-Lyase Activity.Fertility and Sterility 2006;85: 1290-1299.

[52] Geller D H, Auchus R J, Mendonca B B and Miller W L. The Genetic and Functional Basis of Isolated 17,20-Lyase Deficiency. Nature Genetics 1997;17(2): 201-205.

[53] Lee-Robichaud P, Akhtar M E and Akhtar M. Lysine Mutagenesis Identifies Cationic Charges of Human CYP17 That Interact With Cytochrome b_5 to Promote Male Sex-hormone Biosynthesis. Biochemical Journal 1999;342: 309-312.

[54] Van Den Akker E L, Koper J W, Boehmer A L, Themmen A P, Verhoef-Post M, Timmerman M A, Otten B J, Drop S L and De Jong F H. Differential Inhibition of 17α-Hydroxylase and 17,20-Lyase Activities by Three Novel Missense CYP17 Mutations Identified in Patients With P450c17 Deficiency. Journal of Clinical Endocrinology & Metabolism 2002;87(12): 5714-5721.

[55] Sherbet D P, Tiosano D, Kwist K M, Hochberg Z and Auchus R J. CYP17 Mutation E305G Causes Isolated 17,20-Lyase Deficiency by Selectively Altering Substrate Binding. Journal of Biological Chemistry 2003;278(49): 48563-48569.

[56] Miller W L, Auchus R J and Geller D H. The Regulation of 17,20-Lyase Activity. Steroids 1997;62(1): 133-142.

[57] Laughton C A, Neidle S, Zvelebil M J and Sternberg M J. A Molecular Model for The Enzyme Cytochrome $P450_{17\alpha}$, a Major Target for The Chemotherapy of Prostatic Cancer.Biochemical and Biophysical Research Communications 1990;171(3): 1160-1167.

[58] Lin D, Zhang L H, Chiao E and Miller W L. Modeling and Mutagenesis of the Active Site of Human P450c17. Molecular Endocrinology 1994;8(3): 392-402.

[59] Burke D F, Laughton C A and Neidle S. Homology Modelling of the Enzyme P450 17α-Hydroxylase/17,20-Lyase - A Target For Prostate Cancer Chemotherapy - From the Crystal Structure of P450BM-3. Anticancer Drug Design 1997;12(2): 113-123.

[60] Lewis D F and Lee-Robichaud P. Molecular Modelling of Steroidogenic Cytochromes P450 From Families CYP11, CYP17, CYP19 and CYP21 Based on the CYP102 Crystal Structure. Journal of Steroid Biochemistry and Molecular Biology 1998;66(4): 217-233.

[61] Auchus R J and Miller W L. Molecular Modeling of Human P450c17 (17α-Hydroxylase/17,20-Lyase): Insights into Reaction Mechanisms and Effects of Mutations. Molecular Endocrinology 1999;13(7): 1169-1182.

[62] Schappach A and Holtje H D. Molecular Modelling of 17α-Hydroxylase-17,20-Lyase. Pharmazie 2001;56(6): 435-442.

[63] Yang J, Cui B, Sun S, Shi T, Zheng S, Bi Y, Liu J, Zhao Y, Chen J, Ning G and Li X. Phenotype–genotype correlation in eight Chinese 17α-hydroxylase/17,20 lyase-deficiency patients with five novel mutations of CYP17A1 gene. Journal of Clinical Endocrinology & Metabolism 2006;91(9): 3619–3625.

[64] Mendieta M A E P B, Negri M, Jagusch C, Muller-Vieira U, Lauterbach T and Hartmann R W. Synthesis, biological evaluation, and molecular modeling of abiraterone

analogues: novel CYP17 inhibitors for the treatment of prostate cancer. Journal of Medicinal Chemistry 2008;51(16): 5009–5018.

[65] Swart A C, Storbeck K H and Swart P. A single amino acid residue, Ala 105, confers 16α-hydroxylase activity to human cytochrome P450 17α-hydroxylase/17,20 lyase. Journal of Steroid Biochemistry and Molecular Biology 2010;119(3-5): 112–120.

[66] Wang J F, Zhang C C, Chou K C and Wei D Q. Structure of cytochrome P450s and personalized drug. Current Medicinal Chemistry 2009;16(2): 232–244.

[67] Moncada B and Baranda L. Ketoconazole and gynecomastia. Journal of the American Academy of Dermatology 1982;7(4): 557-558.

[68] Pont A, Williams P L, Azhar S, Reitz R E, Bochra C, Smith E R and Stevens D A. Ketoconazole Blocks Testosterone Synthesis. Archives of Internal Medicine 1982;142(12): 2137-2140.

[69] De Felice R, Johnson D G and Galgiani J N. Gynecomastia With Ketoconazole. Antimicrobial Agents and Chemotherapy 1981;19(6): 1073-1074.

[70] Heeres J, Backx L J, Mostmans J H and Cutsem J V. Antimycotic Imidazoles. Part 4. Synthesis and Antifungal Activity of Ketoconazole, a New Potent Orally Active Broad-spectrum Antifungal Agent. Journal of Medicinal Chemistry 1979;22(8): 1003-1005.

[71] Moffat L E, Kirk D, Tolley D A, Smith M F and Beastall G. Ketoconazole as Primary Treatment of Prostatic Cancer. British Journal of Urology 1988;61(5): 439-440.

[72] Mahler C, Verhelst J and Denis L. Ketoconazole and Liarozole in the Treatment of Advanced Prostatic Cancer. Cancer 1993;71(3 Suppl): 1068-1073.

[73] Lake-Bakaar G, Scheuer P J and Sherlock S. Hepatic Reactions Associated With Ketoconazole in the United Kingdom. British Medical Journal 1987;294: 419-422.

[74] Schappach A and Holtje H D. Investigations on Inhibitors of Human 17α-Hydroxylase-17,20-Lyase and Their Interactions With the Enzyme. Molecular Modelling of 17α-Hydroxylase-17,20-Lyase, Part II. Pharmazie 2001;56(11): 835-842.

[75] Arth G E, Patchett A A, Jefopoulus T, Bugianesi R L, Peterson L H, Ham E A, Kuehl F A and Brink N G. Steroidal Androgen Biosynthesis Inhibitors. Journal of Medicinal Chemistry 1971;14(8): 675-679.

[76] Nakajin S, Takahashi K and Shinoda M. Inhibitory Effect and Interaction of Stanozolol With Pig Testicular Cytochrome P-450 (17α-hydroxylase/$C_{17,20}$-lyase). Chemical & Pharmaceutical Bulletin (Tokyo) 1989;37(7): 1855-1858.

[77] Angelastro M R, Laughlin M E, Schatzman G L, Bey P and Blohm T R. 17β-(Cyclopropylamino)-androst-5-en-3β-ol, A Selective Mechanism-based Inhibitor of Cytochrome $P450_{17}\alpha$ (Steroid 17α-Hydroxylase/$C_{17,20}$-Lyase). Biochemical and Biophysical Research Communications 1989;162(3): 1571-1577.

[78] Angelastro M R and Blohm T R. 4-Substituted 17β-(cyclopropyloxy)androst-5-en-3β-ol and Related Compounds Useful as $C_{17,20}$-Lyase Inhibitors. *US Patent* 4,966,897; 1990.

[79] Angelastro M R, Marquart A L, Weintraub P M, Gates C A, Laughlin M E, Blohm T R and Peet N P. Time-dependent Inactivation of Steroid $C_{17(20)}$-Lyase by 17β-Cyclopropyl Ether-substituted Steroids. Bioorganic & Medicinal Chemistry Letters 1996;6(1): 97-100.

[80] Weintraub P M, Gates C, Angelastro M R and Flynn G A. Process For the Preparation of 4-Amino-Δ^4-3-ketosteroids Via Nitro-Δ^4-3-ketosteroids. *WO Patent* 95/29932; 1995.

[81] Weintraub P M, Gates C A, Angelastro M R, Curran T T and Johnston J O. 4-Amino-17β- (Cyclopropyloxy)androst-4-en-3-one, 4-Amino-17β-(Cyclopropylamino)androst-4-en-3-one and Related Compounds as $C_{17,20}$-Lyase and 5α-Reductase Inhibitors. *US Patent* 5,486,511; 1996.

[82] Wilson S R and Miao E. Anti-testosterone compounds and Method of Use Thereof. *WO Patent* 92/15604; 1992.

[83] Burkhart J P, Gates C A, Laughlin M E, Resvick R J and Peet N P. Inhibition of Steroid $C_{17(20)}$-Lyase With C17-Heteroaryl Steroids. Bioorganic & Medicinal Chemistry 1996;4(9): 1411-1420.

[84] Peet N P, Burkhart J P and Gates C. 16-Unsaturated C17 Heterocyclic Steroids Useful as Steroid $C_{17,20}$-Lyase Inhibitors. *US Patent* 5,677,293; 1997.

[85] Peet N P, Burkhart J P and Gates C. Methods and Compositions using Δ^{16}-Unsaturated C17-Heterocyclic Steroids Useful as $C_{17,20}$-Lyase Inhibitors. *US Patent* 5,977,094; 1999.

[86] Potter G A, Barrie S E, Jarman M and Rowlands M G. Novel Steroidal Inhibitors of Human Cytochrome $P450_{17\alpha}$ (17α-Hydroxylase-$C_{17,20}$-Lyase): Potential Agents For the Treatment of Prostatic Cancer. Journal of Medicinal Chemistry 1995;38(13): 2463-2471.

[87] Haidar S, Ehmer P B and Hartmann R W. Novel Steroidal Pyrimidyl Inhibitors of P450 17 (17α-Hydroxylase/$C_{17,20}$-Lyase). Archiv der Pharmazie (Weinheim) 2001;334(12): 373-374.

[88] Haidar S, Ehmer P B, Barassin S, Batzl-Hartmann C and Hartmann R W. Effects of Novel 17α-Hydroxylase/$C_{17,20}$-Lyase (P450 17, CYP 17) Inhibitors on Androgen Biosynthesis *in vitro* and *in vivo*. Journal of Steroid Biochemistry and Molecular Biology 2003;84(5): 555-562.

[89] Ling Y Z, Li J S, Liu Y, Kato K, Klus G T and Brodie A. 17-Imidazolyl, Pyrazolyl, and Isoxazolyl Androstene Derivatives. Novel Steroidal Inhibitors of Human Cytochrome $C_{17,20}$-Lyase ($P450_{17\alpha}$). Journal of Medicinal Chemistry 1997;40(20): 3297-3304.

[90] Brodie A and Yangzhi L. Androgen Synthesis Inhibitors. *US Patent* 6,133,280; 2000.

[91] Nnane I P, Kato K, Liu Y, Lu Q, Wang X, Ling Y Z and Brodie A. Effects of Some Novel Inhibitors of $C_{17,20}$-Lyase and 5α-Reductase *in vitro* and *in vivo* and Their Potential Role in the Treatment of Prostate Cancer. Cancer Research 1998;58(17): 3826-3832.

[92] Klus G T, Nakamura J, Li J S, Ling Y Z, Son C, Kemppainen J A, Wilson E M and Brodie A M. Growth Inhibition of Human Prostate Cells *in vitro* by Novel Inhibitors of Androgen Synthesis. Cancer Research 1996;56(21): 4956-4964.

[93] Long B J, Grigoryev D N, Nnane I P, Liu Y, Ling Y Z and Brodie A M. Antiandrogenic Effects of Novel Androgen Synthesis Inhibitors on Hormone-dependent Prostate Cancer. Cancer Research 2000;60(23): 6630-6640.

[94] Nnane I P, Long B J, Ling Y Z, Grigoryev D N and Brodie A M. Anti-tumour Effects and Pharmacokinetic Profile of 17-(5'-Isoxazolyl)androsta-4,16-dien-3-one (L-39) in Mice: An Inhibitor of Androgen Synthesis. British Journal of Cancer 2000;83(1): 74-82.

[95] Nnane I P, Njar V C O and Brodie A M H. Pharmacokinetics of Novel Inhibitors of Androgen Synthesis After Intravenous Administration in Mice. Cancer Chemotherapy and Pharmacology 2003;51(6): 519-524.

[96] Wolfling J, Oravecz E A, Ondre D, Mernyak E, Schneider G, Toth I, Szecsi M and Julesz J. Stereoselective Synthesis of Some 17β-Dihydrooxazinyl Steroids, as Novel Presumed Inhibitors of 17α-Hydroxylase-$C_{17,20}$-Lyase. Steroids 2006;71: 809-816.

[97] Ondre D, Wölfling J, Iványi Z, Schneider G, Tóth I, Szécsi M and Julesz J. Neighboring group participation. Part 17 Stereoselective synthesis of some steroidal 2-oxazolidones, as novel potential inhibitors of 17α-hydroxylase-C17,20-lyase. Steroids 2008;73: 1375-1384.

[98] Ondre D, Wölfling J, Tóth I, Szécsi M, Julesz J and Schneider G. Steroselective synthesis of some steroidal oxazolines, as novel potential inhibitors of 17α-hydroxylase-C17,20-lyase. Steroids 2009;74: 1025-1032.

[99] Frank E, Mucsi Z, Szecsi M, Zupko I, Wolfling J and Schneider G. Intramolecular approach to some new D-ring-fused steroidal isoxazolidines by 1,3-dipolar cycloaddition: synthesis, theoretical and *in vitro* pharmacological studies. New Journal of Chemistry 2010;34: 2671-2681.

[100] Iványi Z, Wölfling J, Görbe T, Szécsi M, Wittmann T and Schneider G. Synthesis of regioisomeric 17-*N*-phenylpyrazolyl steroid derivatives and their inhibitory effect on 17α-hydroxylase/C17,20-lyase. Steroids 2010;75: 450-456.

[101] Njar V C, Klus G T and Brodie A M H. Nucleophilic Vinylic "Addition-elimination" Substitution Reaction of 3β-Acetoxy-17-chloro-16-formylandrosta-5,16-diene: A Novel and General Route to 17-Substituted Steroids. Part 1 - Synthesis of Novel 17-Azolyl-Δ^{16}-steroids; Inhibitors of 17α-Hydroxylase/17,20-Lyase (17α-Lyase). Bioorganic & Medicinal Chemistry Letters 1996;6(22): 2777-2782.

[102] Njar V C, Kato K, Nnane I P, Grigoryev D N, Long B J and Brodie A M. Novel 17-Azolyl Steroids, Potent Inhibitors of Human Cytochrome 17α-Hydroxylase-$C_{17,20}$-Lyase (P450$_{17}\alpha$): Potential Agents for the Treatment of Prostate Cancer. Journal of Medicinal Chemistry 1998;41(6): 902-912.

[103] Brodie A and Njar V C. 17-Azolyl Steroids Useful as Androgen Synthesis Inhibitors. *US Patent* 6,200,965 B1; 2001.

[104] Handratta V D, Jelovac D, Long B J, Kataria R, Nnane I P, Njar V C and Brodie A M. Potent CYP17 Inhibitors: Improved Syntheses, Pharmacokinetics and Anti-tumor Activity in the LNCaP Human Prostate Cancer Model. Journal of Steroid Biochemistry and Molecular Biology 2004;92(3): 155-165.

[105] Handratta V D, Vasaitis T S, Njar V C, Gediya L K, Kataria R, Chopra P, Newman D, Farquhar R, Guo Z, Qiu Y and Brodie A M. Novel C17-Heteroaryl Steroidal CYP17 Inhibitors/Antiandrogens: Synthesis, *in vitro* Biological Activity, Pharmacokinetics, and Antitumor Activity in the LAPC4 Human Prostate Cancer Xenograft Model. Journal of Medicinal Chemistry 2005;48(8): 2972-2984.

[106] Brodie A and Njar V C. Novel C-17-Heteroaryl Steroidal CYP17 Inhibitors/Antiandrogens: Synthesis, *in vitro* Biological Activities, Pharmacokinetics and Antitumor Activity. *WO Patent* 2006/093993; 2006.

[107] Barrie S E, Jarman M, Potter G A and Hardcastle I R. 17-Substituted Steroids Useful in Cancer Treatment. *US Patent* 5,604, 213; 1997.

[108] Grigoryev D N, Long B J, Nnane I P, Njar V C, Liu Y and Brodie A M. Effects of New 17α-Hydroxylase/C17,20-Lyase Inhibitors on LNCaP Prostate Cancer Cell Growth *in vitro* and *in vivo*. British Journal of Cancer 1999;81(4): 622-630.

[109] Nnane I P, Njar V C, Liu Y, Lu Q and Brodie A M. Effects of Novel 17-Azolyl Compounds on Androgen Synthesis *in vitro* and *in vivo*. Journal of Steroid Biochemistry and Molecular Biology 1999;71(3-4): 145-152.

[110] Brodie A and Jisong L. 20-Substituted Pregnene Derivatives and Their Use as Androgen Inhibitors. *US Patent* 5,264,427; 1993.

[111] Li J S, Li Y, Son C and Brodie A M. Synthesis and Evaluation of Pregnane Derivatives as Inhibitors of Human Testicular 17α-Hydroxylase/$C_{17,20}$-Lyase. Journal of Medicinal Chemistry 1996;39(21): 4335-4339.

[112] Hartmann R W, Hector M, Haidar S, Ehmer P B, Reichert W and Jose J. Synthesis and Evaluation of Novel Steroidal Oxime Inhibitors of P450 17 (17α-Hydroxylase/$C_{17,20}$-Lyase) and 5α-Reductase Types 1 and 2. Journal of Medicinal Chemistry 2000;43(22): 4266-4277.

[113] Haidar S, Klein C D and Hartmann R W. Synthesis and Evaluation of Steroidal Hydroxamic Acids as Inhibitors of P450 17 (17α-Hydroxylase/$C_{17,20}$-Lyase). Archiv der Pharmazie (Weinheim) 2001;334(4): 138-140.

[114] Li J, Li Y, Son C, Banks P and Brodie A. 4-Pregnene-3-one-20β-carboxaldehyde: A Potent Inhibitor of 17α-Hydroxylase/$C_{17,20}$-Lyase and of 5α-Reductase. Journal of Steroid Biochemistry and Molecular Biology 1992;42(3-4): 313-320.

[115] Njar V C, Hector M and Hartmann R W. 20-Amino and 20,21-Aziridinyl Pregnene Steroids: Development of Potent Inhibitors of 17α-Hydroxylase/$C_{17,20}$-Lyase (P450 17). Bioorganic & Medicinal Chemistry 1996;4(9): 1447-1453.

[116] Hartmann R W, Hector M, Wachall B G, Palusczak A, Palzer M, Huch V and Veith M. Synthesis and Evaluation of 17-Aliphatic Heterocycle-substituted Steroidal Inhibitors of 17α-Hydroxylase/$C_{17,20}$-Lyase (P450 17). Journal of Medicinal Chemistry 2000;43(23): 4437-4445.

[117] Neubauer B L, Best K L, Blohm T R, Gates C, Goode R L, Hirsch K S, Laughlin M E, Petrow V, Smalstig E B, Stamm N B, Toomey R E and Hoover D M. LY207320 (6-Methylene-4-pregnene-3,20-dione) Inhibits Testosterone Biosynthesis, Androgen Uptake, 5α-Reductase, and Produces Prostatic Regression in Male-Rats. Prostate 1993;23(3): 181-199.

[118] Njar V C, Klus G T, Johnson H H and Brodie A M. Synthesis of Novel 21-Trifluoropregnane Steroids: Inhibitors of 17α-Hydroxylase/17,20-Lyase (17α-Lyase). Steroids 1997;62(6): 468-473.

[119] Burkhart J P, Weintraub P M, Gates C A, Resvick R J, Vaz R J, Friedrich D, Angelastro M R, Bey P and Peet N P. Novel Steroidal Vinyl Fluorides as Inhibitors of Steroid $C_{17(20)}$-Lyase. Bioorganic & Medicinal Chemistry 2002;10(4): 929-934.

[120] Peet N P, Weintraub P M, Burkhart J P and Gates C. 20-Fluoro-17(20)-Vinyl steroids as Inhibitors of $C_{17,20}$-Lyase and 5α-Reductase. *WO Patent* 02/00681 A1; 2002.

[121] Peet N P, Weintraub P M, Burkhart J P and Gates C. 20-Fluoro-17(20)-Vinyl Steroids. *US Patent* 6,413,951 B2; 2002.

[122] Weintraub P M, Holland A K, Gates C A, Moore W R, Resvick R J, Bey P and Peet N P. Synthesis of 21,21-Difluoro-3β-hydroxy-20-methylpregna-5,20-diene and 5,16,20-Triene as Potential Inhibitors of Steroid $C_{17(20)}$-Lyase. Bioorganic & Medicinal Chemistry 2003;11(3): 427-431.

[123] Deadman J J, McCague R, and Jarman M. Heptafluoro-*p*-tolyl as a protecting group in a synthesis of 3-hydroxy-17a-aza-17a-homopregn-5-en-20-one. A potential inhibitor of androgen biosynthesis. Journal of the Chemical Society, Perkin Transactions 1 1991;(10): 2413-2416.

[124] Curran T T, Flynn G A, Rudisill D E and Weintraub P M. A Novel Route to a 4-Amino Steroid - MDL 19687. Tetrahedron Letters 1995;36(27): 4761-4764.

[125] Li J, Li Y, Son C and Brodie A M. Inhibition of Androgen Synthesis by 22-Hydroximino-23,24-Bisnor-4-cholen-3-one. Prostate 1995;26(3): 140-150.

[126] Barrie S E, Potter G A, Goddard P M, Haynes B P, Dowset M, Jarman M. Pharmacology of novel steroidal inhibitors of cytochrome $P450_{17\alpha}$ (17α-hydroxylase C17-20 lyase). Journal of Steroid Biochemistry and Molecular Biology 1994;50(5-6): 267-273.

[127] Jarman M, Barrie S E and Llera J M. The 16,17-Double Bond Is Needed for Irreversible Inhibition of Human Cytochrome $P450_{17\alpha}$ by Abiraterone (17-(3-Pyridyl)androsta-5,16-dien-3β-ol) andRelated Steroidal Inhibitors. Journal of Medicinal Chemistry 1998;41(27): 5375-5381.

[128] Molina A and Belldegrun A. Novel Therapeutic Strategies for Castration Resistant Prostate Cancer: Inhibition of Persistent Androgen Production and Androgen Receptor Mediated Signaling. Journal of Urology 2011;185: 787-794.

[129] O'Donnell A, Judson I, Dowset M, Raynaud F, Dearnaley D, Mason M, Harland S, Robbins A, Halbert G, Nutley B and Jarman M. Hormonal impact of the 17α-hydroxylase/$C_{17,20}$-lyase inhibitor abiraterone acetate (CB7630) in patients with prostate cancer. British Journal of Cancer 2004;90: 2317–2325.

[130] Eichholz A, Ferraldeschi R, Attard G and de Bono J S. Putting the brakes on continued androgen receptor signaling in castration-resistant prostate cancer. Molecular and Cellular Endocrinology 2012;360: 68–75.

[131] Attard G, Reid AH, Yap TA, Raynaud F, Dowsett M, Settatree S, Barrett M, Parker C, Martins V, Folkerd E, Clark J, Cooper CS, Kaye SB, Dearnaley D, Lee G and de Bono JS. Phase I clinical trial of a selective inhibitor of CYP17, abiraterone acetate, confirms that castration-resistant prostate cancer commonly remains hormone driven. Journal of Clinical Oncology 2008;26(28): 4563–4571.

[132] Ryan CJ, Smith MR, Fong L, Rosenberg JE, Kantoff P, Raynaud F, Martins V, Lee G, Kheoh T, Kim J, Molina A and Small EJ. Phase I clinical trial of the CYP17 inhibitor abiraterone acetate demonstrating clinical activity in patients with castration-resistant prostate cancer who received prior ketoconazole therapy. Journal of Clinical Oncology 2010;28(9): 1481–1488.

[133] Attard G, Reid AH M, A'Hern R, Parker C, Oommen NB, Folkerd E, Messiou C, Molife LR, Maier G, Thompson E, Olmos D, Sinha R, Lee G, Dowsett M, Kaye SB, Dearnaley D, Kheoh T, Molina A and de Bono JS. Selective inhibition of CYP17 with abiraterone acetate is highly active in the treatment of castration-resistant prostate cancer. Journal of Clinical Oncology 2009;27(23): 3742–3748.

[134] Danila DC, Morris MJ, de Bono JS, Ryan CJ, Denmeade SR, Smith MR, Taplin ME, Bubley GJ, Kheoh T, Haqq C, Molina A, Anand A, Koscuiszka M, Larson SM, Schwartz L H, Fleisher M and Scher HI. Phase II multicenter study of abiraterone acetate plus prednisone therapy in patients with docetaxel-treated castration-resistant prostate cancer. Journal of Clinical Oncology 2010;28(9): 1496–1501.

[135] Reid AH, Attard G, Danila DC, Oommen NB, Olmos D, Fong PC, Molife LR, Hunt J, Messiou C, Parker C, Dearnaley D, Swennenhuis JF, Terstappen LW, Lee G, Kheoh T,

Molina A, Ryan CJ, Small E, Scher H I and de Bono JS. Significant and sustained antitumor activity in post-docetaxel, castration-resistant prostate cancer with the CYP17 inhibitor abiraterone acetate. Journal of Clinical Oncology 2010;28(9): 1489–1495.

[136] de Bono JS, Logothetis CJ, Molina A, Fizazi K, North S, Chu L, Chi KN, Jones RJ, Goodman OB Jr, Saad F, Staffurth JN, Mainwaring P, Harland S, Flaig TW, Hutson TE, Cheng T, Patterson H, Hainsworth JD, Ryan CJ, Sternberg CN, Ellard SL, Fléchon A, Saleh M, Scholz M, Efstathiou E, Zivi A, Bianchini D, Loriot Y, Chieffo N, Kheoh T, Haqq C M and Scher HI. Abiraterone and increased survival in metastatic prostate cancer. The New England Journal of Medicine 2011;364(21): 1995–2005.

[137] ClinicalTrials.gov: US National Institute of Health. www.ClinicalTrials.gov (accessed 27 July 2012).

[138] Vasaitis T, Belosay A, Schayowitz A, Khandelwal A, Chopra P, Gediya LK, Guo Z, Fang HB, Njar VC O and Brodie AM H. Androgen receptor inactivation contributes to antitumor efficacy of 17α-hydroxylase/17,20-lyase inhibitor 3β-hydroxy-17-(1H-benzimidazole-1-yl)androsta-5,16-diene in prostate cancer. Molecular Cancer Therapeutics 2008;7(8):2348–2357.

[139] Schayowitz A, Sabnis G, Njar V C O and Brodie A M H. Synergistic effect of a novel antiandrogen, VN/124-1, and signal transduction inhibitors in prostate cancer progression to hormone independence *in vitro*. Molecular Cancer Therapeutics 2008;7(1): 121–132.

[140] Schayowitz A, Sabnis G, Goloubeva O, Njar V C O and Brodie A M H. Prolonging hormone sensitivity in prostate cancer xenografts through dual inhibition of AR and mTOR. British Journal ofCancer 2010;103(7): 1001–1007.

[141] Soifer HS, Souleimanian N, Wu S, Voskresenskiy AM, Collak F K, Cinar B and Stein CA.Direct Regulation of Androgen Receptor Activity by Potent CYP17 Inhibitors in Prostate Cancer Cells. Journal of Biological Chemistry 2012;287(6): 3777-3787.

[142] Bruno RD, Vasaitis TS, Gediya LK, Purushottamachar P, Godbole AM, Ates-Alagoz Z, Brodie AM H and Njar VC O. Synthesis and biological evaluations of putative metabolically stable analogs of VN/124-1 (TOK-001): Head to head anti-tumor efficacy evaluation of VN/124-1 (TOK-001) and abiraterone in LAPC-4 human prostate cancer xenograft model. Steroids 2011;76(12): 1268–1279.

Chapter 13

Intermittent Androgen Suppression Therapy for Prostate Cancer Patients: An Update

Gerhard Hamilton and Gerhard Theyer

Additional information is available at the end of the chapter

http://dx.doi.org/10.5772/53484

1. Introduction

Prostate cancer is the leading cause of cancer and the second leading cause of cancer-related deaths among men in the Western world [1]. For early stage prostate cancer treatment with surgery and radiation is often curative; however, about 10–20% of men with prostate cancer present with metastatic disease at diagnosis, while 20–30% of patients diagnosed with localized disease will eventually develop metastases [2]. Primary tumor involvement outside the prostatic capsule or relapse following radical prostatectomy results generally in incurability [3,4]. Androgen suppression (AS) is the mainstay of initial therapy in these patients, and orchidectomy or use of LHRH analogs and steroidal or nonsteroidal antiandrogens consistently results in a 90–95% reduction in circulating testosterone levels [5]. However, nearly all patients that respond initially will develop progressive disease, termed castration-resistant prostate cancer (CRPC), after a median duration of 18–24 months. Although CRPC may respond to secondary hormonal manipulations (including antiandrogens, estrogens and ketoconazole) this benefit is usually short-lived.

Although continuous androgen suppression [CAS] therapy has been a cornerstone of the management of prostate cancer for more than 50 years, controversy remains regarding its optimum application. Generally, AS is performed as continuous treatment, resulting in apoptotic regression of the tumor cells in a high percentage of cases. The side-effects of CAS are well described and include anaemia, osteoporosis, impotence, cognitive functional effects, gynaecomastia, muscle atrophy, depression, dyslipidaemia and generalized lethargy [5]. Following failure of the antiandrogenic therapy, chemotherapy is used as secondary treatment. However, responses to cytotoxic therapy are low and only recently several studies revealed a possible benefit of incorporating chemotherapeutic agents in treatment regimen for prostate cancer [6]. In the last years new agents were approved by the U.S. Food and Drug Administration (FDA), comprising an immunotherapeutic product (sipuleucel-T), the novel taxane, cabazitaxel, which showed a survival advantage over mitoxantrone in docetaxel-pretreated patients and an androgen synthesis inhibitor, abiraterone acetate, which was also reported to improve survival when evaluated against placebo in docetaxel-pretreated patients [3,7].

In order to reduce side effects of the CAS and to prolong the duration of the hormone-responsive state of prostate cancers intermittent androgen suppression (IAS) was introduced as new clinical concept [8]. Stopping CAS has the hypothetical advantage of reducing the selection pressure which favors the clones that have initiated molecular adaptations to achieve androgen-independent growth. If there is a population of androgen-dependent clones left then these will proliferate and repopulate the gland, and androgen dependence will resume. Experimental animal models involving androgen-dependent xenografts supported the hypothesis that during limited regrowth in the antiandrogenic treatment cessation periods tumorigenic cells are residing in an androgen-responsive state. The concept of IAS was experimentally developed using the androgen-dependent Shionogi mouse mammary tumor, investigating regular phases of growth, regression and recurrence of xenograft tumors during serial transplantation [9]. For the androgen-dependent Shionogi carcinoma regular cycles of treatment cessations and castration-induced regressions were successfully repeated four times before tumor growth became androgen-independent during the fifth cycle [10]. The average duration of one cycle was 30 days and progression to androgen-insensitivity was observed after 150 days. Serial determinations of the proportion of stem cells in the Shionogi tumor revealed a constant part during the first three cycles, but a 15-fold increase between the third and fourth cycles [11]. Therefore, it was concluded that independent of intermittent or continuous androgen withdrawal, conversion to hormone-insensitivity occurs when the tumor has accumulated one-third to one-half of the total stem cell compartment with androgen-independent cells. The next step included the switch to a human prostate cancer xenograft model using the LNCaP androgen-dependent prostate cancer cell line, where serum PSA levels correlated well with tumor volume and decreased rapidly following castration, followed by appearance of androgen-independency after 3-4 weeks [12]. IAS therapy prolonged time to androgen-independent PSA production threefold, from an average of 26 days in the CAS group to 77 days in the IAS group. It was concluded that IAS in the LNCaP model delayed the onset of androgen-independent PSA gene regulation markedly, most likely due to androgen-induced differentiation and/or downregulation of androgen-suppressed gene expression. In summary, the animal experimental data indicated that androgen-dependent tumor xenografts can be subjected to several cycles of androgen withdrawal/replacement and revealed prolonged hormone-dependency compared to CAS.

Since induction of androgen independence may occur early after treatment initiation, cessation of antiandrogen therapy prior to this switch is expected to maintain the apoptotic potential of the tumor cells and keep them sensitive to retreatment. Serial serum PSA determinations are used to decide on AS, treatment cessation and reinitiation of therapy [13]. Generally, IAS consists of an initial androgen suppression period of up to nine months combining LHRH antagonists and antiandrogens, which is followed by treatment cessation until a certain PSA threshold is reached, then AS is reinitiated for the same time period as the initial suppression phase (Figure 1) In initial pilot trials regrowing tumors of patients undergoing IAS were consistently reported to be sensitive to several cycles of androgen withdrawal [14,15]

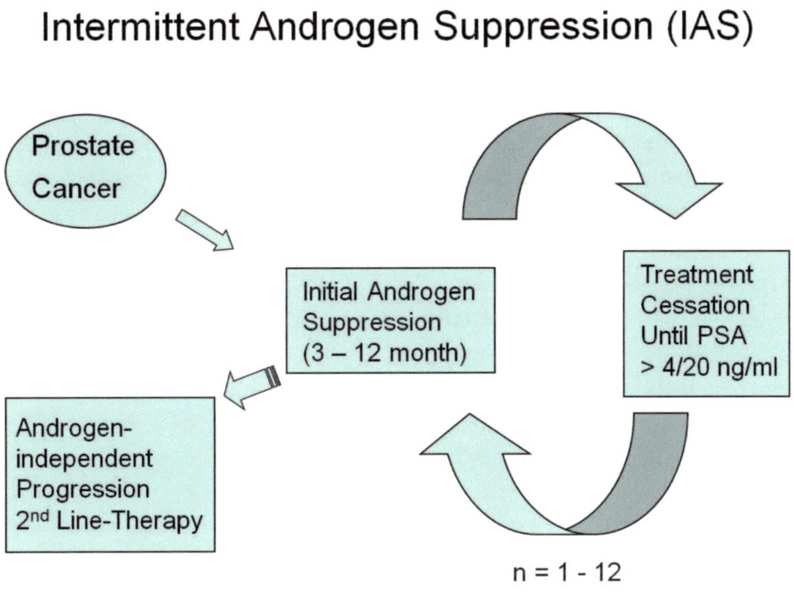

Figure 1. Schematic presentation of IAS. Patients undergo an initial phase of AS. If successful, AS is paused until progression to 4 (localized disease) or 10-20 (metastatic disease) ng/ml PSA. Then AS is resumed and cycles repeated until progression to androgen-independent disease that is treated with diverse regimens second-line.

Therefore, the primary goal of IAS was the prolongation of the hormone-sensitivity of the tumors, which in turn was expected to result in increased survival eventually. Furthermore, IAS was expected to reduce the side effects of CAS, comprising reduced sexual activity, cardiovascular problems, metabolic consequences and osteoporosis among others. Based on the available evidence, IAS nowadays represents a valid treatment option for patients with non-metastatic prostate cancer, including those with locally advanced disease, either with or without lymph node involvement, and those who biochemically relapsed following apparently curative treatment. IAS has been researched since the mid-1980s in a number of clinical phase II and III trials in an effort to prolong hormone-dependency and reduce adverse effects and costs of CAS [16]. With preclinical evidence suggesting a potential benefit for IAS in terms of time to androgen independence, with phase II and phase III studies producing optimistic results, and with the potential for decreased costs and complications IAS has now become a popular modality of therapy worldwide. Quite recently, according to results of a Phase III trial presented in a plenary session at the 2012 ASCO Annual Meeting, IAS was shown to be less effective than CAS for a subgroup of patients with hormone-sensitive metastatic prostate cancer, questioning the use of IAS as standard therapy for these patients [17].

2. Clinical evaluation of intermittent androgen suppression

2.1. Introduction

Maximal androgen ablation through combination therapy increases treatment-related side effects and expenses and fails to prolong time to progression to androgen-independence and, furthermore, preliminary evidence indicates that a low androgen milieu is associated with tumor aggressiveness. Transition to androgen-independence is a complex process and involves both selection and outgrowth of preexisting androgen-resistant clones, as well as adaptative upregulation of genes that enable cancer cells to survive and grow after CAS [18]. CAS in men with prostate cancer increases the risk of osteoporotic fractures, type 2 diabetes and, possibly, cardiovascular events [19]. The benefits of CAS in treating non-metastatic prostate cancer need to be carefully weighed against the risks of CAS-induced adverse events. Management of the metabolic sequelae of CAS includes optimal reduction of cardiovascular risk factors, with particular attention to weight, blood pressure, lipid profile, smoking cessation and glycemic control. Supported by preclinical and first clinical IAS results, several centers tested the feasibility of IAS in non-randomized groups of prostate cancer patients with serum PSA as trigger point followed by a number of extended phase II and III trials [16,20]

2.2. Clinical phase II studies of IAS

2.2.1. Comparison of therapeutic efficacies of IAS and CAS

Following apparently successful pilot studies, a number of phase II IAS trials were conducted (Table 1) [16]. Since the end points of most phase II studies were safety and feasibility of IAS, survival data were not reported in general. Out of the 19 studies reviewed by Abrahamsson only five involved more than 100 patients (102, 103, 146, 250 and 566 patients, respectively) and the other smaller studies employed a mean number of 52 patients [16]. Although patients with advanced, metastatic prostate cancer were included in several studies, most patients treated in phase II IAS trials had localized disease or biochemical progression following prostatectomy/radiation therapy. The number of IAS cycles given ranged from 1 to 12, with an average of 2–3 per patient, and the length of time off therapy generally decreased or remained stable with each succeeding cycle. Most of the studies reported off-treatment periods of approximately 50% of the duration of the IAS cycles, dependent on the tumor stage of the respective prostate cancer patients [16]. A metaanalysis by Shaw et al. involving ten phase II trials reported a median number of two cycles per patient and a median time off-therapy of 15.4 months [21]. Time on treatment also varied but was usually in the region of 6–9 months [16]. The proportion of men in whom serum testosterone normalized was generally high following the first cycle (70–90%) but tended to decrease during subsequent cycles [16]. Factors influencing time to delay in testosterone normalization may include advanced age, low baseline testosterone levels, and duration of AS. Testosterone recovery to baseline values was achieved in 79% during the first and in 65% during the second IAS cycle, respectively [22]. No significant difference was observed up to 1000 days between IAS and CAS with regard to time to androgen-independent tumor progression.

Authors	#	Endpoint(s)	Tumor stage	Androgen suppression
Calais da Silva et al. [13]	626	Time to subjective or objective progression	Locally advanced or metastatic	GnRH agonist + cyproterone acetate
De Leval et al. [36]	68	Time to androgen-independence	Locally advanced, metastatic or recurrent	Goserelin + flutamide
Miller et al. [37]	335	Time to clinical or biochemical progression	Locally advanced or D1/D2	Goserelin + bicalutamide
Mottet et al. [38]	173	Overall survival	Metastatic PCa (D2)	Leuprorelin + flutamide
TULP [39,40]	290	Time to clinical progression or PSA escape	Advanced or locally advanced	Buserelin depot + nilutamide
Tunn et al [22]	184	Clinical or PSA progression	PSA relapse after radical prostatectomy	Leuprorelin + cyproterone acetate
Verhagen et al. [35]	366	QoL	Metastatic	Cyproterone acetate
Klotz et al.[34]	1386	Survival	PSA recurrence after radical Radiotherapy	All types of AS
Salonen et al. [41,42]	554	Progression/Survival	Advanced or locally advanced	Goserelin + cyproterone acetate
Hussain et al. [17]	1345	Survival	Advanced (D2)	Goserelin + bicalutamide

Table 1. Overview of the published phase II IAS trials

In a study by Bruchovsky et al. men who quickly recovered serum testosterone levels experienced a more rapid rise in PSA levels and a shorter time off therapy [23]. Generally, low levels (2–16%) of progression to hormone-refractory prostate cancer have been reported [16,22]. In a review by Zhu et al. there were 16 trials that compared IAS with CAS with a total of 3264 patients (1624 with IAS and 1640 with CAS) [24]. Pooled effects indicated no significant difference between IAS and CAS groups in terms of death and progression rate (hazard ratio HR=0.99, 95% CI 0.80-1.23, and HR=1.03, 95% CI 0.84-1.26 respectively). Calculated results indicated that quality of live (QoL) on sexual activity was significantly higher in the IAS group (HR=0.24, 95% Cl 0.17-0.33, $p<0.00001$). Moreover, IAS could effectively reduce side effects associated with AS. Thus, the therapeutic efficacy was not significantly different between the IAS and CAS groups. However, IAS could effectively preserve the QoL (in particular sexual life) and reduce the side effects.

2.2.2. Comparison of the side effects/QoL of IAS and CAS

Because it became increasingly clear that the time to androgen-independence seems not to be prolonged by IAS, trials focussed on the impact of the intermittent therapy on side effects of AS and QoL. Malone et al estimated that approximately 50% of patients recovered from anaemia during off-therapy periods and that the weight gain normally associated with CAS was prevented [25]. Bouchot et al reported hot flushes in most cases during the on-therapy period, which showed significant improvement during treatment cessation periods and pain significantly improved during on-therapy periods with no new pain occurring once therapy was withdrawn [26]. Goldenberg et al. observed that all patients tolerated therapy well and responded in a positive physical and psychological manner to the cycling approach [27]. The attenuation of spine and hip bone mineral density (BMD) decline after 3-year IAS compared with those reported for CAS appears to be due to testosterone-driven BMD recovery in the cessation period [28]. Failure of testosterone recovery was associated with worse final BMD. Patients experienced the greatest average change in BMD during early treatment periods of IAS with a smaller average change thereafter and fractures were rare [29]. During the first off-treatment period (median duration 37.4 weeks), BMD recovery at the spine was significant; however, subsequent periods had heterogeneous changes of BMD without significant average changes. By reducing the potential risk for adverse bone complications, intermittent therapy may become an important consideration when the therapeutic ratio is narrow [30]. We examined the effect of IAS on bone metabolism by determinations of CrossLaps levels, a biochemical marker of collagen degradation, in blood samples of prostate cancer patients. Measurements of the CrossLaps concentration in patients under IAS revealed that treatment cessation phases rapidly reversed increased bone degradation, which was associated with the AS phases, in good agreement with the clinical observations of reduced loss of BMD in IAS [31]. Since pretreatment concentrations of CrossLaps were restored within several months of treatment cessation and mean duration of the off-treatment periods ranged from 8–16 months in our patients, this protective effect of IAS is expected to be effective for several treatment cycles. Additionally, procollagen I N-terminal peptide (PINP), a parameter of bone synthesis was increased during off-treatment phases in IAS [32].

Improvement of sexual activity was highlighted in several studies and concerned approximately half of the patients [16]. Sato et al reported significant worsening of potency and physical well-being during AS and significant improvements in potency, lack of energy, social/family well-being, and ability to enjoy life during off-therapy periods [33]. In a study by Spry et al. QoL scores also deteriorated during androgen suppression, but had generally achieved baseline levels by the end of the off-treatment period [28]. In summary, IAS showed benefits in the treatment of prostate cancer with respect to QoL in the majority of trials.

2.2.3. IAS phase II studies – conclusion

In phase II studies there has been considerable variation in the particular approaches in regard to medication, duration of AS phases, target PSA nadir and selection of the PSA value for restarting therapy. At that time preliminary results of the the ongoing randomized controlled trials have generated evidence that the use of IAS in patients with advanced or locally advanced disease was at least as safe as CAS [16,24]. In conclusion, phase II studies of IAS demonstrated that several cycles of IAS were feasible, the duration of response was not worse than historical controls of CAS and well-being was better during treatment cessation periods. Patients with localized disease fared superior under IAS compared to patient with extended disease. The need for randomized phase III trials was stressed in order to get firm data on progression-free and overall survival (OS) as well as time to androgen insensitivity for IAS and CAS, respectively.

2.3. Clinical phase III studies of IAS

Nowadays a number of phase III trials have been completed comparing IAS with CAS [16]. Of the ten reported trials, two included patients with relapse after radical prostatectomy or radiation therapy, all others studied locally advanced and metastatic disease [22,34]. The number of patients in these trials varied from 68 to 1386, but only four involved >500 patients; the average age of patients was around 70 years. Full details of trial design are not available for all studies, several reports are available only in abstract form [16]. The treatment regimen in all but one of the trials consisted of a LHRH agonist and an antiandrogen. The exception was Verhagen et al., in which antiandrogen monotherapy (cyproterone acetate/CPA) was the sole regimen studied [35]. Although there was generally consistency in the PSA levels designated for AS discontinuation (0.1/4 ng/ml or 20% of the initial PSA value), the criteria for resuming treatment were less uniform, with 4 ng/ml for biochemical relapses and 10 or 20 ng/ml 20 ng/ml for locally advanced or metastatic disease, respectively. The low PSA nadir and reinitiation values used by Tunn et al. and Klotz et al. are due to the fact that the study involved patients who had relapsed after radical prostatectomy [22,34]. End points in these studies also varied to some degree: whereas the majority had time to progression as the primary end point, three assigned survival and one focussed on QoL outcomes [35]. Average follow-up times in these studies have all been >2 yr, with a maximum of 12 years cited by Calais da Silva et al. [13].

2.3.1. South European uroncological trial [13]

Patients with locally advanced or metastatic with histologically confirmed prostate adenocarcinoma, cT3–cT4 M0, cT3–cT4 M1, PSA >4 ng/ml, were recruited for this study and end point was time to subjective or objective progression. All registered patients had an initial 3-months induction treatment with CPA (200 mg daily for two weeks) followed by monthly depot injections of a LHRH analog plus 200 mg of CPA daily. Patients (n = 626) whose PSA level decreased to <4 ng/ml or by at least 80% of the initial level by the end of the induction were randomized. Time to any progression was slightly longer in the continuous arm, with an HR of progression of 0.81. Both metastatic status and PSA level were independent predictors of progression, with M1 and PSA level > 4 ng/ml associated with a greater hazard of progressing. In the intermittent and continuous arm there was no significant difference in OS (p = 0.84) and the HR was 0.99 for CAS compared with IAS. The greater number of cancer deaths in the IAS treatment group was balanced by a greater number of cardiovascular deaths under CAS. Both PSA level and metastatic status at randomization were independently associated with survival. A significant interaction of metastatic status with treatment was almost reached (p = 0.07). Among M0 patients, the HR for continuous therapy compared with intermittent therapy was 0.86 (95% CI: 0.65–1.14), favouring continuous; among M1 patients, the HR was 1.26 (95% CI: 0.90–1.78), favouring intermittent. It was concluded that IAS should be considered for use in routine practice because it is associated with no reduction in survival, no clinically meaningful impairment in QoL, better sexual activity, and considerable economic benefit to the individual and the community. Since this study used only three months of therapy before stopping treatment in the intermittent arm, without impairing survival, there are significant savings for a patient receiving IAS for one year relative to CAS.

2.3.2. *Study by De Leval et al. [36]*

In this trial, a total of 68 evaluable patients with hormone-naive advanced or relapsing prostate cancer were randomized to receive AS (goserelin and flutamide) according to a continuous (n = 33) or intermittent (n = 35) regimen. The outcome variable was time to androgen-independence and mean follow-up was 30.8 months. The estimated 3-year progression rate was significantly lower in the IAS group (7.0%) than in the CAS group (38.9%). It was concluded that IAS treatment may maintain the androgen-dependent state of advanced human prostate cancer, as assessed by PSA measurements, at least as long as CAS treatment. This study may be regarded as underpowered to assess the full impact of IAS and the authors recommended further studies with longer follow-up times and larger patient cohorts to determine the comparative impacts of CAS and IAS with certainty.

2.3.3. *Study by Miller et al. [37]*

This randomized study compared AS with goserelin + bicalutamide in CAS with IAS. The primary endpoint was time to clinical and/or biochemical progression of the disease and secondary endpoints were survival time, QoL and side effects. Patients had histologically confirmed adenocarcinoma of the prostate in clinical stage T1-4N1-3M0 or T1-4N0-3M1 (D1 or D2). After an induction phase of six months with AS, 335 patients whose PSA decreased under 4 ng/ml or 90% from baseline were randomized. About two-thirds of the patients of both the intermittent and the continuous therapy arm (65% versus 66%, ITT population) experienced a clinical and/or biochemical disease progression. The median time to progression was longer for patients randomised to IAS (16.6 months) compared with patients randomized to CAS (11.5 months; difference not significant). The median time to death from any cause was 51.4 months in the intermittent arm compared and 53.8 months in the continuous therapy arm ($p = 0.658$). There were no differences in the incidence of patients with any safety parameter. Patients' self-assessment of their overall health and of their sexual activity appeared to be favourable in the IAS therapy arm. It was concluded that IAS in D1 and D2 prostate cancer patients seems to be safe and superior in respect to QoL.

2.3.4. *TAP22 investigators group trial [38]*

This study aimed at comparing CAS to IAS with AS consisting of leuproreline and flutamide in patients with newly diagnosed metastatic prostate cancer with bone metastases (stage D2). All patients had a positive bone or CT scan and a PSA > 20 ng/ml. After a 6 months induction period with AS, they were randomized into two groups if the PSA was < 4 ng/ml. CAS was continued after randomization and in the IAS group treatment was discontinued until PSA > 10 ng/ml or clinical progression. AS was then resumed for

3 months periods until the PSA became < 4 ng/ml and then treatment was then stopped again until the next progression for a new cycle. 341 patients were selected and received a 6 months induction AS period, and 173 were randomized: 83 to CAS and 86 to IAS. Patients were off-treatment approximately 50% of the first cycle, without decline in succeeding cycles and most had testosterone recovery. A progression occurred in 127 patients (73.4%). The overall QoL did not differ significantly between both arms. Median OS was 52 months for CAS and 42.2 months for IAS (p=0.74) and the median progression-free survial was 15 months for CAS and 20.7 months for IAS (p=0.73). This randomized trial comparing CAS to IAS in metastatic prostate cancer patients suggests that IAS may be as safe as CAS in D2 prostate cancer patients.

2.3.5. Therapy Upgrading Life in Prostate cancer (TULP) study [39,40]

Eligible patients (n = 290) had histologically proven advanced prostate cancer with positive lymph nodes or distant metastases (T2-4N1-3M0 or T2-4NxM1). They received AS with buserelin and nilutamide for 6 months. Patients who had a normalisation of PSA (< 4 ng/ml) after the course, were randomized between IAS (n=97) or CAS (n=96). Median time to clinical progression or PSA escape was 18.0 months in the IAS arm and 24.1 months in the CAS arm. In particular, the 2-year risk of progression for baseline PSA < 50 ng/ml, 50 to <500 ng/ml, and ≥500 ng/ml was 25%, 55%, and 76% (P = 0.03) in CAS, and 38%, 64%, and 85% (p = 0.006) in IAS, respectively. There was no clinically significant difference in QoL scores between patients. Metastatic prostate cancer patients with high baseline PSA, pain, and high PSA nadir, after a 6-months induction course, have a poor prognosis with hormonal therapy. Overall, in this study patients on IAS seem to do worse than CAS patients. Also, patients receiving IAS with low PSA nadir had significantly higher progression rates than CAS patients. In IAS testosterone recovery during the off-treatment phase was incomplete, explaining the missing benefit for QoL, even though more side effects occurred during CAS. Therefore, it was concluded from this study that IAS constitutes not a good treatment option for most metastatic prostate cancer patients.

2.3.6. European trial EC507 [22]

In this multicentre European prospective randomized phase III trial EC507, testosterone serum concentrations under AS were analyzed in prostate cancer patients with PSA progression after radical prostatectomy. Patients were randomized to either CAS or IAS therapy using a 3-months depot with leuprorelin acetate as microcapsule formulation. In 109 patients testosterone recovery to baseline values was achieved in 79% during the first and in 65% during the second IAS cycle, respectively. Median time to testosterone normalization was 100 days in the first and 115 days in the second cycle, respectively. There also appeared to be a QoL benefit during off-treatment intervals owing to the recovery of serum testosterone levels. No significant difference was observed up to 1000 days between IAS and CAS with regard to time to androgen-independent progression. This was the first prospective study of leuprolide, demonstrating normalization of testosterone levels in the off-treatment period in patients undergoing IAS.

2.3.7. *Study by Verhagen et al. [35]*

This randomized trial compared efficacy and QoL of IAS and CAS treatment by CPA of asymptomatic patients with prostate cancer metastatic to the bone. A total of 366 patients with metastatic prostate cancer received 3 to 6 months CPA (100 mg daily) depending on their PSA response. Patients with a good or moderate response were randomized to continuous or intermittent treatment. Intermittent hormonal therapy of metastatic prostate cancer by CPA has advantages in important QoL domains. However, cognitive function scores appeared reduced in the intermittent group.

2.3.8. *NCIC CTG PR.7/SWOG PR.7/CTSU JPR.7/UK trial [34]*

This Intergroup randomized phase III trial compared IAS vs. CAS to test for non-inferiority of IAS with respect to OS. Patients had rising PSA > 3.0 ng/ml >1 year post radical radiotherapy (RRT), either initial or salvage, for localized prostate cancer. Stratification factors were time since RRT (>1-3 vs >3 years), initial PSA (<15 vs >15), prior radical prostatectomy and prior AS. IAS was delivered for 8 months in each cycle with restart when PSA reached >10 ng/ml off-treatment. Primary endpoint was OS, secondary endpoints included time to hormone refractory state, QoL, duration of treatment/non-treatment intervals, time to testosterone and potency recovery. The trial was halted after a planned interim analysis demonstrated that a prespecified stopping boundary for non-inferiority was crossed. 1,386 patients were randomized to IAS (690) or CAS (696) arms. IAS patients completed a median of 2 x 8 months cycles (range: 1-9) and median follow-up was 6.9 years. 524 deaths were observed (268 on IAS vs. 256 on CAS). Median OS was 8.8 vs. 9.1 years on IAS and CAS arms, respectively (HR 1.02, 95%CI 0.86-1.21; p for non-inferiority [HR IAS vs CAS ≥ 1.25] = 0.009). The IAS arm had more disease related (122 vs. 97) and fewer unrelated (134 vs. 146) deaths. Time to androgen insensitivity was statistically significantly improved on the IAS arm (HR 0.80, 95%CI 0.67-0.98; p = 0.024). IAS patients had reduced hot flashes, but otherwise there was no evidence of differences in adverse events, including myocardial events or osteoporotic fractures. Thus, in men with PSA recurrence after RRT IAS was non-inferior to CAS with respect to OS.

2.3.9. *SWOG 9346 intergroup trial [17]*

The largest trial comparing IAS and CAS in metastatic patients was reported by Hussain et al. [17]. Between 1995 and 2008, the study enrolled 3040 men with newly diagnosed metastatic disease and PSA levels ≥ 5 ng/mL. The study population was preselected for hormone sensitivity and when PSA level fell to ≤ 4 ng/mL, patients were randomized to either IAS (n = 770) stopping treatment at that point until a rise in PSA level was observed (an increase to 20 ng/mL, or for those with baseline value < 20 ng/mL, when PSA returned to baseline) or CAS (n = 765). Hormone therapy consisted of goserelin and bicalutamide for 7 months, which was in use in 1995 when the study was launched. At randomization, patients were stratified according to performance status, extent of disease, and prior exposure to hormone therapy.

At a median follow-up of 9.2 years, median overall survival was 5.1 years with IAS and 5.8 years with CAS, an absolute difference of slightly more than 6 months favoring CAS in the entire study population. The study design specified that survival with IAS would be non-inferior to CAS if the upper 95% confidence bound for the HR did not reach or include 1.2. This specification would rule out with high confidence the possibility of a 20% or greater increase in the relative risk of death with IAS. The difference between the two treatments resulted in a HR of 1.09 in favor of CAS, but the upper boundary of the 95% confidence interval was 1.24, so the conclusion was that the two treatments could not be called equivalent and survival with IAS therapy was regarded inferior to IAS by these authors. For this study, survival in both arms was much better than the expected 3-year median OS. In all examined subgroups, CAS was slightly better than IAS, with exception of extensive disease, where IAS achieved comparable survival (5 years on IAS vs 4.4 years on CAS). In this subgroup analysis, patients with minimal disease had a median overall survival of 5.2 years in the IAS group vs. 7.1 years with CAS, suggesting that the loss of almost two years of life in the intermittent group could not be ruled out. In this study "minimal disease" was defined as disease that had not spread beyond the lymph nodes or the bones of the spine or pelvis and "extensive disease" as disease that had spread beyond the spine pelvis, and lymph nodes or to the lungs or liver.

Trial participants also compared QoL measures across the two study arms during the first 15 months following patient randomization, including measures of sexual function (impotence and libido), physical and emotional function, and energy level. They found improved sexual function in men who received IAS as compared to those on continuous therapy.

2.3.10. FinnProstate study VII [41,42]

The FinnProstate study VII enrolled 852 men with locally advanced or metastatic prostate cancer to receive AS for 24 weeks [41]. Study inclusion criteria were M1 disease at any PSA, M0 disease at PSA 60 ng/ml or greater, or T3-4 M0 prostate cancer at PSA 20 ng/ml or greater, or previously surgically or radiotherapy treated localized prostate cancer and PSA recurrence of 20 ng/ml or greater. Patients in whom PSA decreased to less than 10 ng/ml, or by 50% or more if less than 20 ng/ml at baseline, were randomized to IAS or CAS. In the intermittent therapy arm AS was withdrawn and resumed again for at least 24 weeks based mainly on PSA decrease and increase. Of the 852 men, 554 patients were randomized and observed for a median follow-up of 65.0 months. Of these patients 71% died, including 68% in the intermittent and 74% in the continuous arm ($p = 0.12$). There were 248 prostate cancer deaths, comprised of 43% under IAS and 47% under CAS ($p = 0.29$). Median times to progression were 34.5 and 30.2 months in the intermittent and continuous arms, respectively. Median times to death (all cause) were 45.2 and 45.7 months, to prostate cancer death 45.2 and 44.3 months, and to treatment failure 29.9 and 30.5 months, respectively. Therefore, according to this trial, IAS is a feasible, efficient and safe method to treat advanced prostate cancer compared with CAS. However, the prevalence of adverse events was not significantly lower with IAS [42].

2.3.11. Phase III studies - Summary

In general, the phase III trials comparing IAS with CAS involved a varying number of patients, prostate cancer tumor stages ranging from biochemical relapse to metastatic and recurring disease and widely differing durations of initial AS as well as differing PSA values for the start of treatment cessations and reinitiations. Therefore, conclusions to be drawn are restricted to specific tumor stages and treatment schemes.

2.3.11.1. IAS – phase III – impact on survival

The Miller randomized trial of IAS versus continuous CAS in 335 patients with advanced (lymph node-positive or metastatic) prostate cancer demonstrated equivalent survival [37]. Patients in the intermittent arm were off-treatment >40% of the time. It is important to note that testosterone recovery after discontinuation of the LHRH agonist is often delayed and may depend on treatment duration, age, baseline testosterone, and ethnicity [22,43]. In the TULP trial of IAS versus CAS for advanced prostate cancer, 193 patients were randomized and, after a mean follow-up of 34 months, no difference in survival was observed [40]. The larger de Silva trial randomized 312 men to CAS and 314 men to IAS [13]. With a median follow-up of 51 months from randomization, there were fewer cancer deaths (84 vs. 106), more cardiovascular deaths (52 vs 41), and an equivalent number of total deaths (169 vs. 170) in the continuous versus intermittent arms respectively. Median time off AS was 52 weeks for patients in the intermittent arm [13]. It should be noted that the randomization criteria for all of these trials are a PSA decline of 80–90%, or to <4ng/ml, on initial AS.

In the study by Miller et al. about two thirds of patients receiving either IAS or CAS experienced clinical and/or biochemical progression, with no significant differences between groups with respect to median time to tumour progression or median time to death [37]. Similarly, Mottet et al. reported no significant difference between patients receiving IAS and CAS with respect to median overall survival (OS; 1265 vs 1560 days) and median progression-free survival (PFS) (620 vs 452 days) [38]. Tunn et al. also reported equivalency between IAS and CAS with respect to PFS (91.7 vs 93.6%) and median time to progression (1.86 vs 2.36 yr), although estimated mean PFS was longer in the IAS group compared with the CAS group (1234 vs 1010 days) [22]. In the TULP study, median time to progression was longer in the CAS arm (24.1 vs 18 months; significance not stated); more recent data from this study show no difference in OS between groups (mean follow-up of 66 months) [39,40]. The Intergroup randomized phase III trial demonstrated non-inferiority of IAS with respect to OS and time to hormone refractory state for patients with biochemical relapses after radical radiotherapy [34]. Similarly, the FinnProstate Study VII, found no significant differences in time to progression and OS, concluding that IAS is an efficient method to treat advanced prostate cancer compared with CAS [41].

However, differences in OS between CAS and IAS have been reported in two studies. De Leval et al. reported that the estimated risk of 3-year progression in CAS patients was significantly higher than in the IAS group (38.9% vs. 7%; $p = 0.0052$) [36]. In patients with a Gleason score >6, 3-year progression rates were significantly higher in CAS than in IAS patients ($p = 0.018$) but not in patients with lower Gleason scores. Compared with CAS, the IAS group had better results with respect to the number of deaths from hormone-refractory disease (4 vs. 2), number of patients with disease progression (10 vs. 3), and mean time to progression (21 vs. 28 months) (level of significance not stated for any outcome). In patients without bone metastases at initiation, risk of progression was significantly higher in CAS than IAS patients ($p < 0.001$). The largest trial comparing IAS to CAS is the SWOG 9346 intergroup trial, which included metastatic prostate cancer patients [17]. At a median follow-up of 9.2 years, the median overall survival was six months longer with CAS in the entire study population. This was caused by a comparable survival in extensive disease and an inferior survival in response to IAS in patients with minimal metastatic disease. The results of these two studies point to an inferior clinical results of IAS in metastatic prostate cancer.

2.3.11.2. IAS – phase III – impact on QoL

Early results from the study by Calais da Silva et al. showed no clinically meaningful differences between groups in virtually all QoL parameters and no evidence that IAS carries a significantly higher risk of death [13]. Mottet et al. also reported no significant difference in QoL outcomes in patients receiving either IAS or CAS [38]. However, updated results from a larger cohort of the Calais da Silva study (maximum follow-up of 7 years; median: 2 years) suggest a better tolerability profile for IAS versus CAS, with up to three times as many patients in the CAS arm reporting side effects compared with IAS patients (hot flushes: 23% vs. 7%; gynaecomastia: 33% vs. 10%; headaches: 12% vs. 5%; all $p < 0.0001$) [44]. Levels of sexual activity also increased in the IAS group compared with the CAS group, reported in 28 vs. 10% of patients after 15 months. Similarly, Miller et al. reported that patients' self-assessment of their overall health and sexual activity appeared to favour IAS; however, no differences in incidence of adverse events or other safety parameters were noted in this study [37]. Further evidence of QoL advantages comes from Verhagen et al. who note that EORTC scores on physical and emotional function were significantly better in the IAS group than in the CAS group. Role and social function were equivalent between groups, although cognitive function was surprisingly reduced in the IAS group, but not in the CAS group [35]. AS-related side effects were reported in most patients by de Leval et al., most of which resolved in the IA group on discontinuation of therapy [36]. In the TULP study, 26 preliminary withdrawals were reported due to adverse events, 20 in the CAS group and 6 in the IAS group [39,40]. The FinnProstate Study VII reported no significant difference in the prevalence of adverse with IAS [42]. Improved sexual function in men who received IAS as compared to CAS was confirmed in the SWOG 9346 intergroup trial [17].

2.3.11.3. IAS – phase III trials – Conclusion

Following pilot and phase II clinical trials comparing IAS to CAS, results of phase III studies were awaited eagerly to get a definite judgement of these different regimens of AS. The clinical results, time to progression and OS, seem to be comparable between IAS and CAS for prostate cancer patients with biochemical relapses and localized disease. With the exception of two studies, namely trials performed by the South European Uroncological Group and the SWOG 9346 intergroup, IAS was not inferior to CAS in respect to progression of disease and OS in metastatic prostate cancer. In the two dissenting studies, patients with limited metastatic disease seem to have an impaired OS under IAS. However, the statement that IAS is possibly inferior to CAS and not standard therapy of all prostate cancer patients is an oversimplification [17]. Improvements in QoL parameters were confirmed by most studies, depending on testosterone recovery and extent of disease.

NCI Trial #	Treatment	End point/Study subject	Start	Status
NCT00283803	Exisulind	Duration of off-treatment period	2006	Unknown
NCT00686036	Zactima (18 mo)	Duration of off-treatment period	2008	Terminated
NCT00553878	Dutasteride	Duration of off-treatment period	2007	Ongoing
NCT00668642	Dutasteride	Androgen-Response Gene Expression	2008	Recruiting
NCT00801242	Degarelix (1 mo)	Duration of off-treatment period	2008	Ongoing
NCT00928434	Degarelix IAS	Duration of off-treatment period /QoL	2009	Ongoing
NCT01512472	Degarelix (4 vs 10 mo)	Duration of off-treatment period	2011	Recruiting
NCT00002651	IAS vs. CAS	Survival/QoL Prostate cancer D2	1999	Recruiting
NCT00223665	IAS	Progression/QoL Localized Prostate Cancer	2005	Recruiting
NCT00378690	ELIGARD	Survival/QoL Metastatic Prostate Cancer	2006	Ongoing

Table 2. Overview of the IAS trials currently under investigation

2.4. IAS trials currently under investigation

Table 2. lists the trials comprising IAS treatment of prostate cancer patients registered in the United States National Institute of Health (NIH) clinical studies site. With exception of a few further trials comparing IAS to CAS in metastatic cancer patients, several drugs are investigated for their potential to prolong the off-treatment phase of IAS. Exisulind (Aptosyn or sulindac sulfone) may be useful as a treatment for men with advanced prostate cancer, achieving disease stabilization. This drug increases the rate of programmed cell death in cancer cells without damaging normal tissue by interfering with cyclic GMP phosphodiesterase in abnormally growing precancerous and cancerous cells [45]. Zactima (vandetanib) is an oral inhibitor of vascular endothelial growth factor receptor 2 (VEGFR-2), epidermal growth factor receptor (EGFR) and Ret tyrosine kinases involved in tumor growth, progression and angiogenesis [46]. Although, as single agent, no significant antitumor activity has been observed for Zactima in small cell lung cancer, advanced ovarian, colorectal, breast, prostate cancer and multiple myeloma. Further drugs target the androgen-stimulated growth by exploiting distinct mechanism or new formulations. Dutasteride is a non-selective inhibitor of steroid 5α-reductase, an enzyme responsible for conversion of testosterone to a more potent androgen dihydrotestosterone (DHT) approved for clinical use in treatment of benign prostate hyperplasia (BPH) and currently tested in clinical trials for prevention and treatment of prostate cancer [47]. Degarelix is a GnRH antagonist, that was found to be at least as effective as leuprolide in the ability to suppress serum testosterone to < or =0.5 ng/mL for up to 1 year in prostate cancer patients in different doses and in depot form [48]. Finally, Eligard constitutes a new leuprorelin acetate formulation that appears to achieve a testosterone suppression of 20 ng/dL in 98% of patients, while maintaining a side effect profile comparable to other products in its class [49]. It remains to be investigated, whether this use of drugs targeting androgen-independent mechanisms or improving AS can prolong the duration of the off-treatment periods of IAS and, possibly, contribute to extended survival compared to CAS.

3. Discussion

In many patients with prostate cancer, androgen deprivation therapy is administered over prolonged periods of time. The benefits of long-term AS in patients with advanced disease are well established, nevertheless, because this therapy has potential long-term side effects strategies should be applied that manage or prevent long-term complications [50]. One such strategy is IAS, in which patients receive regular cycles of AS, the duration of which is usually determined by PSA levels [51]. Canadian prostate cancer researchers have led the field of androgen withdrawal therapy for many years, from Nobel prize winner (Halifax born) Charles Huggins in 1940 to Nicholas Bruchovsky's Vancouver team's preclinical and clinical work on intermittent therapy in the early 1990s [52]. The basic premise of IAS is that periods (or cycles) on androgen deprivation for cancer control are followed by periods off therapy for testosterone recovery and improvements in quality of life parameters (such as libido, sexual function, energy, cognition and sense of masculinity). Preclinical studies suggest that the reintroduction of testosterone into the cellular milieu during the off-treatment period keeps the remaining cancer cells androgen-dependent, allowing for the next successful round of AS and delaying progression to hormone-resistant prostate cancer [51]. Accumulating data indicate that this approach improves the tolerability of AS and patients' QoL, without compromising clinical outcomes.

Consequently, the latest European Association of Urology guidelines state that IAS should no longer be considered investigational. Furthermore, given the adverse effects of CAS, there may be beneficial effects and potential cost savings in time off therapy with intermittent treatment, particularly if suppressive effects on prostate cancer are equivalent to CAS [53,54]. Seruga and Tannock, reviewing >1000 randomised patients, concluded that compelling data indicate that IAS should be regarded as standard therapy [54]. Likewise, Spendlove and Crawford put forward a strong argument that IAS has now demonstrated that it is no less effective than CAS and that it clearly reduces the impact of the side effects of hormone therapy on patient QoL [55]. Although current evidence suggests that IAS may be reasonable for some patients with hormone-sensitive prostate cancer, there are still questions about patient selection, timing, and methodology of IAS [56].

Results of the IAS phase III trials were expected to finally give some answers in regard to the clinical applicability and feasibility of this novel form of AS in prostate cancer patients. Phase II trials pointed to a non-inferiority of IAS as compared to CAS and improved tolerability of AS; however, these findings were only partially confirmed in phase III studies. According to the part of these trials involving patients with biochemical progression and confined disease, IAS can be regarded as non-inferior to CAS and superior in respect to QoL. For metastatic prostate cancer patients the situation seems to be different: whereas in patients with extended disease the intermittent and continuous form of AS were equivalent in respect to disease progression and OS, patients with limited metastatic disease fare worse, according to preliminary data stemming from the South European Uroncological Group trial and to definitive data from the SWOG 9346 intergroup trial [13,17]. The latter study could not exclude the loss of two years in OS in patients in which the disease that had not spread beyond the lymph nodes or the bones of the spine or pelvis. The results of Hussain et al. did not apply to men without metastases, who constitute a much larger group getting hormonal therapy. For those men IAS remain a reasonable option and even men with metastatic cancer might still opt for IAS to give their years more live instead of giving their live more years. It should be noted that the metastatic prostate cancer patients in this study had an unusual mean OS and AS consisted of a 7 months course, that may be short of the minimum of 8 months requested by Bruchovsky et al. for full downstaging [57].

The question that needs to be discussed is the selection of the prostate cancer patients who will get an optimal benefit from IAS instead of CAS. Men with local or biochemical failures after radiotherapy would benefit from IAS because they are treatment-free for longer periods of time and so are less likely to develop hormone-refractory disease [58]. De la Taille et al. identified patients >70 years of age with localised prostate cancer, a Gleason score of < 7, and a first off-therapy period of >1 year as the best candidates for IAS [59]. Grossfeld et al. recommend investigation of IAS in patients with clinically localised cancer who are not appropriate for definitive local treatment, but have significant risk of tumour progression, patients who refuse all local treatment options despite risk of progression, and those who have failed prior local therapy [60]. Poor candidates for IAS have been described as those with initial bulky tumors, with numerous lymph nodes or bone metastases, PSA doubling time <9 months, and initial serum PSA >100 ng/ml or severe pain [61]. Gleave et al. suggest that patients who fail to achieve a PSA nadir of <4 ng/ml after 6 months of therapy and most men with TxNxM1 disease should not be offered IAS, whereas those with TxN1-3M0 who are sexually active, compliant, or intolerant of AS side effects make good candidates, as long as they are informed of its investigational status [62]. Patients most likely to benefit are those with locally advanced prostate cancer with or without lymph node metastases but without any evidence of bone metastases. Also, those patients with biochemical failure following radiologic or surgical therapy for prostate cancer, those who cannot tolerate side effects of CAS, and those who wish to remain sexually active would appear to be good candidates. However, treatment should be restricted to those who can comply with close follow-up. Clearly, IAS is impossible in a significant fraction of men who do not respond to an initial course of AS.

Although the American Urological Association has not yet included IAS in its treatment guidelines for prostate cancer, the European Association of Urology acknowledged that IAS is at present widely offered to patients with prostate cancer in various clinical settings and states that its status should no longer be regarded as investigational [63,64]. This is in contrast to the American Society of Clinical Oncology practice guidelines, which state that there are currently insufficient data to support the use of IAS outside of clinical trials [65]. The 2008 UK National Institute for Health and Clinical Excellence (NICE) recommends that IAS be offered as a first-line hormonal therapy option to men with newly diagnosed or relapsing metastatic cancer, provided they are aware of its unproven status [66]. They also note that results from uncontrolled studies have shown satisfactory outcomes and that IAS will probably be more cost effective than CAS, despite the need for close monitoring. Irrespective of official guideline recommendations, IAS is a treatment option used worldwide by both urologists and oncologists outside of clinical trials. Based on available evidence and general clinical opinion, IAS is a valid treatment option in non-metastatic prostate cancer cases, that is, patients with locally advanced disease with or without lymph node involvement and those experiencing relapse following curative treatment. These patients have a higher chance of survival than those with more advanced disease, making QoL a key consideration.

Since the introduction of PSA screening in the late 1980s, more prostate cancers have been detected, and at an earlier stage that are low grade and slow growing and will not need aggressive therapy [67,68]. With this long natural history and a median survival without treatment that often approaches at least 15 to 20 years many patients will die rather with than of prostate cancer. Approximately one-third of patients who undergo radical prostatectomy will develop a detectable PSA level within 10 years [69]. Management of PSA recurrence is controversial, as prostate cancer may take an indolent course, or it may develop aggressively into metastatic disease. Prostate cancer is over-treated at present but a short course of AS might identify those patients for whom the outcome would be good with IAS by identifying those with a good PSA response. Multivariate models show the power of the initial PSA level and PSA nadir, and type of treatment and the PSA threshold for restarting treatment, in predicting outcome [21]. In those patients who rapidly achieve a good PSA nadir it is safe to shorten treatment to < 4 months. In the presence of evidence of metastasis, treatment must be protracted to ≥ 8 months. Restarting treatment when the PSA level approaches 15 ng/mL is associated with improved survival in patients with metastases, indicating the need for a more aggressive treatment strategy in these patients. Maximum androgen blockade or LHRH analog should be the standard for patients treated with IAS. The duration of biochemical remission after a period of IAS is a durable early indicator of how rapidly progression and death will occur, and will make a useful endpoint in future trials. The initial PSA level and PSA nadir allow the identification of patients with prostate cancer in whom it might be possible to avoid radical therapy.

Twenty years ago it was expected that the IAS regimen would be associated with extended survival, mainly through postponing the castration-resistant status [70]. The expected associated benefits were a decrease in the adverse effects of castration, such as hot flushes, decreased libido and erection, bone and muscle problems, depression, and metabolic syndrome (Table 3). Regarding the expected QoL and adverse effects benefits, few prospective data from randomized trials are available comparing IAS to CAS treatment. The report from Salonen et al. shows some benefit in QoL for activity limitation, physical capacity, and sexual functioning [41,42]. Surprisingly, no difference was observed in drug-induced adverse effects, such as hot flushes or night sweats. This lack of a clear sexual benefit is disappointing and a little different from what is observed in other trials, especially the South European Urooncological Group or the Miller trial [13,37]. The different questionnaires might partly explain this difference, as might the different treatment modalities, such as varied duration of treatment cycles and combined treatments or monotherapy. It was also hoped that IAS would decrease the treatment adverse effects; this decrease, at best, has been marginally obtained as the claimed QoL benefit. The thresholds, which were different from trial to trial, were only empirically chosen. The lower the PSA level after the AS induction period, the longer the survival. Therefore, the threshold of 4 ng/ml to stop the treatment in most metastatic trials might be too high and the threshold of 20 ng/ml to resume treatment might also be too high; however, it allows a longer off-treatment period, although not long enough to lead to a clear large QoL benefit [70]. Mottet concludes that apart from treatment cost, IAS does not hold to its promises and should probably be considered with caution in the most advanced situations, even in patients with a clear PSA response.

Initial goals of IAS

- Prolongation of androgen dependence and survival
- Therapy working in most stages of prostate cancer
- Reduction of the side effects of CAS
- Reduction of adverse events associated with CAS
- Reduction of the costs of prostate cancer treatment
-

Current status of IAS

- Survival under IAS not inferior to CAS?
- Prolongation of androgen-dependence of tumor not confirmed
- Most suitable for relapse after prostatectomy/radiation therapy
- Reduction of side effects of AS in most studies?
- Improved quality of life during off treatment dependent on testosterone recovery
- No consistent and optimal scheme for the implementation of IAS?
- Reduced costs of IAS compared to CAS

Table 3. Summary of the achievements and shortcomings of IAS

These findings for IAS are far from what was initially expected, and the presented SWOG 9346 trial added even more questions regarding IAS [17]. It has long been said that IAS does not appear to be inferior to CAS. Those results were obtained from under-powered trials or large trials including heterogeneous patients, such as the FinnProstate Study VII [41] or even the large, recently presented SWOG JPR7 [17] trial in postradiotherapy relapsing patients. None of the trials even suggested increased overall or specific survival. IAS was expected to postpone androgen independence; this finding, however, as well as an increase in OS has never been obtained in any trial. Thus, the marked elongation of hormone-dependency in the Shionogi mouse model could not be materialized in patients, which may be most likely due to increased cycle length of several months in humans compared to one month these animals, allowing for better adaptation to hormone deprivation. Furthermore, the Shionogi study was done on androgen-dependent mouse mammary carcinoma. This animal model may be insufficient to explain homeostasis of human stem cells and their progenies in relation to human prostate cancer. Miki et al. reported that human prostate cancer stem cells had no androgen receptors or PSA [71]. Guzmán-Ramírez and coworkers presented a similar protein expression pattern of prostate cancer stem cells [72]. There is a high probability that human prostate cancer stem cells are really androgen-independent. Another possibility is that two populations of stem cells exist within human prostate cancer and that the first population is androgen-sensitive and the second is androgen-independent. Our knowledge of prostate cancer stem cells is still too immature to support the rational approach for IAS therapy. Furthermore, Pfeiffer and Schalken reported difficulties in finding stem cells within established prostate cell lines in vitro, reflecting their limited use in such research [73].

In the world of medicine it has been estimated that it takes an average of 17 years for practice changing evidence to reach the bedside [52]. The first phase II study of IAS was published in 1995 and after 17 years it was advised to accept that multiple randomized controlled trials have supported its use as a non-inferior option to CAS in defined populations and to reintroduce suitable men with prostate cancer intermittently to the pleasure of their androgens [52]. High-risk patients seem to be poor candidates for any type of androgen suppression. In summary, it can be concluded from the trials that IAS is neither inferior nor superior to CAS with respect to clinical end points, namely the time period until hormone-resistance as well as cancer-specific survival, but offers significant advantages in terms of adverse effects, quality of life and costs. The off-treatment periods particularly offer the possibility to apply drugs, such as finasteride, or chemotherapeutics in order to delay disease progression [74]. However, the clinical lack of prolongation of the hormone-sensitive state of prostate cancers by IAS raises doubts about the underlying hypothesis of keeping the prostate cancer cell in an androgen responsive state by cycling between AS and off-treatment periods. Fundamental tumor biology studies in patients would be needed to clarify this issue. Otherwise IAS may be regarded as treatment regimen aiming simple for AS reduction to a level that does not permit efficient tumor growth and simultaneously lowers the side effects of AS. Patients that respond well to a first cycle of AS may go on off-treatment for years [75]. Clearly, IAS is not standard therapy for all prostate cancer patients, but a valid and favourable regimen for a significant part of selected patients.

Acknowledgment

We thank all the patients and staff involved in our IAS trial.

Author details

Gerhard Hamilton[1] and Gerhard Theyer[2]

*Address all correspondence to: gerhard.hamilton@toc.lbg.ac.at

1 Ludwig Boltzmann Cluster of Translational Oncology, Vienna, Austria

2 LKH Kittsee, Burgenland, Austria

References

[1] Siegel R, Naishadham D, Jemal A. Cancer statistics. CA Cancer J. Clin.2012; 62, 10–29.

[2] Fitzpatrick JM, Schulman C, Zlotta AR, Schroeder FH. Prostate cancer: a serious disease suitable for prevention. BJU Int 2009;103, 864-870.

[3] Felici A, Pino MS, Carlini P. A Changing Landscape in Castration-Resistant Prostate Cancer Treatment.Front Endocrinol (Lausanne). 2012;3:85.

[4] Lassi K. and Dawson NA. Emerging therapies in castrate-resistant prostate cancer.CurrOpinOncol 2009;21, 260-265.

[5] Kollmeier, M.A. and Zelefsky, M.J. What is the role of androgen deprivation therapy in the treatment of locally advanced prostate cancer? Nat ClinPractUrol 2008;5, 584-585.

[6] Chang, S.S., and Kibel, A.S. The role of systemic cytotoxic therapy for prostate cancer. BJU Int 2009;103, 8-17.

[7] Madan, R.A., Pal, S.K., Sartor, O. &Dahut, W.L. Overcoming chemotherapy resistance in prostate cancer. Clin Cancer Res 2011;17(12), 3892-3902.

[8] Bruchovsky, N., Goldenberg, S.L., Rennie, P.S. &Gleave M. Theoretical considerations and initial clinical results of intermittent hormone treatment of patients with advanced prostatic carcinoma. Urologe-A 1995;34, 389-392.

[9] Bruchovsky, N., Rennie, P.S., Coldman, A.J., Goldenberg, S.L., To, M. & Lawson D. Effects of androgen withdrawal on the stem cell composition of the Shionogi carcinoma. Cancer Res 1990;50(8), 2275-2282.

[10] Akakura, K., Bruchovsky, N., Goldenberg, S.L., Rennie, P.S., Buckley, A.R. & Sullivan L.D.Effects of intermittent androgen suppression on androgen-dependent tumors. Apoptosis and serum prostate-specific antigen. Cancer 1993;71(9), 2782-2790.

[11] Rennie, P.S., Bruchovsky, N. &Coldman, A.J. Loss of androgen dependence is associated with an increase in tumorigenic stem cells and resistance to cell-death genes. J Steroid BiochemMolBiol 1990;37(6), 843-847.

[12] Gleave, M., Santo, N., Rennie, P.S., Goldenberg, S.L., Bruchovsky, N. & Sullivan, L.D. Hormone release and intermittent hormonal therapy in the LNCaP model of human prostate cancer. ProgUrol 1996;6(3), 375-385.

[13] Calais da Silva, F.E., Bono, A.V., Whelan, P., Brausi, M., Marques Queimadelos, A., Martin J.A., Kirkali, Z., Calais da Silva, F.M. & Robertson C. Intermittent androgen deprivation for locally advanced and metastatic prostate cancer: results from a randomised phase 3 study of the South European Uroncological Group. EurUrol 2009;55(6), 1269-1277.

[14] Bruchovsky, N., Snoek, R., Rennie, P.S. Akakura, K., Goldenberg, L.S. &Gleave M. Control of tumor progression by maintenance of apoptosis. Prostate 1996;6S, 13-21.

[15] Theyer, G. and Hamilton G. Current status of intermittent androgen suppression in the treatment of prostate cancer. Urology 1998;53, 353-359.

[16] Abrahamsson P.A. Potential Benefits of Intermittent Androgen Suppression Therapy in the Treatment of Prostate Cancer.EurUrol 2010;57(1), 49-59.

[17] Hussain M, Tangen CM, Higano CS, et al. Intermittent (IAD) versus continuous androgen deprivation (CAD) in hormone sensitive metastatic prostate cancer (HSM1PC) patients: results of S9346 (INT- 0162), an international phase III trial. J CliniOncol 2012;30(Suppl), abstract LBA 4.

[18] Corona, G., Baldi, E. & Maggi, M. Androgen regulation of prostate cancer: Where are we now? J Endocrinol Invest 2011;34(3), 232-243.

[19] Grossmann, M., Hamilton, E.J., Gilfillan, C., Bolton, D., Joon, D.L. &Zajac, J.D. Bone and metabolic health in patients with non-metastatic prostate cancer who are receiving androgen deprivation therapy. Med J Aust 2011;194(6), 301-306.

[20] Buchan NC, Goldenberg SL. Intermittent androgen suppression for prostate cancer. Nat Rev Urol. 2010;7(10):552-560.

[21] Shaw GL, Wilson P, Cuzick J, Prowse DM, Goldenberg SL, Spry NA, Oliver T. International study into the use of intermittent hormone therapy in the treatment of carcinoma of the prostate: a meta-analysis of 1446 patients. BJU Int. 2007;99(5):1056-1065.

[22] Tunn UW, Canepa G, Kochanowsky A, Kienle E. Testosterone recovery in the off-treat ment time in prostate cancer patients undergoing intermittent androgen deprivation therapy. Prostate Cancer Prostatic Dis. 2012, in press.

[23] Bruchovsky N, Klotz L, Crook J, Phillips N, Abersbach J, Goldenberg SL.Quality of life, morbidity, and mortality results of a prospective phase II study of intermittent androgen suppression for men with evidence of prostate-specific antigen relapse after radiation therapy for locally advanced prostate cancer. ClinGenitourin Cancer. 2008;6(1):46-52.

[24] Zhu J, Wang Y, Xu S, Sun Z. Intermittent androgen blockade or continuous androgen blockade in advanced prostate cancer: a meta-analysis of efficacy, quality of life and side effects. J BUON. 2012;17(2):350-356.

[25] Malone S, Perry G, Segal R, Dahrouge S, Crook J. Long-term side effects of intermittent androgen suppression therapy in prostate cancer: results of a phase II study. BJU Int 2005;96:514–20.

[26] Bouchot O, Lenormand L, Karam G, et al. Intermittent androgen suppression in the treatment of metastatic prostate cancer. EurUrol 2000;38:543–9.

[27] Goldenberg SL, Gleave ME, Taylor D, Bruchovsky N. Clinical experience with intermittent androgen suppression in prostate cancer: Minimum of 3 years' follow-up. MolUrol 1999;3:287–292.

[28] Spry NA, Kristjanson L, Hooton B, et al. Adverse effects to quality of life arising from treatment can recover with intermittent androgen suppression in men with prostate cancer. Eur J Cancer 2006;42: 1083–1092.

[29] Yu EY, Kuo KF, Gulati R, Chen S, Gambol TE, Hall SP, Jiang PY, Pitzel P, HiganoCS.Long-term dynamics of bone mineral density during intermittent androgen deprivation for men with nonmetastatic, hormone-sensitive prostate cancer. J CliniOncol. 2012;30(15):1864-1870.

[30] Spry NA, Galvão DA, Davies R, La Bianca S, Joseph D, Davidson A, Prince R. Long-term effects of intermittent androgen suppression on testosterone recovery and bone mineral density: results of a 33-month observational study. BJU Int. 2009;104(6): 806-12.

[31] Theyer G, Holub S, Olszewski U, Hamilton G (2010) Measurement of bone turnover in prostate cancer patients receiving intermittent androgen suppression therapy. OA Journal of Urology 2010;2: 155-159.

[32] Hamilton G, Olszewski-Hamilton U, Theyer G. Type I collagen synthesis marker procollagen I N-terminal peptide (PINP) in prostate cancer patients undergoing intermittent androgen suppression. Cancers 2011;3: 3601-3609.

[33] Ng E, Woo HH, Turner S, Leong E, Jackson M, Spry N. The influence of testosterone suppression and recovery on sexual function in men with prostate cancer: observations from a prospective study in men undergoing intermittent androgen suppression. J Urol. 2012;187(6):2162-2166.

[34] L. Klotz, C. J. O'Callaghan, K. Ding, D. P. Dearnaley, C. S. Higano, E. M. Horwitz, S. Malone, S. L. Goldenberg, M. K. Gospodarowicz, J. M. Crook. A phase III random-

ized trial comparing intermittent versus continuous androgen suppression for patients with PSA progression after radical therapy: NCIC CTG PR.7/SWOG PR.7/ CTSU JPR.7/UK Intercontinental Trial CRUKE/01/013. J ClinOncol 29: 2011 (suppl 7; abstr 3).

[35] Verhagen, P.C.M.S.1, Wissenburg, L.D.1, Wildhagen, M.F.1, Bolle, W.A.B.M.1, Verkerk, A.M.1, Schroder, F.H.1, Bangma, C.H.1, Mickisch, G.H.2 Quality of life effects of intermittent and continuous hormonal therapy by cyproterone acetate (CPA) for metastatic prostate cancercancer [abstract 541]. Presented at: 23rd Annual Congress of the European Association of Urology; March 26–29, 2008; Milan, Italy.

[36] de Leval J, Boca P, Yousef E, Nicolas H, Jeukenne M, Seidel L, Bouffioux C, Coppens L, Bonnet P, Andrianne R, Wlatregny D. Intermittent versus continuous total androgen blockade in the treatment of patients with advanced hormone-naive prostate cancer: results of a prospective randomized multicenter trial. Clin Prostate Cancer. 2002;1(3):163-171.

[37] Miller K, Steiner U, Lingnau A, et al. Randomised prospective study of intermittent versus continuous androgen suppression in advanced prostate cancer [abstract 5105]. Presented at: American Society of Clinical Oncology; June 1–5, 2007; Chicago, IL, USA.

[38] Mottet N, Van Damme J, Loulidi S, Russel C, Leitenberger A, Wolff JM, the TAP22 Investigators Group. Intermittent hormonal therapy in the treatment of metastatic prostate cancer: a randomized trial. BJU Int. In press.

[39] Langenhuijsen JF, Schasfoort EMC, Heathcote P, et al. Intermittent androgen suppression in patients with advanced prostate cancer: an update of the TULP survival data [abstract 538]. Presented at: 23rd Annual Congress of the European Association of Urology; March 26–29, 2008; Milan, Italy.

[40] Langenhuijsen JF, Badhauser D, Schaaf B, Kiemeney LA, Witjes JA, Mulders PF. Continuous vs. intermittent androgen deprivation therapy for metastatic prostate cancer.UrolOncol. 2011, in press.

[41] Salonen AJ, Taari K, Ala-Opas M, Viitanen J, Lundstedt S, Tammela TL; FinnProstate Group. The FinnProstate Study VII: Intermittent Versus Continuous Androgen Deprivation in Patients with Advanced Prostate Cancer. J Urol. 2012;187(6):2074-2081.

[42] Salonen AJ, Taari K, Ala-Opas M, Viitanen J, Lundstedt S, Tammela TL; the FinnProstate Group. Advanced Prostate Cancer Treated with Intermittent or Continuous Androgen Deprivation in the RandomisedFinnProstate Study VII: Quality of Life and Adverse Effects. Eur Urol. 2012, in press.

[43] Gulley JL, Figg WD, Steinberg SM, et al. A prospective analysis of the time to normalization of serum androgens following 6 months of androgen deprivation therapy in patients on a randomized phase III clinical trial using limited hormonal therapy. J Urol 2005;173:1567–1571.

[44] Calais da Silva FE, Goncales F, Santos A, et al. Evaluation of quality of life, side effects and duration of therapy in a phase 3 study of intermittent monotherapy versus continuous androgen deprivation [abstract 540]. Presented at: 23rd Annual Congress of the European Association of Urology; March 26–29, 2008; Milan, Italy.

[45] Webster WS, Leibovich BC. Exisulind in the treatment of prostate cancer.Expert Rev Anticancer Ther. 2005;5(6):9579-62.

[46] Morabito A, Piccirillo MC, Costanzo R, Sandomenico C, Carillio G, Daniele G, Giordano P, Bryce J, Carotenuto P, La Rocca A, Di Maio M, Normanno N, Rocco G, Perrone F. Vandetanib: An overview of its clinical development in NSCLC and other tumors. Drugs Today (Barc). 2010;46(9):683-698.

[47] Schmidt LJ, Tindall DJ. Steroid 5 α-reductase inhibitors targeting BPH and prostate cancer. J Steroid BiochemMol Biol. 2011;125(1-2):32-38.

[48] Steinberg M. Degarelix: a gonadotropin-releasing hormone antagonist for the management of prostate cancer. ClinTher. 2009;31Pt 2:2312-2331.

[49] Berges R, Bello U. Effect of a new leuprorelin formulation on testosterone levels in patients with advanced prostate cancer. CurrMed Res Opin. 2006;22(4):649-655.

[50] Schulman C, Irani J, Aapro M. Improving the management of patients with prostate cancer receiving long-term androgen deprivation therapy.BJU Int.2012;109Suppl 6:13-21.

[51] Hamilton G, Olszewski-Hamilton U., Theyer G. Intermittent Androgen Suppression Therapy for Prostate Cancer Patients: A Choice for Improved Quality of Life? Prostate Cancer - Diagnostic and Therapeutic Advances, 2011;18;363-378.

[52] Ischia J, S., Goldenberg L. Intermittent Androgen Suppression—Ready for Prime Time? J Urol, 2012;187(6), 1956–1957.

[53] Seruga B, Tannock F. Intermittent androgen blockade should be regarded as standard therapy in prostate cancer. Nat ClinPractOncol 2008;5:574–576.

[54] Sharifi N, Gulley JL, Dahut WL. Continuous ADT versus intermittent ADT.An update on androgen deprivation therapy for prostate cancer.EndocrRelat Cancer. 2010;17(4):R305-315.

[55] Spendlove J, Crawford D. Intermittent Versus Continuous Androgen Deprivation Therapy. AUA News,2012;16(5), 13-14.

[56] Keizman D, Carducci MA Intermittent androgen deprivation--questions remain. Nat Rev Urol. 2009;6(8):412-414.

[57] Gleave, M.E, Goldenberg, S.L., Jones, E.C., Bruchovsky N. & Sullivan L.D. Maximal biochemical and pathological downstaging requires eight months of neoadjuvant hormonal therapy prior to radical prostatectomy. J Urol 1996;155, 213-219.

[58] Crook JM, Szumacher E, Malone S, Huan S, Segal R. Intermittent androgen suppression in the management of prostate cancer. Urology 1999;53:530–534.

[59] de la Taille A, Zerbib M, Conquy S, et al. Intermittent androgen suppression in patients with prostate cancer. BJU Int 2003;91:18–22.

[60] Goldenberg SL, Gleave ME, Taylor D, Bruchovsky N. Clinical experience with intermittent androgen suppression in prostate cancer: Minimum of 3 years' follow-up. MolUrol 1999;3:287–292.

[61] Grossfeld GD, Small EJ, Carroll PR. Intermittent androgen deprivation for clinically localized prostate cancer: initial experience. Urology 1998;51:137–44.

[62] Gleave M, Klotz L, Taneja SS. The continued debate: intermittent vs.continuous hormonal ablation for metastatic prostate cancer. UrolOncol 2009;27:81–86.

[63] American Urological Association. Guideline for the management of clinically localized prostate cancer: 2007 update. Linthicum, MD: American Urological Association; 2007.

[64] Heidenreich A, Aus G, Bolla M, et al. Guidelines on prostate cancer. European Association of Urology 2007;1–114.

[65] Loblaw DA, Virgo KS, Nam R, et al. Initial hormonal management of androgen- sensitive metastatic, recurrent, or progressive prostate cancer: 2006 update of an American Society of Clinical Oncology practice guideline. J ClinOncol 2007;25:1596–1605.

[66] National Institute for Health and Clinical Excellence. Prostate cancer: diagnosis and treatment. February 2008. http://www.nice.org.uk/CGO58. Accessed on 3 July 2008.

[67] Gjertson CK, Albertsen PC. Use and assessment of PSA in prostate cancer. Med Clin North Am. 2011;95(1):191-200.

[68] Carroll PR. Early stage prostate cancer – do we have a problem with overdetection, overtreatment or both? J Urol 2005; 173:1061–1062.

[69] Tzou K, Tan WW, Buskirk S. Treatment of men with rising prostate-specific antigen levels following radical prostatectomy. Expert Rev Anticancer Ther. 2011;11(1): 125-136.

[70] Mottet N. Intermittent Androgen Deprivation Therapy in Prostate Cancer: Is Everything So Clear?Eur Urol. 2012 in press.

[71] Miki J. Investigations of prostate epithelial stem cells and prostate cancer stem cells. Int J Urol. 2010;17(2):139-147.

[72] Guzmán-Ramírez N, Völler M, Wetterwald A, Germann M, Cross NA, Rentsch CA, Schalken J, Thalmann GN, Cecchini MG. In vitro propagation and characterization of neoplastic stem/progenitor-like cells from human prostate cancer tissue.Prostate. 2009;69(15):1683-1693.

[73] M.J. Pfeiffer, J.A. Schalken. Stem cell characteristics in prostate cancer cell lines. Eur-Urol, 2010;57:246–255.

[74] Locke, J.A. &Bruchovsky, N. Prostate cancer: finasteride extends PSA doubling time during intermittent hormone therapy.Can J Urol 2010;7(3), 5162-5169.

[75] Theyer, G., Ulsperger, E., Baumgartner, G., Raderer, M. & Hamilton, G. Prolonged response to a single androgen suppression phase in a subpopulation of prostate cancer patients. Ann Oncol 2000;11, 877-881.

Section 6

Cell Biology of Prostate Cancer

Chapter 14

Stem Cells and Prostate Cancer

Vildan Bozok Çetintaş, Burçin Tezcanlı Kaymaz and Buket Kosova

Additional information is available at the end of the chapter

http://dx.doi.org/10.5772/52289

1. Introduction

Latest statistics based on GLOBOCAN 2008, the standard set of worldwide estimates of cancer incidence and mortality produced by the International Agency for Research on Cancer (IARC), revealed that prostate cancer (PC) is the most commonly diagnosed malignancy and the second leading cause of cancer-related mortality in male in developed countries [1]. The options in the treatment of PC are surgical tumor resection, hormonal therapy, radiotherapy, and adjuvant chemotherapy. These therapies, alone or in combination, show beneficial effects and a significant curative rate in treating patients with localized PC in the early stages. However, the development of locally advanced and/or metastatic hormone-refractory prostate cancers (HRPCs) eventually results in disease recurrence. Most patients who undergo potentially curative resection for advanced and/or metastatic HRPCs subsequently relapse due to the persistence of foci and micro-metastases. Therefore systemic chemotherapy may represent another option to eradicate the PC cells, including the highly tumorigenic stem/ progenitor cells that can drive tumor growth at primary neoplasms and distant metastatic sites.

The existence of stem cells (SCs) was firstly demonstrated by James Till and the late Ernest McCulloch in 1963 in their earlier work on the radiation sensitivity of mouse bone marrow cells by showing that limited numbers of cells could give rise to clonal colonies of erythroid and myeloid cells in the spleens of the irradiated hosts [2]. Although, much improvement has been achieved in the development of methods to kill cancer cells that form a variety of malignancies; nevertheless, relapse is an ongoing problem along with the development of metastatic tumors at sites remote from that of the original tumor. One suggestion to account for these phenomena is the existence of a stem cell with tumorigenic properties capable of regenerating all the differentiated cell types presented in the original tumor. The key paper supporting the cancer stem cell (CSC) hypothesis from the laboratory of John Dick appeared in 1997, in which they demonstrated that an isolated cell type was capable of initiating acute myeloid leukemia (AML) [3]. With the knowledge provided by the science of stem cell biology, the Nobel Prize in Physiology or Medicine in the year 2007 was awarded jointly to Mario R. Capecchi, Sir Martin J. Evans and Oliver Smithies "for their discoveries of principles for introducing specific gene modifications in mice by the use of embryonic stem cells".

Stem cells possess some unique properties: a) they are undifferentiated and unspecialized; b) they are able to multiply for long periods while remaining undifferentiated (slowly cycling); c) they are capable of differentiating into specialized cells of a particular tissue (produce progeny in at least two lineages); and d) they can be serially transplanted. The combination of these properties is often referred to as "stemness" [4]. Stem cells can divide symmetrically or asymmetrically. A symmetrical division occurs when two daughter cells share the same stem cell features and happens when their numbers (stem cell pool) need to be expanded, such as during embryonic development or after tissue injury. An asymmetrical division occurs when one of the progeny remains undifferentiated, thereby replenishing the pool of SCs, while the other daughter cell can proliferate and differentiate into specialized cells to generate new tissue mass.

Stem cells have long been implicated in prostate gland formation. The prostate undergoes regression after androgen deprivation and regeneration after testosterone replacement. Regenerative studies suggested that those stem cells are found in the proximal ducts and basal layer of the prostate. Many characteristics of PC also indicate that it originates from stem cells. In this chapter, the biological and clinical implications of stem cells in prostatic carcinogenesis and the involvement of prostate cancer stem cells (PCSCs) in the many faces of PC are demonstrated and summarized. The theory of a stem cell origin of cancers represents a major paradigm shift that may completely revamp to diagnosis, monitoring, and therapy of PC.

2. Prostate epithelium and stem cells

Human prostate is an exocrine gland that consists of basal, luminal and neuroendocrine cell types embedded in a fibro-muscular stroma. The basal cells are relatively undifferentiated, not dependent on androgens and hence express low levels of androgen receptors (ARs). Additionally, basal cells generate some secretory products such as CD44 [5], p63 [6], $p27^{kip}$ and c-Met [7], cytokeratin 5 (CK 5) and CK 14 [8]. In contrast to the basal layer of cells, luminal (or secretory) cells are terminally differentiated and specifically secrete the prostate like prostate specific antigen (PSA) and prostatic acid phosphatase (PAP) into the glandular medulla in response to androgens. Because, survival of these luminal cells depend on androgens they express ARs on a high level; whereas, their other specific secretory products are CD57 [5], CK 8 and CK 18 [8]. The third type of cell in the cellular organization of the prostate epithelium is the neuroendocrine (NE) cell. The specific functions of NE cells have not been deduced so far. However, Bonkhoff suggested that they are post-mitotic cells derived from luminal secretory cells [9]. NE cells are terminally differentiated, androgen insensitive and scattered throughout the epithelium. Unlike the luminal cells, NE cells do not express AR or PSA; but, they do express NE-specific markers such as chromogranin A and synaptophysin [10]. Basal and luminal cells can also be distinguished by comparing expression profiles of other genes; like basal cells do mainly express CK 5 and CK 14, whereas luminal cells express CK 8 and CK 18 [8]. Morphologically basal cells are small, flattened cells with condensed chromatin and small amounts of cytoplasm. Luminal cells instead have increased cytoplasm and their chromatin appear more opened [11]. Finally, the stroma is located under the epithelial layer of prostate. Stromal cells are androgen responsive and they do express AR. Development, maintenance and differentiation of epithelial cells are provided by these stromal cells [12].

2.1. Prostate stem cells

Prostate stem cells (PSCs) need to carry following characteristics: they must be castration-resistant, able to renew themselves and regenerate new tissue [13]. In contrast to the epithelial tissue of other adult organs, the prostate and mammary glands exert hormonal-dependence. Therefore, to account for changes in hormone levels the PSCs should be responsive to, but not dependent on, androgen for survival. This property is referred to as castration-resistance. PSCs should have tissue-regenerative capacity to replenish the gland after routine cell death. But, when compared to the hematopoietic stem cells that must generate a vast array of mature lineages, PSCs only must regenerate a relatively simple double-layered epithelium. Eventually, and most importantly, PSCs must be able to self-renew meeting the needs of the organ over the course of a man's lifetime.

2.2. Localization of stem cells within the prostate epithelium

In the 1980s, John Isaacs and colleagues performed classic androgen cycling experiments and suggested that prostate epithelium must contain a SC population. Than, when rodents are deprived of androgen by surgical or medical castration, the gland atrophies due to apoptosis of terminally differentiated cells which are dependent on androgen for their survival [14]. However, when androgen is replaced the gland regenerates and resumes its normal functions. This involution and regeneration can be repeated for many sequential cycles. The regenerative capacity has been attributed to a population of long lived SCs within adult prostate epithelium that are thought not androgen-dependent for survival, but androgen-sensitive and androgen-responsive. Apoptosis occurs mostly in androgen-dependent luminal cell epithelium, while the androgen-independent basal cells generally remain unaffected [15]. In accordance with this, the regenerative capacity is referred to the action of basal SCs, while the harbor of these self-renewing cells is confined to the basal-cell layer [14, 16]. Later, also other observations and studies have supported this hypothesis in many ways; like, that basal cells exhibit a higher proliferation rate in normal and hyperplastic acini than luminal epithelial cells [9]. Or for example, as bromodeoxyuridine (BrdU) labeling studies have suggested that prostatic tumor-initiating cells reside in the basal cell compartment and express a $p63^+$ signature [17]. And, that basal cells preferentially survive after androgen ablation;

whereas, 90% of luminal epithelial cells are lost through programmed cell death [18]. Androgen treatment restores the secretory glandular structure, hinting towards that the basal compartment contains SCs that undergo transit amplification to repopulate the luminal epithelium [19]. Cell types expressing an intermediate phenotype of basal and luminal cell characteristics have been identified in the developing and adult prostate [19].

On the other hand, there are also some studies that do not support the idea that SCs reside in the basal cell compartment. Experiments in mice where SCs were labeled with BrdU, suggested that stem cells are not restricted to the basal cell compartment; but, may also reside in luminal cell layer as a slow proliferating population in the proximal part of prostatic ducts [20]. Using tissue rescue experiments, Gerald R. Cunha and colleagues have demonstrated that the embryonic p63 null urogenital sinus developed into prostate when engrafted under the renal capsule of male mice [21]. Although, basal cells were absent the grafts contained luminal and NE cells, demonstrating that p63 was essential for basal but not for luminal and NE cell differentiation [21].

In human prostate, there is a consistent body of evidence that the SCs reside in the basal layer. Within the basal layer, $CD133^{+}/\alpha_2\beta_1^{hi}$ (high expression of $\alpha_2\beta_1$ integrin) cells represent a small subpopulation of quiescent cells with SC characteristics: they have a high proliferative potential *in vitro* and can reconstruct functional prostate acinar structures *in vivo* [22]. Molecular characterization of these cells revealed that they do not express AR at mRNA level [23], indicating that they are not dependent on androgen for their survival. Using CD49f and tumor-associated calcium signal transducer-2 (TROP2) as markers, Goldstein and collaborators identified basal cells with enhanced sphere-forming and tissue regenerating abilities [24].

2.3. Characterization of prostatic stem cells

Recent studies have revealed that a very small subpopulation of multipotent and undifferentiated PSCs, comprising about 0.1–3.0% of the total prostatic epithelial cell population, principally reside within specialized areas or "niches" localized in the basal cell layer of acinar and ductal regions of the human prostate gland [5]. Anne T. Collins and colleagues isolated and characterized human adult SCs based on the identity of cell surface integrin antigens [25]. They showed that, *in vivo*, putative SCs express higher levels of the α_2-integrin subunit than other cells within the basal layer. Later, it was shown that a subpopulation of $\alpha_2\beta_1^{hi}$ basal cells express the CD133 antigen and that this expression correlates with a high proliferative potential and ability to regenerate a fully differentiated prostatic epithelium with expression of prostatic secretory products *in vivo* [22]. $CD133^{+}$ cells possess three important attributes of epithelial stem cells: they are rare, comprise a high *in vitro* proliferative potential, and are capable of reconstituting highly branched ductal structures. Besides, Patricia E. Burger and colleagues reported that SCs can be purified from isolated proximal duct regions by virtue of their high expression of the cell surface protein stem cell antigen 1 (SCA-1) [26]. Subsequently, it was demonstrated that the Sca-1 surface antigen can be used to enrich for murine prostate cells displaying multiple properties of primitive cells including androgen independence, replication quiescence, multi lineage differentiation, and *in vivo* prostate regenerative capacity [27]. Combined cell surface markers such as $CD45^{-}CD31^{-}Ter119^{-}Sca\text{-}1^{+}CD49f^{+}$ were defined by Devon A. Lawson and colleagues who found that prostate cells can self-renew to form spheres for many generations and can differentiate to produce prostatic tubule structures containing both basal and luminal cells *in vivo*. These cells also localize to the putative PSC niche in the proximal region of the prostate gland [28].

2.4. Prostate stem cell niche

In all epithelial organs, adult SCs are maintained in a tissue niche that regulates stem cell fate decisions. The niche provides structural support, as well as the biological cues that influence the SCs' decision to self-renew or divide into more differentiated progeny. Integrin and junctional proteins play a major role in regulating SC differentiation in the prostate [29]. For instance, integrin α_6 shows a wider distribution amongst SC populations in the prostate tissue [28]. It was also shown that the high surface expression of $\alpha_2\beta_1$ integrin in human prostate epithelium correlates with colony forming ability and the potential to regenerate a fully differentiated prostate epithelium *in vivo* [25]. Additionally, proteins belonging to the connexin, cadherin and catenin families were reported as key molecules mediating cell-cell and cell-extracellular matrix interaction that dictate cell differentiation decisions [30].

Prostate homeostasis is maintained as a result of androgenic regulation of stromal epithelial interactions. Mesenchyme is the key androgen target tissue during development of prostate and many androgenic effects expressed in epithelium are elucidated trough paracrine influences from the mesenchyme [31].

The pathways controlling SC fate in prostate include NOTCH1 and Transforming growth factor beta-1 (TGFβ1) signaling. NOTCH signaling is critical for normal cell proliferation and differentiation in the prostate, and deregulation of this pathway may facilitate prostatic oncogenesis [32]. Increased TGFβ1 signaling has been found in the quiescent proximal region of the ducts in an androgen-replete animal and cells in this region were also overexpressing the B-cell leukemia/lymphoma-2 (Bcl-2) protein, which protects them from apoptosis [33]. This signaling seems to be responsible for a quiescent stem cell niche.

3. Cancer stem cells

The cancer stem cell (CSC) theory has started more than a century ago with the "embryonal rest hypothesis" that was relying on histological similarities between teratocarcinomas and embryonic tissue [34] and later was than accelerated by findings that leukemia could be transferred by a single cell in a mouse model system [35]. Later investigations clarified that when this single cell was transplanted to non-severe combined immunodeficiency (SCID) mice it could induce leukemia that was phenotypically identical to the parental tumor leading to the conclusion that a leukemic tumor stem cell had developed from hematopoietic stem cells [3]. The first CSCs in a solid tumor was discovered for breast cancer in the year 2003 [36]. Following that, CSCs were also found in solid tumors like liver, lung, thyroid, skin, pancreas, colon and prostate cancer [37]. Nevertheless, through the 1960s transplant experiments had proven that cancers were composed of heterogeneous cell populations with some differences in their self-renewal capability and potential for reconstituting a tumor following transplantation [38-40]. These early investigations made the researchers think that the actual tumor cell population could be arisen from a small group of CSCs and two theories were suggested upon this idea [39]. In the stochastic theory, every cell in a tumor population is believed to be a potentially tumor initiating cell; but, each cell's possibility of entering the cell cycle is low and controlled stochastically. Whereas, the hierarchy theory assumes that the tumor is functionally heterogeneous and only a small subpopulation of cells in it have the ability to initiate tumor growth [40]. Regardless of the theories, CSC is generally accepted as the original cell of a tumor that generates an accumulation of self-sustaining cells with unlimited self-renewal capability. Meaning it is that one cell that later raises the formation of a heterogeneous bulk tumor which differentiates, comprises metastatic ability, preserves itself by activating anti-apoptotic pathways, and is responsible of tumor relapse. In this context, the self-renewal capability is very important to SCs; *i.e.* the one or both daughter cells -that result after cell division- that keep the ability to replicate and form the same differentiated cell lineage as the parental cell. CSCs have the capability of creating the generations of a constantly growing tumor and can either arise from the stem cells of a corresponding tissue or from mutation bearing tissue cells that dedifferentiate to become cancerous SCs [41].

3.1. Cell division in cancer stem cells

Stem cells can divide symmetrically or asymmetrically: while the symmetric division results in two new SCs; asymmetric division gives rise to a new stem cell and a daughter cell that undergoes a differentiation process. Stem cells alternate between these two division types. Asymmetric cell division is regulated by some intrinsic factors such as the specific arrangement of cell polarity and/or cell fate factors like Numb or PAR-aPKC, and by extrinsic mechanism like the stem cell niche. Thus, asymmetric division is not necessary for stem-cell identity but rather is a tool that stem cells can use to maintain appropriate numbers of progeny. The facultative use of symmetric or asymmetric divisions by stem cells may be a key adaptation that is crucial for adult regenerative capacity [42]. The result of each division is different; since symmetric cell division gives rise to induce new tumors, the machinery that promotes asymmetric cell divisions has an evolutionarily conserved role in tumor suppression [43, 44].

3.2. Regulatory mechanisms of CSCs

Regulatory proteins and pathways establish a balance between a CSC's self-renewal ability and its death by apoptosis. The WNT, SHH, NOTCH, and PI3K/AKT/mTOR signaling pathways are especially important in this regulation and are often found be impaired in tumors. The WNT signaling pathway is mainly involved in cell proliferation and differentiation. A mutation in one of its components resulting either in an up-regulation or disruption of the signaling cascade can accelerate tumorigenesis; dysregulation of the WNT pathway component E-cadherin can also lead to metastasis [45, 46]. Differentiation and self-renewal of adult SCs is usually controlled by the SHH pathway and disruption of it results in their aberrant differentiation and proliferation [47]. The NOTCH signaling pathway also regulates the differentiation, proliferation and self-renewal of adult SCs. Dysregulation of this pathway affects specific tissues and often leads to basal cell carcinoma, breast-, kidney- and prostate cancer [48-50]. In mouse models a significant inhibition of tumor growth could be achieved when the NOTCH signaling cascade was blocked [51]. The PTEN, a tumor suppressor protein with function in cell cycle regulation, is acting on the PI3K/AKT/mTOR signaling pathway. Inactivating mutations of PTEN can cause uncontrolled growth and cell division and are often found in tumors such as brain, bladder, prostate and kidney cancers [52-54].

3.3. Therapeutic approaches to target CSCs

Searching for powerful therapeutic approaches that specifically target CSCs is an accelerating area of research, after the discovery that CSCs significantly influence metastatic diseases and drug resistance. For instance, relapse is a result of a small CSCs population's survival which has self-renewal ability. If these CSCs are not exterminated by chemotherapy or targeted disruption of the SHH or NOTCH signaling pathways, they stay dormant in the target organs or bone marrow until triggered to regenerate the heterogeneous cell populations of a tumor [55]. But, attention should be focused on whether all solid tumors are sustained by CSCs and whether cell surface specific markers could be found that differentiate between normal SCs and CSCs. A great improvement will be achieved in cancer therapy when CSCs are selectively eliminated, while normal SCs are spared and thus left unaffected. Identification of a specific CSC marker in cancer of interest would simplify the development of anticancer drugs that eliminate the CSCs from the tumor cell population [56].

4. Prostate cancer stem cells

4.1. Origin of PCSCs

The origin of PCSCs continues to stay as a controversial issue. Different cells in origin may generate clinically relevant subtypes with different prognosis and outcome. There are two possible cell origin resources in PC: the basal and luminal cell-of-origin.

4.1.1. Basal cell-of-origin

Much stronger studies came from several independent laboratories that used different PC models to support the view that basal stem cells provide the cell-of-origin for PC. When CD49f^{hi}Trop2^{hi} cells were selected from the basal fraction, transfected with Akt/Erg vectors and transplanted to induce initiation of prostatic intraepithelial neoplasia [57]; these basal cells derived from primary benign human prostate tissue initiated PC in immunodeficient mice [24]. It was also reported that Lin^-Sca-1^+CD49f^{hi} cells isolated from the basal fraction of murine prostate produced luminal-like disease characteristics of human PC after transplantation [58]. Recently, Norman J. Maitland and colleagues reported that selected cells with basal phenotypes are tumor initiating and basal SCs are the source of a luminal progeny [23]. In addition, a small population of TRA-1-60$^+$ CD151$^+$ CD166$^+$ tumor initiating cells (TICs) isolated from human prostate xenograft tumors exhibited stem-like cell characteristics and recapitulated the cellular hierarchy of the original tumor in serial xenotransplantation experiments [59]. Moreover, these cells expressed basal cell markers and showed increased Nuclear factor-κB (NF-κB) signaling.

4.1.2. Luminal cell-of-origin

Luminal cells are believed to be the cells of origin for human PC, because the disease is characterized by AR$^+$ luminal cell expansion. That is why pathologists diagnose PC based on the absence of basal cell markers. It is known, that rare luminal cells which express the homeobox gene Nkx3.1 in the absence of testicular androgens (castration-resistant Nkx3.1-expressing cells, CARNs) are bipotential with self-renewal capability *in vivo* [60]. Single-cell transplantation of CARNs can reconstitute prostate ducts in renal grafts. Besides, targeted deletion of PTEN in CARNs results in rapid formation of carcinoma following androgen-mediated regeneration. Hanneke Korsten and colleagues [61] showed that genetic alterations are first seen in a subset of luminal cells expressing the progenitor markers TROP2 and SCA-1, implying that the luminal cells are the cell-of-origin in this model.

The reason why the origin of PC and the cell type of origin remains a controversial issue is in part of the distinct functional assays that were employed. Furthermore, since PC is a very heterogeneous disease it is plausible that different PCs are derived from different originating cell types.

4.2. Characterization and markers of PCSCs

Every stem cell does not express the defined markers that are used to isolate SCs from various cancerous or normal tissues. Although the CD133, CD44, SCA1 and THY1 cell surface markers are commonly used to enrich CSCs; they are also expressed in normal stem cells as well as in many non-stem cells in various tumors and tissues. Eventually, the majority of cells expressing these markers are not SCs. Apart from that, a marker that is found to be functional in identifying a SC from one tissue may not be useful for identifying the SC in another tissue. Another feasible way of identifying SCs, besides searching for specific cell surface markers, is by label retention (BrdU incorporation) assays [62]. This DNA labeling assay depends on the label retaining characteristics of the seldom dividing SCs [63]. Finally, CSCs can be isolated by the detection of a "side population (SP)" of cells that actively transport lipophilic dyes out of the cells by drug-transporting proteins [64]. Margaret A. Goodell and colleagues first observed that a small population of bone marrow-derived cells that were incubated with the lipophilic dye Hoechst 33342 failed to accumulate an appreciable amount of this dye [65]. This subpopulation was identified by dual-wavelength flow cytometry analysis as the Hoechst^{low}SP. Remarkably, the SP was highly enriched for hematopoietic stem cells. Subsequently, the SP technique was widely employed to enrich stem-like cells from solid cancers. This technique was also used for PC cells and the SP of cells derivable from this primary prostate tumors was ~1% [66]. Since the gold standard to confirm CSCs is *in vivo* tumor development, analyzed and sorted SP cells were inoculated into immune-deficient mice and tested for tumor producing ability. By this, it was found out that cell surface markers combined with SP analysis are a more accurate way in identifying the real SC population.

The density of CSCs in a tumor is probably less than 0.1% [37]. Therefore, to obtain a good yield after isolation these cells certainly should be specified first. So far, identification can be achieved *via* characteristic cell surface markers, DNA labeling, and the cells' ability to expel dyes. Table 1 presents the expression profiles of cell surface proteins that are specific for SCs or tumors. But, it should kept in mind, that many cell surface proteins are not too specific to CSCs, because they are also expressed on physiological stem cells; and thus, using antibodies to detect them can lead to false-positive results due to non-specific cross reactivity.

Tumor type	Cancer stem cell marker
Acute myeloid leukemia	CD34/CD38
Breast carcinoma	CD44/CD24-/ALDH
Bladder carcinoma	Side Population [67]
Colorectal carcinoma	CD133, CD44, EPCM, ALDH
Ewing's sarcoma	CD133
Gastric carcinoma	CD44
Medulloblastoma, Glioma	CD133
Pancreatic carcinoma	CD133, CD44, CD24, ALDH, EPCM
Prostate carcinoma	CD133, CD44, ALDH
Hepatocellular carcinoma	CD133, CD44, ALDH
Lung carcinomas (non-small cell and small cell)	CD133, Side Population [67], ALDH
Head and neck carcinoma	CD44, Side Population [67], ALDH
Endometrial carcinoma	CD133, Side Population [67]

Table 1. Established CSC markers expressed in tumors of different tissues in human [56]

4.3. Methods for assaying PCSCs

Although, a SC in any type of adult tissue has the common self-renewal and differentiation abilities, it will be wrong to generalize the results obtained from one tissue while defining a SC in another tissue. SCs in different tissues can differ significantly from one another. The actual assay to identify a CSC that has self-renewal and tumor progression capability is an *in vivo* model known as the serial transplantation in animal models. Other assays are usually generated in an *in vitro* environment and to be ideal, they have to full-fill the following criteria: they should be quantitative, highly specific in measuring only the cells of interest, sufficiently sensitive to measure candidate stem cells even at low frequencies, and fast [37].

For SC studies, human primary cells are the optimal tools to mimic and represent the original characteristics of tissues; however, it is quite difficult to get primary cell cultures from PC tissues due to limited access. Furthermore, cell lines can serve as a resource for CSC studies, but there are several disadvantages in utilization of this *in vitro* model: it cannot replicate exact *in vivo* conditions during the long-term culture process and some cell property changes might take place like gene alterations; the *in vitro* cultured cells often lose their original differentiated function; and it cannot stably maintain the exact properties of the original organ. Nevertheless, primary PC cells, established PC cell lines, xenograft and animal models have all been utilized to identify PCSCs with different surface markers.

4.3.1. *In vivo systems*

Gerald R. Cunha and Ben Lung have developed tissue recombination of a rodent model for the growth of normal epithelial cells in 1978 [68]. In this system, tissue fragments of fetal urogenital sinus mesenchyme were used to support the growth of normal prostate epithelial tissue fragments when implanted in collagen under the renal capsule of immunodeficient mice. This system was later modified to evaluate the growth activities of different prostate cell subpopulations using mechanical and enzymatic digestion to dissociate both, the urogenital sinus mesenchyme and adult murine prostate tissue into single cell suspensions [69]. Dissociated prostate epithelia regenerate ductal structures that histologically resemble normal murine prostate. Matrigel transplantation method was described that provides a reconstitution assay of prostatic cells. It was shown that the prostate contains stem cells capable of reconstituting the whole prostate and this method can be used to analyze prostate stem cells, epithelial mesenchymal interactions, and prostate cancer stem cells [70]. Ken Goto and colleagues performed serial transplantation that was analogous to the serial reconstitution method to investigate PSCs self-renewal [71]. They showed that regenerated prostate tissue could be dissociated and transplanted to regenerate prostate tissue at least three times.

4.3.2. *In vitro culture systems and assays*

There are two types of culture system to study CSCs: primary cell cultures and cell lines. Primary cell cultures are directly established from human tissues and have the advantage that their cells represent the original features of the tissue. However, difficulties including the limited access to biopsy materials, the need for the exclusion of contamination by cancer or normal cells, their limited lifespan, and the small population of the putative SCs are its disadvantages [72]. Cell lines are permanent cell cultures with unlimited proliferation capacity. They are widely used in many aspects of research as the most common *in vitro* culture model, because they have a big advantage in being easy to handle for their infinite reproducible quantities. So far, most of the human PC cell lines have been established from metastatic lesions or from xenograft tumors.

Prostate colony assay: The clonal and population analyses of mammalian stem cells was first accomplished by using two dimensional culture conditions [73]. Co-culture with irradiated fibroblast feeder layer is now also used to cultivate human prostate epithelial cells. In this assay, the feeder layer contains serum free medium (but, growth factors added) and low calcium [74]. Under these conditions, murine prostate epithelial cells form colonies of cells that express epithelial cytokeratins when cultured with irradiated 3T3 feeder cells [28].

Prostate sphere assay: Colonies that are derived from primitive cells cannot be passaged efficiently, since culture conditions promote cell differentiation. The three dimensional sphere is a non-adherent culture system that has been used as a useful model to elucidate stem cell characteristics [75]. A suspension culture system like this is thought to keep cancer stem cells in their undifferentiated state facilitating their enrichment; like for AR-negative and AR-positive PC cell lines that both can form prostaspheres [76]. Actually, all PC cell lines can form prostaspheres; but, because heterogeneity exists only a subpopulation of cells in each cell line can form these prostaspheres. The expression of stem cell markers, such as CD133 and CD44, is also significantly enhanced in a prostasphere.

In contrast to the suspension sphere culture systems 3-D culture in Matrigel, which is a widely used commercially available basement membrane, has been demonstrated to promote the differentiation of PSCs. It was possible to induce morphological and phenotypical differentiation in normal and malignant prostate epithelial cell lines with Matrigel [72].

4.4. Alterations in signaling pathways of PCSCs

Alterations in the signaling pathways are probably one of the reasons why cancer stem cells gain a tumorigenic potential. Thus, disclosing the signaling pathways' expressional regulations might provide potential therapeutic targets. The WNT, JAK/STAT, NF-κB, NOTCH, and PI3K/AKT/mTOR signaling pathways were found to be the regulators of CSC biology in prostate tissue and therefore are candidate targets. The idea of inhibiting signaling that induces proliferation and survival could mean an effective therapy for PC [77].

Proteins acting in the WNT signaling pathway are usually over-expressed in PCSCs. Hence, tumorigenesis is promoted and prostaspheres which have self-renewal capacity exhibit proliferation, differentiation, and heterogeneous expression of stem cell-associated markers such as CD44, ABCG2 and CD133. When WNT inhibitors are applied the size of prostaspheres and their self-renewal ability can be reduced; plus, the CD133 and CD44 expressions are down-regulated. WNT activity also regulates the self-renewal capacity of PC cells that have stem cell-like features and inhibition of WNT signaling potentially reduces the self-renewal ability of PCSCs with an enviable therapeutic outcome [76].

The JAK/STAT signaling pathway seems to be important in PCSC biology. Than, when PCSCs expressing aldehyde dehydrogenase ($ALDH^+$), which is involved in the formation of bone metastasis, were treated *via* a galiellactone- a specific STAT3 signaling inhibitor-; apoptosis of cancerous cells could be induced [78]. Besides, *in vivo* targeting of STAT3 in a drug treated DU145 xenograft gave also desired results. Therefore, targeting of JAK/STAT signaling pathway components might be a promising therapeutic resulting in ALDH1A1 expressional down-regulation in PSCSs [78]. The importance of the NF-κB signaling pathway came up after the finding of enhanced functional signaling in purified naïve stem-like human prostatic TICs. When cells were treated with small molecular inhibitors that targeted the NF-κB signaling pathway secondary sphere formation *in vitro* and tumor-initiation *in vivo* could be inhibited [59].

Cell fate specification, initiation of differentiation, and SC maintenance is regulated by the NOTCH signaling pathway in many tissues [79]. The over-expression of various proteins that function in the NOTCH signaling cascade has been found in a number of different tumors including PC. For example JAGGED-1, a NOTCH receptor ligand, has been found to be significantly more expressed in metastatic PC when compared with localized PC or benign prostatic tissue samples. This up-regulation also correlated with clinical features like recurrence, progression and metastasis of PC [80]. When Jagged-1 expression was down-regulated with small interfering RNAs (siRNAs) cell growth was inhibited and cell cycle arrest achieved in the S phase of cell division [81].

The PI3K/AKT/mTOR signaling pathway member PTEN was first identified as a candidate tumor suppressor gene that was frequently mutated in brain, breast, and prostate tumors [82]. Introduction of PTEN into cancer cells that lack PTEN function down-regulated cell migration and survival, and induced cell cycle arrest and apoptosis [82]. PTEN is the most mutated gene in metastatic PC that is advanced and has an aggressive tumor phenotype; and has been associated with cancer progression in 30–60% of PC cases [83]. An association between androgen-independent tumor growth and PTEN mutations has also been discovered [84]. A number of mouse models for PC suggested that PTEN might play a role in the initiation or early progression of this disease. PTEN heterozygous mice are likely to develop epithelial dysplasia and hyperplasia resembling high-grade PIN and adenocarcinoma [53, 85]. While PTEN mutations lead to a predisposition for PC in mouse models, such an association could not be shown for human yet [83, 84].

4.5. Endocrine effects on PCSCs

In PC, the stromal niche or microenvironment plays a critical role in regulating differentiation of CSCs, probably by altered endocrine and/or paracrine signaling. Direct androgen binding to epithelial ARs is not required for epithelial differentiation, but is essential for the induction and maintenance of a secretory activity [11].

AR is a member of the steroid hormone receptor family and its over-expression is involved prostate tumorigenesis. Consequently, androgen deprivation therapy (ADT) has been used to treat locally advanced and metastatic PC [86]. Despite initial regression of the tumor the majority of patients inevitably develop castrate-resistant prostate cancer (CRPC), which establishes metastases relatively rapidly and is subsequently incurable by current treatment strategies. Mouse model studies revealed that androgen ablation can select for more aggressive and metastatic disease, which means that current hormonal therapies do not affect the AR^--CSCs [87]. ADT may promote disease progression by causing an increase in the castrate-resistant SC pool and/or activating quiescent SCs to repopulate the tumor with androgen-independent SCs. Vander *et al.* reported that unlike normal adult human prostate SCs, $CD133^+$ PCSCs are AR^+ and suggested that AR^+ prostate TICs are derived from a malignantly transformed intermediate cell that acquired "stem-like activity". The AR signaling pathway might therefore comprise another therapeutic target, especially for prostate TICs [88].

In addition to androgens, estrogens play key roles in prostate carcinogenesis and progression. However, the mechanisms are not fully understood. Although there is still no direct evidence that estrogens initiate PC in humans, there is accumulating evidence pointing towards a central role for estrogens in PC [89]. To give just some examples are the rising E2:T ratio in aging men, association of estrogen metabolizing gene polymorphisms and elevated urine hydroxy-estrone ratios with higher PC risk, progressive increase in aromatase expression in PCs upon advancement to metastatic disease, and marked alterations in estrogen receptor expression with cancer progression. Normal human prostate progenitor cells are responsive to estrogens with increased rates of self-renewal, implicating them as direct estrogen targets.

The importance of estrogen receptor (ER) expression, *e.g.* ERα and ERβ, is unknown; but, is of interest based on the integral role of estrogens in prostate carcinogenesis. The expression of ERα is low and hard to detect in prostatic epithelial cells, where ERβ is predominantly expressed. An ERβ agonist compound could selectively induce apoptosis in castrate-resistant CD133$^+$ basal cells, providing a rationale for further exploring the role of ERβ in PC and PCSCs [90].

Prolactin (PRL) is a peptide hormone that is secreted by the pituitary gland. It regulates several physiological functions, many of which relate to male and female reproduction. In humans PRL is also produced by prostate epithelial cells under normal physiological conditions. Local PRL profoundly affects the prostate epithelial compartment, with dramatic expansion of basal and stem-like epithelial cells, markedly enhanced epithelial cell proliferation, and strong activation of the STAT5 pathway as three hallmarks of tumorigenesis [91].

4.6. Potential role of PCSCs in metastasis

PC is the second leading cause of cancer death in male; but, because of the progress made in the diagnosis and treatment of primary PC, mortality in 70 - 80% of the patients is increasingly linked to its metastatic disease. The bone marrow is the most frequent site for metastasis in PC; and stem cells, besides their role in tumorigenicity, are highly migratory cells that are involved in bone metastasis formation [92].

CSCs contain a subpopulation of cells that are exclusively capable of disseminating and subsequently providing the substrate for tumor metastasis; *e.g.* CD44$^+$ PC cells are more tumorigenic and metastatic than the corresponding CD44$^-$ cells [93]. Stromal cell derived factor and its C-X-C chemokine receptor type 4 (CXCR4) form a critical regulatory axis for SC migration, engraftment and homing, and also function in the metastasis of breast and prostate cancer [94]. Using a mouse/human comparative translational genomics approach an 11-gene signature that consistently displays a stem cell–like expression pattern in metastatic lesions of prostate carcinomas could be recovered from multiple distant target organs [95].

On the other hand, some incidents do not support the CSC involvement in metastasis. For example, CD44$^+$CD24$^-$ and CD44$^+$CD24$^+$ breast CSCs have same metastatic potential [96]. Then, in an orthotopic pancreatic cancer model CD133$^+$ cells were not metastatic, whereas CD133$^+$CXCR4$^+$ cells showed strong metastasis [97]. Also, CD133$^-$ colon cancer cells were more aggressive and metastatic than their CD133$^+$ counterparts [98]. In conclusion, metastasis and tumor initiation might be processed by distinct cancer cell populations, probably by metastatic CSCs.

Tumor microenvironment facilitates cancer metastasis by several mechanisms. When human PC cells were injected into the dorsal prostate of a nude mouse more metastasis was generated, than when cells were injected subcutaneous [99]. Later, it was shown that dorsal prostate-implanted human PC cells over-express many CSC genes including osteoponin, CXCR4, CD133, ABCG2, CD44 and CD24. Some of these genes clearly have functional roles in PC metastasis [100]. But, the exact molecular mechanisms that account for the microenvironment regulated PC cell metastasis are still not known.

4.7. MicroRNA-mediated regulation of PCSCs

For the identification of novel PC therapeutic targets it is important to evaluate functional genes that are related with CSCs self-renewal and survival abilities. The experiences with PC therapy showed that PC recurs frequently; meaning that chemotherapy, radiotherapy, androgen-ablation therapy, and radical prostatectomy are not sufficient enough to eliminate TICs or metastatic cells. PCSCs are androgen independent and therapy resistant cells. Thus, generating novel therapies that specifically target PCSCs may be more effective than those that target differentiated PC cells. New approaches depend on CSC exterminating rather than total tumor decay. The limitation for these studies is to be able to specifically target CSCs in normal tissue that also contains its specific SCs; since, they have similar expressional and antigenic profiles [101]. Consequently, new markers are needed to distinguish CSCs from tissue specific SCs. microRNAs (miRNA) can be considered as such novel therapeutic target molecules for distinguishing PCSCs from normal SCs. MicroRNAs are 21- to 25-nucleotide (nt)–long, noncoding RNAs that induce the target mRNA degradation or repress mRNA translation by imperfect binding to their 3'-untranslated region (UTR) [102].

Depending on their expressional profiles and their target-mRNA types miRNAs can be divided into two classes: one that act like oncogenes (oncomiRs) and the other that act like tumor suppressor genes. OncomiRs are commonly up-regulated in tumors and target tumor suppressor mRNA transcripts, causing a decrease of tumor suppressor protein syntheses and thus function. Tumor suppressor miRNAs on the other hand are mostly down-regulated in tumors and therefore cannot target and inhibit the syntheses of the specific oncogene mRNA transcripts into oncoproteins. When tumor suppressor miRNAs are experimentally over-expressed in cancer cells they inhibit their proliferation, invasion and proliferation capacity [103].

Expression profiling of miRNAs in PC have showed that some miRNAs were significantly up- or down-regulated when compared to normal prostate tissue, pointing to the importance of miRNAs in tumor progression and pathogenesis; *e.g.* miR-34a and miR-34c were found to have an important role in AR-dependent and p53-mediated apoptosis [104, 105]. miR-125b was an up-regulated miRNA in clinical PC samples and androgen independent cell lines; thus, its up-regulation might be related with androgen-independence and survival [103]. Another up-regulated miRNA in PC was miR-21; but, it affected tumorigenesis, invasion and metastasis by inhibiting the synthesis of proteins that normally function in these

http://dx.doi.org/10.5772/52289

pathways. miR-21 also inhibits apoptosis [103]; and, contributes to drug resistance of PC to docetaxel treatment [106, 107]. miR-148a was defined as an androgen-responsive microRNA that promoted growth when up-regulated in the PC cell line LNCaP and one if its mRNA targets was found to be the cullin associated and neddylation-dissociated 1 (CAND1) transcript, coding for a tumor suppressor protein [108].

In contrast, miRNAs like miR-15a and miR-16-1 were found to be down-regulated in PC; their over-expression achieved by intra-cell delivery methods showed significant tumor regression capacity *in vivo* [103]. Other down-regulated miRNAs with tumor suppressor function in PC were miR-125b, miR-99a, miR-99b and miR-100. Again, when their expressions were restored, PSA expressions could be reduced and PC cell proliferation was inhibited [109].

miR-145 and miR-143 are tumor suppressor miRNAs that are commonly dysregulated in all cancer types. miR-145 and miR143 are also first transcribed together on a cluster and cleaved off during the miRNA maturation process. In PC miR-145 is down-regulated and over-expression of it has an anti-tumorigenic effect, resulting with the inhibition of migration and invasion of PC cells [103].

Some miRNAs take part in formation of androgen-independent PC; and, by comparing androgen-dependent and -independent PC samples, miR-146a has been revealed as such [110]. Finally, an example of a miRNA that is regulated by its target is miR-34a. The tumor suppressor and transcription factor p53 directly regulates the expression of miR-34a, which is decreased in $CD44^+$ PC cells. When normally expressed it could inhibit PC regeneration and metastasis by directly repressing CD44 [111, 112]. The list of miRNAs which expressions are most significantly altered in PC are given in Table 2.

4.8. New therapeutic approaches in targeting PCSCs

Despite progress in the therapeutic approaches that significantly increased the survival rate of PC patients, most prostate aggressive tumors become resistant to currently used treatment protocols. PC that initially responded well to a standard chemotherapy often recur with selective outgrowth of tumor cell subpopulations and get resistant not only to the original chemotherapeutic agent but also to other therapeutics. Thus, for most patients with relapse of castration-resistant metastatic PC currently no curative treatment exists. It has been suggested that AR expression in PC is modulated by CSCs and the CSC model may be responsible for the degree of sensitivity to anti-androgen therapy [114], [115].

The majority of studies to date have focused on the identification of characteristics that potentially could define CSCs. However, more questions have been raised on the issue which of these characteristics would be better suited as target and now research has seemed to shift towards identifying the way these CSCs behave that make them different from bulk tumor cells. Two important features of acute myeloid leukemia (AML) that allowed to discovery of new therapeutic agents were $CD34^+/CD38^-$ and $CD33^+$. Anti-CD33 antibodies have become an important aspect of CSCs targeted therapy. A drug called Gemtuzumab ozogamacin or Mylotarg, approved by the FDA in 2000, combines the cytotoxic antibiotic calicheamicin with the monoclonal anti-CD33 antibody [116].

Androgen-Independent miRNAs	
Up-regulated	*Down-regulated*
miR-184	miR-128b
miR-361	miR-221
miR-424	miR-222
miR-616	miR-146a/b
	miR-148a
	miR-663
Cancer Stem Cell, Invasion or Metastasis Related miRNAs	
Up-regulated	*Down-regulated*
miR-377	miR-34a
miR-141	miR-143
	miR-145
	miR-15
	miR-16
Common Cancer Related miRNAs	
Up-regulated	*Down-regulated*
miR-182	miR-125b
miR-96	miR-15a/16-1
miR-375	miR-34a
	miR-205
	miR-145
	miR-221
	miR-222
	miR-181b
	miR-31
	miR-200c

Table 2. Up- and down-regulated microRNAs in postate cancer [113]

Novel therapeutic strategies against locally advanced and/or metastatic hormone-refractory prostate cancers (HRPCs) by targeting different oncogenic signaling cascade elements are listed in Table 3. Recent studies have revealed that the blockade of these tumorigenic signaling cascades could be beneficial as adjuvant therapy in the early phases of PC for decreasing the risk of relapse as well as in the late stages for improving the efficacy of current androgen deprivation therapy, radiotherapy, and/or systemic chemotherapy and patient survival rates [117]. Inhibition of the epidermal growth factor (EGFR) pathway by anti-EGFR antibody or EGFR tyrosine kinase inhibitor causes a cell cycle arrest, inhibits invasion and/ or induces apoptosis in metastatic PC cells when applied *in vitro* or *in vivo* [118-120]. Blockade of the SHH signaling pathway, which is important in stem cell self-renewal, by cyclopamine leads to long-term PC regression without recurrence, strongly suggesting a connection between this pathway and PCSCs [121]. Salinomycin, a structurally related compound to monensin, was recently identified as a potent PCSC inhibitor [122]. It inhibited the growth of PCs, but did not affect non-malignant prostate epithelial cells. That salinomycin impaired PCSC growth and function was evident by the findings of reduced $CD44^+$ cell fraction and ALDH activity. Moreover, salinomycin reduced the expression of MYC, AR and ERG; induced oxidative stress; and, inhibited NF-κB activity and cell migration.

Regulation of the cell cycle is frequently altered in PC, in part, by the interplay of activation of oncogenic cascades with diverse hormones, growth factors, and cytokines. Thus, inhibitors of cell cycle regulatory proteins have become an area of increased interest in targeting CSCs [123]. The cyclin-dependent kinase inhibitor VMY-1-103 inhibited at very low concentrations the Erb-2/Erb-3/heregulin-induced cell proliferation in LNCaP PC cells. [124]. It was also observed that VMY-1-103 induced apoptosis *via* decreased mitochondrial membrane polarity; and induced p53 phosphorylation, caspase-3 activation, and PARP cleavage in these PC cells, which do express endogen wild type p53. But, VMY-1-103 failed to induce apoptosis in the p53-null PC cell line PC3 [124]. These results, strongly suggest that VMY-1-103 may be an effective therapeutic agent, either alone or in combinations with other drugs, in treating PC.

Adhesion receptors of the integrin family, particularly α_v-integrins, have functions including bone homing by cancer cells, tumor-induced angiogenesis, and osteoclastic bone resorption. Targeting of integrins by an α_v-integrin antagonist (GLPG0187) could inhibit the *de novo* formation and progression of bone metastases in PC by antitumor (including inhibition of epithelial-to-mesenchymal transition and the size of the PCSC population), antiresorptive, and antiangiogenic mechanisms [125].

Targeting the local microenvironment niche and stromal components of the CSCs would comprise two other promising therapeutic approaches. For instance, it is known that particularly the combined use of antiangiogenic agents with cytotoxic drugs inhibits tumor growth and invasion. Combining docetaxel with the EGFR-targeting agent cetuximab and the antiangiogenic agent sunitinib (SUTENT) inhibits tumor growth approximately 50% at the end of the 3rd week dosing schedule [126]. Targeting the fibroblast-to-myofibroblast transition with halofuginone (inhibitor of collagen type I) may also synergize with low doses of chemotherapy in achieving a significant antitumor effect, avoiding the need of high-dose chemotherapy and its toxicity without impairing treatment efficacy [57]. These results all support the idea that targeting PCSCs, their further differentiated progenies, and microenvironment could be more effective to counteract PC transition to invasive and metastatic stages.

Target	Effect	Molecules	Reference
EGFR signaling pathway	Anti-EGFR antibody	Cetuximab, Erbitux, mAb-C225, IMCC225	[118, 120]
	EGFR tyrosine kinase inhibitor	Gefinib, Erlotinib, EKB-569	
SHH signaling pathway	Signaling inhibition	GDC-0449	[127]
		Cyclopamine	[121]
		Anti-SHH antibody	[128]
Cell signaling pathway	Reducing ALDH activity and CD44+ cell fraction	Salinomycin	[122]
STAT3 signaling pathway	STAT3 signaling inhibitor	Galiellalactone	[78]
WNT/β-Catenin signaling pathway	Suppression of the WNT co-receptor LRP6 expression	Silibinin	[129]
Cell cycle	Cyclin-dependent kinase inhibitor	VMY-1-103	[124]
Adhesion receptors	α_v-integrin antagonist	GLPG0187	[125]
Niche and stromal components	Collagen type I inhibitor	Halofuginone	[57]
	Anti-angiogenic agent	Sunitinib, SUTENT	[126]
	Telomerase reverse transcriptase (hTERT) promoter-induced CXCR4 knockdown	siRNA	[130]

Table 3. Novel targets for therapy against advanced prostate cancer

5. Conclusion

Despite all recent developments in cancer diagnosis and therapy, PC still remains one of the leading causes of cancer related deaths in men. Nevertheless, designed new tools for precise diagnosis will enable researchers to distinguish patients "who will be recurred earlier, but will require more extensive treatments" from those "who will have lifespan less effected from their disease". Unlike some other solid tumors, PC is one of these tumor types in which limited treatment options are available so far and gain of drug-resistance is seen more often. That is why there is an urgent need for alternative and novel therapies.

CSCs are believed to be a subpopulation of cancer cells that modulate malignancy and show resistance to current anticancer treatments, which make them indicators of poor prognosis. There are still many aspects of CSCs that remain to be discovered; like, which main mechanisms regulate normal SC function and how are they used by malignant cells to propagate the disease? A careful dissection of the main differences between normal adult SCs and CSCs as well as of their overlapping aspects are important to distinguish how cancers proceed. Transforming the gained knowledge in CSC biology into effective therapies would then help patients to regain their health much earlier. Altogether, that is the reason why the relation between the expressed CSC markers and resulting malignant behavior needs to be sufficiently understood, as they are primarily relevant with the prognosis of cancer.

Author details

Vildan Bozok Çetintaş, Burçin Tezcanlı Kaymaz and Buket Kosova

Department of Medical Biology, Ege University Medical Faculty, Izmir, Turkey

References

[1] Jemal A, Bray F, Center MM, Ferlay J, Ward E,Forman D. Global cancer statistics. CA Cancer J Clin 2011;61: 69-90.

[2] Becker AJ, Mc CE,Till JE. Cytological demonstration of the clonal nature of spleen colonies derived from transplanted mouse marrow cells. Nature 1963;197: 452-4.

[3] Bonnet D,Dick JE. Human acute myeloid leukemia is organized as a hierarchy that originates from a primitive hematopoietic cell. Nat Med 1997;3: 730-7.

[4] Mikkers H,Frisen J. Deconstructing stemness. EMBO J 2005;24: 2715-9.

[5] Liu AY, True LD, LaTray L, Nelson PS, Ellis WJ, Vessella RL, Lange PH, Hood L,van den Engh G. Cell-cell interaction in prostate gene regulation and cytodifferentiation. Proc Natl Acad Sci U S A 1997;94: 10705-10.

[6] Signoretti S, Waltregny D, Dilks J, Isaac B, Lin D, Garraway L, Yang A, Montironi R, McKeon F,Loda M. p63 is a prostate basal cell marker and is required for prostate development. Am J Pathol 2000;157: 1769-75.

[7] van Leenders GJ, Gage WR, Hicks JL, van Balken B, Aalders TW, Schalken JA,De Marzo AM. Intermediate cells in human prostate epithelium are enriched in proliferative inflammatory atrophy. Am J Pathol 2003;162: 1529-37.

[8] Sherwood ER, Theyer G, Steiner G, Berg LA, Kozlowski JM,Lee C. Differential expression of specific cytokeratin polypeptides in the basal and luminal epithelia of the human prostate. Prostate 1991;18: 303-14.

[9] Bonkhoff H, Stein U,Remberger K. The proliferative function of basal cells in the normal and hyperplastic human prostate. Prostate 1994;24: 114-8.

[10] Palapattu GS, Wu C, Silvers CR, Martin HB, Williams K, Salamone L, Bushnell T, Huang LS, Yang Q,Huang J. Selective expression of CD44, a putative prostate cancer stem cell marker, in neuroendocrine tumor cells of human prostate cancer. Prostate 2009;69: 787-98.

[11] Taylor RA, Toivanen R,Risbridger GP. Stem cells in prostate cancer: treating the root of the problem. Endocr Relat Cancer 2010;17: R273-85.

[12] Berry PA, Maitland NJ,Collins AT. Androgen receptor signalling in prostate: effects of stromal factors on normal and cancer stem cells. Mol Cell Endocrinol 2008;288: 30-7.

[13] Goldstein AS, Stoyanova T,Witte ON. Primitive origins of prostate cancer: in vivo evidence for prostate-regenerating cells and prostate cancer-initiating cells. Mol Oncol 2010;4: 385-96.

[14] English HF, Santen RJ,Isaacs JT. Response of glandular versus basal rat ventral prostatic epithelial cells to androgen withdrawal and replacement. Prostate 1987;11: 229-42.

[15] Montpetit M, Abrahams P, Clark AF,Tenniswood M. Androgen-independent epithelial cells of the rat ventral prostate. Prostate 1988;12: 13-28.

[16] Evans GS,Chandler JA. Cell proliferation studies in the rat prostate: II. The effects of castration and androgen-induced regeneration upon basal and secretory cell proliferation. Prostate 1987;11: 339-51.

[17] Wang S, Garcia AJ, Wu M, Lawson DA, Witte ON,Wu H. Pten deletion leads to the expansion of a prostatic stem/progenitor cell subpopulation and tumor initiation. Proc Natl Acad Sci U S A 2006;103: 1480-5.

[18] De Marzo AM, Nelson WG, Meeker AK,Coffey DS. Stem cell features of benign and malignant prostate epithelial cells. J Urol 1998;160: 2381-92.

[19] De Marzo AM, Meeker AK, Epstein JI,Coffey DS. Prostate stem cell compartments: expression of the cell cycle inhibitor p27Kip1 in normal, hyperplastic, and neoplastic cells. Am J Pathol 1998;153: 911-9.

[20] Tsujimura A, Koikawa Y, Salm S, Takao T, Coetzee S, Moscatelli D, Shapiro E, Lepor H, Sun TT,Wilson EL. Proximal location of mouse prostate epithelial stem cells: a model of prostatic homeostasis. J Cell Biol 2002;157: 1257-65.

[21] Kurita T, Medina RT, Mills AA,Cunha GR. Role of p63 and basal cells in the prostate. Development 2004;131: 4955-64.

[22] Richardson GD, Robson CN, Lang SH, Neal DE, Maitland NJ,Collins AT. CD133, a novel marker for human prostatic epithelial stem cells. J Cell Sci 2004;117: 3539-45.

[23] Maitland NJ, Frame FM, Polson ES, Lewis JL,Collins AT. Prostate cancer stem cells: do they have a basal or luminal phenotype? Horm Cancer 2011;2: 47-61.

[24] Goldstein AS, Huang J, Guo C, Garraway IP,Witte ON. Identification of a cell of origin for human prostate cancer. Science 2010;329: 568-71.

[25] Collins AT, Habib FK, Maitland NJ,Neal DE. Identification and isolation of human prostate epithelial stem cells based on alpha(2)beta(1)-integrin expression. J Cell Sci 2001;114: 3865-72.

[26] Burger PE, Xiong X, Coetzee S, Salm SN, Moscatelli D, Goto K,Wilson EL. Sca-1 expression identifies stem cells in the proximal region of prostatic ducts with high capacity to reconstitute prostatic tissue. Proc Natl Acad Sci U S A 2005;102: 7180-5.

[27] Xin L, Lawson DA,Witte ON. The Sca-1 cell surface marker enriches for a prostate-regenerating cell subpopulation that can initiate prostate tumorigenesis. Proc Natl Acad Sci U S A 2005;102: 6942-7.

[28] Lawson DA, Xin L, Lukacs RU, Cheng D,Witte ON. Isolation and functional characterization of murine prostate stem cells. Proc Natl Acad Sci U S A 2007;104: 181-6.

[29] Knox JD, Cress AE, Clark V, Manriquez L, Affinito KS, Dalkin BL,Nagle RB. Differential expression of extracellular matrix molecules and the alpha 6-integrins in the normal and neoplastic prostate. Am J Pathol 1994;145: 167-74.

[30] Habermann H, Ray V, Habermann W,Prins GS. Alterations in gap junction protein expression in human benign prostatic hyperplasia and prostate cancer. J Urol 2002;167: 655-60.

[31] Cunha GR, Alarid ET, Turner T, Donjacour AA, Boutin EL,Foster BA. Normal and abnormal development of the male urogenital tract. Role of androgens, mesenchymal-epithelial interactions, and growth factors. J Androl 1992;13: 465-75.

[32] Wang XD, Leow CC, Zha J, Tang Z, Modrusan Z, Radtke F, Aguet M, de Sauvage FJ,Gao WQ. Notch signaling is required for normal prostatic epithelial cell proliferation and differentiation. Dev Biol 2006;290: 66-80.

[33] Salm SN, Burger PE, Coetzee S, Goto K, Moscatelli D,Wilson EL. TGF-{beta} maintains dormancy of prostatic stem cells in the proximal region of ducts. J Cell Biol 2005;170: 81-90.

[34] Virchow R. Cellular pathology. Arch Pathol Anat Physiol Klin Med 1855;8: 3-39.

[35] J. Furth KM. The transmission of leukemia in mice with a single cell. Am J Cancer Res 1937;31: 276-82.

[36] Al-Hajj M, Wicha MS, Benito-Hernandez A, Morrison SJ,Clarke MF. Prospective identification of tumorigenic breast cancer cells. Proc Natl Acad Sci U S A 2003;100: 3983-8.

[37] Moltzahn FR, Volkmer JP, Rottke D,Ackermann R. "Cancer stem cells"-lessons from Hercules to fight the Hydra. Urol Oncol 2008;26: 581-9.

[38] Bruce WR,Van Der Gaag H. A Quantitative Assay for the Number of Murine Lymphoma Cells Capable of Proliferation in Vivo. Nature 1963;199: 79-80.

[39] Hamburger AW,Salmon SE. Primary bioassay of human tumor stem cells. Science 1977;197: 461-3.

[40] Sabbath KD, Ball ED, Larcom P, Davis RB,Griffin JD. Heterogeneity of clonogenic cells in acute myeloblastic leukemia. J Clin Invest 1985;75: 746-53.

[41] Clarke MF,Becker MW. Stem cells: the real culprits in cancer? Sci Am 2006;295: 52-9.

[42] Morrison SJ,Kimble J. Asymmetric and symmetric stem-cell divisions in development and cancer. Nature 2006;441: 1068-74.

[43] Clevers H. Stem cells, asymmetric division and cancer. Nat Genet 2005;37: 1027-8.

[44] Humbert P, Russell S,Richardson H. Dlg, Scribble and Lgl in cell polarity, cell proliferation and cancer. Bioessays 2003;25: 542-53.

[45] Menke A, Philippi C, Vogelmann R, Seidel B, Lutz MP, Adler G,Wedlich D. Downregulation of E-cadherin gene expression by collagen type I and type III in pancreatic cancer cell lines. Cancer Res 2001;61: 3508-17.

[46] Reya T,Clevers H. Wnt signalling in stem cells and cancer. Nature 2005;434: 843-50.

[47] Taipale J,Beachy PA. The Hedgehog and Wnt signalling pathways in cancer. Nature 2001;411: 349-54.

[48] Gallahan D,Callahan R. Mammary tumorigenesis in feral mice: identification of a new int locus in mouse mammary tumor virus (Czech II)-induced mammary tumors. J Virol 1987;61: 66-74.

[49] Reedijk M, Odorcic S, Chang L, Zhang H, Miller N, McCready DR, Lockwood G,Egan SE. High-level coexpression of JAG1 and NOTCH1 is observed in human breast cancer and is associated with poor overall survival. Cancer Res 2005;65: 8530-7.

[50] Sjolund J, Manetopoulos C, Stockhausen MT,Axelson H. The Notch pathway in cancer: differentiation gone awry. Eur J Cancer 2005;41: 2620-9.

[51] Sjolund J, Johansson M, Manna S, Norin C, Pietras A, Beckman S, Nilsson E, Ljungberg B,Axelson H. Suppression of renal cell carcinoma growth by inhibition of Notch signaling in vitro and in vivo. J Clin Invest 2008;118: 217-28.

[52] Cantley LC,Neel BG. New insights into tumor suppression: PTEN suppresses tumor formation by restraining the phosphoinositide 3-kinase/AKT pathway. Proc Natl Acad Sci U S A 1999;96: 4240-5.

[53] Di Cristofano A,Pandolfi PP. The multiple roles of PTEN in tumor suppression. Cell 2000;100: 387-90.

[54] Tsuruta H, Kishimoto H, Sasaki T, Horie Y, Natsui M, Shibata Y, Hamada K, Yajima N, Kawahara K, Sasaki M, Tsuchiya N, Enomoto K, Mak TW, Nakano T, Habuchi T,Suzuki A. Hyperplasia and carcinomas in Pten-deficient mice and reduced PTEN protein in human bladder cancer patients. Cancer Res 2006;66: 8389-96.

[55] Kasper S. Exploring the origins of the normal prostate and prostate cancer stem cell. Stem Cell Rev 2008;4: 193-201.

[56] Kasper S. Identification, characterization, and biological relevance of prostate cancer stem cells from clinical specimens. Urol Oncol 2009;27: 301-3.

[57] Sheffer Y, Leon O, Pinthus JH, Nagler A, Mor Y, Genin O, Iluz M, Kawada N, Yoshizato K,Pines M. Inhibition of fibroblast to myofibroblast transition by halofuginone contributes to the chemotherapy-mediated antitumoral effect. Mol Cancer Ther 2007;6: 570-7.

[58] Lawson DA, Zong Y, Memarzadeh S, Xin L, Huang J,Witte ON. Basal epithelial stem cells are efficient targets for prostate cancer initiation. Proc Natl Acad Sci U S A 2010;107: 2610-5.

[59] Rajasekhar VK, Studer L, Gerald W, Socci ND,Scher HI. Tumour-initiating stem-like cells in human prostate cancer exhibit increased NF-kappaB signalling. Nat Commun 2011;2: 162.

[60] Wang X, Kruithof-de Julio M, Economides KD, Walker D, Yu H, Halili MV, Hu YP, Price SM, Abate-Shen C,Shen MM. A luminal epithelial stem cell that is a cell of origin for prostate cancer. Nature 2009;461: 495-500.

[61] Korsten H, Ziel-van der Made A, Ma X, van der Kwast T,Trapman J. Accumulating progenitor cells in the luminal epithelial cell layer are candidate tumor initiating cells in a Pten knockout mouse prostate cancer model. PLoS One 2009;4: e5662.

[62] Clarke MF, Dick JE, Dirks PB, Eaves CJ, Jamieson CH, Jones DL, Visvader J, Weissman IL,Wahl GM. Cancer stem cells--perspectives on current status and future directions: AACR Workshop on cancer stem cells. Cancer Res 2006;66: 9339-44.

[63] Lee JT,Herlyn M. Old disease, new culprit: tumor stem cells in cancer. J Cell Physiol 2007;213: 603-9.

[64] Hirschmann-Jax C, Foster AE, Wulf GG, Nuchtern JG, Jax TW, Gobel U, Goodell MA,Brenner MK. A distinct "side population" of cells with high drug efflux capacity in human tumor cells. Proc Natl Acad Sci U S A 2004;101: 14228-33.

[65] Goodell MA, Brose K, Paradis G, Conner AS,Mulligan RC. Isolation and functional properties of murine hematopoietic stem cells that are replicating in vivo. J Exp Med 1996;183: 1797-806.

[66] Bhatt RI, Brown MD, Hart CA, Gilmore P, Ramani VA, George NJ,Clarke NW. Novel method for the isolation and characterisation of the putative prostatic stem cell. Cytometry A 2003;54: 89-99.

[67] Gurden MD, Holland AJ, van Zon W, Tighe A, Vergnolle MA, Andres DA, Spielmann HP, Malumbres M, Wolthuis RM, Cleveland DW,Taylor SS. Cdc20 is required for the post-anaphase, KEN-dependent degradation of centromere protein F. J Cell Sci 2010;123: 321-30.

[68] Cunha GR,Lung B. The possible influence of temporal factors in androgenic responsiveness of urogenital tissue recombinants from wild-type and androgen-insensitive (Tfm) mice. J Exp Zool 1978;205: 181-93.

[69] Xin L, Ide H, Kim Y, Dubey P,Witte ON. In vivo regeneration of murine prostate from dissociated cell populations of postnatal epithelia and urogenital sinus mesenchyme. Proc Natl Acad Sci U S A 2003;100 Suppl 1: 11896-903.

[70] Azuma M, Hirao A, Takubo K, Hamaguchi I, Kitamura T,Suda T. A quantitative matrigel assay for assessing repopulating capacity of prostate stem cells. Biochem Biophys Res Commun 2005;338: 1164-70.

[71] Goto K, Salm SN, Coetzee S, Xiong X, Burger PE, Shapiro E, Lepor H, Moscatelli D,Wilson EL. Proximal prostatic stem cells are programmed to regenerate a proximal-distal ductal axis. Stem Cells 2006;24: 1859-68.

[72] Miki J,Rhim JS. Prostate cell cultures as in vitro models for the study of normal stem cells and cancer stem cells. Prostate Cancer Prostatic Dis 2008;11: 32-9.

[73] Reynolds BA,Weiss S. Clonal and population analyses demonstrate that an EGF-responsive mammalian embryonic CNS precursor is a stem cell. Dev Biol 1996;175: 1-13.

[74] Litvinov IV, Vander Griend DJ, Xu Y, Antony L, Dalrymple SL,Isaacs JT. Low-calcium serum-free defined medium selects for growth of normal prostatic epithelial stem cells. Cancer Res 2006;66: 8598-607.

[75] Fan X, Liu S, Su F, Pan Q,Lin T. Effective enrichment of prostate cancer stem cells from spheres in a suspension culture system. Urol Oncol 2012;30: 314-8.

[76] Bisson I,Prowse DM. WNT signaling regulates self-renewal and differentiation of prostate cancer cells with stem cell characteristics. Cell Res 2009;19: 683-97.

[77] Barnhart BC,Simon MC. Metastasis and stem cell pathways. Cancer Metastasis Rev 2007;26: 261-71.

[78] Hellsten R, Johansson M, Dahlman A, Sterner O,Bjartell A. Galiellalactone inhibits stem cell-like ALDH-positive prostate cancer cells. PLoS One 2011;6: e22118.

[79] Zhang Y, Wang Z, Ahmed F, Banerjee S, Li Y,Sarkar FH. Down-regulation of Jagged-1 induces cell growth inhibition and S phase arrest in prostate cancer cells. Int J Cancer 2006;119: 2071-7.

[80] Santagata S, Demichelis F, Riva A, Varambally S, Hofer MD, Kutok JL, Kim R, Tang J, Montie JE, Chinnaiyan AM, Rubin MA,Aster JC. JAGGED1 expression is associated with prostate cancer metastasis and recurrence. Cancer Res 2004;64: 6854-7.

[81] Li H, Yu B, Zhang Y, Pan Z,Xu W. Jagged1 protein enhances the differentiation of mesenchymal stem cells into cardiomyocytes. Biochem Biophys Res Commun 2006;341: 320-5.

[82] Li J, Yen C, Liaw D, Podsypanina K, Bose S, Wang SI, Puc J, Miliaresis C, Rodgers L, McCombie R, Bigner SH, Giovanella BC, Ittmann M, Tycko B, Hibshoosh H, Wigler MH,Parsons R. PTEN, a putative protein tyrosine phosphatase gene mutated in human brain, breast, and prostate cancer. Science 1997;275: 1943-7.

[83] Chow LM,Baker SJ. PTEN function in normal and neoplastic growth. Cancer Lett 2006;241: 184-96.

[84] Dong JT. Chromosomal deletions and tumor suppressor genes in prostate cancer. Cancer Metastasis Rev 2001;20: 173-93.

[85] Podsypanina K, Ellenson LH, Nemes A, Gu J, Tamura M, Yamada KM, Cordon-Cardo C, Catoretti G, Fisher PE,Parsons R. Mutation of Pten/Mmac1 in mice causes neoplasia in multiple organ systems. Proc Natl Acad Sci U S A 1999;96: 1563-8.

[86] Denmeade SR,Isaacs JT. A history of prostate cancer treatment. Nat Rev Cancer 2002;2: 389-96.

[87] Gingrich JR, Barrios RJ, Morton RA, Boyce BF, DeMayo FJ, Finegold MJ, Angelopoulou R, Rosen JM,Greenberg NM. Metastatic prostate cancer in a transgenic mouse. Cancer Res 1996;56: 4096-102.

[88] Vander Griend DJ, Karthaus WL, Dalrymple S, Meeker A, DeMarzo AM,Isaacs JT. The role of CD133 in normal human prostate stem cells and malignant cancer-initiating cells. Cancer Res 2008;68: 9703-11.

[89] Hu WY, Shi GB, Hu DP, Nelles JL,Prins GS. Actions of estrogens and endocrine disrupting chemicals on human prostate stem/progenitor cells and prostate cancer risk. Mol Cell Endocrinol 2012;354: 63-73.

[90] McPherson SJ, Hussain S, Balanathan P, Hedwards SL, Niranjan B, Grant M, Chandrasiri UP, Toivanen R, Wang Y, Taylor RA,Risbridger GP. Estrogen receptor-beta activated apoptosis in benign hyperplasia and cancer of the prostate is androgen independent and TNFalpha mediated. Proc Natl Acad Sci U S A 2010;107: 3123-8.

[91] Rouet V, Bogorad RL, Kayser C, Kessal K, Genestie C, Bardier A, Grattan DR, Kelder B, Kopchick JJ, Kelly PA,Goffin V. Local prolactin is a target to prevent expansion of basal/stem cells in prostate tumors. Proc Natl Acad Sci U S A 2010;107: 15199-204.

[92] van den Hoogen C, van der Horst G, Cheung H, Buijs JT, Lippitt JM, Guzman-Ramirez N, Hamdy FC, Eaton CL, Thalmann GN, Cecchini MG, Pelger RC,van der Pluijm G. High aldehyde dehydrogenase activity identifies tumor-initiating and metastasis-initiating cells in human prostate cancer. Cancer Res 2010;70: 5163-73.

[93] Patrawala L, Calhoun T, Schneider-Broussard R, Li H, Bhatia B, Tang S, Reilly JG, Chandra D, Zhou J, Claypool K, Coghlan L,Tang DG. Highly purified CD44+ prostate cancer cells from xenograft human tumors are enriched in tumorigenic and metastatic progenitor cells. Oncogene 2006;25: 1696-708.

[94] Li F, Tiede B, Massague J,Kang Y. Beyond tumorigenesis: cancer stem cells in metastasis. Cell Res 2007;17: 3-14.

[95] Glinsky GV, Berezovska O,Glinskii AB. Microarray analysis identifies a death-from-cancer signature predicting therapy failure in patients with multiple types of cancer. J Clin Invest 2005;115: 1503-21.

[96] Hurt EM,Farrar WL. Cancer stem cells: the seeds of metastasis? Mol Interv 2008;8: 140-2.

[97] Hermann PC, Huber SL, Herrler T, Aicher A, Ellwart JW, Guba M, Bruns CJ,Heeschen C. Distinct populations of cancer stem cells determine tumor growth and metastatic activity in human pancreatic cancer. Cell Stem Cell 2007;1: 313-23.

[98] Shmelkov SV, Butler JM, Hooper AT, Hormigo A, Kushner J, Milde T, St Clair R, Baljevic M, White I, Jin DK, Chadburn A, Murphy AJ, Valenzuela DM, Gale NW, Thurston G, Yancopoulos GD, D'Angelica M, Kemeny N, Lyden D,Rafii S. CD133 expression is not restricted to stem cells, and both CD133+ and CD133- metastatic colon cancer cells initiate tumors. J Clin Invest 2008;118: 2111-20.

[99] Stephenson RA, Dinney CP, Gohji K, Ordonez NG, Killion JJ,Fidler IJ. Metastatic model for human prostate cancer using orthotopic implantation in nude mice. J Natl Cancer Inst 1992;84: 951-7.

[100] Li H,Tang DG. Prostate cancer stem cells and their potential roles in metastasis. J Surg Oncol 2011;103: 558-62.

[101] Lawson DA,Witte ON. Stem cells in prostate cancer initiation and progression. J Clin Invest 2007;117: 2044-50.

[102] Bartel DP. MicroRNAs: genomics, biogenesis, mechanism, and function. Cell 2004;116: 281-97.

[103] Sevli S, Uzumcu A, Solak M, Ittmann M,Ozen M. The function of microRNAs, small but potent molecules, in human prostate cancer. Prostate Cancer Prostatic Dis 2010;13: 208-17.

[104] Mashima T, Okabe S,Seimiya H. Pharmacological targeting of constitutively active truncated androgen receptor by nigericin and suppression of hormone-refractory prostate cancer cell growth. Mol Pharmacol 2010;78: 846-54.

[105] Rokhlin OW, Taghiyev AF, Bayer KU, Bumcrot D, Koteliansk VE, Glover RA,Cohen MB. Calcium/calmodulin-dependent kinase II plays an important role in prostate cancer cell survival. Cancer Biol Ther 2007;6: 732-42.

[106] Zhang HL, Yang LF, Zhu Y, Yao XD, Zhang SL, Dai B, Zhu YP, Shen YJ, Shi GH,Ye DW. Serum miRNA-21: elevated levels in patients with metastatic hormone-refractory prostate cancer and potential predictive factor for the efficacy of docetaxel-based chemotherapy. Prostate 2011;71: 326-31.

[107] Shi GH, Ye DW, Yao XD, Zhang SL, Dai B, Zhang HL, Shen YJ, Zhu Y, Zhu YP, Xiao WJ,Ma CG. Involvement of microRNA-21 in mediating chemo-resistance to docetaxel in androgen-independent prostate cancer PC3 cells. Acta Pharmacol Sin 2010;31: 867-73.

[108] Murata T, Takayama K, Katayama S, Urano T, Horie-Inoue K, Ikeda K, Takahashi S, Kawazu C, Hasegawa A, Ouchi Y, Homma Y, Hayashizaki Y,Inoue S. miR-148a is an androgen-responsive microRNA that promotes LNCaP prostate cell growth by repressing its target CAND1 expression. Prostate Cancer Prostatic Dis 2010;13: 356-61.

[109] Sun D, Lee YS, Malhotra A, Kim HK, Matecic M, Evans C, Jensen RV, Moskaluk CA,Dutta A. miR-99 family of MicroRNAs suppresses the expression of prostate-specific antigen and prostate cancer cell proliferation. Cancer Res 2011;71: 1313-24.

[110] Lin SL, Chiang A, Chang D,Ying SY. Loss of mir-146a function in hormone-refractory prostate cancer. RNA 2008;14: 417-24.

[111] Liu C, Kelnar K, Liu B, Chen X, Calhoun-Davis T, Li H, Patrawala L, Yan H, Jeter C, Honorio S, Wiggins JF, Bader AG, Fagin R, Brown D,Tang DG. The microRNA miR-34a inhibits prostate cancer stem cells and metastasis by directly repressing CD44. Nat Med 2011;17: 211-5.

[112] Suzuki HI, Yamagata K, Sugimoto K, Iwamoto T, Kato S,Miyazono K. Modulation of microRNA processing by p53. Nature 2009;460: 529-33.

[113] Ozen M, Sevli S. The Role of Cancer Stem Cells and MicroRNAs in Human Prostate Cancer. Edited by Philippe E. Prostate Cancer – From Bench to Bedside, In Tech, 2011; 411-422. Available from: http://www.intechopen.com/books/prostate-cancer-from-bench-to-bedside/the-role-of-cancer-stem-cells-and-micrornas-in-human-prostate-cancer (accessed 08.08.2012)

[114] Schalken JA. Validation of molecular targets in prostate cancer. BJU Int 2005;96 Suppl 2: 23-9.

[115] Maitland NJ,Collins AT. Prostate cancer stem cells: a new target for therapy. J Clin Oncol 2008;26: 2862-70.

[116] Clayton S,Mousa SA. Therapeutics formulated to target cancer stem cells: Is it in our future? Cancer Cell Int 2011;11: 7.

[117] Mimeault M, Mehta PP, Hauke R,Batra SK. Functions of normal and malignant prostatic stem/progenitor cells in tissue regeneration and cancer progression and novel targeting therapies. Endocr Rev 2008;29: 234-52.

[118] Angelucci A, Gravina GL, Rucci N, Millimaggi D, Festuccia C, Muzi P, Teti A, Vicentini C,Bologna M. Suppression of EGF-R signaling reduces the incidence of prostate cancer metastasis in nude mice. Endocr Relat Cancer 2006;13: 197-210.

[119] Kharait S, Dhir R, Lauffenburger D,Wells A. Protein kinase Cdelta signaling downstream of the EGF receptor mediates migration and invasiveness of prostate cancer cells. Biochem Biophys Res Commun 2006;343: 848-56.

[120] Normanno N,Gullick WJ. Epidermal growth factor receptor tyrosine kinase inhibitors and bone metastases: different mechanisms of action for a novel therapeutic application? Endocr Relat Cancer 2006;13: 3-6.

[121] Zhou Y, Yang J,Kopecek J. Selective inhibitory effect of HPMA copolymer-cyclopamine conjugate on prostate cancer stem cells. Biomaterials 2012;33: 1863-72.

[122] Ketola K, Hilvo M, Hyotylainen T, Vuoristo A, Ruskeepaa AL, Oresic M, Kallioniemi O,Iljin K. Salinomycin inhibits prostate cancer growth and migration via induction of oxidative stress. Br J Cancer 2012;106: 99-106.

[123] Malumbres M,Barbacid M. Cell cycle, CDKs and cancer: a changing paradigm. Nat Rev Cancer 2009;9: 153-66.

[124] Ringer L, Sirajuddin P, Yenugonda VM, Ghosh A, Divito K, Trabosh V, Patel Y, Brophy A, Grindrod S, Lisanti MP, Rosenthal D, Brown ML, Avantaggiati ML, Rodriguez O,Albanese C. VMY-1-103, a dansylated analog of purvalanol B, induces caspase-3-dependent apoptosis in LNCaP prostate cancer cells. Cancer Biol Ther 2010;10: 320-5.

[125] van der Horst G, van den Hoogen C, Buijs JT, Cheung H, Bloys H, Pelger RC, Lorenzon G, Heckmann B, Feyen J, Pujuguet P, Blanque R, Clement-Lacroix P,van der Pluijm G. Targeting of alpha(v)-integrins in stem/progenitor cells and supportive microenvironment impairs bone metastasis in human prostate cancer. Neoplasia 2011;13: 516-25.

[126] Guerin O, Formento P, Lo Nigro C, Hofman P, Fischel JL, Etienne-Grimaldi MC, Merlano M, Ferrero JM,Milano G. Supra-additive antitumor effect of sunitinib malate (SU11248, Sutent) combined with docetaxel. A new therapeutic perspective in hormone refractory prostate cancer. J Cancer Res Clin Oncol 2008;134: 51-7.

[127] Shaw A,Bushman W. Hedgehog signaling in the prostate. J Urol 2007;177: 832-8.

[128] Sanchez P, Hernandez AM, Stecca B, Kahler AJ, DeGueme AM, Barrett A, Beyna M, Datta MW, Datta S,Ruiz i Altaba A. Inhibition of prostate cancer proliferation by interference with SONIC HEDGEHOG-GLI1 signaling. Proc Natl Acad Sci U S A 2004;101: 12561-6.

[129] Lu W, Lin C, King TD, Chen H, Reynolds RC,Li Y. Silibinin Inhibits Wnt/beta-catenin Signaling by Suppressing Wnt Co-receptor LRP6 Expression in Human Prostate and Breast Cancer Cells. Cell Signal 2012.

[130] Xing Y, Liu M, Du Y, Qu F, Li Y, Zhang Q, Xiao Y, Zhao J, Zeng F,Xiao C. Tumor cell-specific blockade of CXCR4/SDF-1 interactions in prostate cancer cells by hTERT promoter induced CXCR4 knockdown: A possible metastasis preventing and minimizing approach. Cancer Biol Ther 2008;7: 1839-48.

Chapter 15

Salinomycin-Induced Apoptosis in Human Prostate Cancer Cells

Hak-Jong Choi, Kwang-Youn Kim, Sun-Nyoung Yu,
Sang-Hun Kim, Sung-Sik Chun, Hak-Sun Yu,
Yeong-Min Park and Soon-Cheol Ahn

Additional information is available at the end of the chapter

http://dx.doi.org/10.5772/52783

1. Introduction

Salinomycin is a carboxylic polyether ionophore which was isolated from the culture supernatant of the bacterium *Streptomyces albus* in 1974 [1]. Structurally, it is composed of a pentacyclic molecule with a unique tricyclic spiroketal ring system and a unsaturated six-membered ring (Fig. 1). Its lipophilic property enables salinomycin to act in cytoplasmic and mitochondrial membranes as an ionophore with a strong preference for potassium. Therefore, it promotes cellular and mitochondrial potassium efflux and inhibits mitochondrial oxidative phosphorylation [2, 3].

Salinomycin exhibits a broad antimicrobial spectrum against gram-positive bacteria including mycobacteria, *Bacillus subtilis, Staphylococcus aureus* and some filamentous fungi, but not against gram-negative bacteria and yeast [1]. Moreover, salinomycin has been shown to kill protozoan parasites, such as *Plasmodium falciparum* and *Eimera* spp., that cause severe coccidiosis in the livestock and poultry industries. Owing to its anti-parasite properties, salinomycin has been used to control coccidiosis in parasite-infected chickens and cows [4, 5].

More recently, the anticancer property of salinomycin has been recognized based on its ability to induce apoptosis and cause growth inhibition in diverse types of apoptosis- and chemotherapeutic-resistant cancer cells [6]. Salinomycin-mediated apoptosis in these cells is independent of known mediators of the cell death signal pathway, such as the p53 tumor suppressor protein, the 26S proteasome and the CD95/DC95 ligand system. This drug also triggers apoptosis by overcoming ATP-Binding Cassette (ABC) transporter-mediated multidrug resistance, as was observed in the case of KG-1a human leukemia cells [7, 8]. Salinomycin caused massive tumor cell apoptosis and associated regression of breast tumor growth and metastasis in vivo in a mouse xenograft tumor model [9]. In fact, in high-throughput screening of ~16,000 small molecule chemicals, breast cancer stem cells (CSCs) were found to be inhibited selectively by salinomycin [9]. CSCs are a subpopulation of cells within the tumor mass that are thought to account for cancer recurrence by virtue of their refractivity to cytotoxic cancer treatment agents such as radiation and a wide variety of chemotherapeutic agents. Susceptibility of CSCs to salinomycin bolsters the possibility that this drug may target treatment-resistant advanced human cancers. Delineation of the mechanism(s) that underlies cancer cell apoptosis by salinomycin is needed in order to rigorously evaluate the potential of this drug as a novel cancer therapeutic.

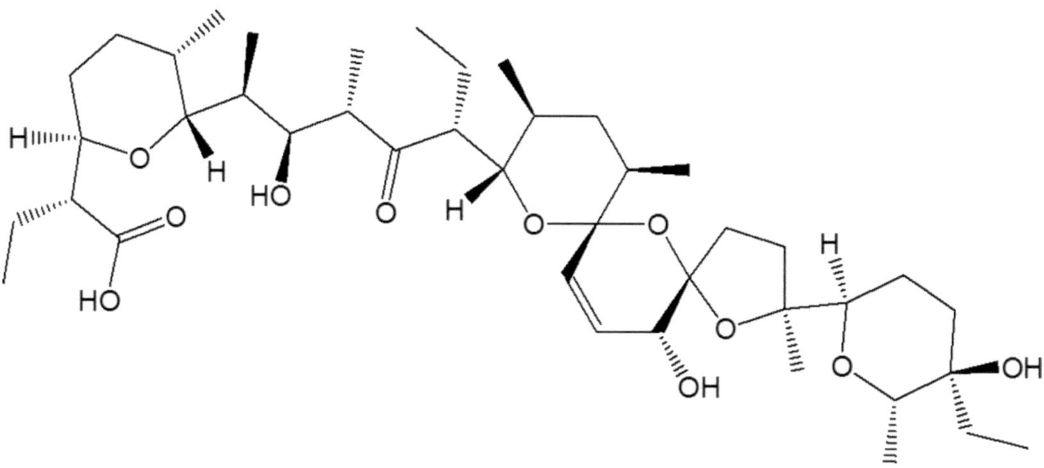

Figure 1. Structural formula of salinomycin. It has a molecular mass of 751 Da and a molecular formula of $C_{42}H_{70}O_{11}$.

Apoptosis is a regulated cell death process that requires the cascaded activation and execution of a series of regulatory molecules and cysteine-aspartic proteases, known as caspases [10]. Stress agents, such as reactive oxygen species (ROS), ultraviolet radiation, viral infections, and anticancer agents are well-characterized apoptosis triggers. Mitochondria are the primary site of origin for the initiating signals of apoptosis, although a death receptor-dependent extramitochondrial apoptotic pathway also exists. Mitochondrially originated apoptotic signals include a change in the electron transport system, loss of mitochondrial membrane potential (MMP, $\Delta\Psi m$), failure of Ca^{2+} flux homeostasis, generation of ROS, and release of caspase activators. Early apoptosis is invariantly marked by a breakdown in the MMP, which precedes DNA fragmentation in all cell types and under all types of apoptotic stimuli [11]. Production of endogenous ROS as mitochondrial byproducts of respiration is tightly controlled by MMP. Disruption in the ROS homeostasis plays a critical role in the regulation of mitochondrial dysfunction and apoptotic events [12].

Prostate cancer initially responds to androgen deprivation, which is a standard-of-care therapy when the androgen-dependent malignant cells meet with apoptotic death in an environment of low, castrate-level circulating androgens. Relapse, however, is a common occurrence at which point the recurrent cancer cells are castration resistant and have the ability to progress on chemotherapeutics to become completely therapy resistant [13-15].

In this chapter, we describe our recent findings that salinomycin induces apoptosis of prostate cancer cells by elevating oxidative stress through intracellular ROS production, which leads to the disruption of mitochondrial function and subsequent release of cytochrome c to the cytosol, activation of caspase-3, and cleavage of PARP-1 in androgen-independent, chemotherapeutic-refractive PC-3 human prostate cancer cells [16].

2. Salinomycin in human prostate cancer cells

Prostate cancer is the most frequently diagnosed cancer and the second leading cause of cancer death among men in the United States. Considerable progress has been made in the early detection and treatment of prostate cancer over the last two decades. Nevertheless, mortality from prostate cancer remains a significant health care problem [17]. Androgen deprivation therapy is increasingly becoming a central component in the management of prostate cancer. Although initially effective, patients acquire resistance and eventually develop metastatic castration-resistant prostate cancer (CRPC) [18-20]. For treatment in patients with CRPC, chemotherapy with docetaxel represents the standard first-line treatment. However, in order to prolong overall survival time after treatment with docetaxel, development of novel therapeutic strategies is essential.

2.1. Salinomycin reduced viability of prostate cancer cells at a lower dose than non-malignant prostate epithelial cells

Our recent study has revealed that salinomycin induces apoptosis in human prostate cancer cells by accumulated reactive oxygen species and mitochondrial membrane depolarization [20]. Using androgen-independent PC-3 and DU-145, the androgen-dependent LNCaP prostate cancer cells and non-malignant RWPE-1 prostate epithelial cells, we examined the effects of salinomycin on the viability of prostate cancer cells. When the cells were treated with increasing concentrations of salinomycin for different time periods, the viability of prostate cancer cells were reduced in a dose- and time-dependent manner (Fig. 2A, 2B and 2C). By comparison, RWPE-1 cells were relatively less sensitive to salinomycin, since at 0.15 μM concentration, the drug did not significantly inhibit viable cell number (Fig. 2D), unlike the all three cancer cells, which showed significant drop in viability in MTT assay. To some extent, differential sensitivity to the drug was also seen for LNCaP vs PC3 and DU-145 cells, since at 1.33 μM of the drug, LNCaP cells manifested a stronger inhibition -- viability reduced to ~55%, 38%, 35% and 22% (after 12 h, 24 h, 36 h and 48 h, respectively), whereas >50% of PC-3 and DU-145 cells remained viable after 36 h treatment of the drug (at 1.33 μM), and even at 48 h, >30% of PC-3 cells and >50% of DU-145 cells remained viable (Fig. 2B vs. Figs 2A & 2C). At 0.15 μM salinomycin, the three cell lines showed approximately similar sensitivity to the drug. To summarize, these results indicate that the chemo-resistance of the hormone-independent cancer cells to salinomycin is higher than that of the hormone-dependent cells, and compared to the cancer cells, non-malignant prostate epithelial cells (such as RWPE-1) are relatively more resistant to salinomycin. We next focused on the PC-3 cell model to investigate the molecular events associated with the salinomycin-induced loss of cell viability [20].

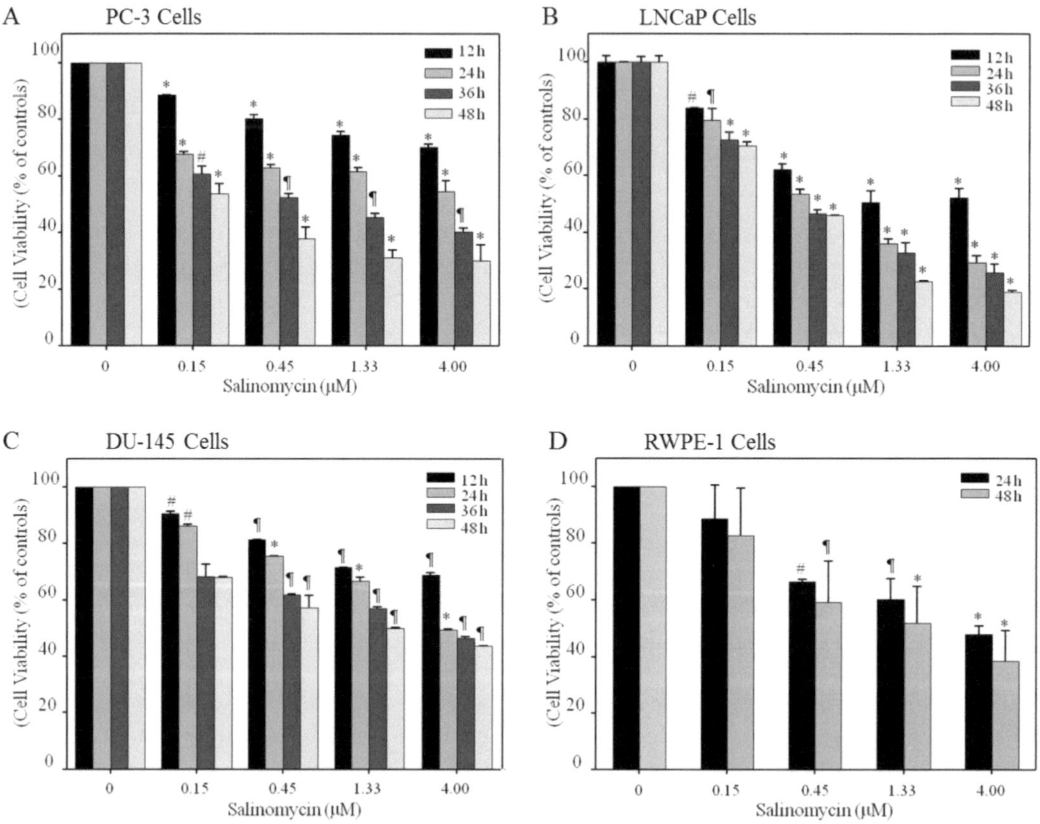

Figure 2. Salinomycin inhibited viability of prostate cancer cells. (A) PC-3 (B) LNCaP (C) DU-145 (D) RWPE-1 cells. 5×10^4 cells/ml were treated with salinomycin (0.15–4.00 μM) at different time points (12 h, 24 h, 36 h and 48 h). Cell viability was determined by MTT assay. Data are presented as mean ± SD (n = 3 in each group). #p<0.05, p<0.01, *p<0.001 vs. the control group.

2.2. Salinomycin induced PC-3 cell apoptosis

To examine if the salinomycin effect is due to apoptosis, we examined PC-3 cells for the nuclear morphology, annexin V staining and induction of various apoptosis-related molecular events before and after salinomycin treatment [20]. Laser scanning confocal microscopy of DAPI-stained PC-3 cells showed that in the absence of the drug, the nuclei were round and homogeneous, whereas salinomycin treatment caused a reduction of cell volume, nuclear condensation (a hallmark feature of apoptotic cells), and increased non-adherence of the cells to the culture surface (Fig. 3A). Induction of apoptosis was rigorously substantiated by examining the flow cytometry pattern of annexin V stained cells (Fig. 3B). Apoptotic cells accounted for 27.13% and 34.61% of the cells in early apoptosis plus late apoptosis, and necrotic cells were 13.03% and 21.24% of total cells, in response to salinomycin treatment at 1.33 μM and 4.00 μM, respectively (Fig. 3B). Taken together, these results show that salinomycin induced apoptotic cell death; at higher doses necrosis may also account for cell death.

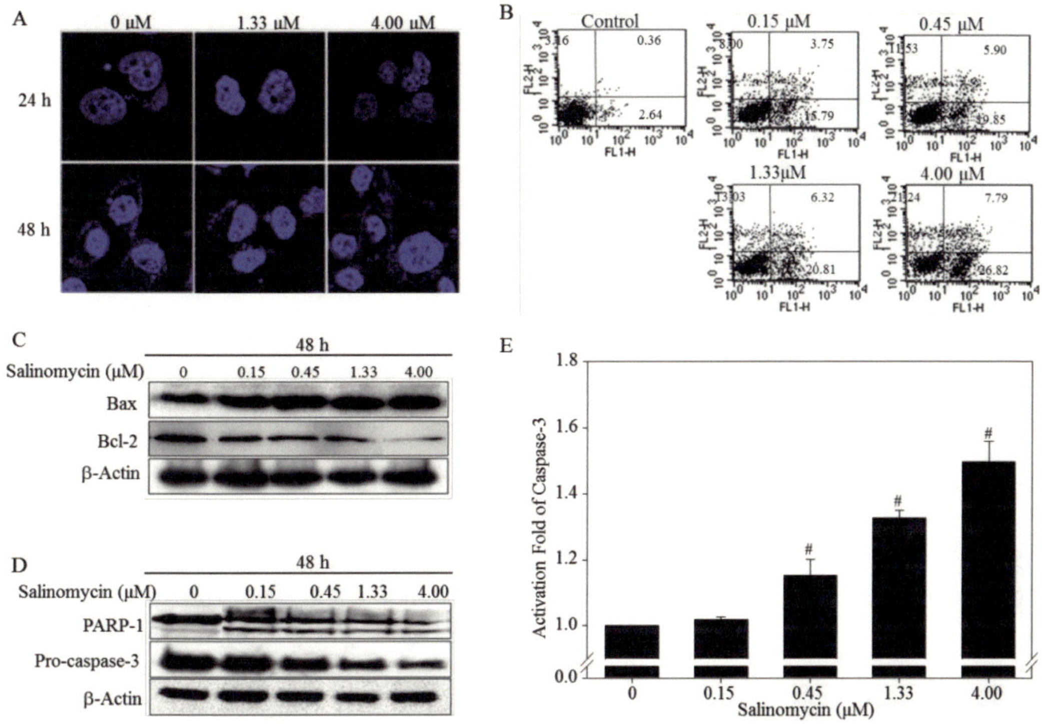

Figure 3. Salinomycin induced apoptosis in PC-3 cells. (A) Morphological changes. After treatment with salinomycin (1.33 and 4.00 μM) for 24 h and 48 h, nuclear fragmentation was observed by laser scanning confocal microscopy. Magnification, at × 1,800. (B) Flow cytometric analysis of annexin V/propidium iodide (PI) staining. PC-3 cells were treated with various concentrations of salinomycin for 48 h. The dual parameter dot plots combining annexin V and PI show the viable cell population in the lower left quadrant (annexin V^-PI^-), apoptotic cells in the lower right quadrant (annexin V^+PI^-) and the upper right quadrant (annexin V^+PI^+), and necrotic cells in the upper left quadrant (annexin V^-PI^+). (C) Bax and Bcl-2 expression in total cell lysates, detected by western blotting. (D) Pro-caspase-3 and poly (ADP-ribose) polymerase (PARP-1, cleaved and uncleaved) levels. (E) Caspase-3 activity, determined by a colorimetric assay kit using the specific substrate Ac-DEVD-pNA. Data show mean ± SD (n = 3 in each group). #p<0.01 vs. the control group.

Recently, a similar study has been performed by Ketola et al., describing that salinomycin is capable of inhibiting the growth of prostate cancer cells, but not affecting non-malignant prostate epithelial cells [21]. However, in contrast to our results that salinomycin induces apoptosis in PC-3 cells, the authors were not able to detect caspase-3- and 7-mediated apoptosis in prostate carcinoma cells, VCaP and LNCaP, by salinomycin treatment (see below). This discrepancy is probably due to the different prostate cell lines were used in each study.

2.3. Salinomycin differentially altered the levels of Bcl-2 family proteins and induced caspase-3 activation and PARP-1 cleavage in PC-3 cells

In addition, we examined the expression of Bax and Bcl-2, the apoptosis and cell survival related protein, respectively, and also cleavage of pro-caspase-3, and PARP-1 (a caspase-3 substrate) using western blotting [16]. Salinomycin increased Bax expression and decreased Bcl-2 expression in a dose-dependent manner within total cell lysates (Fig. 3C). Furthermore, declining pro-caspase-3 levels and increasing cleavage of PARP-1 were evident with increasingly higher salinomycin concentrations (Fig. 3D). Caspase-3 activity assay using an in vitro colorimetric method further confirmed caspase-3 activation in the presence of salinomycin. Treatment of PC-3 cells with the drug for 48 hr resulted in a dose-dependent increase of caspase-3 activity (Fig. 3E). Thus, salinomycin mediated a cascaded series of molecular events that led to an attenuated level of Bcl-2, augmented level of the pro-apoptotic protein Bax, and activation of the executer apoptosis enzyme caspase-3.

2.4. Intracellular production of ROS in PC-3 cells increased markedly after salinomycin treatment

Cancer chemotherapy is known to induce tumor cell death in a variety of cell types in part by promoting the production of intracellular ROS [21]. In order to demonstrate whether ROS production is associated with salinomycin-induced apoptosis of PC-3 cells, we assessed the state of ROS at various time points after salinomycin treatment by examining the fluorescence intensity of DCHF-DA-incubated cells. A representative fluorescence pattern from flow cytometry (Fig. 4A, upper panel) shows that the intracellular ROS level increased after 4 h of salinomycin treatment, and pretreatment of the cells with the antioxidant N-acetylcysteine (NAC), a known quencher of ROS, left shifted the fluorescence peak closer to the peak generated by cells with no treatment or NAC treatment without subsequent exposure to salinomycin. The number of DCF-positive cells increased as early as 15 min following exposure to 1.33 μM salinomycin, and the peak production of ROS was after 4 h incubation of the drug (Fig. 4A, lower panel). As expected, pretreatment of the cells with NAC reduced the number of DCF-positive cells. NAC also increased the cell viability from 41.96% to 57.08% for 1.33 μM and from 25.4% to 41.21% for 4.00 μM of salinomycin (Fig. 4B). Salinomycin-induced caspase-3 activation in PC-3 cells was also inhibited by NAC (Fig. 4C). These findings suggest that intracellular ROS production is closely linked to caspase-3 activation and to the viability of PC-3 cells [20]. Consistent with these data, similar results has observed that salinomycin induces oxidative stress in VCaP and LNCaP cells detemined by the expression level of oxidative stress markers and intracellular level of ROS [22].

http://dx.doi.org/10.5772/52783

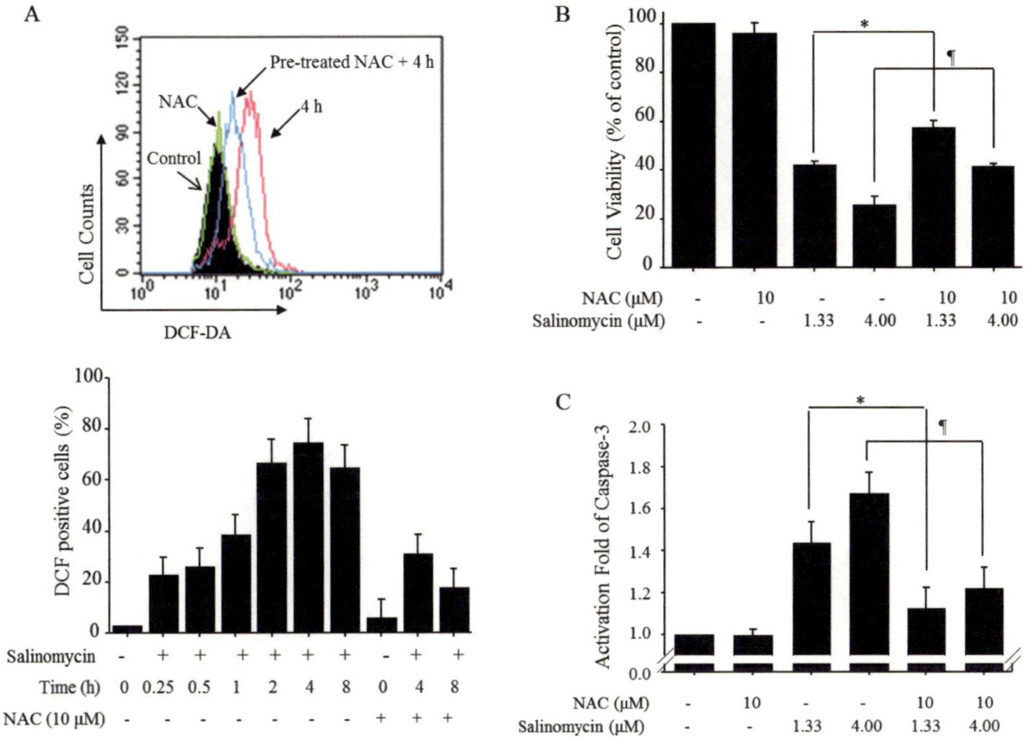

Figure 4. Salinomycin mediated ROS-induced apoptosis. (A) The intracellular ROS level. Cells were treated with salinomycin (1.33 μM) for indicated time periods with or without prior 1 h incubation with N-acetylcysteine (NAC; 10 mM). The dichlorodihydrofluorescein (DCF) fluorescence intensity in the cells was detected by flow cytometry. (B) Cytotoxicity. Cells were treated with salinomycin for 48 h with or without pre-treatment for 1 h with NAC (10 mM). (C) Caspase-3 activity. Cells were treated with salinomycin for 48 h with or without NAC (10 mM, 1 h). Data are presented as mean ± SD (n = 3 in each group). $p<0.01$, $^*p < 0.001$ vs. the control group.

2.5. Salinomycin induced loss of mitochondrial membrane potential in PC-3 cells

ROS is known to be involved in specific aspects of mitochondrial dysfunctions such as opening of the mitochondrial permeability transition pore that causes depolarization of the mitochondrial transmembrane potential (MMP; $\Delta\Psi m$), release of apoptogenic factors and loss of oxidative phosphorylation. Flow cytometry of DiOC6 fluorescence dye-labeled PC-3 cells showed progressive left shift of fluorescence intensity, indicating reduction in MMP, after treatment with 1.33 μM and 4.00 μM salinomycin (Fig. 5A, upper panel). Reduction in MMP was also prevented in NAC-pretreated cells, as shown in the results of intracellular ROS level (Fig. 5A, lower panel). These data suggest that dissipation of MMP in salinomycin-treated PC-3 cells is dependent on intracellular ROS production [20].

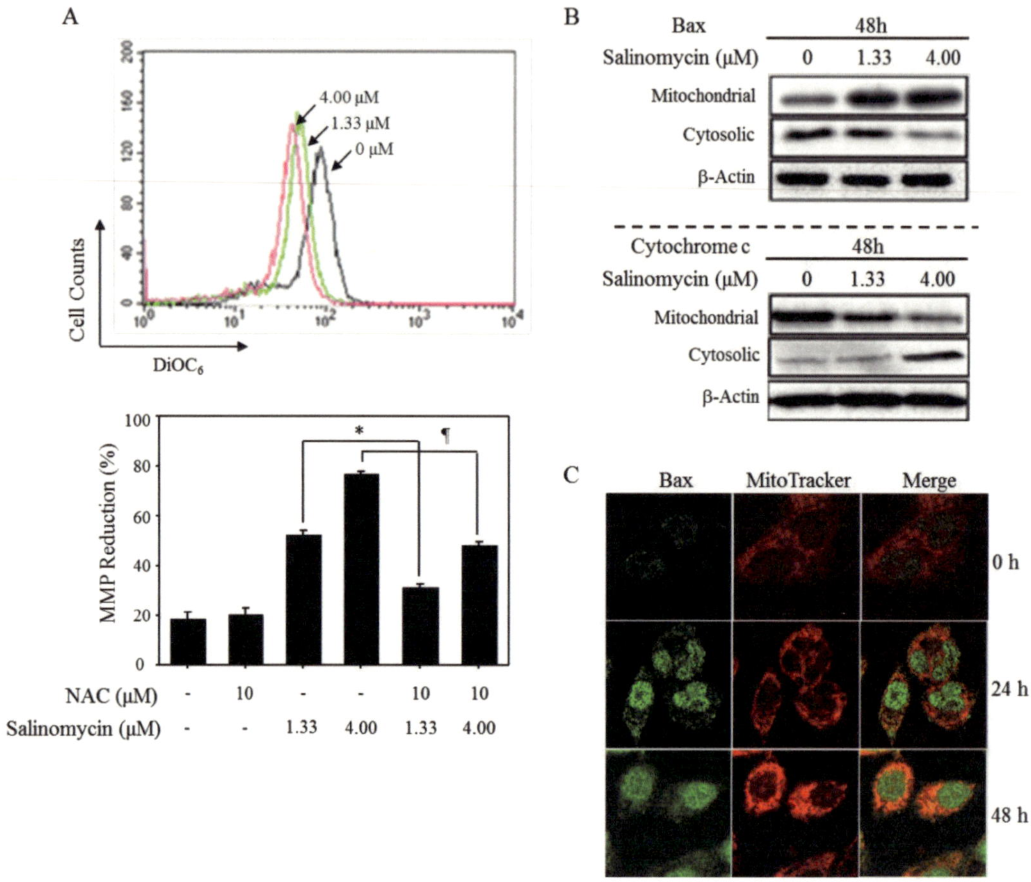

Figure 5. Salinomycin induced dysfunctions of mitochondrial membrane in PC-3 cells. (A) Mitochondrial membrane potentials (MMP). Cells were treated with salinomycin (1.33 and 4.00 µM) for 48 h in the presence or absence of 1 h pre-incubation with NAC (10 mM). MMP changes were determined from DiOC6 fluorescence, measured by flow cytometry analysis. Data are presented as mean ± SD (n = 3 in each group). $p<0.01$, *$p<0.001$ vs. the control group. (B) Bax translocation and release of cytochrome c. The levels of Bax and cytochrome c in the cytosol fraction and mitochondrial fraction were determined by western blotting. (C) Mitochondrial Bax translocation. Confocal microscopic images were observed by using the mitochondria staining dye Mitotracker Red CMXROS and anti-Bax antibody. Magnification, at × 1,800.

2.6. Salinomycin promoted Bax translocation to mitochondria and cytosolic release of cytochrome c

Participation of mitochondrial components in salinomycin-induced apoptosis was determined by assessing the subcellular localization of Bax and cytochrome c before and after salinomycin treatment. The drug triggered Bax translocation onto the mitochondrial membrane (Fig. 5B, upper panel) and mitochondrial cytochrome c release into the cytosol (Fig. 5B, lower panel), revealed from western blot assay. Bax translocation to mitochondria was visually confirmed by confocal microscopy (Fig. 5C), which showed a greatly enhanced staining for Bax in the mitochondrial compartment after treatment with salinomycin (1.33 μM) for 24 h or 48 h. These data suggest that salinomycin plays a pivotal role in the mitochondrial uptake of Bax and concomitant release of cytochrome c [20].

3. Salinomycin in human cancer stem cells and cancer cells

Anticancer activity of salinomycin was first described by Gupta et al. [9]. They developed an automated high-throughput screening method to discover compounds showing selective toxicity for breast CSCs. Among more than 16,000 small molecule chemicals, only one compound, salinomycin, was identified as a selective inhibitor of breast CSCs, and salinomycin pretreatment resulted in a >100-fold decrease in tumor-seeding ability relative to paclitaxel, a commonly used breast cancer chemotherapeutic drug [23], indicating that CSCs within breast cancer cell populations are resistant to paclitaxel but sensitive to treatment with salinomycin [9].

Salinomycin has been validated for its anticancer effects on $CD4^+$ T-cell leukemia cells from from the peripheral blood of a patient with acute T-cell leukemia [7]. While salinomycin failed to induce apoptosis in normal $CD4^+$ T cells, various human leukemia and lymphoma cells undergo apoptosis by salinomycin treatment. Interestingly, salinomycin induces apoptosis selectively in human cancer cells that exhibit resistance to apoptosis by lacking p53 expression and anticancer agents by overexpression of Bcl-2, P-glycoprotein or 26S proteasomes with enhanced proteolytic activity [7, 24]. Although the exact mechanism of salinomycin-induced apoptosis is unknown, this study highlights that salinomycin activates a distinct apoptotic pathway in cancer cells that is not accompanied by cell cycle arrest and that is independent of p53, caspase activation, the CD95/CD95L system and the 26S proteasome [7]. In addition, a new study demonstrated that salinomycin massively induces apoptosis in human leukemia stem cell-like cells which is expressing various ABC transporters conferring resistance to a broad spectrum of chemotherapeutic drugs [8].

In order to identify and improve conditions for increasing sensitivity of cancer cells to doxorubicin (DOX) or etoposide (ETO), various human cancer cells were co-treated with salinomycin and DOX- or ETO-pretreated cells [25]. The authors has shown that salinomycin is able to sensitize cancer cells to the effects of DOX or ETO. Intriguingly, they also has demonstrated for the first time that salinomycin sensitizes cancer cells with two different pathways, which mediated by increased DNA damage and reduced p21 protein levels through increased proteasome activity [25]. These findings suggest that salinomycin may be used for combination chemotherapy with DOX or ETO to reduce the viability of cancer cells.

The in vitro effects of salinomycin on aldehyde dehydrogenase (ALDH)-positive lung cancer cell line A549 has been observed [26]. ALDH is highly expressed in several tumor types including brain, breast, liver, colon, pancreas and lung [27], and ALDH positive cells from these tumors has been shown to enrich for tumor initiating cells with increased proliferation rate, migration and adhesion ability, and more recently with metastatic potential [28]. Treatment of salinomycin not only ruptured the lung cancer tumorospheres from ALDH positive

A549 lung cells but also reduced the expression of stem cell markers such as OCT-4, NANOG and SOX2 [26]. This study suggests that salinomycin may be a promising agent for lung cancer chemotherapy.

Anticancer effects of salinomycin on cancer stem-like cells in human colorectal cancers (CRC) have been described [29]. $CD133^+$ cell subpopulations within CRC have been identified as cancer stem-like cells, which are resistant to many current cancer therapies [30]. Salinomycin reduced the proportion of CRC $CD133^+$ cell subpopulations and upregulated expression of E-cadherin in CRC cells, suggesting that salinomycin may induce the mesenchymal-epithelial transition in the CRC cells. Furthermore, treatment of salinomycin reduced clonogenicity and mobility of the CRC cells [29].

A recent study has shown that salinomycin is active against human squamous cell carcinomas (SCCs) [31]. Based on the expression level of surface E-cadherin, SCCs can be classified into mesenchymal-like (Ecad-lo) cells and epithelial-like (Ecad-hi) cells, and upon down-regulating surface expression of E-cadherin, SCCs acquire mesenchymal-like phenotypes increasing resistance to both cytotoxic and targeted agents [32]. In contrast to cisplatin which selectively depleted Ecad-hi cells, salinomycin displayed comparable efficacy against both Ecad-hi and Ecad-lo cells [31].

More recently, the biochemical mechanism of anticancer effects of salinomycin has been demonstrated in chronic lymphocytic leukemia cells and osteosarcoma cells [33, 34]. As an inhibitor of Wnt/β-catenin signaling which plays a crucial role in embryonic development and cancer [35-37], salinomycin has been shown to block the phosphorylation of the Wnt coreceptor lipoprotein receptor related protein 6 (LRP6) and induce its degradation [33, 34]. These findings suggest that the anticancer properties of salinomycin may be mediated by Wnt inhibition, and targeting Wnt receptors LRP6 could represent a novel therapeutic treatment for cancers [37].

Using human ovarian cancer cell line OV2008, Dong et al. [38] very recently has reported that salinomycin inhibits the growth of ovarian cancer cells by inducing apoptosis in vitro and in vivo. To examine the signal pathway involved in salinomycin-induced growth inhibitory effect and apoptosis in OV2008 cells, the authors determined the phosphorylation of p38 MAPK which is implicated in cancer cell apoptosis and is induced by several chemotherapeutic drugs [39]. They observed that salinomycin treatment to OV2008 cells increases in the phosphorylation of p38 MAPK in a time-dependent and a concentration-dependent mode, suggesting that the activation of p38 MAPK appears to contribute to the proapoptotic effect of salinomycin in OV2008 cells [38].

4. Conclusion

The pharmacologic action of salinomycin has garnered increased attention in recent years in view of its potential as a new cancer chemotherapeutic based on its activity as a selective inhibitor of breast cancer stem cells. Salinomycin treatment also reduced formation of metastatic nodules by CSCs [6, 40]. Since CSCs are inert to all current cancer therapy interventions, they are likely to drive tumor recurrence and progression. The absence of androgen receptor expression in the putative CSCs in prostate cancer suggests that targeting of the androgen receptor pathway will not yield lasting therapy for advanced prostate cancer. A recent finding that salinomycin is detrimental to the viability of androgen-dependent and androgen-independent prostate cancer cells due to the onset of apoptosis hints at the possibility that this drug or more likely, a significantly less cytotoxic derivative of this drug activity, may have clinical utility as part of a future treatment strategy for advanced prostate cancer [20].

Our present study shows 1) salinomycin decreased viability of the androgen-dependent LNCaP and androgen-independent PC-3 and DU-145 prostate cancer cells in MTT assay in a time- and dose-dependent manner. The non-malignant RWPE-1 prostate epithelial cells were resistant to the drug-induced lethality at a lower salinomycin dose, which was still effective in inhibiting LNCaP, PC-3 and DU-145 cells; 2) Early and late apoptosis and necrosis in salinomycin-treated PC-3 cells was revealed from the nuclear morphology of DAPI-stained cells and from flow cytometry of annexin V-labeled cells; 3) Biochemical evidence of apoptosis came from the results that salinomycin activated caspase-3, induced cleavage of PARP-1 and caused a dose-dependent decreased expression of the survival protein Bcl-2 and increased expression of the pro-apoptotic protein Bax; 4) Bax was translocated to the mitochondria and cytochrome c was released into the cytosol of salinomycin-treated PC-3 cells, in agreement with the known coordinated events in the apoptosis pathway in which translocated Bax forms a transmembrane pore across the outer mitochondrial membrane, which in turn helps the cytosolic release of cytochrome c; 5) Finally, new evidence presented here shows that salinomycin promotes escalation of intracellular ROS levels which is accompanied by decreased mitochondrial membrane potential and increased caspase-3 activity of PC-3 cells and these effects of salinomycin were prevented by pretreatment of the cells with the antioxidant NAC (Fig. 6).

Previously it was reported that cancer chemopreventive agents induce apoptosis in part through ROS generation and disruption of redox homeostasis [41]. It is also known that the pro-apoptotic signal(s) emanating from accumulated ROS triggers the mitochondrial release of caspase-activating proteins, such as cytochrome c, apoptosis inducting factor (AIF) and Smac/DIABLO to the cytosol [42]. ROS shows secondary messenger function because of its ability to influence MMP and mitochondrial function and to induce intracellular Ca^{2+} flux and eventual activation of the caspase cascade [43]. Although our results provide clear evidence of salinomycin-induced ROS generation, mitochondrial membrane depolarization and augmentation of caspase-3 activity in PC-3 cells, we did not detect any change in the intracellular Ca^{2+} level [20].

The mechanistic implication of our data is that salimomycin-mediated ROS production, initiated upstream of mitochondrial dysfunction, is a determining event that commits the cancer cells to apoptotic death subsequent to the loss of MMP, cytosolic release of cytochrome c and activation of the caspase zymogen cascade. The link between ROS and apoptosis in salinomycin-exposed cells was also evident from the inhibition of apoptosis in NAC-pretreated PC-3 cells [20]. The NAC inhibition hints at the possibility that the extent of salinomycin-induced cytotoxicity in a therapeutic setting may be controlled with the intermittent use of an antioxidant in the therapeutic regimen of prostate cancer treatment. In contrast, however, a recent study has shown that salinomycin inhibits growth and migration of prostate cancer cell lines, VCaP and LNCaP, by reducing the expression of some prostate cancer oncogenes such as *MYC, AR* and *ERG,* inducing oxidative stress, decreasing the antioxidative capacity and the proportion of CSCs, but not by inducing apoptosis [21]. Nevertheless, these studies suggest that salinomycin may have multiple mechanisms to inhibit prostate cancer cell growth.

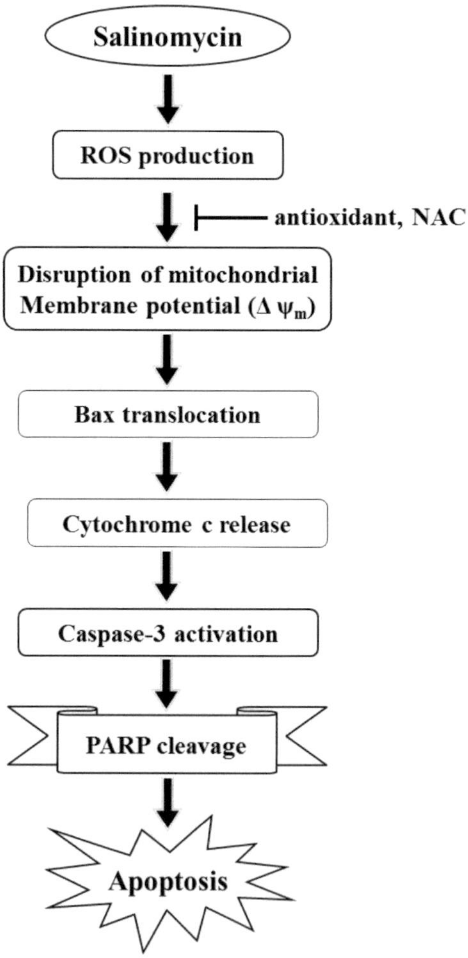

Figure 6. Schematic representation of salinomycin-induced apoptosis in human prostate cancer cells.

Future extension of the studies will constitute evaluating the anticancer efficacy of salinomycin on human prostate cancer xenograft models and on patient-derived primary prostate tumor cells, and the investigation of a group of salinomycin derivatives which are more effective and less toxic for humans is a challenge in the near future.

Acknowledgements

This research was supported by Basic Science Research Program through the National Research Foundation of Korea (NRF) funded by the Ministry of Education, Science and Technology (2012R1A1A2022587).

Author details

Hak-Jong Choi[1], Kwang-Youn Kim[2], Sun-Nyoung Yu[2], Sang-Hun Kim[2], Sung-Sik Chun[3], Hak-Sun Yu[4], Yeong-Min Park[2] and Soon-Cheol Ahn[2,5]

1 Globalization Research Department, World Institute of Kimchi, Gwangju, Republic of Korea

2 Department of Microbiology and Immunology, Pusan National University School of Medicine, Yangsan, Republic of Korea

3 Division of Food Science, International University of Korea, Jinju, USA

4 Department of Parasitology, Pusan National University School of Medicine, Yangsan, Republic of Korea

5 Medical Research Institute, Pusan National University, Yangsan, Republic of Korea

References

[1] Miyazaki Y, Shibuya M, Sugawara H, Kawaguchi O, Hirsoe C. Salinomycin, a new polyether antibiotic. J Antibiot 1974;27(11) 814-821.

[2] Mitani M, Yamanishi T, Miyazaki Y. Salinomycin: a new monovalent cation ionophore. Biochem Biophys Res Commun 1975;66(4) 1231-1236.

[3] Mitani M, Yamanishi T, Miyazaki Y, Otake N. Salinomycin effects on mitochondrial ion translocation and respiration. Antimicrob Agents Chemother 1976;9(4) 655-660.

[4] Mahmoudi N, de Julián-Ortiz JV, Ciceron L, Gálvez J, Mazier D, Danis M, Derouin F, García-Domenech R. Identification of new antimalarial drugs by linear discriminant analysis and topological virtual screening. J Antimicrob Chemother 2006;57(3) 489-497.

[5] Danforth HD, Ruff MD, Reid WM, Miller RL. Anticoccidial activity of salinomycin in battery raised broiler chickens. Poult Sci 1977;56(3) 926-932.

[6] Naujokat C, Fuchs D, Opelz G. Salinomycin in cancer: a new mission for an old agent. Mol Med Report 2010;3(4) 555-559.

[7] Fuchs D, Heinold A, Opelz G, Daniel V, Naujokat C. Salinomycin induces apoptosis and overcomes apoptosis resistance in human cancer cells. Biochem Biophys Res Commun 2009;390(3) 743-749.

[8] Fuchs D, Daniel V, Sadeghi M, Opelz G, Naujokat C. Salinomycin overcomes ABC transporter-mediated multidrug and apoptosis resistance in human leukemia stem cell-like KG-1a cells. Biochem Biophys Res Commun 2010;394(4) 1098–1104.

[9] Gupta PB, Onder TT, Jiang G, Tao K, Kuperwasser C, Weinberg RA, Lander ES. Identification of selective inhibitors of cancer stem cells by high-throughput screening. Cell 2009;138(4) 645-659.

[10] Degterev A, Yuan J. Expansion and evolution of cell death program. Nat Rev Mol Cell Biol 2008;9(5) 378-390.

[11] Liu MJ, Wang Z, Li HX, Wu RC, Liu YZ, Wu QY. Mitochondrial dysfunction as an early event in the process of apoptosis induced by woodfordin I in human leukemia K562 cells. Toxicol Appl Pharmacol 2004;194(2) 141-155.

[12] Simon HU, Haj-Yehia A, Levi-Schaffer F. Role of reactive oxygen species (ROS) in apoptosis induction. Apoptosis 2000;5(5) 415-418.

[13] Seruga B, Ocana A, Tannock IF. Drug resistance in metastatic castration-resistant prostate cancer. Nat Rev Clin Oncol 2011;8(1) 12-23.

[14] Kassi E, Moutsatsou P. Glucocorticoid receptor signaling and prostate cancer. Cancer Lett 2011;302(1) 1-10.

[15] Yang H, Dou QP. Targeting apoptosis pathway with natural terpenoids: implications for treatment of breast and prostate cancer. Curr Drug Targets 2010;11(6) 733-744.

[16] Feroze-Merzoug F, Schober MS, Chen YQ. Molecular profiling in prostate cancer. Cancer Metastasis Rev 2001;20(3-4) 165-171.

[17] Foley R, Marignol L, Keane JP, Lynch TH, Hollywood D. Androgen hypersensitivity in prostate cancer: molecular perspectives on androgen deprivation therapy strategies. The Prostate 2011;71(5) 550-557.

[18] Higano CS, Crawford ED. New and emerging agents for the treatment of castration-resistant prostate cancer. Urol Oncol 2011;29(6) S1-S8.

[19] Garcia JA, Rini BI. Castration-resistant prostate cancer: many treatments, many options, many challenges ahead. Cancer 2012;118(10) 2583-2593.

[20] Kim KY, Yu SN, Lee SY, Chun SS, Choi YL, Park YM, Song CS, Chatterjee B, Ahn SC. Salinomycin-induced apoptosis of human prostate cancer cells due to accumulated

reactive oxygen species and mitochondrial membrane depolarization. Biochem Biophys Res Commun 2011;413(1) 80-86.

[21] Ketola K, Hilvo M, Hyötyläinen T, Vuoristo A, Ruskeepää AL, Orešič M, Kallioniemi O, Iljin K. Salinomycin inhibits prostate cancer growth and migration via induction of oxidative stress. Br J Cancer 2012;106(1) 99-106.

[22] Wellen KE, Thompson CB. Cellular metabolic stress: considering how cells respond to nutrient excess. Mol Cell 2010;40(2) 323-332.

[23] Fitzpatrick FA, Wheeler R. The immunopharmacology of paclitaxel (Taxol), docetaxel (Taxotere), and related agents. Int Immunopharmacol. 2003;3(13-14) 1699-1714.

[24] Riccioni R, Dupuis ML, Bernabei M, Petrucci E, Pasquini L, Mariani G, Cianfriglia M, Testa U. The cancer stem cell selective inhibitor salinomycin is a p-glycoprotein inhibitor. Blood Cells Mol Dis 2010;45(1) 86-92.

[25] Kim JH, Chae M, Kim WK, Kim YJ, Kang HS, Kim HS, Yoon S. Salinomycin sensitizes cancer cells to the effects of doxorubicin and etoposide treatment by increasing DNA damage and reducing p21 protein. Br J Pharmacol 2011;162(3) 773-784.

[26] Wang Y. Effects of salinomycin on cancer stem cell in human lung adenocarcinoma A549 cells. Med Chem 2011;7(2) 106-111.

[27] Jiang F, Qiu Q, Khanna A, Todd NW, Deepak J, Xing L, Wang H, Liu Z, Su Y, Stass SA, Katz RL. Aldehyde dehydrogenase 1 is a tumor stem cell-associated marker in lung cancer. Mol Cancer Res 2009;7(3) 330-338.

[28] Su Y, Qiu Q, Zhang X, Jiang Z, Leng Q, Liu Z, Stass SA, Jiang F. Aldehyde dehydrogenase 1 A1-positive cell population is enriched in tumor-initiating cells and associated with progression of bladder cancer. Cancer Epidemiol Biomarkers Prev 2010;19(2) 327-337.

[29] Dong TT, Zhou HM, Wang LL, Feng B, Lv B, Zheng MH. Salinomycin selectively targets 'CD133+' cell subpopulations and decreases malignant traits in colorectal cancer lines. Ann Surg Oncol 2011;18(6) 1797-1804.

[30] Eyler CE, Rich JN. Survival of the fittest: cancer stem cells in therapeutic resistance and angiogenesis. J Clin Oncol 2008;26(17) 2839–2845.

[31] Basu D, Montone KT, Wang LP, Gimotty PA, Hammond R, Diehl JA, Rustgi AK, Lee JT, Rasanen K, Weinstein GS, Herlyn M. Detecting and targeting mesenchymal-like subpopulations within squamous cell carcinomas. Cell Cycle 2011;10(12) 2008-2016.

[32] Basu D, Nguyen TT, Montone KT, Zhang G, Wang LP, Diehl JA, Rustgi AK, Lee JT, Weinstein GS, Herlyn M. Evidence for mesenchymal-like sub-populations within squamous cell carcinomas possessing chemoresistance and phenotypic plasticity. Oncogene 2010;29(29) 4170-4182.

[33] Lu D, Choi MY, Yu J, Castro JE, Kipps TJ, Carson DA. Salinomycin inhibits Wnt signaling and selectively induces apoptosis in chronic lymphocytic leukemia cells. Proc Natl Acad Sci USA 2011;108(32) 13253-13257.

[34] Tang QL, Zhao ZQ, Li JC, Liang Y, Yin JQ, Zou CY, Xie XB, Zeng YX, Shen JN, Kang T, Wang J. Salinomycin inhibits osteosarcoma by targeting its tumor stem cells. Cancer Lett 2011;311(1) 113-121.

[35] Clevers H. Wnt/beta-catenin signaling in development and disease. Cell 2006;127(3) 469–480.

[36] Moon RT, Kohn AD, De Ferrari GV, Kaykas A. WNT and beta-catenin signalling: Diseases and therapies. Nat Rev Genet 2004;5(9) 691–701.

[37] King TD, Suto MJ, Li Y. The Wnt/β-catenin signaling pathway: a potential therapeutic target in the treatment of triple negative breast cancer. J Cell Biochem 2012;113(1) 13-18.

[38] Zhang B, Wang X, Cai F, Chen W, Loesch U, Bitzer J, Zhong XY. Effects of salinomycin on human ovarian cancer cell line OV2008 are associated with modulating p38 MAPK. Tumour Biol DOI 10.1007/s13277-012-0445-9 (accessed 7 July 2012).

[39] Wagner EF, Nebreda AR. Signal integration by JNK and p38 MAPK pathways in cancer development. Nat Rev Cancer 2009;9(8) 537–549.

[40] Maitland NJ, Collins AT. Prostate cancer stem cells: a new target for therapy. J Clin Oncol 2008;26(17) 2862-2870.

[41] Hail N Jr, Lotan R. Cancer chemoprevention and mitochondria: targeting apoptosis in transformed cells via the disruption of mitochondrial bioenergetics/redox state. Mol Nutr Food Res 2009;53(1) 49-67.

[42] Circu ML, Aw TY. Reactive oxygen species, cellular redox systems, and apoptosis. Free Radic Biol Med 2010;48(6) 749-762.

[43] Ly JD, Grubb DR, Lawen A. The mitochondrial membrane potential (Δψm) in apoptosis; an update. Apoptosis 2003;8(2) 115-128.

Chapter 16

Natural Compounds, Antioxidant and Antiandrogens in the Prevention of Prostate Cancer: *In vivo* Evidences from Murine Models and Human Clinical Studies

Rossano Lattanzio, Alessia Lamolinara,
Mauro Piantelli and Manuela Iezzi

Additional information is available at the end of the chapter

http://dx.doi.org/10.5772/45948

1. Introduction

Prostate cancer (PCa)is the most frequent malignant neoplasia in men. The number of cases has continuously increased over the past decades, partly due to the higher life expectancy. Additional factors are the high caloric diet and lack of physical exercise, typically seen in the Western countries. Notably, up to 40% of cancer incidents are preventable by consuming a healthy diet, regular physical activity, and maintenance of optimum body weight, and more than 20% by consuming vegetables and fruits. PCa represents an ideal candidate disease for chemoprevention. It is typically diagnosed in elderly men and even a modest delay in the neoplastic development could result in substantial reduction in the incidence of the clinically detectable disease.In this chapter we will review the history, the development, and the applications of some of the most common animal models of PCa,and we will discuss of the role of animal models in translational research.

2. Body

Prostate cancer (PCa) is the most common non-cutaneous malignant neoplasm in men in Western countries, responsible for the deaths of approximately 30,000 and 85,000 men per year in the United States and Europe, respectively [1,2].The number of cases is increasing rapidly in step with the growing number of men >50 worldwide, strategies for the prevention of PCa and its progression are urgently required. Since studies of chemopreventive agents in humans are hampered by the long latency period and challenging epidemiological problems, reliable preclinical models can be useful to overcome these problems. Early prostate tumorigenesis is apparently characterised by dysplasia that starts with proliferative inflammatory atrophy as the prelude to low-grade Prostatic Intraepithelial Neoplasia (PIN), high-grade PIN, primary cancer, metastatic cancer, and hormone-refractory cancer. During this progression, genetic damage accumulates within cancer cells [3,4]. Animal modelling has made a significant contribution to the study of prostate development and disease. Identification of the molecular features of PCa pathogenesis and progression could be greatly facilitated by laboratory and clinical models. However, a prerequisite for the elaboration of useful models is a better understanding of the molecular characteristics of human PCa. This puzzle, in addition to the well-known inter- and intra-individual heterogeneity of the disease itself and its multi-faceted nature, has necessitated the development of several complementary model systems. The most effective animal models will be those that most closely mimic the phenotypic and genetic changes accompanying the progression of the human disease. Systems shown to be promising include the dog, the rat, the human xenograft, and the genetically manipulated mouse. They have been widely employed to test preventive regimens, combinations of chemopreventive agents and/or drugs, cancer vaccines, and targeted treatments [5-12].This paper reviews the history, development, and applications of some of the most common animal models, and discusses their pros and cons in translational research.

3. Canine models

The dog is the animal known to commonly develop high-grade PIN and PCa spontaneously in a human-like manner [13]. The many similarities between the canine and the human form include the morphologic and phenotypic heterogeneity of the tumoral lesions, the age-dependency of tumor occurrence, and the propensity to metastasize to bones in an osteoblastic manner [14,15]. Androgen-dependency, on the other hand, is ruled out by a similar incidence in castrated animals [15], while a relatively long latency, the low incidence of spontaneous disease, the impracticability of genetic manipulation, and the high expense of maintaining dog colonies [16,17] are other limitations of canine systems.

4. Rat models

Spontaneous PCa is sometimes observed in some strains of rats [18]. The Dunning model [19] is the most popular. The original R-3327 tumor arose spontaneously in an inbred Copenhagen rat, and was translated into a syngenic Copenhagen x Fisher F1 rat. It is a slow growing, well differentiated and non-metastatic form. Several sublines with different characteristics mimicking some aspects of the human disease have since been developed [20-23]. Copenhagen and Wistar rats also develop a wide range of PCa phenotypes [24,25]. This variability, however, coupled with the rarity and long latency of these tumors, and their lack of metastases, bar the realistic employment of such models [12], though the recent elaboration of knockout methods [26-28] indicates that greater use could be made of genetically engineered rats in the future [29].

5. Xenograft models

In immunodeficient nude mice tumors grow after injection of cancer cells or xenograft implantation with no evidence of a graft-versus-host response. In function of the number of cells injected, or the size of the xenograft, the tumor will develop over 1–8 weeks, 1–4 months, or longer, and its response to treatment can be studied [30]. By comparison with in vitro studies, this approach offers several advantages, especially a 3D structure complete with tumor-induced angiogenesis, hormonal, paracrine/autocrine factors, and metastasis [12]. Xenografting of human PCa began in the 1970s [31]. Thereafter several cell lines that displayed different PCa phenotypes when injected into athymic nude mice have been developed [32,33]. This model has been used to show the ability of tumor xenografts to metastasize to the lymph node and bone, the two most common human sites [34].

Mice with an autosomal recessive Severe Combined Immuno Deficiency mutation (SCID mice) were identified in 1983 [35]. This mutation results in a lack of T- and B-lymphocyte function. However, normal natural killer (NK) cells and myeloid function are present, and in some SCID mice, some B and T cells are still present [36]. In this model subcutaneous injection of HER2/neu overexpressing human CLNCaP cells has shown that HER2/neu induces androgen-independent tumor growth through modulation of the androgen receptor signalling pathway[37].

In 1995, the features of this model were improved by crossing SCID mice with nonobese diabetic (NOD) mice, which lack in NK cells, antigen-presenting cells, and circulating complement [38]. NOD-SCID mice accepted foreign tissue more successfully and were more immunodeficient than SCID mice. This strain has been used to elaborate a model for orthotopic implantation of PC-3 and DU145 cells with a tumor take efficacy of >80% for both lines [39]. Some xenograft models result in metastasis to bone after intracardiac injection of bone cells that probably survive in a niche whose microenvironment is optimal for their seeding and growth. However intracardiac injection is not an ideal procedure and attention has thus been focused on xenografts to orthotopic sites such as the prostate. The success rates depend on the host strain and the use of hormones or Matrigel to provide adequate growth factors and a scaffold for cell growth [40-42].

The immunodeficiency mouse model has been further improved by crossing NOD-SCID mice with interleukin-2 receptor gamma null mice (NOG/NSG mice). These long-living mice (median 90 weeks) totally lack B, T, and NK cell activities, and cytokine signaling, together with no age-related "leakiness". They have a higher xenograft success rate and are more effective than other models, particularly in long-term studies involving prostate and non prostate cancer cells [43-45].

For preclinical prostate studies, most laboratories employ human PCa cell lines xenografted in mice. Many excellent reviews of the characteristics of these lines have been published [46-50]. The most widely used, each with thousands of studies published according to PubMed, are the classic three lines PC-3, LNCaP, and DU145, while each of the other lines has less than 200 citations [8]. These cell lines do not represent the steps of PCa progression. For example, almost all cell lines, including the most popular, were obtained from metastatic deposits: PC-3 from bone, LNCaP from lymph node, and DU145 from dural metastasis. In addition, PC-3 and DU145 are androgen receptor (AR) negative and LNCaP expresses a mutated AR. Again, cell lines, and their sublines in particular, are not fully genetically, functionally and phenotypically characterized, nor is there a method for standardization [8,46-48].

6. Transgenic mouse models

The last ten years have witnessed a remarkable shift in animal-based cancer research from xenograftedtumor to transgenic models since it is believed that they will recapitulate the complete course of carcinogenesis more accurately[48].This assumption stems from the recognition of several advantages that transgenic models offer when compared to xenograft systems. Among these are that the process of carcinogenesis begins with normal cells, progresses through distinct genetic and histological stages, occurs in an immuno-competent host and in its own cellular microenvironment, and that metastasis can occur along routes and to sites relevant to the clinical disease. A perhaps unrecognized attribute lies in the fact that, because the disease is not initiated by human action but by a genetic program that passes through the germline, the disease process is ''reset'' each generation. Statistically, the progression of a transgenic model of cancer should therefore be precisely recapitulated across time and between colonies. Given appropriate record keeping and data analysis, this feature should allow epidemiological- style investigations of great statistical power, free from both the mathematical noise of genetic and environmental variation, and from many of the economic and ethical constraints of human medicine.

Genetically engineered mouse (GEM) models have been utilized to identify pathways involved in carcinogenesis and investigate the role of particular gene mutations/deletions, and validate key genes as therapeutic targets. These models have been widely employed to test preventive regimens, combinations of chemopreventive agents and/or drugs, cancer vaccines, and targeted PCa treatments [5-12]. To mimic the human disease, GEMs could be generated through several mechanisms, such as overexpression or activation of oncogenes, elimination of target suppressor genes (Knock-outs), or generating dominant negative proteins that disrupt the function of regulatory genes.

The methods initially reported for genetic mouse modification involved the introduction of DNA constructs designed to induce the expression of proteins under the control of strong tissue-specific promoters, such as probasin and PSA. Simian virus 40 (SV40) large T antigens (Tag) were widely used because of their transforming ability. They interact with and sup-

http://dx.doi.org/10.5772/45948

press the tumor suppressor protein p53 and retinoblastoma [51,52]. In addition, the small t antigen interacts with the serine/threonine-specific protein phosphatase 2α to induce transformation [53].

The first model involving the expression of SV40 tumor antigens to develop PCa in the mouse was the C3(1)-Tag model[54].Targeting the Tag expression to the prostate was achieved by using a region of the C3 (1) gene, the rat prostatic steroid binding protein gene. Most C3(1)-Tag mice developed PIN after about eight weeks of age. Invasive adenocarcinomas followed after 28 weeks in about 40%. These tumors rarely metastasized (<4%), and always to the lungs. However, SV 40 expression was also detected in the mammary and salivary gland, while all females develop mammary intraepithelial neoplasia that may progress to mammary carcinomas[55].More effective prostate targeting was obtained in later models. Relatively few studies have used the C3 (1)/Tag model.

The transgenic adenocarcinoma of the mouse prostate (TRAMP) mouse [56,57] is the best known and most widely used PCa model because it closely mimics the human disease.In this model, expression of both large and small SV40 early genes (T and t antigen, Tag) are driven by the prostate-specific promoter probasin that leads to cell transformation within the prostate. In this model, Tag are under the control of the minimal rat probasin –426/+C28 fragment. All male TRAMP mice develop PCa spontaneously: as in humans, they develop PIN, and well- or moderately- differentiated adenocarcinomas (between 10 and 20 weeks of age) and undifferentiated carcinomas (expressing or not AR) as well as phyllode tumors in the seminal vesicles [58,59]. Most adenocarcinomas arose in the dorsolateral lobe, which is considered most analogous to the peripheral zone where the human disease originates [10]. TRAMP was the first mouse model to display distant organ metastases, albeit rarely to the skeleton. Metastatic progression can be observed after 28 weeks of age, when almost all mice display lymphatic and >60% lung metastases from AR-, poorly differentiated (PD) tumors that constitute the main "lethal phenotype" in the TRAMP mouse on account of their fast growth and consequent acute renal damage due to compression, and also because they are the source of distant metastases and systemic cachexia [60]. These phenomena can also occur in the absence of other physiologic sequelae of metastatic disease [61]. An issue with the TRAMP model is that its most frequent lethal and metastatic malignancy (i.e. the PD tumor), has been reported to be of neuroendocrine nature and origin, while the simultaneous loss of p53 and Rb could increase susceptibility to neuroendocrine cancer [62-64].

The TRAMP mouse has become a popular preclinical model for studying chemoprevention/ treatment of PCa, and elucidation of the antitumorigenic effects of many classes of chemopreventive/therapeutic regimens, including anti-androgen, anti-estrogen, anti-angiogenic, ornithine decarboxylase inhibitors, green tea polyphenols, COX-2 inhibitors, phytoestrogens, retinoic acid, grape seed extract, flavonolignans, etc (Table 1).This model enables comparison of the efficacy of treatments. A significant decrease of incidence and a delay of tumor progression was observed following anti angiogenic treatment (endostatin and angiostatin gene therapy), and lycopene and tomato supplementation. Other promising antioxidant agents include green tea, soy, resveratrol, crucifers, curcumin, tocotrienols, triterpenoids and methyl-selenium.

Regimen	Compound	Reference	Year
Anti-androgen	Flutamide	108	2000
Ornithine decarboxylase inhibition	alpha-difluoromethylornithine	109	2000
Green tea	Polyphenolic extract	110	2001
Soy	Genistein	111	2001
Anti-estrogen	Toremifene	112	2002
Anti-inflammatory	Celecoxib	113	2004
Anti-inflammatory	Celecoxib, exisulind	114	2004
Soy	Genistein	115	2004
Differentiative, antiangiogenic	Retinoic acid	116	2004
Green tea	Polyphenolic extract	117	2004
Green tea	Epigallocatechin-3-gallate (EGCG)	118	2004
Green tea	Polyphenolic extract	119	2004
Green tea	Polyphenolic extract	120	2005
Anti-inflammatory	Etodolac	121	2005
Block of the α1-adrenergic receptors	Doxazosin	122	2005
Rye	Bran	123	2005
Soy	Genistein	124	2005
Anti-inflammatory	Celecoxib	125	2006
Anti-oxidative	Spinach extract, EGCG, acetylcysteine	126	2006
DNA methyltransferase inhibition	5-aza-2'-deoxycytidine	127	2006
Estrogen metabolite	2-Methoxyestradiol	128	2006
Grape seeds	Polyphenolicextracy	129	2007
Anti-β-Catenin	Apigenin	130	2007
Soy	Genistein	131	2007
Anti-angiogenic	Endostatin and angiostatin gene therapy	132	2007
Green tea	Epigallocatechin-3-gallate (EGCG)	133	2007
Milk thistle(Silybummarianum) seeds	Silibin	134	2007
Combined immunoprophylaxis	Allogeneic cells and recombinant IL-12	135	2007
Saw palmetto	Liposterolic extract	136	2007
Grape	Resveratrol	137	2007
Plant flavonoid	Apigenin	138	2007
Milk thistle(Silybummarianum) seeds	Silibin	139	2008
Milk thistle(Silybummarianum) seeds	Silibin	140	2008

http://dx.doi.org/10.5772/45948

Regimen	Compound	Reference	Year
Cruciferous vegetables	Sulphoraphane	141	2009
Green tea	Polyphenolic extract	142	2009
Milk thistle(Silybummarianum) seeds	Silibin	143	2009
Anti-oxidative	γ-Tocopherol	144	2009
Systemic buffers		145	2012
Anti-oxidative	γ-Tocopherol	146	2012
Anti-inflammatory	Ursolic acid	147	2012
High-fat diet	Whole walnuts	148	2012
Pomegranate	Fruit exctract	149	2012
Plant flavonoid	Apigenin	150	2012
Cancer therapy	Docetaxel, Dexametasone, Octeotride	151	2012
Bitter melon	Fruit exctract	152	2011
Diet	Folate deficiency	153	2011
Anti-inflammatory	Ursolic acid	154	2011
Anti-inflammatory + anti-hormonal	Celecoxib, Hormone ablation	155	2011
Garlic	Diallyltrisulfide	156	2011
Anti-oxidative	Indolole-3-carbinole	157	2011
Anti-oxidative	Whole tomatoes	158	2010
Anti-oxidative	Lycopene beadlet, tomato paste	159	2010
Diet	Western diet	160	2010
Anti-oxidative	Seleniun	161	2011
Triterpenoids	Synthetic CDDO	162	2011
Mitocondrial Hsp90 inhibition		163	2011
Arginine metabolism	Modulators	164	2011
Anti-oxidative	Methyl-seleniun	165	2009
Hormonal	Methoxyestradiol	166	2009
Interferon-alpha		167	2009
3,3'-Diindolylmethane		168	2010
Anti-oxidative	Mixed tocotrienols	169	2010
Diet	Zinc	170	2010
Cancer therapy	Treatment targeting HIF-a and Stat3	171	2011
Crucifers	Indole-3-carbinol	172	2011

Table 1. Preventive/Therapeutic Regimens Tested in the TRAMP Model of Prostate Cancer

To increase the transgene expression beyond that obtained with the minima probasin promoter, as in the TRAMP mouse, an 11.5 kb 5′ flanking fragment of the prostate-specific probasin promoter (large probasin) has since been isolated [65], and used to direct large T-antigen expression to the dorsolateral and ventral prostate (Lady mouse model). The second key difference in this model is that the large probasin promoter was linked to a deletion mutant of the SV40 T-antigen that expressed only the large T-antigen [66,67]. The Lady model is advantageous because expression is high, but the PCa progression is less aggressive, beginning with low to high-grade PIN and proceeding to carcinoma with neuroendocrine features. However, metastatic progression was not seen [5,67]. Several other trangenic mouse models have been developed with or without the involvement of SV40 antigens and with different strategies (reviewed in ref. [12]). In summary, while T antigen expression generally induces castration-resistant, aggressive and metastatic PCas, often with a neuroendocrine phenotype, the specific expression of other oncogenes in the prostate results in a mild phenotype that rarely progresses to adenocarcinoma.

7. Knockout mice

7.1. Whole body models

The roles of genes significant in prostate carcinogenesis can also be studied in, whole-body knockout models. Here, however, the gene involved is knocked out ubiquitously, and its specific role in a given organ cannot be readily determined. Estrogen receptor b knockout mice display hyperplastic foci in the prostate or even no pathological changes [68]. Deletion of retinoic acid receptor γ determines squamous metaplasia of prostate and seminal vesicles, but not carcinomas [69]. p27knockout mouse display prostatic hyperplasia histologically similar to that observed in human BPH, but not PIN, and a pathogenetic role of p27 loss in BPH development in both mice and humans has been suggested [70]. Inactivation of T (phosphatase and tensin homolog deleted on chromosome 10) prevents activation of AKT and apoptosis resulting in embryonic lethality. However, haploinsufficiency leads to early stages (PIN) of prostatic carcinogenesis [71]. Double-knockout models in which loss of PTEN is associated with loss of other tumor suppressors (p27, Nkx3.1, and p53), are characterized by more aggressive tumor phenotype.The highest stage of tumor progression was adenocarcinoma (PTEN x p27 mouse) [72], lymph node metastases (PTEN x Nkx3.1 mouse) [73], and high grade PIN (PTEN x p53 mouse) [74]. In addition, several mouse models with up to 5 genetic hits demonstrated, as expected, the complexity of the events required for a complete progression of prostatic tumors from low-grade PIN to metastatic disease (see review [75]).

7.2. Conditional models

The "old" (1979) [76] Cre-loxP system was used to produce mice with prostate-specific alterations. Cre is a recombinase that promotes specific genetic recombination in trans at loxP sites. The Cre-loxP system was developed and used for genetic recombination first in yeast and later in mice [77,78]. Many genes knocked out with the whole body strategy were also knocked out by using a conditional approach that results in higher prostate tumor severity. As an example, tissue-specific deletion indicated that homozygous loss of prostatic PTEN led to most stages of prostate tumor progression (metastatic disease) when compared to whole-body haploinsufficiecy, where only PIN was present [79]. At present, the Cre-lox system is diffusely employed to generate mouse models characterized by cell-type-specific and tissue-specific genetic modification (see recent review in ref. [12]). The probasin and the prostate specific antigen (PSA) promoters were extensively utilized to induce targeted Cre expression in the prostate. PB-Cre and PSA-Cre mice have been employed to delete the intraprostatic expression of PTEN, Rb, p53, APC, IGF1 and PTEN, Nkx3, respectively.

E-Resources for mouse models of human cancer, including PCa, are also available online (http://emice.nci.nih.gov/,http://cancermodels.nci.nih.gov/,andhttp://cancerimages.nci.nih.gov/).

8. Clinical trials

Mouse models have significantly contributed to our understanding of PCa biology through their identification of new cancer genes and biomarkers, and their illustration of the molecular and cellular mechanisms underlying tumor initiation and progression. They have also been employed in a preclinical setting to test novel preventive and/or therapeutic strategies [5,6,8-12,80]. Mice, in fact, offer several advantages. They are small, relatively inexpensive, and reproduce rapidly with large litters. More importantly, technical advances have facilitated the generation of defined genetic modifications that can also be spatially controlled, to mimic human prostate carcinogenesis. In general, and perhaps not surprisingly, a variety of phenotypes are obtained depending on the specific genetically engineered mouse model, but none exactly mimics the human disease. Although preclinical studies and the epidemiological evidence suggest that specific dietary components or nutritional supplements influence overall mortality and/or reduce the risk of PCa, randomized, controlled clinical trials provide high-quality evidence of benefit, no effect, or even harm. Examples of ongoing clinical trials are reported in Table 2. In the last ten years, several primary prevention trials have been reported (reviewed in ref. [11,81]). Preventive strategies in a clinical setting have focused on two approaches: antioxidant regimens to reduce DNA damage and suppression of androgenic stimulation [82]. Since a wealth of preclinical and epidemiologic data indicated that selenium and vitamin E reduce PCa, these compounds were evaluated in humans. The Nutritional Prevention of Cancer (NPC) trial found a 63% reduction of PCa incidence (secondary endpoint) following the administration of selenized yeast [83]. The Alpha-Tocopherol Beta-Carotene Cancer prevention study (ATBC), one of the first large studies (14,569 subjects enrolled), investigated the prevention of lung cancer among male smokers. The results indicated that beta carotene supplements increased the risk of lung cancer, rather than preventing it, and that vitamin E had no effect [84-86]. However, a significantly lower risk of PCa was observed for participants receiving vitamin E alone. The NPC and ATBC findings underpinned the NCI-sponsored selenium and vitamin E cancer prevention trial (SELECT). This randomized 35,533 men into four groups: (1) selenium/placebo, (2) vitamin E/placebo, (3) both agents, and (4) placebo alone [87]. At a mean of 5.5 years neither agent reduced risk of PCa. However, at a mean of 7 years and with an additional person-year of follow-up, men receiving vitamin E alone had a significantly increased the risk of PCa (Hazard Ratio 1.17, 99% CI 1.004– 1.36, P = 0.008) [88]. Does vitamin E prevent or promote cancer? More research on the biological activities of the forms and mixtures of tocopherols (alpha, gamma, and delta), and their baseline serum levels should be considered (analyses and discussion in ref. [81,89,90]).

The most promising agents for preventing PCa are probably the 5-alpha reductase inhibitors (5-ARIs). Five-alpha reductase catalyzes the conversion of testosterone to the more active dihydrotestosterone. The Prostate Cancer Prevention Trial (PCPT) and the Reduction by Dutasteride of Prostate Cancer Events (REDUCE) Trial evaluated the activities of two 5-ARIs, finasteride and dutasteride, respectively (reviewed in ref. [81,91]). 5-ARI use for 4-7 years reduced the overall risk of biopsy-detectable PCa by 23-25%. All the prevented cases are either low-grade (PCPT) or GS ≤3 + 4 = 7 prostatic carcinoma (REDUCE). It is unclear whether the slightly increased risk of high-grade cancers in both trials is real or an artifact. In addition to the risk of androgen-independent tumors, the side effects of 5-ARI such as neurodegeneration, osteoporosis, cardiovascular diseases, genitourinary dysfunctions, and hormonal disarrangement limit their use as primary chemopreventive drugs [92-94].

Clinical translation has thus proved to be a general failure when viewed against the optimism aroused by preventive treatments (antioxidant, anti-hormonal, anti-inflammatory, anti-angiogenic etc agents) in the preclinical setting. It has been proposed that species-specific differences, and differences in time of treatment intervention age, trial design enrolment criteria, genetic variation, and the choice, dose, and bioavailability of preventive/therapeutic agents are lie behind for the discrepancy [11]. The most substantial challenge posed by mouse models of PCa, as for other tumors, is their species-specific differences. The lifespan of a mouse is 25-50 times shorter than that of humans, and mice are 3000 times smaller, with consequent differences in pharmacokinetics [95,96]. Anatomically, the human prostate is a single alobular organ with a central, a transitional, and a peripheral zone, whereas the murine prostate comprises four paired lobes located around the urethra, namely the anterior (or coagulating gland), dorsal, lateral, and ventral prostate. The dorsal and lateral lobes are treated as one (the dorsolateral lobe) as they share a ductal system. This lobe has been described as the most similar to the human peripheral zone where most carcinomas arise [97,98]. According to the Bar Harbor Pathology Panel consensus opinion, however, there is no direct relationship between any mouse lobe and any of the human zones [58]. Histologically, the mouse and the human prostate display similar cell types (secretory, basal and neuroendocrine), but their ratio varies from one species to another [99,100]. Mice have fewer basal cells and a discontinuous layer on the basal membrane, whereas in humans, this layer is continuous between secretory cells and the basal membrane. Neuroendocrine cells, rare in humans, are even more rare in mice. The human prostate is characterized by an abundant fibromuscular stoma, whereas the murine gland has a small stromal component. Mice are susceptible to malignancies. By comparison with humans, however, they tend to have more sarcomas and lymphomas and very few epithelial tumors, probably due to differences in relative telomere activity [101-103]. Telomerase, mostly inactive in cells from adult humans, is present in mouse cells, which can thus be transformed/immortalized more easily than their human counterparts, and fewer genetic hits are required to bring about neoplastic transformation in mice than in men. Inactivation of telomerase in the mouse model may be necessary to more accurately recapitulate human cancer phenotypes [80,104].

Most primary PCa prevention studies used mice with an average age of 4-8 weeks, by which time they are considered to have attained sexual maturity and are unlikely to have sustained hormone-induced oxidative stress. In the mouse, a delay in the start of treatment results in a reduced or even no effect. Most human PCa prevention trials were conducted on men aged 50 or more. In addition, the agent dose in animals is 50-80% of the maximally tolerated dose, whereas in humans lower doses may be required for bioethical reasons. The excellent review of Pienta et al. (Prostate Cancer Model Working Group) offers a list of limitations of preclinical models that have hampered the translation of their findings to human clinical trials [8].

Agent*	Trial No.	Type	Institution	Phase	Status
Green tea	NCT00685516	Therapy	Jonsson Comprehensive Cancer Center	II	Recruiting
	NCT00253643	Prevention	Oregon Health and Science University		Recruiting
	NCT00003367	Therapy	Memorial Sloan-Kettering Cancer Center	III	Active
	NCT00676780	Basic science	Louisiana State University Active	II	Active
	NCT00744549	Therapy	University Health Network, Toronto	II	Recruiting
Genistein	NCT00546039	Basic science	University Hospital, Aker Active	II	
	NCT00005827	Therapy	North Carolina University LinebergerCenter	I	Completed
	NCT00058266	Therapy	Robert H. Lurie Cancer Center	II	Active
	NCT00584532	Therapy	University of California, Davis	II/III	Completed
	NCT00376948	Therapy	Barbara Ann Karmanos Cancer Institute	II	Suspended
	NCT00499408	Therapy	Wake Forest University	II	Recruiting
Pomegranate	NCT00413530	Therapy	M. D. Anderson Cancer Center		Recruiting
	NCT00719030	Prevention	University of California, Los Angeles		Recruiting
	NCT00732043	Prevention	Radiant Research	II	Recruiting
	NCT00731848	Therapy	Radiant Research	II	Recruiting

Agent*	Trial No.	Type	Institution	Phase	Status
	NCT00336934	Therapy	Roll International Corporation	III	Recruiting
	NCT00060086	Therapy	Jonsson Comprehensive Cancer Center	II	Active
	NCT00433797	Therapy	University of Oslo	I/II	Recruiting
Lycopene	NCT00042731	Therapy	H. Lee Moffitt Cancer Center		Completed
	NCT00416325	Prevention	University of Illinois	I	Completed
	NCT00178113	PIN Prevention	University of Pittsburgh	I	Completed
	NCT00093561	Prevention	University of Illinois Completed	I	Completed
	NCT00450749	Therapy	M. D. Anderson Cancer Center	II	Recruiting
	NCT00006078	Prevention	University of Illinois	I	Completed
	NCT00322114	Prevention	University of Illinois	II	Recruiting
	NCT00402285	Therapy	University of California San Francisco		Active
	NCT00450957	Prevention	University of Illinois	I	Active
	NCT00068731	Therapy	North Central Cancer Treatment Group	II	Active
	NCT00744549	Therapy	University Health Network, Toronto	II	Recruiting
	NCT00669656	Therapy	Norris Comprehensive Cancer Center	II	Recruiting
n-3 poly	NCT00458549	Therapy	Dana-Farber Cancer Institute		Recruiting
unsaturated fatty acids	NCT00402285	Therapy	California San Francisco Helen Diller Center		Active

* Data from ref. [105]

Table 2. Clinical Trials of Preventive/Therapeutic Regimens for Prostate Cancer

9. Conclusions

Genetically engineered mouse models of PCa have paved the way to many important discoveries and helped to define the molecular events of prostate tumorigenesis. However, no single model precisely recapitulates all the molecular or cellular features of the progression of PCa from the normal gland to metastatic, hormone-refractory carcinoma, especially since its early stages are not those of single-cell-type disease, but must be viewed as a complex system of epithelial cells that display dysregulated growth within both a microenvironment composed of many cells which support such growth, and the host macroenvironment with its unique genotype and immune system. Further research is needed to better define these

http://dx.doi.org/10.5772/45948

interactions, many of which are potential therapeutic targets. Several in vivo models can be utilized to study specific components of tumor initiation and progression. Meaningful interpretation of their results, however, demands a full understanding of the properties and limits of each model, along with employment of the model most consonant with the subject to be studied. Preclinical models have been poorly predictive of results in human studies because of both their inadequacy and their inappropriate use leading to the designing of clinical trials that do not mirror the preclinical model testing [106]. However, the chemoprevention field is particularly challenging since discrepancies have also been found between initial findings in several trials, secondary analyses and epidemiologic data, and subsequent randomized studies in humans [107]. These inconsistencies may reasonably be supposed to stem from the fact that dietary agents may act long before the scheduled commencement of a chemoprevention trial. Since such trials need to find outcomes (cancers), they invariably start with populations at higher risk of developing clinically detectable cancer, namely middle-aged and older subjects. However, dietary elements may either have a lifelong effect in their changes to the baseline risk for cancer or act at key points by priming the pump for its future development. In either case, dietary chemoprevention might be possible, but its indisputable demonstration in a trial would be highly unlikely. Do these discrepancies mean that all the preclinical and epidemiologic studies are wrong? It must primarily be considered that the timing of such interventions is unclear. Their employment in very high risk subjects, indeed, may actually be too late to significantly prevent cancer formation. Future studies will require both the use of other models founded on our increased understanding of human cancer proteomic genetics and epigenetics to define the very first steps in the progression of the disease and the ability of agents to impair or retard it, and a better "translational approach" achieved through preclinical studies that utilize the appropriate agent doses, and pharmacokinetic and pharmacodynamic parameters to take into account the differences in metabolism between mice and humans, together with clinical trials whose design takes account of how the preclinical testing was accomplished.

Acknowledgments

We wish to thank Prof. John Iliffe for reading the manuscript and critical suggestions. The work of the authors is supported by the Italian Ministry for the Universities and Research.

Author details

Rossano Lattanzio[1], Alessia Lamolinara[2], Mauro Piantelli[1] and Manuela Iezzi[2]

1 Departement of Biomedical Sciences, University "G. D'Annunzio" Chieti, Italy

2 Department of Medicine and Aging Sciences, University "G. D'Annunzio" Chieti, Italy

References

[1] Ferlay J, Autier P, Boniol M, Heanue M, Colombet M, Boyle P. Estimates of the cancer incidence and mortality in Europe in 2006. Ann Oncol 2007;18(3):581-592.

[2] Jemal A, Murray T, Ward E, Samuels A, Tiwari RC, Ghafoor A, Feuer EJ, Thun MJ. Cancer statistics, 2005. CA Cancer J Clin 2005;55(1):10-30.

[3] Dasgupta S, Srinidhi S, Vishwanatha JK. Oncogenic activation in prostate cancer progression and metastasis: Molecular insights and future challenges. J Carcinog;11:4.

[4] Nelson WG, De MarzoAM, Isaacs WB. Prostate cancer. N Engl J Med 2003;349(4): 366-381.

[5] Lamb DJ, Zhang L. Challenges in prostate cancer research: animal models for nutritional studies of chemoprevention and disease progression. J Nutr 2005;135(12 Suppl):3009S-3015S.

[6] Nguewa PA, Calvo A. Use of transgenic mice as models for prostate cancer chemoprevention. CurrMol Med;10(8):705-718.

[7] Ozten-Kandas N, Bosland MC. Chemoprevention of prostate cancer: Natural compounds, antiandrogens, and antioxidants - In vivo evidence. J Carcinog;10:27.

[8] Pienta KJ, Abate-Shen C, Agus DB, Attar RM, Chung LW, Greenberg NM, Hahn WC, Isaacs JT, Navone NM, Peehl DM, Simons JW, Solit DB, Soule HR, VanDyke TA, Weber MJ, Wu L, Vessella RL. The current state of preclinical prostate cancer animal models. Prostate 2008;68(6):629-639.

[9] Roy-Burman P, Wu H, Powell WC, Hagenkord J, Cohen MB. Genetically defined mouse models that mimic natural aspects of human prostate cancer development. EndocrRelat Cancer 2004;11(2):225-254.

[10] Sharma P, Schreiber-Agus N. Mouse models of prostate cancer. Oncogene 1999;18(38):5349-5355.

[11] Thapa D, Ghosh R. Antioxidants for prostate cancer chemoprevention: challenges and opportunities. Biochem Pharmacol;83(10):1319-1330.

[12] Valkenburg KC, Williams BO. Mouse models of prostate cancer. Prostate Cancer; 2011:895238.

[13] Waters DJ, Sakr WA, Hayden DW, Lang CM, McKinney L, Murphy GP, Radinsky R, Ramoner R, Richardson RC, Tindall DJ. Workgroup 4: spontaneous prostate carcinoma in dogs and nonhuman primates. Prostate 1998;36(1):64-67.

[14] Leroy BE, Northrup N. Prostate cancer in dogs: comparative and clinical aspects. Vet J 2009;180(2):149-162.

[15] Winter SF, Cooper AB, Greenberg NM. Models of metastatic prostate cancer: a transgenic perspective. Prostate Cancer Prostatic Dis 2003;6(3):204-211.

[16] Ghoniem GM, VandenBerg TL. Dollars and sense: considerations for experimental model design. NeurourolUrodyn 1994;13(2):91-96.

[17] Maini A, Archer C, Wang CY, Haas GP. Comparative pathology of benign prostatic hyperplasia and prostate cancer. In Vivo 1997;11(4):293-299.

[18] Rosol TJ, Tannehill-Gregg SH, LeRoy BE, Mandl S, Contag CH. Animal models of bone metastasis. Cancer 2003;97(3 Suppl):748-757.

[19] Dunning WF. Prostate Cancer in the Rat. Natl Cancer InstMonogr 1963;12:351-369.

[20] Isaacs JT, Isaacs WB, Feitz WF, Scheres J. Establishment and characterization of seven Dunning rat prostatic cancer cell lines and their use in developing methods for predicting metastatic abilities of prostatic cancers. Prostate 1986;9(3):261-281.

[21] Isaacs JT, Weissman RM, Coffey DS, Scott WW. Concepts in prostatic cancer biology: Dunning R-3327 H, HI, and AT tumors. ProgClinBiol Res 1980;37:311-323.

[22] Lubaroff DM, Canfield L, Feldbush TL, Bonney WW. R3327 adenocarcinoma of the Copenhagen rat as a model for the study of the immunologic aspects of prostate cancer. J Natl Cancer Inst 1977;58(6):1677-1689.

[23] Lubaroff DM, Canfield L, Rasmussen GT, Reynolds CW. An animal model for the study of prostate carcinoma. Natl Cancer InstMonogr 1978(49):275-281.

[24] Jeet V, Russell PJ, Khatri A. Modeling prostate cancer: a perspective on transgenic mouse models. Cancer Metastasis Rev;29(1):123-142.

[25] Pollard M. Animal models for prostate cancer. Prostate 1980;1(2):207-213.

[26] Geurts AM, Cost GJ, Freyvert Y, Zeitler B, Miller JC, Choi VM, Jenkins SS, Wood A, Cui X, Meng X, Vincent A, Lam S, Michalkiewicz M, Schilling R, Foeckler J, Kalloway S, Weiler H, Menoret S, Anegon I, Davis GD, Zhang L, Rebar EJ, Gregory PD, Urnov FD, Jacob HJ, Buelow R. Knockout rats via embryo microinjection of zinc-finger nucleases. Science 2009;325(5939):433.

[27] Izsvak Z, Frohlich J, Grabundzija I, Shirley JR, Powell HM, Chapman KM, Ivics Z, Hamra FK. Generating knockout rats by transposon mutagenesis in spermatogonial stem cells. Nat Methods;7(6):443-445.

[28] Tong C, Li P, Wu NL, Yan Y, Ying QL. Production of p53 gene knockout rats by homologous recombination in embryonic stem cells. Nature;467(7312):211-213.

[29] Hamra FK. Gene targeting: Enter the rat. Nature;467(7312):161-163.

[30] Morton CL, Houghton PJ. Establishment of human tumorxenografts in immunodeficient mice. Nat Protoc 2007;2(2):247-250.

[31] Schroder FH, Jellinghaus W. Prostatic adenoma and carcinoma in cell culture and heterotransplantation. ProgClinBiol Res 1976;6:301-312.

[32] Hoehn W, Schroeder FH, Reimann JF, Joebsis AC, Hermanek P. Human prostatic adenocarcinoma: some characteristics of a serially transplantable line in nude mice (PC 82). Prostate 1980;1(1):95-104.

[33] van Weerden WM, Romijn JC. Use of nude mouse xenograft models in prostate cancer research. Prostate 2000;43(4):263-271.

[34] Thalmann GN, Anezinis PE, Chang SM, Zhau HE, Kim EE, Hopwood VL, Pathak S, von Eschenbach AC, Chung LW. Androgen-independent cancer progression and bone metastasis in the LNCaP model of human prostate cancer. Cancer Res 1994;54(10):2577-2581.

[35] Bosma GC, Custer RP, Bosma MJ. A severe combined immunodeficiency mutation in the mouse. Nature 1983;301(5900):527-530.

[36] Bosma MJ, Carroll AM. The SCID mouse mutant: definition, characterization, and potential uses. Annu Rev Immunol 1991;9:323-350.

[37] Craft N, Shostak Y, Carey M, Sawyers CL. A mechanism for hormone-independent prostate cancer through modulation of androgen receptor signaling by the HER-2/neu tyrosine kinase. Nat Med 1999;5(3):280-285.

[38] Shultz LD, Schweitzer PA, Christianson SW, Gott B, Schweitzer IB, Tennent B, McKenna S, Mobraaten L, Rajan TV, Greiner DL, et al. Multiple defects in innate and adaptive immunologic function in NOD/LtSz-scid mice. J Immunol 1995;154(1): 180-191.

[39] Bastide C, Bagnis C, Mannoni P, Hassoun J, Bladou F. A Nod Scid mouse model to study human prostate cancer. Prostate Cancer Prostatic Dis 2002;5(4):311-315.

[40] Nemeth JA, Harb JF, Barroso U, Jr., He Z, Grignon DJ, Cher ML. Severe combined immunodeficient-hu model of human prostate cancer metastasis to human bone. Cancer Res 1999;59(8):1987-1993.

[41] Wainstein MA, He F, Robinson D, Kung HJ, Schwartz S, Giaconia JM, Edgehouse NL, Pretlow TP, Bodner DR, Kursh ED, et al. CWR22: androgen-dependent xenograft model derived from a primary human prostatic carcinoma. Cancer Res 1994;54(23): 6049-6052.

[42] Yonou H, Yokose T, Kamijo T, Kanomata N, Hasebe T, Nagai K, Hatano T, Ogawa Y, Ochiai A. Establishment of a novel species- and tissue-specific metastasis model of human prostate cancer in humanized non-obese diabetic/severe combined immunodeficient mice engrafted with human adult lung and bone. Cancer Res 2001;61(5): 2177-2182.

[43] D'Antonio JM, Vander Griend DJ, Antony L, Ndikuyeze G, Dalrymple SL, Koochekpour S, Isaacs JT. Loss of androgen receptor-dependent growth suppression by prostate cancer cells can occur independently from acquiring oncogenic addiction to androgen receptor signaling. PLoS One;5(7):e11475.

[44] Ito M, Hiramatsu H, Kobayashi K, Suzue K, Kawahata M, Hioki K, Ueyama Y, Koyanagi Y, Sugamura K, Tsuji K, Heike T, Nakahata T. NOD/SCID/gamma(c)(null) mouse: an excellent recipient mouse model for engraftment of human cells. Blood 2002;100(9):3175-3182.

[45] Quintana E, Shackleton M, Sabel MS, Fullen DR, Johnson TM, Morrison SJ. Efficient tumour formation by single human melanoma cells. Nature 2008;456(7222):593-598.

[46] Sobel RE, Sadar MD. Cell lines used in prostate cancer research: a compendium of old and new lines--part 1. J Urol 2005;173(2):342-359.

[47] Sobel RE, Sadar MD. Cell lines used in prostate cancer research: a compendium of old and new lines--part 2. J Urol 2005;173(2):360-372.

[48] Sobel RE, Wang Y, Sadar MD. Molecular analysis and characterization of PrEC, commercially available prostate epithelial cells. In Vitro Cell DevBiolAnim 2006;42(1-2): 33-39.

[49] van Bokhoven A, Caires A, Maria MD, Schulte AP, Lucia MS, Nordeen SK, Miller GJ, Varella-Garcia M. Spectral karyotype (SKY) analysis of human prostate carcinoma cell lines. Prostate 2003;57(3):226-244.

[50] vanBokhoven A, Varella-Garcia M, Korch C, Johannes WU, Smith EE, Miller HL, Nordeen SK, Miller GJ, Lucia MS. Molecular characterization of human prostate carcinoma cell lines. Prostate 2003;57(3):205-225.

[51] DeCaprio JA, Ludlow JW, Figge J, Shew JY, Huang CM, Lee WH, Marsilio E, Paucha E, Livingston DM. SV40 large tumor antigen forms a specific complex with the product of the retinoblastoma susceptibility gene. Cell 1988;54(2):275-283.

[52] Lane DP, Crawford LV. T antigen is bound to a host protein in SV40-transformed cells. Nature 1979;278(5701):261-263.

[53] Pallas DC, Shahrik LK, Martin BL, Jaspers S, Miller TB, Brautigan DL, Roberts TM. Polyoma small and middle T antigens and SV40 small t antigen form stable complexes with protein phosphatase 2A. Cell 1990;60(1):167-176.

[54] Maroulakou IG, Anver M, Garrett L, Green JE. Prostate and mammary adenocarcinoma in transgenic mice carrying a rat C3(1) simian virus 40 large tumor antigen fusion gene. ProcNatlAcadSci U S A 1994;91(23):11236-11240.

[55] Yoshidome K, Shibata MA, Maroulakou IG, Liu ML, Jorcyk CL, Gold LG, Welch VN, Green JE. Genetic alterations in the development of mammary and prostate cancer in the C3(1)/Tag transgenic mouse model. Int J Oncol 1998;12(2):449-453.

[56] Gingrich JR, Barrios RJ, Kattan MW, Nahm HS, Finegold MJ, Greenberg NM. Androgen-independent prostate cancer progression in the TRAMP model. Cancer Res 1997;57(21):4687-4691.

[57] Greenberg NM, DeMayo F, Finegold MJ, Medina D, Tilley WD, Aspinall JO, Cunha GR, Donjacour AA, Matusik RJ, Rosen JM. Prostate cancer in a transgenic mouse. ProcNatlAcadSci U S A 1995;92(8):3439-3443.

[58] Shappell SB, Thomas GV, Roberts RL, Herbert R, Ittmann MM, Rubin MA, Humphrey PA, Sundberg JP, Rozengurt N, Barrios R, Ward JM, Cardiff RD. Prostate pathology of genetically engineered mice: definitions and classification. The consensus report from the Bar Harbor meeting of the Mouse Models of Human Cancer Consortium Prostate Pathology Committee. Cancer Res 2004;64(6):2270-2305.

[59] Tani Y, Suttie A, Flake GP, Nyska A, Maronpot RR. Epithelial-stromal tumor of the seminal vesicles in the transgenic adenocarcinoma mouse prostate model. Vet Pathol 2005;42(3):306-314.

[60] Gingrich JR, Barrios RJ, Foster BA, Greenberg NM. Pathologic progression of autochthonous prostate cancer in the TRAMP model. Prostate Cancer Prostatic Dis 1999;2(2):70-75.

[61] Wood RW, Baggs RB, Schwarz EM, Messing EM. Initial observations of reduced uroflow in transgenic adenocarcinoma of murine prostate. Urology 2006;67(6):1324-1328.

[62] Bono AV, Montironi R, Pannellini T, Sasso F, Mirone V, Musiani P, Iezzi M. Effects of castration on the development of prostate adenocarcinoma from its precursor HGPIN and on the occurrence of androgen-independent, poorly differentiated carcinoma in TRAMP mice. Prostate Cancer Prostatic Dis 2008;11(4):377-383.

[63] Chiaverotti T, Couto SS, Donjacour A, Mao JH, Nagase H, Cardiff RD, Cunha GR, Balmain A. Dissociation of epithelial and neuroendocrine carcinoma lineages in the transgenic adenocarcinoma of mouse prostate model of prostate cancer. Am J Pathol 2008;172(1):236-246.

[64] Huss WJ, Gray DR, Tavakoli K, Marmillion ME, Durham LE, Johnson MA, Greenberg NM, Smith GJ. Origin of androgen-insensitive poorly differentiated tumors in the transgenic adenocarcinoma of mouse prostate model. Neoplasia 2007;9(11): 938-950.

[65] Yan Y, Sheppard PC, Kasper S, Lin L, Hoare S, Kapoor A, Dodd JG, Duckworth ML, Matusik RJ. Large fragment of the probasin promoter targets high levels of transgene expression to the prostate of transgenic mice. Prostate 1997;32(2):129-139.

[66] Kasper S, Sheppard PC, Yan Y, Pettigrew N, Borowsky AD, Prins GS, Dodd JG, Duckworth ML, Matusik RJ. Development, progression, and androgen-dependence of prostate tumors in probasin-large T antigen transgenic mice: a model for prostate cancer. Lab Invest 1998;78(6):i-xv.

[67] Kasper S, Tu W, Roberts RL, Shappell SB. Transgenic mouse models for prostate cancer. Identification of an androgen-dependent promoter and creation and characterization of the long probasin promoter-Large T antigen (LPB-Tag) model. Methods Mol Med 2003;81:113-147.

[68] Weihua Z, Makela S, Andersson LC, Salmi S, Saji S, Webster JI, Jensen EV, Nilsson S, Warner M, Gustafsson JA. A role for estrogen receptor beta in the regulation of growth of the ventral prostate. ProcNatlAcadSci U S A 2001;98(11):6330-6335.

[69] Lohnes D, Kastner P, Dierich A, Mark M, LeMeur M, Chambon P. Function of retinoic acid receptor gamma in the mouse. Cell 1993;73(4):643-658.

[70] Cordon-Cardo C, Koff A, Drobnjak M, Capodieci P, Osman I, Millard SS, Gaudin PB, Fazzari M, Zhang ZF, Massague J, Scher HI. Distinct altered patterns of p27KIP1 gene expression in benign prostatic hyperplasia and prostatic carcinoma. J Natl Cancer Inst 1998;90(17):1284-1291.

[71] Podsypanina K, Ellenson LH, Nemes A, Gu J, Tamura M, Yamada KM, Cordon-Cardo C, Catoretti G, Fisher PE, Parsons R. Mutation of Pten/Mmac1 in mice causes neoplasia in multiple organ systems. ProcNatlAcadSci U S A 1999;96(4):1563-1568.

[72] Di Cristofano A, De Acetis M, Koff A, Cordon-Cardo C, Pandolfi PP. Pten and p27KIP1 cooperate in prostate cancer tumor suppression in the mouse. Nat Genet 2001;27(2):222-224.

[73] Abate-Shen C, Banach-Petrosky WA, Sun X, Economides KD, Desai N, Gregg JP, Borowsky AD, Cardiff RD, Shen MM. Nkx3.1; Pten mutant mice develop invasive prostate adenocarcinoma and lymph node metastases. Cancer Res 2003;63(14):3886-3890.

[74] Couto SS, Cao M, Duarte PC, Banach-Petrosky W, Wang S, Romanienko P, Wu H, Cardiff RD, Abate-Shen C, Cunha GR. Simultaneous haploinsufficiency of Pten and Trp53 tumor suppressor genes accelerates tumorigenesis in a mouse model of prostate cancer. Differentiation 2009;77(1):103-111.

[75] Kasper S. Survey of genetically engineered mouse models for prostate cancer: analyzing the molecular basis of prostate cancer development, progression, and metastasis. J Cell Biochem 2005;94(2):279-297.

[76] Sternberg N. Demonstration and analysis of P1 site-specific recombination using lambda-P1 hybrid phages constructed in vitro. Cold Spring HarbSymp Quant Biol 1979;43Pt 2:1143-1146.

[77] Metzger D, Chambon P. Site- and time-specific gene targeting in the mouse. Methods 2001;24(1):71-80.

[78] Sauer B, Henderson N. Cre-stimulated recombination at loxP-containing DNA sequences placed into the mammalian genome. Nucleic Acids Res 1989;17(1):147-161.

[79] Wang S, Gao J, Lei Q, Rozengurt N, Pritchard C, Jiao J, Thomas GV, Li G, Roy-Burman P, Nelson PS, Liu X, Wu H. Prostate-specific deletion of the murine Ptentumor suppressor gene leads to metastatic prostate cancer. Cancer Cell 2003;4(3):209-221.

[80] Cheon DJ, Orsulic S. Mouse models of cancer. Annu Rev Pathol;6:95-119.

[81] Klein EA, Thompson IM. Chemoprevention of prostate cancer: an updated view. World J Urol;30(2):189-194.

[82] Walsh PC. Chemoprevention of prostate cancer. N Engl J Med;362(13):1237-1238.

[83] Clark LC, Dalkin B, Krongrad A, Combs GF, Jr., Turnbull BW, Slate EH, Witherington R, Herlong JH, Janosko E, Carpenter D, Borosso C, Falk S, Rounder J. Decreased incidence of prostate cancer with selenium supplementation: results of a double-blind cancer prevention trial. Br J Urol 1998;81(5):730-734.

[84] Albanes D, Heinonen OP, Taylor PR, Virtamo J, Edwards BK, Rautalahti M, Hartman AM, Palmgren J, Freedman LS, Haapakoski J, Barrett MJ, Pietinen P, Malila N, Tala E, Liippo K, Salomaa ER, Tangrea JA, Teppo L, Askin FB, Taskinen E, Erozan Y, Greenwald P, Huttunen JK. Alpha-Tocopherol and beta-carotene supplements and lung cancer incidence in the alpha-tocopherol, beta-carotene cancer prevention study: effects of base-line characteristics and study compliance. J Natl Cancer Inst 1996;88(21):1560-1570.

[85] Virtamo J, Pietinen P, Huttunen JK, Korhonen P, Malila N, Virtanen MJ, Albanes D, Taylor PR, Albert P. Incidence of cancer and mortality following alpha-tocopherol and beta-carotene supplementation: a postintervention follow-up. Jama 2003;290(4): 476-485.

[86] Weinstein SJ, Wright ME, Lawson KA, Snyder K, Mannisto S, Taylor PR, Virtamo J, Albanes D. Serum and dietary vitamin E in relation to prostate cancer risk. Cancer Epidemiol Biomarkers Prev 2007;16(6):1253-1259.

[87] Lippman SM, Klein EA, Goodman PJ, Lucia MS, Thompson IM, Ford LG, Parnes HL, Minasian LM, Gaziano JM, Hartline JA, Parsons JK, Bearden JD, 3rd, Crawford ED, Goodman GE, Claudio J, Winquist E, Cook ED, Karp DD, Walther P, Lieber MM, Kristal AR, Darke AK, Arnold KB, Ganz PA, Santella RM, Albanes D, Taylor PR, Probstfield JL, Jagpal TJ, Crowley JJ, Meyskens FL, Jr., Baker LH, Coltman CA, Jr. Effect of selenium and vitamin E on risk of prostate cancer and other cancers: the Selenium and Vitamin E Cancer Prevention Trial (SELECT). Jama 2009;301(1):39-51.

[88] Klein EA, Thompson IM, Jr., Tangen CM, Crowley JJ, Lucia MS, Goodman PJ, Minasian LM, Ford LG, Parnes HL, Gaziano JM, Karp DD, Lieber MM, Walther PJ, Klotz L, Parsons JK, Chin JL, Darke AK, Lippman SM, Goodman GE, Meyskens FL, Jr., Baker LH. Vitamin E and the risk of prostate cancer: the Selenium and Vitamin E Cancer Prevention Trial (SELECT). Jama;306(14):1549-1556.

[89] McNeil C. Vitamin E and prostate cancer: research focus turns to biologic mechanisms. J Natl Cancer Inst;103(23):1731-1734.

[90] Yang CS, Suh N, Kong AN. Does vitamin E prevent or promote cancer? Cancer Prev Res (Phila);5(5):701-705.

[91] Azzouni F, Mohler J. Role of 5alpha-reductase inhibitors in prostate cancer prevention and treatment. Urology;79(6):1197-1205.

[92] Feldman BJ, Feldman D. The development of androgen-independent prostate cancer. Nat Rev Cancer 2001;1(1):34-45.

[93] Jones TH. Cardiovascular risk during androgen deprivation therapy for prostate cancer. Bmj;342:d3105.

[94] Taylor LG, Canfield SE, Du XL. Review of major adverse effects of androgen-deprivation therapy in men with prostate cancer. Cancer 2009;115(11):2388-2399.

[95] de Jong M, Maina T. Of mice and humans: are they the same?--Implications in cancer translational research. J Nucl Med;51(4):501-504.

[96] Rangarajan A, Weinberg RA. Opinion: Comparative biology of mouse versus human cells: modelling human cancer in mice. Nat Rev Cancer 2003;3(12):952-959.

[97] Powell WC, Cardiff RD, Cohen MB, Miller GJ, Roy-Burman P. Mouse strains for prostate tumorigenesis based on genes altered in human prostate cancer. Curr Drug Targets 2003;4(3):263-279.

[98] Xue L, Yang K, Newmark H, Lipkin M. Induced hyperproliferation in epithelial cells of mouse prostate by a Western-style diet. Carcinogenesis 1997;18(5):995-999.

[99] Garabedian EM, Humphrey PA, Gordon JI. A transgenic mouse model of metastatic prostate cancer originating from neuroendocrine cells. ProcNatlAcadSci U S A 1998;95(26):15382-15387.

[100] Marker PC, Donjacour AA, Dahiya R, Cunha GR. Hormonal, cellular, and molecular control of prostatic development. DevBiol 2003;253(2):165-174.

[101] Artandi SE, DePinho RA. Telomeres and telomerase in cancer. Carcinogenesis;31(1): 9-18.

[102] Harvey M, McArthur MJ, Montgomery CA, Jr., Butel JS, Bradley A, Donehower LA. Spontaneous and carcinogen-induced tumorigenesis in p53-deficient mice. Nat Genet 1993;5(3):225-229.

[103] Jacks T, Remington L, Williams BO, Schmitt EM, Halachmi S, Bronson RT, Weinberg RA. Tumor spectrum analysis in p53-mutant mice. CurrBiol 1994;4(1):1-7.

[104] Maser RS, Choudhury B, Campbell PJ, Feng B, Wong KK, Protopopov A, O'Neil J, Gutierrez A, Ivanova E, Perna I, Lin E, Mani V, Jiang S, McNamara K, Zaghlul S, Edkins S, Stevens C, Brennan C, Martin ES, Wiedemeyer R, Kabbarah O, Nogueira C, Histen G, Aster J, Mansour M, Duke V, Foroni L, Fielding AK, Goldstone AH, Rowe JM, Wang YA, Look AT, Stratton MR, Chin L, Futreal PA, DePinho RA. Chromosomally unstable mouse tumours have genomic alterations similar to diverse human cancers. Nature 2007;447(7147):966-971.

[105] Amin AR, Kucuk O, Khuri FR, Shin DM. Perspectives for cancer prevention with natural compounds. J ClinOncol 2009;27(16):2712-2725.

[106] Gupta S. Prostate cancer chemoprevention: current status and future prospects. ToxicolApplPharmacol 2007;224(3):369-376.

[107] Strope SA, Andriole GL. Update on chemoprevention for prostate cancer. CurrOpin Urol;20(3):194-197.

[108] Raghow S, et al. Cancer Res 2000;60:4093–7;

[109] Gupta S, et al. Cancer Res 2000;60:5125-33;

[110] Gupta S, et al. Proc NatlAcadSci USA 2001;98:10350-5;

[111] Mentor-Marcel R, et al. Cancer Res 2001;61:6777-82;

[112] Raghow S, et al. Cancer Res 2002;62:1370-6;

[113] Gupta S, et al. Cancer Res 2004;64:3334-43;

[114] Narayanan BA, et al. Clin Cancer Res 2004;10:7727-37;

[115] Wang J, et al. Mol CellEndocrinol 2004;219:171-80;

[116] Huss WJ, et al. Prostate 2004;61:142-52;

[117] Adhami VM, et al. Cancer Res 2004;64:8715-22;

[118] Sartor L, et al. Int J Cancer 2004; 112, 823-9;

[119] Caporali A, et al. Carcinogenesis 2004;25:2217-24;

[120] Saleem M, et al. Clin Cancer Res 2005;11:147-53;

[121] Kolluri SK, et al. ProcNatlAcadSci USA 2005;102:2525-30;

[122] Chiang CF, et al. Prostate 2005;64:408-18;

[123] Wikstrom P, et al. Nutr Cancer 2005;53:111-6;

[124] Mentor Marcel R, et al. J Nutrition 2005;135:989-95;

[125] Narayanan BA, et al. Prostate 2006;66:257-65;

[126] Tam NN, et al. Prostate 2006;66:57-69;

[127] McCabe MT, et al. Cancer Res 2006;66:385-92;

[128] Garcia GE, et al. Clin Cancer Res 2006;12:980-7;

[129] Raina K, et al. Cancer Res 2007;67:5976-82;

[130] Shukla S, et al. Cancer Res 2007;67:6925-35;

[131] Wang J, et al. J Carcinog. 2007;6:3;

[132] Isayeva T, et al. Cancer Res 2007;67:5789-97;

[133] Harper CE, et al. Prostate 2007;67:1576-89;

[134] Raina K, et al. Cancer Res 2007;67:11083-91;

[135] De Giovanni C Croci S, et al. Int J Cancer 2007;121:88-94;

[136] Harper CE, et al. Prostate 2007;67:1576-89;

[137] Shukla S, et al. Cancer Res 2007;67:6925-35;

[138] Wadsworth TL, et al. Prostate 2007;67:661-73;

[139] Raina K, et al. Cancer Res 2008;68:6822-30;

[140] Singh RP, et al. Clin CanceRes 2008;14:7773-80;

[141] Singh SV, et al. Cancer Res 2009;69:2117-25;

[142] Adhami VM, et al. Clin Cancer Res 2009;15:1947-53;

[143] Raina K, et al. Cancer Res 2009;69:3731-5;

[144] Barve A, et al. Int J Cancer 2009;124:1693-9;

[145] Ibrahim-Hashim A, et al. J Urol 2012;Jun 14 [Epubahead of print];

[146] Huang Y, et al. J Nutr 2012;142:818-23;

[147] Shanmugam MK, et al. PLoS One 2012;7:e32476 [Epub ahead of print];

[148] Davis PA, et al. Br J Nutr 2012;16:1-9 [Epub ahead of print];

[149] Adhami VM, et al. Carcinogenesis 2012;33:644-51;

[150] Shukla S, et al. Pharm Res 2012;29:1506-17;

[151] Dalezis P, et al. In Vivo 2012;26:75-86;

[152] Ru P, et al. Cancer Prev Res (Phila) 2011;4:2122-30;

[153] Bistulfi G, et al.Cancer Prev Res (Phila) 2011;4:1825-34;

[154] Shanmugam MK, et al. Int J Cancer 2011;129:1552-63;

[155] Abedinpour P, et al. Prostate 2011;71:813-23;

[156] Kim SH, et al. Cancer Prev Res (Phila) 2011;4:897-06;

[157] Wu TY, et al. Mol Carcinog 2011;

[158] Pannellini et al. Cancer PrevRes 2010;3:1284-91;

[159] Konijeti R, et al. Prostate 2010;70:1547-54;

[160] Llaverias G, et al. Am J Pathol 2010;177:3180-91;

[161] Wang L, et al. Prostate 2011;71:1429-40;

[162] Deeb D, et al. Carcinogenesis 2011;32:757-64;

[163] Kang BH, et al. Br J Cancer 2011;104:629-34;

[164] Rigamonti N, et al. Clin Cancer Res 2011;17:1012-23;

[165] Wang L, et al. Cancer Prev Res (Phila) 2009;2:484-95;

[166] Ganapathy M, et al. Clin Cancer Res 2009;15:1601-11;

[167] Persano L, et al. Carcinogenesis 2009;30:851-60;

[168] Cho HJ, et al. MolCarcinog 2011;50:100-12;

[169] Barve A, et al. Nutr Cancer 2010;62:789-94;

[170] Prasad AS, et al. J Med Food 2010;13:70-6;

[171] Reddy KR, et al. Prostate 2011;71:1796-09;

[172] Wu TY, et al. Mol Carcinogenesis Aug 2011.

Chapter 17

Prostate Cancer, Inflammation and Antioxidants

Marika Crohns, Tuomas Westermarck and
Faik Atroshi

Additional information is available at the end of the chapter

http://dx.doi.org/10.5772/53296

1. Introduction

Prostate cancer (PCa) is a long latency type of tumour that usually develops in men older than 50 years of age. Prostate epithelial neoplasia (PIN), the initial malignant lesion, progresses to invasive carcinoma over the course of years. Because of the particular features of prostate carcinogenesis, this type of tumour may represent a paradigm for cancer prevention. The lack of a comprehensive aetiology for prostate cancer and the need for an effective and inexpensive biological treatment modality, devoid of side effects, has resulted in a multitude of therapeutic trials. Present evidence suggests that chemo preventive agents may be used in cancer treatment (Tallberg et al. 2008; Crohns et al. 2009). Because they are considered pharmacologically safe and derived from natural sources, most chemo preventive agents can be used in combination with chemotherapeutic agents to enhance the effect at lower doses and thus minimize chemotherapy-induced toxicity. There are various therapies that can successfully reduce the size of tumours, however, often patients suffer a relapse and the tumour re-grows. Some researchers believe that this happens because the therapies fail to eradicate a small proportion of cells that drive tumour growth known as cancer stem cells. They believe that these are the cells that should be targeted to eliminate the tumour forever.

Today, cancer is considered to be a complex multistep disorder, the result of a combination of factors including exposure to radiation and/or carcinogens (damage to DNA), infection, genetics, aging, immune function disorders, and lifestyle factors such as smoking (Nelson et al. 2003; Mahan et al. 2004). Several clinical trials have evaluated the effect of dietary nutrients on prostate tumour development. These dietary agents may help to suppress the transformative, hyper proliferative and inflammatory processes that initiate carcinogenesis. The curative effect does not seem to involve apoptosis (Tallberg and Atroshi, 2011).

Most human diseases are due to chronic inflammation resulting in loss of function of a joint, a blood vessel or an entire organ. In some organs, such as the heart and brain, acute inflammation can be fatal. Oxidative stress is a major by-product of cellular metabolism and its regulation is critical for preventing disease and aging. Levels of reactive oxygen species (ROS) are generally higher in proliferating tumour cells than in normal cells, and this may explain why ROS is a key component in the efficacy of chemotherapeutic drugs (Crohns et al. 2009).

This review focuses on the mechanisms of free radical formation and ROS signalling in prostate cancer on the basis of current literature. We also highlight the mechanisms by which inflammatory processes contribute to prostatic carcinogenesis and how antioxidants react to neutralize free radicals.

2. Prostate cancer as an age-related disease

Prostate cancer is the common among men in the developed world. The risk increases after the age of 50 (Sakr et al., 1994; Abate-Shen and Shen, 2000; Schaeffer, 2003; Yancik 2005). Aggressive treatment for older men is not advisable because of an increased risk of short-term and long-term treatment-related adverse effects (Lu-Yao et al. 1999). The development of cancer lesions can be in two different regions of the prostate gland, in the peripheral zone, which is most common, and the remaining lesions are found in the transition zone located in the periurethral region (McNeal, 1988). Prostatic cancer multifocality makes accurate clinical staging difficult, and repeated revisions have been undertaken in an effort to optimize prognostic accuracy (McNeal, 1988; Andreoiu and Cheng, 2010).

Normal aging is associated with changes in body composition. While treatments for the disease continue to improve with each passing decade, the disease itself has likely been around since ancient times. Recently it was documented that a mummy - thought to be a man in his 50s - had numerous sclerotic spots throughout the bones of his pelvis and lower spine that were most consistent in appearance with metastases from prostate cancer (Prates et al., 2011).

3. Risk factors for prostate cancer

The etiological factors associated with prostate cancer are poorly studied compared to other common cancers. It is suggested that diet (Fair et. 1997; Schulman et al. 2001) and environmental differences (Muir et al. 1991) play important roles (Shimizu et al., 1991; Minami et al., 1993). For example, it is not known whether decreasing fat or increasing fruits and vegetables in the diet helps to decrease the risk of prostate cancer or death from prostate cancer. High intake of fat, especially total fat and saturated fat, is a risk factor for prostate cancer (Andersson et al. 1996; Kolonel, 2001). This has been explained by the evidence indicating that fat may be mediated through endogenous hormones

(Bosland, 2000). Phytoestrogen metabolites have been studied, and dietary habits are probably an important factor contributing to the geographic variations observed in some Asian men compared to European men, which may explain the low incidence of prostate cancer in Asia (Adlercreutz et al., 1993).

4. Mechanism of prostate cancer cell

Living cells have three main systems for protection and repair under oxidative stress: (1) direct antioxidant enzymes (Superoxide dismutase (SOD), catalase, peroxidises), (2) proteases and phospholipases activated by oxidative modification of membranes, (3) lipid and water soluble antioxidants (Sies, 1997; Finkel and Holbrook, 2000). Normalization of malignant gene transcription in an organ requires dietary correction of the etiologic long-standing metabolic deficiency involving six or more inter-linked natural factors aided by hormonal equilibrium, enhanced by specific autologous immunotherapy. In bio-immunotherapy this therapeutic bio-modulation is aims to simulate specific leukaemia, adenocarcinoma or sarcoma regulatory codes, leading to cancer cure by forcing tumour cells back into healthy gene transcription, without apoptosis. According to Lukacs et al. (2010), prostate cancer can be initiated by so many different mutations, and if a key regulator of self-renewal can be found, then partially one may control the growth of the cancer, no matter what the mutation is. Their approach, which aims to attack the process that allows the cancer cells to grow indefinitely, may provide an alternative way of treating cancer by targeting the core mechanism of cancer cell self-renewal and proliferation (Lukacs et al.2010).

Cells are often exposed to a high load of oxidants and free radicals. Oxidative stress can occur as a result of increased metabolic rate, increased oxygen tension, compromise of normal cellular antioxidants and many others endogenous and exogenous factors (Figure 1). Cell motility is a complex biological process, involved in development, inflammation, homeostasis, and pathological processes such as the invasion and metastatic spread of cancer (Collins et al. 2006). Cancer metabolism is a factor that might be exploited as a potential therapeutic target for drug discovery also on how a cancer cell differs in its metabolism to that of a rapidly proliferating normal cell (Vander Heiden et al. 2009). By small interfering RNA–based functional screening of over 200 metabolic enzymes, transporters, and regulators to identify those selectively required for prostate cancer cell survival. Ros and co-workers showed that treatment with a chemical antioxidant rescued the viability of PFKFB4 (one of the genes identified) -deficient prostate cancer cells, further suggesting that PFKFB4 mediates ROS detoxification in cancer cells. Together, these findings reveal that prostate cancer cells are exquisitely sensitive to metabolic perturbations that affect the balance between glucose and the pentose phosphate pathway and implicate PFKFB4 as a potential therapeutic target (Ros et al 2012).

Under normal conditions, the antioxidant defence systems are probably capable of maintaining a low steady-state level of damage and thus protecting the cells (Zhou et al.2003). Among the risk factors for the development of prostate cancer are ageing and lifestyle. Under situations of oxidative stress and with increasing age the organism may not be able to maintain homeostasis with deleterious and potentially unfortunate consequences.

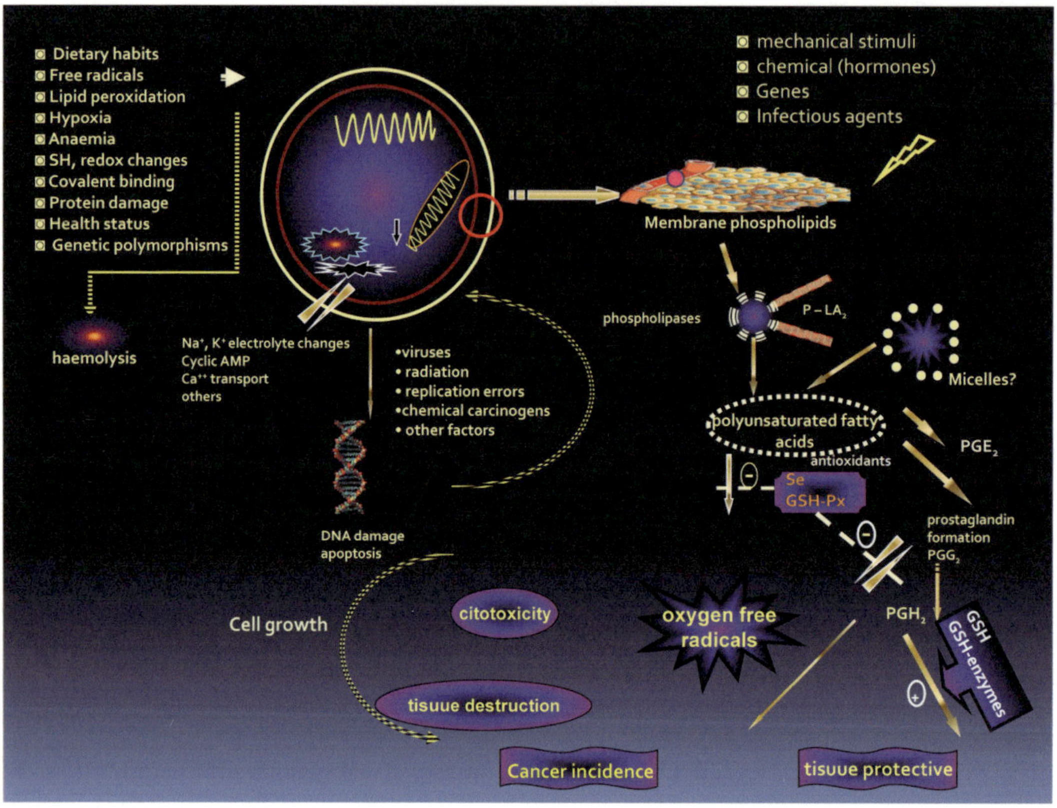

Figure 1. The prostanoid system may belong to the adaptive mechanisms by which the cell reacts to its environment. The reaction may be triggered by chemical, mechanical and other stimuli. Prostacyclin (PGI_2) and PGE_2 stimulate ATPases and the formation of intracellular cyclic AMP, which usually stabilize the cell membrane. TXA_2 among others may activate calcium-related processes which may lead to smooth muscle contraction, platelet aggregation and secretory events. PGE_2 has the capacity for both excitatory and inhibitory activities and it is often released in stressful situations. (Parantainen et al.1988)

5. Inflammation and prostate cancer

Inflammation involves the induction of complex, coordinated chemical signals and associated physiological processes following injury that promote "healing" of damaged tissues (Balkwill and Mantovani, 2001; Rakoff-Nahoum, 2006; Mantovani et al, 2008). Early responses include increases in vascular permeability and activation, together with the directed migration of leukocytes (neutrophils, monocytes and eosinophils) towards the site of injury, where the ground-work is being laid for the formation of a new extracellular matrix. The directional migration is mediated by secreted chemokines that form a concentration gradient towards the site of inflammation (Koopmann and Krangel, 1997). The extracellular matrix provides the structure upon which cells (fibroblasts and endothelial cells) can migrate and proliferate, regenerating new tissue and a vascular network. In later stage of the inflammatory response, the macrophages are the dominant cell type, orchestrating and directing the healing process. Normally, inflammation is a self-limiting process due to the production of anti-inflammatory cytokines, which buffer the effect of pro-inflammatory cytokines. The cytokine/chemokine pattern persisting at the inflammatory site is important in the development of chronic disease. Deregulation of any of the cooperating factors can lead to prolonged inflammation with chronic exposure to cytotoxic mediators (Coussens and Werb, 2002). Chronic inflammation can be caused by a variety of factors, including bacterial, viral, and parasitic infections, chemical irritants, and non-digestible particles, but often the underlying cause is unknown. The longer the inflammation persists, the higher the risk of associated carcinogenesis (Shacter *et al.*, 2002, Coussens and Werb, 2002).

At the site of inflammation, caused by either wounding or infection, phagocytic cells (e.g. neutrophils and macrophages) generate reactive oxygen and nitrogen substances (Atroshi et al. 1988; Gallin, 1992), but these cells also synthesize and secrete large quantities of growth factors and a number of potent angiogenic factors, cytokines, and proteases, all of which are important mediators in the tissue regeneration, but can also potentiate neoplastic tumorigenesis. Prostaglandins, cytokines, nuclear factor NFkB, chemokines and angiogenic factors are the main molecular players that link inflammation to genetic alterations. However, free radical species derived from oxygen (ROI) and nitrogen (RNI) are the main chemical effectors (Jackson et al. 1997; Baron and, Sandler, 2000; Federico et al. 2007). Various carcinomas (including cancers of the liver, bladder, colon, stomach, and oesophagus) have been shown to arise from areas of infection and inflammation (Federico et al. 2007). Over 15% of all malignancies worldwide are attributable to infectious agents, and inflammation is a major component of these chronic infections (Kuper et al., 2000; Ibrahim and Makkiya, 2011). Colon cancers arising in individuals with inflammatory bowel disease (e.g. chronic ulcerative colitis or Crohn's disease) and stomach cancers caused by chronic Helicobacter pylori infection are among the most intensively studied and well established types of cancer associated with inflammation of different origins (Coussens and Werb, 2002).

6. The role of inflammation in the pathogenesis of prostate

Although it has been established that chronic inflammation plays a causative role in the development of many human cancers, the contribution of inflammatory processes to the development of prostate cancer has not been extensively studied. Bioactive food components are increasingly being evaluated as potential prostate chemopreventive agents (Barqawi et al. 2004; Chong and Rashid, 2005; Sonn, et al. 2005; Hsu et al 2010; Schellhammer, 2012). One such agent is resveratrol, a phytochemical which has been considered as a chemopreventive for human prostate cancer (Ratan et al. 2002; Stewart et al. 2003).

The contribution of inflammatory intermediates such as eicosanoids in cancer initiation and progression is another area of interest. These intermediates might form the link between inflammation and cancer. Interest in the relationship between chronic prostatic inflammation and prostate cancer is increasing. Proliferative inflammatory atrophy, or proliferative inflammatory atrophy (PIA), consists of lesions in the prostate characterized by atrophy of the epithelium and by an increased proliferative index (De Marzo et al. 1999). These lesions are common in older men and have been hypothesized to be a precursor of prostate cancer (Nelson et al. 2004; De Marzo et al. 2007). More knowledge about the risk factors could lead to better preventive measures together with better treatments.

Evidence suggests that inflammation is vital for the aetiology of prostate cancer and the pathogenesis of PCa reflects both hereditary and environmental components. These evidence stems from epidemiological, histopathological and molecular pathological studies (Ames et al., 1995; De Marzo et al. 1999; Coussens and Werb, 2002). More general evidence of a relationship between inflammation and prostate cancer has been provided by reports indicating that daily use of non-steroidal anti-inflammatory drugs (NSAIDs) may be associated with a reduce incidence of prostate cancer (Gupta et al. 2000). The exact mechanism whereby inflammation might act in tumour development and progression remains to be elucidated, but is likely to be complex.

Some studies have suggested that prostatitis, inflammation of the prostate gland that includes acute or chronic bacterial infection, may be linked to an increased risk of prostate cancer (Dennis et a. 2002; Roberts et al. 2004). This link was explained that chronic inflammation within the prostate due to the exposure of microbial agents stimulates the production of ROS and inflammatory cytokines leading to carcinogenesis (Coussens and Werb, 2002; De Marzo et al. 2007).

Chronic inflammation has been associated with the development of malignancy in several other organs such as the oesophagus, stomach, colon, liver and urinary bladder. Inflammation is thought to incite carcinogenesis by causing cell and genome damage, promoting cellular turnover, and creating a tissue microenvironment that can enhance cell replication, angiogenesis and tissue repair. Epidemiological data have correlated prostatitis and sexually transmitted diseases with an increased risk of prostate cancer and intake of anti-inflammatory drugs and antioxidants with a decreased risk. Evidence from genetic and molecular studies also supports the hypothesis that prostate inflammation and/or infection may be a cause of prostate cancer. In 1999 De Marzo et al proposed that proliferative inflammatory atrophy (PIA) is a precursor to PIN and cancer. Further research will provide opportunities for the discovery and development of strategies for treatment and prevention of prostate cancer (Sugar, 2006).

Accumulating epidemiologic and molecular evidence suggests that inflammation is an important component in the aetiology of prostate cancer. Supporting this hypothesis, population studies have found an increased risk of prostate cancer in men with a prior history of certain sexually transmitted infections or prostatitis. More general evidence of a relationship between inflammation and prostate cancer has been provided by reports indicating that daily use of non steroidal anti-inflammatory drugs (NSAIDs) may be associated with a lower incidence of prostate cancer. The exact mechanism whereby inflammation might act in tumour development and progression remains to be elucidated, but is likely to be complex.

http://dx.doi.org/10.5772/53296

Cancer lesions can develop in two different regions of the prostate gland, most commonly (in ~80% of cases) in the periphery zone, while most of the remaining lesions are found in the transition zone, which is located in the periurethral region (McNeal, 1968, 1988).

7. Possible interaction between prostaglandins and glutathione metabolism in prostate cancer

Prostaglandins (PGs) constitute a whole family of peroxidized lipids formed in most cells. Almost any kind of stimuli be it mechanical, chemical, physiological or traumatic, may initiate the formation of different kinds of PGs (Atroshi et al. 1986). Thus the particular importance of the local PG-impact is usually very difficult to evaluate. Some PGS, like PGEs and PGI_2 (prostacyclin), are potent triggers of inflammatory symptoms. The main roles for PGEs and PGI_2 in inflammation may in fact be in the generation of hyperalgesia, sensitization of the tissue to the irritant and pain producing activity of the amine and peptide type of mediators of inflammation (Ferreira and Nakamura, 1979; Ferreira 2002). On the other hand, these PGs have a marked tissue protective function, e.g. in preventing vasoconstriction and platelet aggregation. Other prostanoids (PG-like substances), like PGD_2, $PGF_2\alpha$ and thromboxane A_2 (TXA_2), are mostly vasoconstrictors. Their formation may be associated with allergic and other reactions of hypersensitivity, and TXA_2 is a very potent aggregator of platelets.

Prostaglandins play a role in the regulation of several important physiological and pathological processes, and evidence (Marnett, 1992; Thun et al., 1991; Taketo, 1998; Samuelsson et al., 2007) suggests that they could be involved in tumour progression. Studies have demonstrated that PGE_2 and its EP receptors are implicated in promoting carcinogenesis in different types of cancer (Wang and Klein, 2007). Arachidonic acid (AA) is the precursor for prostaglandin E_2 (PGE_2) synthesis and increases growth of prostate cancer cells (Van et al., 1998). However, the real sources of PGs are not well known and are a matter of speculation. For example we do not know for sure if the PGs originate in the blood, inflamed tissue, etc. There are several possibilities:

1. Bacterial toxins might contribute to the PG-release (figure 2). This was clearly demonstrated by Giri and coworkers (1984), and similar mechanisms might operate in the spontaneous disease as well (Liu et al. 2011; Sanz-Motilva et al. 2012).

2. The production of PGs is greatly increased by polymorphonuclear leukocytes. Neutrophil invasion is a typical feature in inflammation (Atroshi et al. 1988).

3. Changes in tissue protein and electrolyte contents are factors that have marked effects on PG-production (atroshi et al. 1988). Albumin is a typical factor increasing the formation of PGs, particularly that of $PGF_2\alpha$.

4. Inflammatory mediators are factors that might contribute to the formation of PGs. (e.g. monoamines and peptide hormones).

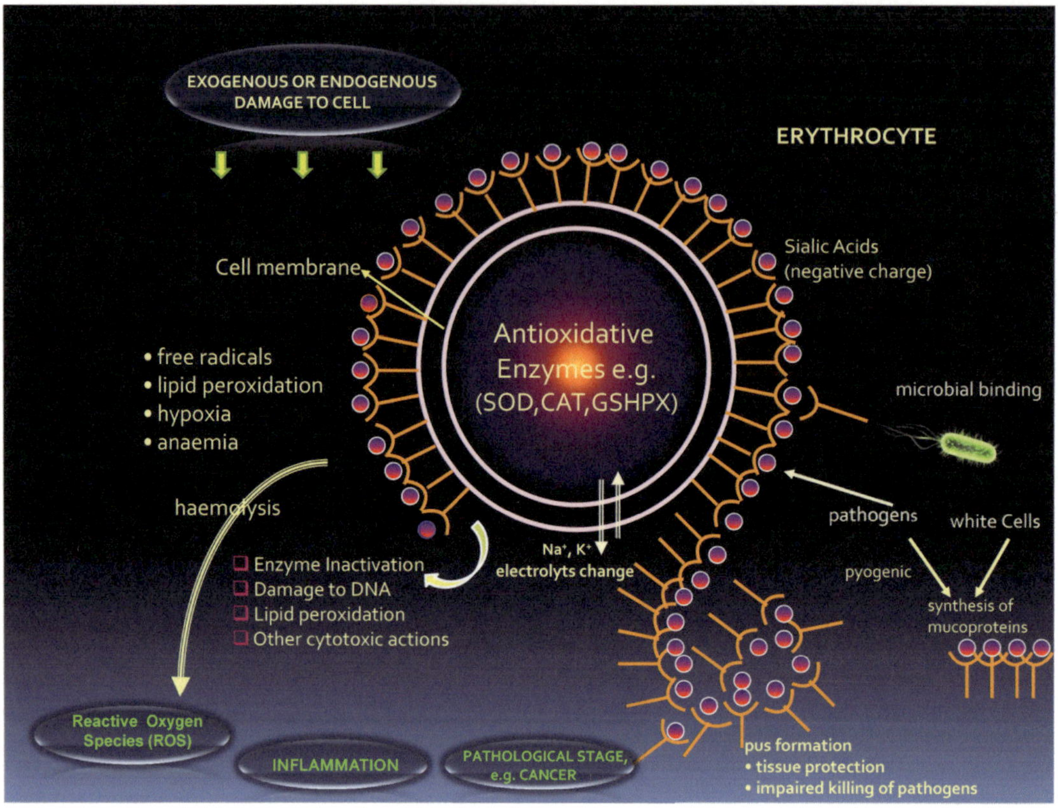

Figure 2. Possible interaction between erythrocyte and inflamed tissue during infection/inflammation. Oxygen free radicals produced by hypoxia, bacterial toxins and phagocytosis increase lipid peroxidation and peroxidative stress in the erythrocyte. Pyogenic bacteria as well as white cells may stimulate the synthesis of mucoproteins. The pus formed has antioxidant activity and the formation of oxygen free radicals is needed. GSH and other antioxidant enzymes represent the intracellular charged compounds, potential sources of reducing equivalents. The intracellular enzymes (GSH, GSHPX etc.) may greatly affected by oxygen free radicals and lipid peroxidation associated e.g. in infection, hypoxia and cancer. Destruction of erythrocytes is one possible source of GSH and other antioxidant enzymes which are elevated in the inflamed tissue. (Atroshi et al.1986)

8. Possible importance of leukotrienes

Leukotrienes (LTs) are biologically active fatty acids derived from the oxidative metabolism of arachidonic acid through the 5-lipoxygenase pathway (Matsuyama et al. 2010; Haeggström and Funk, 2011). Leukotrienes and other lipoxygenase products are synthesized from the same precursor fatty acids as PGs, and substantial changes in PG/LT balance are possible during inflammation and infection (Figure 3). LTs are highly vasoactive, and together with PGs they may contribute to the local haemodynamic changes in the inflamed tissue. Moreover, some LTs are very active leukotactic agents, and LTB_4 in particular could contribute to the massive invasion of neutrophils in the inflammatory area. PGE_2 and LTB_4 are involved

http://dx.doi.org/10.5772/53296

in inflammation and carcinogenesis in several tissues. PGE_2 and inflammation may be associated to stromal benign prostatic hyperplasia whereas LTB_4 may play a role in prostate carcinogenesis; cancerous samples had higher LTB_4 levels than pericancerous samples, but there was no difference in PGE_2 levels (Larré et al. 2008).

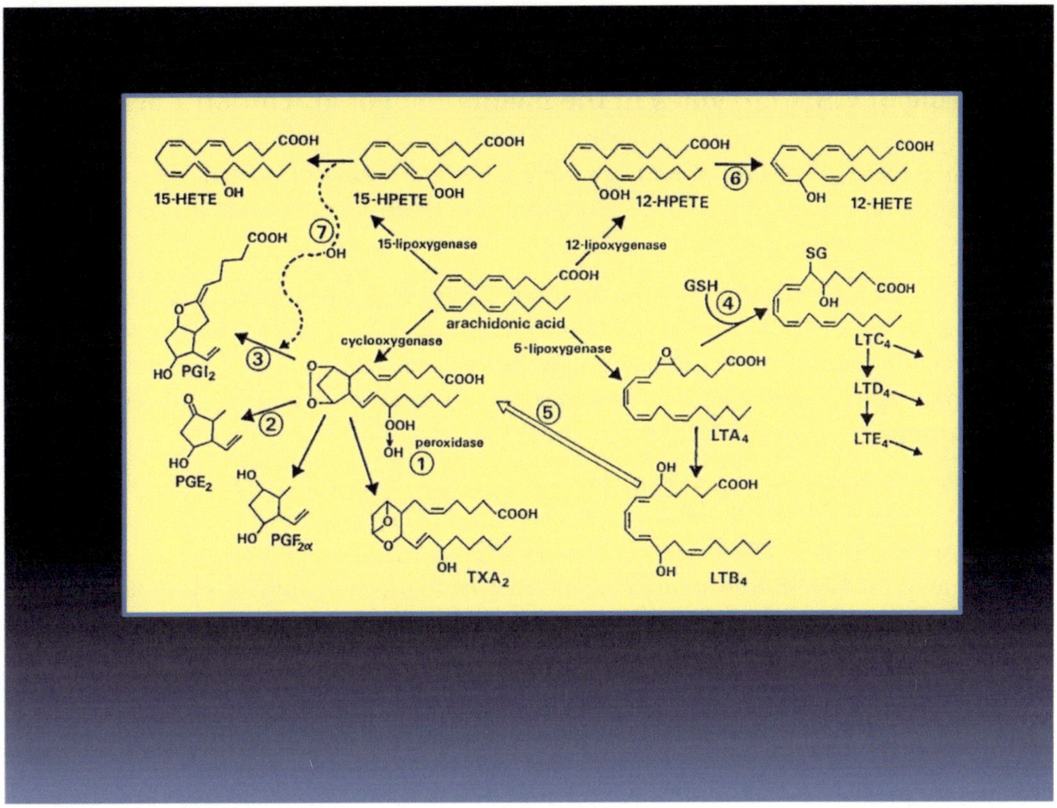

Figure 3. Enzymes with peroxidase activity are needed to reduce the endoperoxide PGG2 to PGH2 (1), and specific isomerases resembling GSH-S-transferase (2) reduce PGH2 further to PGs and prostacyclin (3). GSH and GSH-enzymes are involved in the formation of leukotrienes as well. One molecule of GSH (4) is attached to LTA 4 to form LTC4, the first of the cysteinyl leukotrienes (C, D, E). The peroxidative capacity of erythrocytes may participate in the conversion of LTA 4 to LTB4. Peroxidases are also needed to reduce other lipid hydroperoxides to corresponding alcohols (6) to prevent the enzyme destruction caused by oxygen free radicals (7). The activity of LTB4 may be mediated by PGs (5). (Atroshi et al. 1986)

Lipoxygenase-like activities are seen in the phagocytosis and bacterial killing. Lipid peroxidation as such is a source of oxygen free radicals. On the other hand, the radicals are among the most potent triggerers of lipid peroxidation. Some free radicals, particularly the hydroxyl radical (•OH) are very toxic to the tissues. During reduction of the 15-hydroperoxide, to the corresponding alcohol •OH is formed and the enzyme systems that form PGI_2 may be injured. Leukotriene B_4 (LTB_4) has been implicated in prostate and colon carcinogenesis. The anticancer effect of celecoxib is COX-2-independent in HT-29 and PC-3 cells and in HT-29 cells primarily via down-regulating LTB_4 production (Gao et al., 2010). Matsuyama and co-workers (2010) have demonstrated that CysLT1R expressed in urological cancer may play a crucial role in carcinogenesis and may therefore be a novel target in the treatment of urological cancer. An increasing body of evidence supports an acute role for 5-LO products already during the earliest stages of pancreatic, prostate, and colorectal carcinogenesis (Steinhilber et al., 2010).

9. The role of GSH-enzymes in the metabolism of arachidonic acid

The tissue content of GSH is normally very high, in some tissues the level is up to the 5 mM. The functions of GSH are often tissue protective, and there are numerous enzymes in which GSH plays a central role as a cofactor.

Typical GSH-enzymes include GSH-peroxidase (GSH-Px), located in the circulation almost exclusively in the red cells, various GSH-transferases that have peroxidise-like activity and bind chemicals and γ-glutamyl transferase which reflects the function of the liver and is involved in the transport of amino acids across the cell membrane. GSH is also consumed by some cytochromes, most notably cytochrome P-450.

Several steps in the metabolism of arachidonic acid may be normally regulated by GSH-enzymes (Rouzer et al. 1982). It was an early observation that GSH may function as a chemical cofactor or coenzyme in the formation of some PGs, particularly PGEs (Mimata et al. 1988). Specific, atypical GSH-S-transferases are needed in the isomeration of PG-endoperoxides (the intermediary step) to PGEs and PGDs (Hubatsch et al. 2002). Ghosh (2004) demonstrated that selenium significantly reduced the incidence of clinical prostate cancer. A high intake of dietary fat containing arachidonic acid or its precursor fatty acids should be administered when selenium is used for the management of prostate cancer, as it has been suggested that a combination of selenium and 5-lipoxygenase inhibitors may be an effective regimen for prostate cancer control (Ghosh and Myers, 1998; Ghosh, 2004). A low prostatic arachidonic acid level was found in patients undergoing prostate surgery for either benign or malignant disease. Showed a low prostatic arachidonic acid level, which was explained as a result of the increased use of arachidonic acid for the production of prostaglandins and/or leukotrienes (Faas et al. 2003; Tilg and Moschen, 2006; Calder 2012).

There is little data available on these parameters in the prostate. Richie et al (2012), working with age related changes in selenium and glutathione levels in different lobes of the rat prostate found an increased level of oxidative stress together with decreases in selenium and the major cellular antioxidant glutathione (GSH). They compared the levels of selenium, GSH and protein-bound GSH (GSSP) in blood and prostate tissues in rats. Their findings of age-related changes in GSSP and selenium in the DL prostate are consistent with the sensitivity of this lobe to carcinogenesis and, thus, may be playing a mechanistic role (Richie et al. 2012). Selenium is an integral part of GSH peroxidase, the enzyme that mediates antioxidants by glutathione (Parantainen et al. 1988). Studying the metabolic profiles of human prostate cancer tissues it was shown a significant decrease in reduced glutathione (GSH) during cancer progression from low- to high-grade Gleason scores (Sreekumar et al. 2009; Pavlou and Diamandis, 2009). Some studies found a lower Se concentration in the whole blood and plasma in benign prostatic hyperplasia (BPH) patients compared to healthy controls was observed by Eichholzer et al. (2012); also they found a lower activity of erythrocyte GPx. A significant inverse association between serum Se concentrations and the risk of BPH was shown (Eichholzer et al. 2012).

The formation of PGs is a very specific form of lipid peroxidation, and in these processes GSH-Px may have a central regulatory role. Some pGs inhibit the formation of lipid peroxides, while a certain level of peroxides is needed to maintain normal PG-production (Hemler and Land, 1980; Sugino et al. 2001). Such a "peroxide tone" is a crucial factor in the regulation of the metabolism of arachidonic acid in toto. Peroxidases may have a key role in eliminating the oxygen free radical during the conversion of endoperoxides to corresponding alcohols. The hydroxyl radical formed from 15-HPETE may thus be trapped (Chance et al. 1979; Flohé and Ursini, 2008).

Considering the circulatory peroxides, the functioning of the erythrocyte GSH-Px may have a crucial role. During infection and inflammation there may be a marked reduction in the erythrocyte count. Such anaemia may be due to haemolytic processes in which lipid peroxidation and the formation of free radicals may be the key event.

In the formation of leukotrienes, the GSH-enzymes γ-GT and GSH-S-transferases have a key role. The whole group of **cysteinyl leukotrienes** are formed by adding GSH to LTA_4, which gives rise to LTC_4 and, when the GSH is split, to LTD_4, LTE_4 and LTF_4. In the formation of the other type, LTB_4, GSH does not have a direct role (Morris et al.1981). However, LTA_4 is reduced to LTB_4 on contact with erythrocytes, which points to a certain importance of the peroxidise-like mechanisms, possibly GSH-Px, so abundant in the red cell. Leukotriene B_4 (LTB_4) is a potent lipid mediator of inflammation, implicated in numerous diseases including prostate cancer. An LTB_4 tissue level was shown to play a role in in benign and cancerous prostates. Cancerous from patients' sample had higher LTB_4 than pericancerous samples (Larre et al. 2008).

10. Diet, inflammation and prostate cancer

The causes of cancer have been largely attributed to genetic and environmental factors, including lifestyle, and are generally thought of as either avoidable or unavoidable. Dietary habits have been considered for years in epidemiological and case controlled studies to have an impact on cancer development and prevention. However, this association between diet and cancer has never been as clear as the correlation between smoking and cancer. Differences in diet and lifestyle may account for the variability of prostate cancer rates in different countries (Manolio et al. 2009). Good nutrition may reduce the incidence of prostate cancer and help reduce the risk of prostate cancer progression (Miller et al 2012). Several studies suggest a relationship between diet and prostate cancer risk; however, nutritional studies are difficult to perform because of the inherent heterogeneity of any study population (Klein et al.2006), the variations in individual lifestyles, and the quantitative and qualitative complexity in food and food products (Giovannucci et al, 1993; Huang, 2006). Therefore, randomized and carefully controlled studies can address the relation between prostate cancer and nutrition.

The importance of nutrition in disease prevention and treatment has gained much attention in recent years. Diet may represent a modifiable prostate cancer risk factor, but a vegetable-based prostate-healthy diet is a major change for most men (Carmody et al. 2008). Other study suggest that keeping the appropriate body mass and level of cholesterol by proper diet and physical exercises may be the prophylaxis of prostate cancer (Pilch et al 2012). The cancer preventive activity of vitamin E has been suggested by many epidemiologic studies. Yang and co-workers suggested that vitamin E, as ingested in the diet or in supplements that are rich in γ- and δ-tocopherols, is cancer preventive; whereas supplementation with high doses of α-tocopherol is not (Yang et al 2012). It has been suggested that intake of vegetables and fruit plays a role in protecting against prostate cancer development (Chan and Giovannucci, 2001; Key et al., 2004). Furthermore, vitamins and trace elements have been studied for their roles in prostate cancer pathogenesis (Chanand Giovannucci, 2001; Moyad et al. 2002; Tallberg and Atroshi, 2011).

In order to disentangle the association of diet and prostate carcinogenesis better understanding of the human genome will further accelerate nutrigenomics applications and the development of nutritional modifications including personalized nutrition for our well-being and will also present a strong influence on future drug discovery (Lundstrom,2012). However, antioxidant supplements so far tested seem to offer little improvement over a well-balanced diet, possibly because of the choice of the substances tested or of an excessive dosage (Fair and Wynder, 1996; Dolara et al. 2012). Future trials of nutritional medication might help to disentangle the association of diet and prostate carcinogenesis.

The effect of diet can be direct, via the cumulative effect of exposure to nutrients and carcinogens in foods; in this case, the balance of cancer-promoting and -protective substances may contribute in defining cancer risk (Antila et al. 1996; Adhami and mukhtar, 2012; Adhami et al.2012). There are also indirect ways by which diet affects the cancer process. These include the effects of diet on energy balance and risk of obesity and the hormonal and metabolic responses related to energy balance.

There is an emerging consensus that situations of acute or chronic imbalance between the antioxidative capacity of cells and tissues, and the production of pro oxidative species, is associated with the development of a number of human diseases. Despite enormous interest in the area of antioxidants as therapeutic tools, the development of foreign compounds as therapeutic antioxidants has provided little therapeutic benefit.

1. Many important physiological functions, such as the regulation of cell cycle (mitogenesis and apoptosis), are known to be tightly coupled to the induction of controlled episodes of oxidative stress in biological systems. This entails problems in terms of potential side effects for antioxidant therapy, which have been largely ignored in most clinical use of antioxidants. This may have serious implications for the choice of antioxidant principle to be used.

2. The actual choice of antioxidant therapy is it xenobiotic or endogenous, should be indicated based on sound molecular knowledge of the involvement of oxidative stress in the actual pathology.

3. Dietary habits are probably an important factor that contributes to the geographic variations in prostate cancer rates. A large number of epidemiological studies have investigated the association between dietary factors and prostate cancer. Epidemiologic studies on prostate cancer have extensively investigated dietary risk factors (Kolonel, 2001; Park et al. 2007). Suggesting that diet and environmental differences play important roles in prostate cancer (Shimizu et al., 1991; Minami et al.,1993).

11. Conclusion

Cancer is due to the accumulation of DNA mutations that confer a growth advantage and invasive properties on clones of cells. A variety of external factors including nutrients in the environment interacting with genetic susceptibility influence the accumulation of mutations in cells. Nutrition is important at every stage of carcinogenesis from initiation to promotion to progression and metastasis. In spite of the fact that prostate cancer is the most common male cancer in many countries in the developed world, little is known of risk factors and predisposing conditions.

The number of prostate cancer cases around the world is increasing. Its incidence has been associated with ageing, environmental factors and changes in lifestyle. Based on some research in animals and people, certain dietary measures have been suggested to prevent the progression of prostate cancer. However, there is no solid evidence that a healthy diet can prevent people from developing prostate cancer. The reasons that patients with prostate cancer are using the dietary supplements are to enhance their health. Such dietary elements may also limit drug efficiency.

Oxidative stress has been suggested to play a key role in carcinogenesis. Free radicals have been shown to mediate the anti-cancer actions of many chemotherapeutic regimens. Despite active investigation, knowledge is lacking concerning the local and systemic effects of free radical-generating treatments in cancer. Free radicals are among the environmental factors that might contribute to cancer process (Atroshi et al. 2010). While it has not been conclusively determined whether free radicals are a cause or an effect of prostate cancer, it is clear that characteristic types of free radical damage increase with cancer. However, understanding the nature of that particular tumour can help us to optimize therapy or to design therapeutic approaches. Recently, Maddams and co-workers have shown that a large increase in cancer can be expected in the oldest age groups in the coming decades, and therefore there is an increased demand upon the right treatment and health services (Maddams et al. 2012).

Author details

Marika Crohns[1], Tuomas Westermarck[2] and Faik Atroshi[3]

1 Sanofi - Aventis Oy, Helsinki, Finland

2 Rinnekoti Research Foundation, Espoo, Finland

3 Pharmacology & Toxicology, ELTDK, University of Helsinki, Finland

References

[1] Abate-Shen C and Shen MM. Molecular genetics of prostate cancer. Genes Dev. 2000 14: 2410-2434.

[2] Adhami VM, Mukhtar H. Human Cancer Chemoprevention: Hurdles and Challenges. Top Curr Chem. 2012 Jul 12. [Epub ahead of print.

[3] Adhami VM, Syed DN, Khan N, Mukhtar H. Dietary flavonoid fisetin: A novel dual inhibitor of PI3K/Akt and mTOR for prostate cancer management. Biochem Pharmacol. 2012 Jul 25. [Epub ahead of print

[4] Adlercreutz H, Markkanen H, Watanabe S. Plasma concentrations of phytooestrogens in Japanese men. Lancet, 1993, 342:1209-1210.

[5] Ames, B. N., Gold, L. S. & Willett, W. C. The causes and prevention of cancer. Proc. Natl Acad. Sci. USA ,92, 5258–5265, 1995.

[6] Andersson SO, Wolk A, Bergstrom R, et al. Energy, nutrient intake and prostate cancer risk: a population-based case-control study in Sweden. Int J Cancer 1996;68:716–22.

[7] Andreoiu M, Cheng L. Prostatic cancer multifocality makes accurate clinical staging difficult, and repeated revisions have been undertaken in an effort to optimize prognostic accuracy. Hum Pathol. 2010 ;41(6):781-93.

[8] Antila E, Mussalo-Rahamaa H, Kantola M, Atroshi F, Westermarck T. Association of cadmium in human breast cancer. Sci. Total Environ. 1996, 186:251-256.

[9] Atroshi F, Parantainen J, Sankari S, Österman,T. Prostaglandin and glutathione peroxidase in bovine mastitis. Res. Vet. Sci., 1986, 40:361-366.

[10] Atroshi F., Sankari S., Työppönen J. and Parantainen J. Inflammation related changes in trace elements, GSH-metabolism, prostaglandins and sialic acid. In: Trace Elements in Man and Animals 6 (Hurly LS ; Keen CL; Lonnerdal Bo, & Rucker RB, Editors), Plenum Press, New York & London, 1988, pp.97-99.

[11] Atroshi, F., Tallberg Th, Abdulla VM, Westermarck T. The Impact of Heavy Metals on Health with special emphasis on Cadmium Carcinogenesis. In: Natural Resource Conservation and Environment Management (Bhagirathi Behera, S.P.Panda, Editors), APH Publishing Corporation, New Delhi, pp. 1-12,2010

[12] Balkwill F.& Mantovani A. Inflammation and cancer: back to Virchow? Lancet 357, 539-545,2001.

[13] Baron JA, Sandler RS. Nonsteroidal anti-inflammatory drugs and cancerprevention. Annu Rev Med 2000; 51: 511–23.

[14] Barqawi, A., Thompson, I. M., Crawford, E. D.: Prostate cancer chemoprevention, an overview of United States trials. J. Urol., 2004, 171 , 5–9.

[15] Bosland MC. The role of steroid hormones in prostate carcinogenesis. Journal of the National Cancer Institute Monographs, 2000, 27:39-66.

[16] Calder PC. Omega-3 polyunsaturated fatty acids and inflammatory processes: Nutrition or pharmacology? Br J Clin Pharmacol. 2012 Jul 6. doi: 10.1111/j. 1365-2125.2012.04374.x

[17] Carmody J, Olendzki B, Reed G, Andersen V, Rosenzweig P. A dietary intervention for recurrent prostate cancer after definitive primary treatment: Results of a randomized pilot trial. Urology. 2008;72(6): 1324-1328.

[18] Chan JM, Giovannucci EL. Vegetables, fruits, associated micronutrients, and risk of prostate cancer. Epidemiol Rev, 2001, 23:82-86.

[19] Chance B, Sies H, Boveris A. Hydroperoxide Metabolism in Mammalian Organs. PHYSIOLOGICAL REVIEWS, 1979, 59 (3): 527-605.

[20] Chong, P. and Rashid, P. Can we prevent prostate cancer? Aust Fam Physician, 34: 265-267, 2005.

[21] Collins CS, Jiyong Hong J, Sapinoso L, Zhou Y, Liu Z, Micklash K, Schultz PG, and Hampton GM. A small interfering RNA screen for modulators of tumor cell motility identifies MAP4K4 as a promigratory kinase. Proc Natl Acad Sci U S A. 2006; 103(10): 3775–3780.

[22] Coussens, L. M. & Werb, Z. Inflammation and cancer. Nature, 2002, 420, 860–867.

[23] Crohns M, Saarelainen S, Kankaanranta H, Moilanen E, Alho H, Kellokumpu-Lehtinen P. Local and systemic oxidant/antioxidant status before and during lung cancer radiotherapy. Free Radic Res 2009;43:646–657.

[24] Crohns M, Saarelainen S, Erhola M, Alho H, Kellokumpu-Lehtinen P. Impact of radiotherapy and chemotherapy on biomarkers of oxidative DNA damage in lung cancer patients. Clin Biochem 2009;42:1082–1090.

[25] De Marzo AM, Platz EA, Sutcliffe S, Xu J, Gronberg H, et al. Inflammation in prostate carcinogenesis. Nat Rev Cancer 2007; 7: 256–69.

[26] De Marzo AM, Marchi VL, Epstein JI, NelsonWG. Proliferative inflammatory atrophy of the prostate. Am J Path 1999;155:1985–92.

[27] Dolara P, Bigagli E, Collins A. Antioxidant vitamins and mineral supplementation, life span expansion and cancer incidence: a critical commentary. Eur J Nutr. 2012 Jun 9. [Epub ahead of print]cancer. Urology 60: 78–83

[28] Eichholzer M, Steinbrecher A, Kaaks R, Teucher B, Linseisen J, Rohrmann S. Effects of selenium status, dietary glucosinolate intake and serum glutathione S-transferase α activity on the risk of benign prostatic hyperplasia. BJU Int. 2012 Aug 9. doi: 10.111148–54

[29] Faas FH, Dang AQ, White J, Schaefer RF, Johnson DE. Decreased prostatic arachidonic acid in human prostatic carcinoma. BJU Int. 2003;92(6):551-4.

[30] Fair WR, Wynder EL (1996) Editorial: prostate cancer—nutrition adjunct therapy. J Urol 156:1364–1365

[31] Fair WR, Fleshner NE, Heston W. Cancer of the prostate: a nutritional disease? Urology 1997;50:840–8.

[32] Federico A, Morgillo F, Tuccillo C, Ciardiello F & Loguercio C. Chronic inflammation and oxidative stress in human carcinogenesis .Inter J Cancer. 121(11): 2381–2386, 2007.

[33] Finkel, T; Holbrook, NJ. "Oxidants, oxidative stress and the biology of ageing". Nature,2000, 408 (6809): 239–47

[34] Ferreira SH. Peripheral analgesic sites of action of anti-inflammatory drugs. Int J Clin Pract Suppl. 2002;(128):2-10

[35] Ferreira SH and Nakamura MI (1979) Prostaglandin hyperalgesia, a cAMP/å2+ dependent process. Prostaglandins 18: 179-190.

[36] Flohé L and Ursini F. Peroxidase: A Term of Many Meanings. Antioxid. Redox Signal. 10 (9), 1485–1490, 2008.

[37] Gao P, Guan L, Zheng J. Role of leukotriene B4 in celecoxib-mediated anticancer effect. Biochem Biophys Res Commun. 2010;402(2):308-11

[38] Gallin JJ (eds.): Disorders of phagocytic cells, in Inflammation: Basic Principles and Clinical Correlates, 2d ed, edited by JJ Gallin et al, pp. 859–875. Raven Press, New York, 1992.

[39] Giri, S.N., Z. Chen, E.J. Carroll, R. Mueller, M.J. Schiedt, and L. Panico. 1984. Role of prostaglandins in pathogenesis of bovine mastitis induced by Escherichia coli endotoxin. Am. J.Vet. Res. 45: 586.

[40] Ghosh J. Rapid induction of apoptosis in prostate cancer cells by selenium: reversal by metabolites of arachidonate 5-lipoxygenase. Biochem Biophys Res Commun. 2004;315(3):624-35

[41] Ghosh J, Myers CE. Inhibition of arachidonate 5-lipoxygenase triggers massive apoptosis in human prostate cancer cells. Proc Natl Acad Sci U S A. 1998;95(22):13182-7.

[42] Giovannucci E, Rimm EB, Colditz GA, Stampfer MJ, Ascherio A, Chute CC, et al. A prospective study of dietary fat and risk of prostate cancer. J Natl Cancer Inst, 1993;85(19):1571-9.

[43] Gupta S, Srivastava M, Ahmad N, Bostwick DG, Mukhtar H. Overexpression of cyclooxygenase-2 in human prostate adenocarcinoma. Prostate 42:73–78, 2000.

[44] Haeggström JZ, Funk CD. Lipoxygenase and leukotriene pathways: biochemistry, biology, and roles in disease. Chem Rev. 2011;111(10):5866-98.

[45] Hemler, M.E., Lands, W.E.M., 1980. Evidence of peroxide-initiated free radical mechanism of prostaglandin. biosynthesis. J. Biol. Chem. 225, 6253–6261.

[46] Huang HY. Customized diets for cancer prevention according to genetic polymorphisms: are we ready yet? J Natl Cancer Inst, 2006; 98(22):1590-1.

[47] Hubatsch I, Mannervik B, Gao L, Roberts LJ, Chen Y, Morrow JD. The cyclopentenone product of lipid peroxidation, 15-A(2t)-isoprostane (8-isoprostaglandin A(2)), is efficiently conjugated with glutathione by human and rat glutathione transferase A4-4. Chem Res Toxicol. 2002;15(9):1114-8

[48] Hsu A, Bray TM, Ho E. Anti-inflammatory activity of soy and tea in prostate cancer prevention. Exp Biol Med (Maywood). 2010 ;235(6):659-67.

[49] Ibrahim MA and Makkiya A . Consequences of Chronic Bacterial Infections on Development of Cancer. Research Journal of Microbiology,2011, 6: 310-321.and roles in disease. Chem. Rev., 111, 5866–5898 (2011).

[50] Jackson JR, Seed MP, Kircher CH, Willoughby DA,Winkler JD. The codependence of angiogenesis and Chronic inflammation. FASEB J 1997; 11: 457–65.

[51] Key TJ, Allen N, Appleby P, Overvad K, Tjonneland A, Miller A, Boeing H, Karalis D, Psaltopoulou T, Berrino F, Palli D, Panico S, Tumino R, Vineis P, Bueno-De-Mesquita HB, Kiemeney L, Peeters PH, Martinez C, Dorronsoro M, Gonzalez CA, Chirlaque MD, Quiros JR, Ardanaz E, Berglund G, Egevad L, Hallmans G, Stattin P, Bingham S, Day N, Gann P, Kaaks R, Ferrari P, Riboli E. Fruits and vegetables and prostate cancer: no association among 1104 cases in a prospective study of 130544 men in the European Prospective Investigation into Cancer and Nutrition (EPIC). Int J Cancer, 2004, 109:119-124.

[52] Klein EA, Casey G, Silverman R. Genetic susceptibility and oxidative stress in prostate cancer: integrated model with implications for prevention. Urology, 2006;68(6): 1145-51.

[53] Kolonel LN. Fat, meat, and prostate cancer. Epidemiol Rev, 2001, 23:72-81.

[54] Koopmann W and Krangel MS. Identification of a Glycosaminoglycan-binding Site in Chemokine Macrophage Inflammatory Protein-1α. The Journal of Biological Chemistry, 1997, 272: 10103-10109.

[55] Kuper, H., Adami HO and Trichopoulos D . Infections as a major preventable cause of human cancer. J. Intern. Med.,2000, 248: 171-183.

[56] Larré S, Tran N, Fan C, Hamadeh H, Champigneulles J, Azzouzi R, Cussenot O, Mangin P, Olivier JL. PGE2 and LTB4 tissue levels in benign and cancerous prostates. Prostaglandins Other Lipid Mediat. 2008;87(1-4):14-9.

[57] Liu YW, Su YW, Ong WK, Cheng TH, Tsai YC. Oral administration of Lactobacillus plantarum K68 ameliorates DSS-induced ulcerative colitis in BALB/c mice via the anti-inflammatory and immunomodulatory activities.Int Immunopharmacol. 2011;11(12):2159-66.

[58] Lukacs RU, Goldstein AS, Devon A Lawson DA, Cheng D & Witte ON. Isolation, cultivation and characterization of adult murine prostate stem cells. Nature Protocols 5,702 –713,2010.

[59] Lundstrom K. Past, Present and Future of Nutrigenomics and its Influence on Drug Development. Curr Drug Discov Technol. 2012 Jun 25. [Epub ahead of print]

[60] Lu-Yao GL, Albertsen P, Warren J, Yao SL. Effect of age and surgical approach on complications and short-term mortality after radical prostatectomy—a population-based study. Urology 1999;54:301–7.

[61] Maddams J, Utley M and Møller H. Projections of cancer prevalence in the United Kingdom, 2010–2040. British Journal of Cancer advance online publication 14 August 2012; doi: 10.1038/bjc.2012.366.

[62] Mahan L.K., Escott-Stump S. Krause's Food, Nutrition & Diet Therapy. 11th. Saunders; Philadelphia, PA, USA: 2004.

[63] Mantovani A, Allavena P, Sica A, Balkwill F. Cancer-related inflammation. Nature, 2008, 454(7203):436-44.

[64] Marnett LJ. Aspirin and the potential role of prostaglandins in colon cancer. Cancer Res 1992;52:5575-89.

[65] Matsuyama M, Yoshimura R. Cysteinyl-leukotriene1 receptor is a potent target for the prevention and treatment of human urological cancer. Mol Med Report. 2010 ; 3(2):245-51.

[66] McNeal JE: Regional morphology and pathology of the prostate. Am J Clin Pathol 1968, 49:347-357

[67] McNeal JE. Normal histology of the prostate. Am J Surg Pathol. 1988 Aug;12(8):619–633.

[68] Miller PE, Morey MC, Hartman TJ, Snyder DC, Sloane R, Cohen HJ, Demark-Wahnefried W. Dietary patterns differ between urban and rural older, long-term survivors

of breast, prostate, and colorectal cancer and are associated with body mass index.J Acad Nutr Diet. 2012;112(6):824-31

[69] Mimata H, Tanigawa T, Ogata J, Takeshita M. Regulation of prostaglandin synthesis by reduced glutathione in urinary bladder epithelium. J Urol. 1988;139(3):616-20.

[70] Minami Y, Staples MP, Giles GG. The incidence of colon, breast and prostate cancer in Italian migrants to Victoria, Australia. Eur J Cancer, 1993, 29A:1735-1740.

[71] Manolio TA, Collins FS, Cox NJ, Goldstein DB, Hindorff LA, Hunter DJ, McCarthy MI, Ramos EM, Cardon LR, Chakravarti A, Cho JH, Guttmacher AE, Kong A, Kruglyak L, Mardis E, Rotimi CN, Slatkin M, Valle D, Whittemore AS, Boehnke M, Clark AG, Eichler EE, Gibson G, Haines JL, Mackay TF, McCarroll SA, Visscher PM..Finding the missing heritability of complex diseases. Nature 2009; 461: 747–753.

[72] Muir CS, Nectoux J, Staszewski J. The epidemiology of prostatic cancer: geographical distribution and time-trends. Acta Oncol 1991; 30:133–40.

[73] Nelson WG, De Marzo AM, and Isaacs WB . Prostate Cancer. N Engl J Med 2003; 349:366-381.

[74] Parantainen J., Sankari S. & Atroshi F. (1988) Biological functions of silicon, selenium and glutathione peroxidase (GSH-Px) explained in terms of semicoduction. In: Trace Elements in Man and Animals 6 (Hurly LS ; Keen CL; Lonnerdal Bo, & Rucker RB, Editors), Plenum Press, New York & London, pp.359-360.

[75] Park S, Murphy SP, Wilkens LR, Henderson BE, Kolonel LN. Fat and meat intake and prostate cancer risk: the multiethnic cohort study. Int J Cancer 2007;1339–45.

[76] Pavlou M and Diamandis EP. The Search for New Prostate Cancer Biomarkers Continues. Clinical Chemistry, 2009, 55(7): 1277-1279.

[77] Pilch P, Radziszewski P, Maciukiewicz P. Prostate cancer dependance upon cholesterol, statins and diet. Wiad Lek. 2012;65(1):31-7.

[78] Prates C , Sousa S, Oliveira C, Ikram S. Prostate metastatic bone cancer in an Egyptian Ptolemaic mummy, a proposed radiological diagnosis. International Journal of Paleopathology, 1(2): 98–103,2011

[79] Rakoff-Nahoum S. Why Cancer and Inflammation? Yale journal of biology and medicine, 2006, 79: 123-130

[80] Ratan, H. L., Steward, W. P., Gescher, A. J., and Mellon, J. K. Resveratrol—a prostate cancer chemopreventive agent? Urol Oncol, 7: 223-227, 2002.

[81] Richie JP Jr, Das A, Calcagnotto AM, Aliaga CA, El-Bayoumy K. Age related changes in selenium and glutathione levels in different lobes of the rat prostate. Exp Gerontol. 2012;47(3):223-8.

[82] Ros S, Santos CR, Moco S, Baenke F, Gavin Kelly G, Howell M, Zamboni N and Schulze A. Functional Metabolic Screen Identifies 6-Phosphofructo-2-Kinase/Fruc-

tose-2,6-Biphosphatase 4 as an Important Regulator of Prostate Cancer Cell Survival. Cancer Discovery 2012 2; (4):328-43.

[83] Rouzer CA, Scott WA, Griffith OW, Hamill AL, and Cohn ZA. Arachidonic acid metabolism in glutathione-deficient macrophages. Proc Natl Acad Sci U S A. 1982; 79(5): 1621–1625.

[84] Samuelsson B, Morgenstern R and Jakobsson P-J. Membrane Prostaglandin E Synthase-1: A Novel Therapeutic Target. Pharmacological Reviews ,2007 , 59(3): 207-224.

[85] Sanz-Motilva V, Nagore E, Martorell-Calatayud A. Non-Steroidal Anti-Inflammatory Drugs and Melanoma. Curr Pharm Des. 2012

[86] Schaeffer AJ (2003) Epidemiology and demographics. of prostatitis. Andrologia 35:252-257.

[87] Schulman CC, Ekane S, Zlotta AR. Nutrition and prostate cancer: evidence or suspicion? Urology 2001;58:318–34.

[88] Shacter E, Weitzman SA. Chronic inflammation and cancer. Oncology. 2002;16:217–226.

[89] Sies, Helmut. "Oxidative stress: Oxidants and antioxidants". Experimental physiology, 1997,82 (2): 291–5.

[90] Shimizu H, Ross RK, Bernstein L, Yatani R, Henderson BE, Mack TM. Cancers of the prostate and breast among Japanese and white immigrants in Los Angeles County. Br J Cancer, 1991, 63:963-966.

[91] Sakr WA, Grignon DJ, Crissman JD, Heilbrun LK, Cassin BJ, Pontes JJ, Haas GP. High grade prostatic intraepithelial neoplasia (HGPIN) and prostatic adenocarcinoma between the ages of 20-69: an autopsy study of 249 cases. In Vivo. 1994 May-Jun; 8(3):439-43.

[92] Schellhammer P. Life after failure of traditional androgen deprivation therapy. Urol Oncol. 2012 ;30(4 Suppl):S10-4

[93] Sonn, G. A., Aronson, W., Litwin, M. S., Chong, P., and Rashid, P. Impact of diet on prostate cancer: a review Can we prevent prostate cancer? Prostate Cancer Prostatic Dis, 8: 304-310, 2005.

[94] Sreekumar A, Poisson LM, Rajeniran TM, Khan AP, Cao Q, Yu J, et al. Metabolomic profiles delineate potential role for sarcosine in prostate cancer progression. Nature 2009;457:910-914

[95] Steinhilber D, Fischer AS, Metzner J, Steinbrink SD, Roos J, Ruthardt M, Maier TJ. 5-lipoxygenase: underappreciated role of a pro-inflammatory enzyme in tumorigenesis. Front Pharmacol. 2010;1:143

[96] Stewart, J. R., Artime, M. C., and O'Brian, C. A. Resveratrol: a candidate nutritional substance for prostate cancer prevention. J Nutr, 133: 2440S-2443S, 2003.

[97] Sugar LM. Inflammation and prostate cancer. Can J Urol. 2006 Suppl 1:46-7

[98] Sugino N, Karube-Harada A, Kashida S, Takiguchi S and Kato H. Reactive oxygen species stimulate prostaglandin F2α production in human endometrial stromal cells in vitro. Human Reproduction, 2001, 16(9): 1797-1801.

[99] Tallberg Th and Atroshi F. Prostate Cancer, the Long Search for Etiologic and Therapeutic Factors: Dietary Supplementation Avoiding Invasive Treatment. In "Prostate Cancer: From Bench to Bedside"(Philippe E. Spiess ed.), pp. 33-52, 2011. INTECH Publisher, Croatia.

[100] Tallberg T, Westermarck T, Atroshi F. Cancer Treatment, Based on Active Nutritional Bio-Modulation, Hormonal Therapy and Specific Autologous Immunotherapy.In: Heavy Metals in the Environment (editors: Zueng-Sang Chen, Dar-Yuan Lee, Tser-Sheng Lin). Publisher, National Taiwan University Taipei, Taiwan, November 2008.

[101] Taketo MM. Cyclooxygenase-2 inhibitors in tumorigenesis (part 1). J Natl Cancer Inst 1998;90:1529-36.

[102] Thun MJ, Namboodiri MM, Heath CW Jr. Aspirin use and reduced risk of fatal colon cancer. N Engl J Med 1991;325:1593-6.

[103] Tilg H, Moschen AR. Adipocytokines: mediators linking adipose tissue, inflammation and immunity. Nat Rev Immunol 2006; 6: 772-83.

[104] Vander Heiden, MG, Cantley, LC and Thompson, CB. Understanding the Warburg effect: the metabolic requirements of cell proliferation. Science, 2009. 324(5930): p. 1029-33

[105] Vane JR, Bakhle YS, Botting RM. Cyclooxygenases 1 and 2. Annu Rev Pharmacol Toxicol 1998; 38: 97–120.

[106] Wang X, Klein RD. Prostaglandin E2 induces vascular endothelial growth factor secretion in prostate cancer cells through EP2 receptor-mediated cAMP pathway. Mol Carcinog. 2007 ;46(11):912-23.

[107] Yancik R. Population aging and cancer: a cross-national concern.Cancer J 2005; 11(6): 437-441.

[108] Yang CS, Suh N, Kong AN. Does vitamin E prevent or promote cancer? Cancer Prev Res (Phila). 2012;5(5):701-5.

[109] Zhou Y,Elizabeth EO. Hileman, HW, Keating MJ, and Huang P. Free radical stress in chronic lymphocytic leukemia cells and its role in cellular sensitivity to ROS-generating anticancer agents. Blood, 2003, 101 (10): 4098-4104.

Chapter 18

Inflammatory Microenvironment in Prostate Carcinogenesis

Geraldine Gueron, Javier Cotignola and
Elba Vazquez

Additional information is available at the end of the chapter

http://dx.doi.org/10.5772/52636

1. Introduction

The association between prostate cancer and inflammation was first formally addressed in the nineteen century and since then many authors have confirmed the biological and clinical evidence of this association. However, the molecular mechanism involved is yet to be deciphered.

There are two well established pathways linking inflammation and cancer: the extrinsic pathway from conditions that cause non-resolving smouldering inflammatory responses and the intrinsic pathway where the misregulation of oncogenes and tumor suppressor genes switch on the expression of inflammation-related programs.

Prostate cancer is a complex and progressive disease. Over time the cells become resistance to hormonal therapies that are designed to block the release and/or the uptake of androgens. During this stage androgen receptor (AR) mutants are able to bind promiscuous steroids, and may convert AR antagonists to agonists. Other hormones and their receptors are involved in the abnormal growth of the gland. Particularly, oestrogens and oestrogen receptors defined a subclass of prostate cancer with a very aggressive clinical phenotype (such as the TMPRSS2-ERG fusion). In addition, other signaling cascades are switched on bypassing the androgen/AR axis and favoring tumor progression. Among them, cyclooxygenase-2 (COX-2), neuroendocrine differentiation and the loss of the tumor suppressor phosphatase and tensin homolog (PTEN), with the concomitant inhibition of the PI3K/Akt, resulting in Bcl-2 overexpression and the burst of pro-inflammatory cytokines, chemokines and other growth factors production, contributing all to the progression to the hormonal-resistance disease. As in other malignancies in prostate cancer, reactive oxygen species (ROS) cause oxidative damage to macromolecules in epithelial cells and can react with other cellular components initiating a free radical chain reaction, thus sustaining the prostate carcinogenic process and its progression.

The molecular mechanisms that prime the pathogenesis of cancer-related inflammation are complex and involve a delicate interplay between tumor and its microenvironment. In prostate tumors, the switch to an angiogenic phenotype is known to be critical for its progression. Unless a tumor can stimulate the formation of new blood vessels, it remains restricted to a microscopic size. Inflammation and hypoxia are widely accepted as key elements in the induction of angiogenesis.

Dissection of the diversity of cancer-related inflammation is critical for the design of innovative diagnostic and therapeutic strategies in prostate cancer.

Specifically, the following topics and molecular events are reviewed and discussed in this chapter:

- The cytokine and chemokine orchestration and the associated downstream genetic events that cause neoplastic transformation in the prostatic tissue.
- Acknowledging the oxidative stress imbalance in the tumoral niche as key mediators of signaling cascades.
- The relevance of microRNAs as oncogenes and tumor suppressor genes and how microRNA expression profiles can be used for markers of prostate cancer prevention and therapeutics.
- The potential of prostate tumoral cells in the inflammatory microenvironment to express an endothelial-like phenotype and mimic vasculogenic networks.

2. Body

2.1. The cytokine & chemokine orchestration in prostate cancer: Strategies, avenues and traits

Cytokines are a family of cell-signaling protein molecules that are secreted by various cell types and are a category of signaling molecules used extensively in intercellular communication. Cytokines can be classified as proteins, peptides, or glycoproteins. A variety of cytokines are secreted by cells in the tumor microenvironment and can impact on prostate cancer growth. These cytokines can then act in a paracrine fashion on tumor cells to stimulate a variety of physiological activities including cell proliferation, invasion, migration, chemoresistance, etc.

The tumor inflammatory microenvironment is characterized by immune cell infiltration: tumor-associated macrophages, mast cells, dendritic cells, natural killer cells, neutrophils, eosinophils and lymphocytes. These cells produce a variety of cytotoxic mediators such as ROS and reactive nitrogen species (RNS), serine and cysteine proteases, matrix metalloproteinase (MMP), tumor necrosis factor α (TNFα), interleukins, interferons and enzymes, as COX-2, lipooxygenase-5 and phospholipase A2, which activate or are activated by transcription factors such as nuclear factor κB (NF-κB) and signal transducers and activators of transcription-3 (STAT3), activator protein 1 and hypoxia-inducible factor 1α (HIF-1α) that mediate tumor cell proliferation, transformation, metastasis, survival, invasion, angiogenesis, chemoresistance and radioresistance.

Present discoveries highlight chemokines and their receptors as relevant factors for inflammation. The directed migration of a cell toward the source of a secreted protein signal, known as chemotaxis, has been commonly associated to the leukocyte trafficking triggered by infection and to secondary lymphoid organs. Although extensively studied as part of the immune system, chemokines have lately been investigated as mediators of tumor development. Chemokines, the executors of chemotactic signals, are constitutively expressed in destined cell types and tissues maintaining the homeostasis of the hematopoietic and the immune system. However, inflammatory chemokines, either produced by the tumor cells or by tumor-associated cells, behave differently and their expression is induced upon inflammatory stimuli promoting proliferation and angiogenesis, contributing to the malignant progression. They certainly modify the sensitivity of prostate cancer cells to environmental stresses such as hypoxia, oxidative stress, DNA damage, altering several pathways crosstalk and producing hormone-refractory aggressive tumors. In addition to the classical roles described above, their pleiotropic effects include: potentiating the production of growth factors, inducing growth signals, attenuating apoptosis, further linking the cytokine signaling to the hypothesis that inflammation and inflammatory mediators rise as the seventh hallmark of cancer [1]. In this section we will focus on some of the several cytokines implicated in the prostate cancer microenvironment given that there are too many factors to describe.

2.1.1. The chemokine family acquaintance

To date, over 50 chemokines and 20 chemokine receptors have been recollected. These are grouped into four categories, C, CC, CXC and CX3C, according to the location of the main cysteine residues near the N-terminal domain of these proteins [2]. Chemokine binding to their corresponding seven transmembrane-domain G-protein-coupled receptors causes the activation of signal transduction networks leading to chemotaxis. These receptors have been implicated in the migration of breast, prostate and lung cells to secondary sites in the bone [3]. Up to date the most relevant chemokine receptors in prostate cancer dissemination, are CXCR4, CXCR7 and CXCR6 [3].

The CXCR4/CXCL12 axis exerts multifactorial effects and has been related to both, the homing of tumor cells to specific organs and the growth of tumor cells at specific locations. CXCL12, also known as SDF-1 (stromal derived factor 1), is considered a homeostatic chemokine which regulates the hematopoietic cell trafficking and secondary lymphoid tissue architecture. It is constitutively expressed in several organs including lung, liver, skeletal muscle, brain, kidney, heart, skin, bone marrow and its secretion is linked to tissue damage. CXCR4 is expressed in endothelial cells and pericytes of hypoxic, injured, or pathological tissues. Of note, endothelial precursor cells also express and secrete CXCL12. In turn,

CXCR4 is widely expressed on hematopoietic cells including CD34+ hematopoietic stem cells, T- and B-lymphocytes, monocytes and macrophages, neutrophils and eosinophils as well as by brain, lung, colon, heart, kidney, liver endothelial and epithelial cells, microglia, astrocytes, neuronal cells, and progenitor cells including endothelial and smooth muscle progenitors. Functional CXCR4 is expressed on embryonic pluripotent stem cells and several types of tissue-committed stem cells. These cells with functional CXCR4 expression migrate and/or invade along CXCL12 gradients. CXCR4+ pro-angiogenic cells include immature and mature hematopoietic cells, endothelial precursor cells, and smooth muscle cell progenitors, which have direct or indirect pro-angiogenic properties. Interestingly, CXCL12 plays a role in the mobilization and recruitment of these cells to the neo-angiogenic niches supporting revascularization of ischemic tissue and tumor growth [4]. This axis has been strongly implicated in prostate cancer tumorigenesis and progression [5].

2.1.2. Chemokines and their relevance in the metastatic behavior of prostate cancer

Metastases is a multistep process including: invasion of the primary tumor cells to adjacent tissue, intravasation, dissemination through the blood or lymph, extravasation and seeding, adapting to a different tissue microenvironment and finally proliferating in such distant organs. This process involves both the selection of features that favor cancer cells growth and the concomitant alteration of the stroma generating a "fertile soil" which facilitates invasion, anchoring and survival of metastatic cells [6].

Prostate neoplasms have a striking tendency to metastasize to bone. The molecular mechanisms underlying the bone homing behavior have yet to be decoded. However, such mechanisms may include signaling cascades that induce a vascular pathway, that produce the trigger of chemotactic factors by bone marrow stromal cells and the production of growth factors within the bone, reinforcing the survival and proliferation of tumoral cells. It is of common knowledge that hematopietic stem cells are directed to the bone during bone marrow transplantation and human fetal development [7, 8] and CXCL12/CXCR4 appears in this scene as key molecules in bone seeding. Metastatic prostate cancer cells may use a similar pathway to localize to the bone. Several human prostate cancer cell lines express functional CXCR4 and differential levels of its ligand alter physiological processes of these cells such as adhesion, migration and invasion, assigning a role for this axis in prostate advanced disease. It is worth mentioning some controversial reports regarding the expression of this receptor and its ligand in prostate cancer. Mochizuki *et al.* [9] reported that the expression of CXCR4, but not its ligand, was increased in prostate carcinoma indicating that prostate cancer cells may also be affected by exogenous SDF-1. However, other authors showed high expression of both, ligand and receptor [10].

Interestingly, the blockade of CXCR4 inhibited the expression of vascular endothelial growth factor (VEGF) and the concomitant angiogenesis and even reduced significantly bone metastasis *in vivo* [11]. Furthermore, CXCR4 is positively regulated by AR [12]. Androgen-induced CXCR4 expression was functional in TMPRSS2-ERG-positive prostate cancer cells, further indicating the relevance of this chemokine in prostate cancer metastasis [13]. The immunohistochemical pattern of CXCR4 expression in patients with metastatic prostate cancer has shown that high expression of this chemokine in tumors had poorer cancer-specific survival than patients with low expression of CXCR4. This receptor expression has proved to be a useful prognostic factor for patients with metastatic prostate cancer treated with androgen-withdrawal therapy [14].

Strikingly, regulation of CXCL12 expression in the tumor microenvironment has been poorly studied. Some reports indicate that hypoxia may induce its expression in endothelial cells and in prostate tumor cells [5]. Could CXCL12 have an additional role to its chemo-attractant properties? Could it also act as a growth factor or prevent the apoptosis of tumoral cells enabling metastasis to take place? These questions still need to be answered.

CXCR7 (RDC1), a second receptor for CXCL12, regulates a spectrum of normal and pathological processes but fails to couple to G-proteins and to induce the typical chemokine receptor mediated cellular responses. It also binds to CXCL11 and dimerizes with CXCR4. This receptor with dual specificity is up-regulated in many tumors, but its function within the tumoral niche needs further clarification [15]. Studies show that CXCR7 expression provides proliferation and survival advantages and increased adhesion properties between prostate cancer cells and the host endothelial cells. It is also more highly expressed in prostate metastases (specially those to the bone) compared to primary tumors and elevated levels of CXCR7 correlate with the aggressiveness of the disease. In the vasculature, the expression of CXCR7 is elevated in endothelial cells associated with tumors [16] and this chemokine receptor has been further linked to tumor angiogenesis *in vivo* [17].

Other inflammatory mediators may regulate CXCR7 function. Of note, high serum levels of IL8 have been reported in patients with advanced metastatic prostate cancer. In primary prostate carcinoma tissues, IL8 strongly correlates with biochemical prostate specific antigen (PSA) recurrence and CXCR7 expression is induced by IL8 in prostate tumor cells. As survival following androgen deprivation is a critical step in the emergence of castration-resistant tumors, IL8–induced up-regulation of CXCR7 may enhance the survival and proliferation properties of those tumor cells. Thus the up-regulation of CXCR7 induced by IL8 emerges as a promoter of castration-resistant tumors survival [15]. Moreover, CXCR7-depleted tumors showed significantly reduced levels of relevant factors for prostate tumorigenesis like cyclin D1, VEGF and phosphorylated epidermal growth factor receptor [15]. There is also additional evidence for a potential role of CXCR7 as a CXCL12 scavenger, suggesting that this receptor in turn modulates the activity of CXCR4 in tumor formation and is critical for the fine-tuning of the motility of hematopoietic cells in the bone marrow and lymphoid organs.

However, the blockade of the CXCR4 and CXCR7 only partially impaired the metastatic behavior of prostate cancer *in vivo,* arguing that other functional chemokine/chemokine receptor pairs may be envolved in prostate cancer progression [18].

The third chemokine receptor noteworthy in prostate cancer is CXCR6, displaying high expression not only in prostate cancer cell lines but also in prostate tissues [19]. This receptor is also known as Bonzo, STRL33 or TYMSTR. In humans, Bonzo is expressed by small subsets of T cells and CD16+ cells, but not by B cells, monocytes or dendritic cells [20].

CXCL16 is one of the two known transmembrane chemokines. It is also constitutively expressed on fibroblasts, keratinocytes and cancer cells of various origin tissues [19]. CXCL16 was identified as the ligand for this receptor and was found to signal through NF-κB via heterotrimeric G proteins/PI3K/PDK-1/Akt/IKK/IκB [21]. It was also reported to signal through the Akt/mTOR pathway [22]. A variety of chemokines contain a conserved sequence motif (ELR, glutamic acid-leucine-arginine) that precedes the first cysteine residue near the amino-terminal end which is critical for the receptor binding, for the chemotactic activity and for the promotion of angiogenesis. Intriguingly, although lacking an ELR motif in the chemokine domain, CXCL16 appears as proangiogenic. CXCR6 was shown to regulate blood vessel formation by an autocrine/paracrine loop established between prostate cancer and endothelial cells and was observed that both IL8 and IL6 levels were altered in response to changes in CXCR6 expression [18]. The striking similarities between CXCL16 and CXCL12 are likely to result in additive effects [23]. Moreover, CXCL12 and CXCL16 were observed in tissues enriched with plasma cells and in cultured human bone marrow stromal cells [23]. Thus, plasma cells are likely to be recruited to bone marrow and other target tissues via CXCR4 and CXCR6 [18]. CXCL16 not only attracts T cells and natural killer T cells toward dendritic cells but also supports their firm adhesion to dendritic cells [24]. Taken together, high CXCL16/CXCR6 expression may be strongly related to aggressive cancer behavior, and particularly, high-secreted ligand expression to bone metastases of prostate cancer [19].

While it is well accepted that chemokines promote tumor development, these molecules may in turn be used to the benefit of cancer patients, acting in the recruitment of dendritic cells and /or effector cells or for their angiostatic properties. However, chemokine-mediated recruitment of immature dendritic cells within tumors, due to factors produced by the tumor milieu, may induce immune tolerance. In this context, the balance between positive and negative effects should be examined when designing novel strategies to eradicate tumors based on chemokine targeting.

2.1.3. Role of IL8 and IL6 in the transition to hormone refractory prostate cancer

Prostate cancer cells and the surrounding stroma are exposed to a plethora of interleukins and chemokines, receiving their signaling stimuli, re-enforcing tumor-promoting functions. Similar to other chemokines that recognize and bind G-protein-coupled receptors, IL8 acts through CXC receptors. The expression of CXCL8 (also known as IL8), one of the best-characterized members of the chemokine family, has been described as a key effector in prostate cancer. Normal prostate epithelial cells and tissues produce low amount of IL8, whereas prostate cancer cells from primary and metastatic tumors produce progressively greater amounts [25]. High levels of CXCL8 also correlate to an elevated adherence of the prostate tumor cells to the endothelium, hence increasing angiogenesis, tumorigenicity and lymph node metastasis *in vivo* [26, 27]. Even more, CXCL8 is a transcriptional target of NF-κB and its expression is elevated in androgen independent prostate cancer, contributing to the transition to a castration-resistant state and to resistance to standard chemotherapeutic drugs [28]. To date, the chemotherapy strategy utilized for advanced prostate cancer disease is based on the combination of docetaxel (a cytostatic drug) with prednisone (a glucocorticoid prodrug). However, this therapeutic strategy shows a modest survival benefit over palliative care, where many patients respond initially, but eventually develop a resistance to docetaxel. Among other factors, increased IL8 production decreases the sensitivity of hormone-resistant cells to the cytotoxic chemotherapeutic agents and also reduces prostate cancer cell apoptosis induced by tumor necrosis factor-related apoptosis-inducing ligand (TRAIL). In experimental prostate cancer a naphthalimide was shown to decrease IL8 expression and to enhance taxol activity when co-administered with this compound. Thus, negative regulators of this chemokine could emerge as second line treatment for patients with docetaxel-resistant advanced prostate cancer [29].

One of the most interesting mediators clearly implicated in prostate cancer is IL6, a multifunctional cytokine, produced by inflammatory cells, osteoblasts and even prostate cancer cells. There are multiple lines of clinical and experimental evidence preponderantly showing that IL6 contributes to prostate cancer progression. Both, patients with prostate cancer and patients with advanced metastatic disease display high expression levels of IL6 and its soluble receptor in the circulating plasma [30]. These observations have led to study whether this axis could predict biochemical recurrence in radical prostatectomy patients [31] providing a rationale for the clinical relevance of IL6 as a prognostic factor. In particular, a phase II study assessed the efficacy of siltuximab, in men with castrate resistant prostate cancer that had been treated with one prior chemotherapy with the primary endpoint being PSA response rate (defined by a 50% reduction of PSA) [32]. This drug, also known as CNTO 328, is a human-mouse chimeric monoclonal neutralizing IL6 antibody. The response rate was small and no men with disease had a Response Evaluation Criteria in Solid Tumors (RECIST) response. This criterion defines a set of rules that assesses whether a patient improves ("responds"), stays the same ("stabilizes"), or worsens ("progression") during treatments. The results obtained evidenced the lack of a beneficial therapeutic effect of IL6 neutralization in patients with advanced androgen resistant disease. However, there are still some positive prospects for IL6 neutralization, providing an additional benefit to other chemotherapy regimes, especially in light of its anti-apoptotic effects [33].

In addition to the clinical observations, *in vitro* studies have provided evidence that IL6 modulates prostate cancer cell growth of hormone-refractory cells, but had no effect on the growth of hormone-dependent cell lines [33].

IL6 has also been implicated in other aspects of prostate cancer pathophysiology such as tumorigenesis in the prostate microenvironment. IL6 foremost effect is the activation of Janus kinase (JAK) signaling and of signal transducers and activators of transcription (STAT) proteins, especially STAT3. Through this signaling pathway, IL6 stimulates autocrine activation of insulin-like type I growth factor receptor (IGF-IR) to confer tumorigenesis [34]. Depending on the cellular context, IL6 can also signal through MAPK and phosphatidylinositol-3 kinase (PI3K) pathways [35, 36].

This cytokine can be produced autocrinaly in castrate resistant prostate cells and can transactivate the AR in those cells. However, the AR status as well as other interacting signaling cascades will define the role of IL6 on ligand-independent AR activation, tumor formation, and subsequent growth. Additionally, IL6 has been proposed to initiate an intracrine signaling pathway, alternative to the androgen receptor axis, affecting metabolic enzyme levels. Surprisingly, testosterone plasma levels were significantly increased when IL6 overexpressing prostate cancer cells were inoculated in castrated mice, showing that this cytokine regulates the expression of esteroidogenic genes in tumoral cells [5].

Overall, IL6 strongly correlates with more advanced stages of the disease, therapy resistance, poor prognosis and can be predictive of recurrence after treatment of localized cancer. Based on all the clinical and preclinical evidence, further exploration for IL6 inhibition is justified; however, its efficacy may greatly depend on the stage of disease or other individualized factors.

2.1.4. Tumor Necorsis factor: Linking inflammation to prostate cancer

TNF was named for its ability to induce rapid haemorrhagic necrosis of experimental cancers [37]. However, it soon became noticeable that this cytokine presented anti-tumoral activity and cytotoxicity against several tumoral cells [38]. Currently, TNF is considered as a relevant player in host defense and inflammation with several activities extending far beyond its original anti-tumoral action. Among its effects, TNF signaling may lead to both, cell apoptosis and necrosis, and also to tumor progression and metastasis by switching on survival genes [39].

TNF signals through TNF receptor 1 (TNF-R1) and TNF-R2. While TNF-R1 is expressed constitutively in most tissues, TNF-R2 is modulated and is mostly found on immune system cells. TNF binds to the death domain containing TNF-R1 to recruit TNF receptor-associated death domain (TRADD), Fas-associated death domain (FADD) and caspase-8, forming the death-inducing signaling complex [40]. Interestingly, when TNF-R1 is activated, it also recruits receptor-interacting protein (RIP) and TNF receptor-associated factor 2 (TRAF2) and activates NF-κB, involved in cell survival, proliferation, anti-apoptotic activity and highly implicated in the inflammatory response [41].

TNFα plays critical roles in cancer pathophysiology building an elaborate association between inflammation and cancer. It functions as a key regulator of the tumor microenvironment, promoting tumor progression, even in the absence of invading inflammatory cells [42]. It facilitates cancer development acting directly on neoplastic cells or indirectly through endothelial and other inflammatory cells [43]. However, the mechanisms by which TNFα enables these events are not fully described. A recent publication from Davis *et al.* [44] explains the dichotomy of TNFα effect on the control of apoptosis in prostate cancer cells. These authors propose a physiologic role for TNFα in prostate regression after androgen withdrawal. This factor is required for castration-induced prostate regression, but membrane-bound TNFα protein and stromal cell specific TNFα mRNA levels increase in rat prostate after castration, which is coincident with a paracrine effect of TNFα in prostate cancer regression. However, when wild-type non-castrated mice were treated with TNFα no regression of the gland was observed [44]. All these evidences showed that this cytokine acts in the context of supplemental castration-induced signals.

Summarizing, the chemokine scene displays a vast crosstalk of pathways involved in the day-to-day dialogue between the cancer cells and the inflammatory microenvironment. The challenge relies in identifying the homeostatic target/targets that govern this setting in order to successfully re-direct the therapeutic efforts against prostate cancer.

2.2. The oxidative stress imbalance in the prostate tumor: Gearing the journey to cancer

The development of cancer is a complex process. Cancer cells associate, both in primary as well as in secondary colonization sites with resident stromal fibroblasts, smooth muscle cells, macrophages, endothelium, neurons and migrating cells at metastatic niches and phenotypically and genotypically activate them, triggering different signaling mechanisms. During this process, the cancer cells and cells in the cancer microenvironment "co-evolve" in part due to oxidative stress, and acquire the ability to mimic other cell types (which can be termed osteomimicry, vasculomimicry, neuromimicry and stem cell mimicry), and undergo transition from epithelium to mesenchyme with definitive behavioral modifications. Prostate cancer cells co-evolve in their genotypic and phenotypic characters with stroma and acquire osteomimetic properties allowing these cells to proliferate and survive in the skeleton as bone metastasis [45]. ROS, RNS and other factors implicated in oxidative and nitrosative stress alters the homeostatic milieu, affecting macromolecules and damaging cell membranes, altering organelles permeability and function. Thus co-targeting different players in this complex scenario will be an effective treatment alternative for prostate cancer progression.

2.2.1. The prostate and its oxidative defense barriers

The normal prostate epithelium consists of prostatic ducts that contain basal cells, stem cells, secretory luminal cells and neuroendocrine cells. The stromal component consists of smooth muscle, fibroblasts, vascular endothelial cells, nerve cells, inflammatory cells, insoluble matrix and soluble factors. Inflammation is clearly associated to the early stages of prostate carcinogenesis [46]. The macrophages in the tumor microenvironment produce ROS and RNS. The increase in reactive radicals such as superoxide ($O2^{\bullet -}$), hydrogen peroxide (H_2O_2), hydroxyl radical ($HO^{\bullet}$), etc. produces DNA damage, causes genetic mutations and initiates/promotes cancer progression. Some molecules implicated in prostate atrophy include p53 and AR mutations, hypermethylation of the CpG island of the promoter of gluthathione S tranferase-P1 (GSTP1), decreased activity of manganese superoxide dismutase (MnSOD) and increased expression of NADPH oxidase 1, which initiate high grade prostatic intraepithelial neoplasia (PIN) and progressive prostate cancer [45].

The prostate gland depends on the androgen/AR signaling for growth. Activation of this axis in advanced prostate cancer has been attributed to various mechanisms, including AR hypersensitivity, *de novo* intraprostatic androgen synthesis, promiscuous AR activation via adrenal androgens, non-androgenic steroids and non-canonical AR activation via growth factors and cytokines through intracellular signal-transduction pathways [47]. These mechanisms may result from abnormalities in the AR status (e.g., mutation, splice variants) and/or in the levels of its co-regulators. Furthermore, some AR splice variants have been identified with constitutive effects in the absence of ligands [48].

ROS are endogenously generated during cellular metabolic processes. It can also come from external sources. Thus, excessive ROS production or impairment of antioxidant defense systems can induce oxidative stress. This increase in ROS levels may contribute to the initiation and development of various cancers, including prostate cancer, because oxidative stress regulates cellular fate in various systems. ROS are considered to be tumor initiators/promoters given the potential for induction of DNA damage. Furthermore, signaling pathways in response to intracellular changes in ROS levels may trigger proliferation, apoptosis and senescence, events highly implicated in all the stages of the carcinogenic process. However, little is known about the exact molecular machinery that mediates ROS function in the tumorigenic process. Several transcription factors that regulate AR activity/transcription are implicated in oxidative stress, among them, NF-κB, c-Myc, CREB, Sp1 and Foxo3a [49]. Interestingly, castration-induced oxidative stress in prostate cancer cell lines increased AR levels through the overexpression of an oncogene member of the basic helix-loop-helix transcription factor Twist 1, which regulates the expression of AR by binding to E-boxes in its promoter, resulting in a gain of castration resistant phenotype [50] and being responsible of metastasis [51]. Evidently, there is a connection between oxidative stress and androgen deprivation in prostate cancer, which is also supported by previous observations of increased oxidative damage associated to the development of malignancies [52]. Of interest, when comparing the expression profile of castration resistant prostate cancer gene with the genetic landscape of hormonal sensitive tumors, the endogenous antioxidant defense system is clearly repressed, in particular MnSOD, which regulates ROS production by converting superoxide to a less reactive species, acting as a ROS scavenger. Hence, MnSOD in advanced prostate cancer could be mechanistically linked to AR reactivation. An array for transcription factor DNA binding activity showed that AR (among other transcription factors) binds to DNA after MnSOD knocked-down [53]. These findings correlate with a clear transcriptional repression of stress-related genes [54].

2.2.2. Is oxidative stress governing the co-regulators of nuclear receptors?

Co-regulators of transcription orchestrate the action of nuclear receptors. Each tissue has a "quantitative finger print" of co-activators based on the relative inherited concentrations of these molecules. When the cellular concentration of a co-activator is altered, genetic dysfunction usually leads to a pathologic outcome. Co-regulators contain the potential to efficiently promote cellular pathologies by coordinately misdirecting multiple independent functions such as oncogenesis. During the development and progression of prostate tumors there are a misregulation of AR co-activators, many of them play a critical role in redox maintenance protecting cells from cytotoxicity produced by oxidative stress. That is the case with peroxiredoxin (Prx), a gene elevated in cancer with anti-oxidant capacity. Prx1, a co-activator that facilitates the binding of androgen to the AR, is regulated by nuclear factor (erythroid-derived 2)-related factor 2 (Nrf2), a transcription factor also induced by oxidative stress. Another member of this family, Prx2, is also regulated by oxidative stress but in this case through Foxo3a, another transcription factor implicated in AR transcription and cellular responses to oxidative stress and overexpressed in the castrate resistant-disease. Remarkably, the subcellular distribution of co-regulators seems to be relevant in the regulation of the AR activity. While cytoplasmic Prx2 enhances AR transactivation, its nuclear localization decreases the receptor activity, suggesting that the redox status of the nucleus and cytoplasm might affect AR signaling through this co-regulator [55].

2.2.3. *Oxidative stress and tumor-stroma co-evolution*

Since the initial seed and soil hypothesis elaborated by Paget in 1889 [56], the relevance of the tumor microenvironment in the carcinogenic process is continuously on scene. Tissue recombination experiments with mixed prostate stromal/epithelial cell xenografts surprisingly revealed that transformation of epithelial cells is accompanied by a transdifferentiation of fibroblasts. Prostate stroma is mainly composed of fibroblasts and smooth muscle cells, and an intermediate cell type described as myofibroblast. The highly proliferative stromal cells immediately surrounding malignant glands have been described as "reactive stroma" or "carcinoma-associated fibroblast" (CAF) [57]. Wound repair exhibits a fibroblastic switch to a myofibroblast-like phenotype, with the subsequent extracellular matrix (ECM) remodeling through angiogenesis and increased protease activity [58]. The "reactive stroma" of a malignant tumor may parallel the granulation tissue of a healing wound in many ways, behaving as wounds that never heal. This "reactive stroma" comprises multiple cell types, which have been altered from their original state to become permissive of prostate cancer cell progression. In human prostate cancers, the "reactive stroma" displays increased number of myofibroblasts, amplification of ECM proteins, and increased local vascular density, properties almost identical to those seen in granulation tissue. Intriguingly, there is still no effective marker of "reactive stroma" available. The receptors activated by serine proteases (PARs) are good candidates as PARs play key roles in tissue remodeling and cancer invasion. Other key signaling mediators also involved in the "reactive stroma" phenoptype include tumor growth factor beta (TGFβ), partly responsible for fibroblast transdifferentiation. Other fibroblastic and smooth muscle markers participate in the transformation phenomena, such as vimentin and smooth muscle α-actin. However, TGFβ also affects the cancer cell itself, accomplishing contrary roles in the different stages of cancer evolution. Even in precancerous PIN lesions elevated TGFβ expression was detected in epithelial cells. In addition to TGFβ, chronic inflammation has also been the focus in the development of prostate cancer. Several characteristics of chronic inflammation are increased, such as the induction of the proinflammatory enzyme COX-2 and production of ROS and RNS. In turn, the infiltration of macrophages and leukocytes together with COX-2 activation, further enhances the burst of oxidative stress, promoting a more aggressive phenotype.

2.2.4. *Oxidative stress triggers metabolic reprogramming*

Mounting evidence recollected in the last paper of Hanahan and Weinberg [59] display compelling data on oxidative stress as a scaffold of the well-established hallmarks of cancer. Oxidative stress players are expressed abnormally in tumors, positively affecting compulsory stages of the carcinogenic process, by stimulating cell proliferation and anchorage independent cell growth, causing insensitivity to apoptosis, sustaining *de novo* angiogenesis, and by altering the migration/invasion program through metabolic and epigenetic mechanisms. ROS mediates ligand-independent transactivation of receptor tyrosine kinase and ERK activation affecting proliferation, promoting tissue invasion and metastatic dissemination due to MMP secretion/activation. Furthermore, ROS induce the release of VEGF and angiopoietin promoting angiogenesis and evading apoptosis/anoikis [60-62].

In cancer cells, high levels of ROS can result from increased basal metabolic activity, mitochondrial dysfunction due to hypoxia or mitophagy, peroxisome activity, uncontrolled growth factor of cytokines signaling and oncogene activity, as well as from enhanced activity of known ROS sources as NADPH oxidase, COX or lipoxygenases [62]. It is well accepted that the activity of oxidants on tumors depends on their mutagenic potential, their capacity to rule the intracellular signaling pathways governing cellular homeostasis and their recognized role in stromal reactivity, mandatory for cancer development and dissemination [63, 64].

Cell vulnerability appears as a consequence of the oxidative status of their constituents promoting spontaneous and therapy induced cell death. Thus, resistance to oxidative stress is positioned as a major mechanism of tumor chemo- and radio-defense.

The tumor hypoxic microenvironment as well induces this "reactive stroma", affecting the cancer cells motility, and consequently generating a more aggressive tumor, which can metastasize to the bone. Hypoxia generates ROS production and likewise anti-oxidants agents have shown to suppress hypoxia induced epithelial to mesenchymal transition (EMT), impairing the metastatic phenotype [65]. The "reactive stroma" recruitment to the cancer foci begins early during carcinogenesis and its co-evolution is predictive of human cancer progression, which is facilitated by tumor-stroma interactions.

It is of particular significance that many genes, which are regulated by oxidative stress, are targets of NF-κB [66]. NF-κB is constitutively activated in human prostate carcinoma and correlates with disease progression [67]. NF-κB is an inducible transcription factor that belongs to the Rel/NF-κB family. Increasing evidence suggests that inhibition of NF-κB activity in prostate cancer cells can suppress angiogenesis, invasion and metastasis by down-regulating the expression of NF-κB downstream target genes, such as VEGF, plasminogen activator type urokinase and MMP-9 [68]. Additionally, heme-oxygenase 1 (HO-1), the rate-limiting enzyme in heme degradation, confers cytoprotection against oxidative stress and inflammation [69]. This protein exerts vital metabolic functions limiting the axis of heme degradation and maintaining the cellular homeostasis. Several signaling molecules are implicated in the cytoprotection conferred by HO-1, including NF-κB and PI3K/Akt [70]. Although classical recognized as a microsomal protein, its presence has been detected in other subcellular compartments [71, 72]. Recent studies have reported that HO-1 suffers a proteolytic degradation in its hydrophobic C-terminal domain, which would facilitate its entrance to the nucleus [73]. It has been proposed that HO-1 possesses in the nucleus a non-catalytic canonical function participating in the regulation of the activity of several nuclear transcription factors and also regulating its own transcription [72,

73]. Moreover, it has been documented HO-1 nuclear expression in human primary prostate carcinomas [71]. It has also been reported that it impairs prostate tumor growth *in vivo* and down-regulates the expression of target genes associated with inflammation and angiogenesis [74, 75]. However, clinical data demonstrated a statistically significant difference in HO-1 epithelial expression between benign, high-grade PIN, localized prostate cancer, and advanced prostate cancer, where castration resistant disease presented the highest HO-1 expression followed by benign tissue. This work provides experimental evidence for a cross talk between epithelial HO-1 expression and PTEN deletions, which are associated with adverse clinical outcome [76].

Altogether these findings may indicate that the oxidative stress imbalance may strongly influence the prostate carcinogenic process and may also cooperate in the bone homing of prostate cancer, the most clinically significant aspect of this disease. The stromal–epithelial interaction gains therapeutic relevance, as prostate carcinoma cells must induce the hospitality of bone cells in order to take up residence in an osseous microenvironment.

2.3. MicroRNAs as emerging key players in the etiology and progression of prostate cancer – Clinical implications

MicroRNAs (miRNAs o miRs) are short non-coding RNAs (18-24 nucleotides) regarded as a novel class of regulatory molecules that suppress gene expression at the post-transcriptional level. miRNA genes are, in general, regulated and transcribed in the same manner as a protein-coding gene. They are transcribed by the RNA polymerase II into long primary transcripts (pri-miRNAs) that can contain the precursors of one to several clustered miRNAs. These primary transcripts are then cleaved by endonucleases (Drosha) to produce the pre-miRNAs which consist of ~70-nucleotide hairpin structures. The pre-miRNAs are further processed in the cytoplasm by the Dicer complex into the mature miRNAs which are incorporated into the RNA-induced silencing complex (RISC) that execute the regulatory activity through the binding to the 3′ untranslated region (3′UTR) of target mRNAs having complementary sequences. The formation of the mRNA/miRNA duplexes, lead to mRNA degradation, inhibition of translation, or a combination of both.

At present, there are more than 1,600 human miRNAs entries in the miRBase release 19 [77]. Each of these molecules may regulate the expression of hundreds of genes within one cell, and one particular target may be regulated by several miRNAs via different binding sites, creating an extremely complex regulatory network for gene expression. Indeed, it has been estimated that about 60% of the protein-coding genes are targets of miRNAs [78]. In recent years, rapidly growing evidence has established the significance of miRNAs in different physiological processes such as development and differentiation, cell cycle, metabolism, hemostasis and apoptosis [79].

On the contrary, an altered expression of these regulators play an important role in diseases, including carcinogenesis [80]. Quantitative alterations, either genetic or epigenetic, may modify the expression levels of miRNAs, and are associated with tumor development and progression in various tumors. More than half of the deregulated miRNAs map at, or near to, cancer-associated *loci* prone to deletions, amplifications and translocations [81]. Qualitative changes can also arise when there are mutations that disrupt or create miRNA recognition sites. Therefore, miRNAs may contribute to carcinogenesis acting as oncogenes, called oncomirs, if they promote tumor growth when they are over-expressed. They may also act as tumor suppressors when they stimulate cancer development and progression when they are down-regulated. As a general rule, oncomirs target tumor-suppressor gene mRNAs (e.g. miR-21 regulates PTEN), and tumor-suppressor miRNAs target proto-oncogene mRNAs (e.g. let-7 regulates KRAS).

miRNAs, as well as mRNAs, display tissue-specific expression profiles and, therefore, they may have different roles in cells from different origins. An example of this disparity is miR-125b which can have a tumor suppressor activity in ovarian and breast cancers but act as an oncomir in prostate cancer, thyroid cancer, neuroblastoma and glioblastoma [82]. The study of the global miRNA expression levels (miRNAome) has been rising in the past years and abundant miRNAome data are currently available for several cancers. The miRNA expression patterns in different types of tissues have been reported to be more predictive of tumor origin and differentiation status than mRNA profiles because, unlike mRNA expression, a modest number of miRNAs (~200 in total) might be sufficient to classify human cancers [83]. In prostate cancer, the expression of several miRNAs and their target mRNAs are altered and involved in development, invasion and metastasis. Nevertheless, the data on miRNA expression in prostatic tumors are still conflicting and, at present, a conclusive miRNA profile cannot be recognized. In this section we describe miRNAs that have been studied in the context of prostate cancer and summarize their possible application in disease diagnosis and prognosis.

2.3.1. miRNAs associated to prostate cancer

The expression of miR-21 is up-regulated in many types of cancers, including prostate cancer, glioblastoma, lymphoma, pancreatic cancer, and lung cancer, among others [84, 85]. miR-21 can act as an oncomir that contributes to prostate tumor growth, resistance to apoptosis, invasiveness and metastasis. Its regulatory activity probably involves the down-regulation of the tumor-suppressor gene PTEN (commonly lost or down-regulated) programmed cell death 4 (PDCD4), tropomyosin 1 alpha (TPM1), and myristoylated alanine-rich proteinase kinase C substrate (MARCKS), among other genes. miR-21 was found to be over-expressed in androgen-independent prostate cancer cell lines but its expression is low in androgen-dependent prostate cancer cells; therefore, it may be responsible, at least in part, for the development of castrate-resistant tumors. AR can bind to miR-21 promoter resulting in an androgen-dependent transcriptional regulation of miR-21; consequently androgen-dependent miR-21 expression may contribute to prostate cancer pathogenesis. In support of these findings, an *in vivo* study showed that miR-21 is over-expressed in human prostate tumor samples compared to the matching normal tissue, and tumor growth was accelerated in xenograph models when miR-21 expression was elevated [86].

miR-221 and miR-222 are two highly homologous oncomirs that are frequently over-expressed in different cancers. In primary prostate carcinomas and cell lines, these two miRNAs inversely correlate with the expression of the tumor suppressor gene p27, which is a well-established marker of poor prognosis in prostate cancer and other types of tumors [87]. *In vitro* and *in vivo* experiments link these two miRNAs to prostate cancer development and progression. Furthermore, miR-221 and miR-222 contribute to the growth and maintenance of castration-resistant prostate cancer (CRPC) through mechanisms that comprise the AR signaling.

Another oncomir, miR-125b, was reported to be over-expressed in androgen-independent prostate cancer lines and was also implicated in the hormone independent growth. The mRNA of the pro-apoptotic protein Bak1, which was found down-regulated in CRPC, is a target of miR-125b. However, this miRNA was also suggested to act as a tumor suppressor in a different context because it was found to be down-regulated in CRPC and in breast cancer where it silences the expression of HER-2/*neu* [88]. Interestingly, it was also reported that HER-2/*neu* is over-expressed in the progressing prostate tumors [89]. Therefore, the relevance of miR-125b in prostate cancer progression needs further investigation to assess its role in prostate carcinogenesis.

miR-101-1 and miR-101-2 map in two *locus* (1p31.3 and 9p24.2, respectively) that are commonly deleted in localized and metastatic prostate cancer. In addition, the loss of miR-101-1 or -2 is associated with the over-expression of EZH2, a histone methyltransferase enzyme that is a direct target of miR-101. The up-regulation of this miRNA reduced the proliferation and the invasive potential of the DU145 cell line. COX-2 is another target of miR-101, linking the miRNAs portray to chronic inflammation and tumor development via the COX-2/prostaglandins pathway [90]. *In vitro* studies have shown that there is an inverse correlation between miR-101 and COX-2 in different prostate-derived cell lines, and the over-expression of miR-101 reduces the proliferation rate of the COX-2-associated benign prostatic hyperplasia cell line [91]. Similarly, experimental models by inoculation of cells into BALB/c athymic nude mice demonstrated that the miR-101 over-expressing clone showed a slower tumor growth. Furthermore, the treatment of the tumorigenic BPH1 cell line (BPH^{CAFTD}) with exogenous miR-101 resulted in an inhibition of prostate cancer growth *in vitro* and *in vivo* [91]. Similarly, the over-expression of miR-128a reduced invasion capability of the androgen independent prostate tumor cell line, DU145, and was found to be progressively decreased in tissues from benign prostatic hyperplasia, to localized prostate cancer and to distant metastasis [92].

Another tumor suppressor miRNA that was reported to play a role in prostate cancer progression to CRPC is miR-146. This miRNA is down-regulated in androgen-independent cell lines and CRPC tissues compared to androgen-dependent cell lines and non-tumor epithelial tissues [93]. The mechanism of action of miR-146 consists of the inhibition of the expression of ROCK1 (Rho-activated protein kinase 1), which is a member of the hyaluronan/CD168 pathway involved in prostate cancer invasion and metastasis.

PKCε (protein kinase C epsilon) and ZEB2 (zinc finger E-box binding homeobox 2) are two proteins involve in the migration and invasion capabilities of prostate cancer cells and their expression is regulated, at least in part, by miR-205. This miRNA was reported to be down-regulated in prostate cancer cell lines and carcinomas compared to the non-tumorigenic cell line RWPE-1 and normal prostate tissues, respectively. miR-205 also induces genes involved in cell-cell junctions and down-regulates genes associated with prostate cancer progression such as IL6, caveolin-1, EZH2, ERBB3, E2F1 and E2F5.

This list is just a small part of all miRNA alterations found in prostate cancer (For a more complete list of miRNAs in prostate cancer, the reader may refer to the review written by Coppola *et al.*[85] and Pang *et al.*[94]), but other players cannot be discarded.

2.3.2. miRNAs as biomarkers for prostate cancer diagnosis and prognosis

Based on the evidence that miRNAs may be deregulated in different pathologies in a tissue-specific manner, multiple studies have investigated the potential use of the miRNAome as a biomarker. As a consequence, a growing amount of evidence proposes that the miRNAome can be used as a tool to better define pathological signatures and, in turn, to accurately differentiate tumors according to their origin and cellular linage. In addition, miRNAs meet other important requisites that may allow their use as biomarkers for cancer diagnosis and prognosis: 1) miRNAs are remarkably stable molecules in different types of clinical samples, including formalin-fixed paraffin-embedded (FFPE) tissues which is the standard technique used for long-term conservation of biological samples, 2) they can be analyzed by simple methods such as quantitative retro-transcriptase polymerase chain reaction (qRT-PCR), and 3) the lack of intricate transcriptional and translational regulation compared to mRNA.

The tumoral expression of miR-1 and miR-133a correlates with tumor progression. Interestingly, the relapse-free survival of patients with prostate cancer can be predicted by the expression of miR-1 in the tumor specimens. Patients with tumors having low miR-1 expression are more likely to have a biochemical relapse than patients with tumors having high miR-1 expression [95].

Besides their intracellular function, miRNAs can also be released by cells and circulate in the blood stream. Consequently, miRNAs can be isolated from serum and plasma; evenmore, they can be isolated from other body fluids such as urine, saliva and semen. The discovery of circulating miRNAs opened up intriguing possibilities to use the circulating miRNAome as one additional biomarker to improve cancer diagnosis, determine tumor staging more accurately and predict prognosis. Some reports demonstrate that miRNA levels in body fluids may change under certain pathological conditions, including prostate cancer [96]. For this reason, within the past years, studies on miRNAs in cancer have burst onto the scene, and evidence that miRNAs may represent new diagnostic and prognostic molecules in human cancers is rapidly accumulating. However miRNA levels as tools for diagnosis and prognosis in prostate cancer are still limited [96].

Although, serum and plasma levels of miR-141 seems to be one of the most promising markers for prostate cancer diagnosis because they are consistently increased in men diagnosed with this carcinoma compared to healthy individuals; the differences are statistical significant only when the comparisons are made between healthy persons and advanced prostate cancer patients [96]. miR-141 is also elevated in prostatic tumor specimens, suggesting that the raise of this molecule in the body fluids is originated by the tumor cells and increases as disease progresses. Serum levels of other miRNAs are also altered in specimens from men with prostate cancer when compared to healthy individuals (e.g. miR-21, miR-200, miR-221, miR-375, and others), but results are inconsistent among reports.

miR-141 was also studied as a predictor factor for prostate cancer classification. One study showed increased levels of serum miR-141 and miR-375 in high-risk patients (Gleason score ≥8 or N1) compared to low-risk patients (Gleason score 7 or N0) [97]. Another study found that serum miR-21 is increased in patients with CRPC resistant to docetaxel, opening the possibility to use serum miRNAs as markers of therapeutic response as well [98]. Unfortunately, the specificity and sensitivity of miRNAs when used as single markers for prostate cancer diagnosis and prognosis are similar to the specificity and sensitivity of other markers currently used (e.g. PSA).

In summary, miRNAome from serum or plasma samples may not add much information for prostate cancer diagnosis, outcome and response to therapy when used as a single biomarker. In addition, it is unlikely to achieve the desire level of accuracy for prostate cancer diagnosis or prognosis, because one miRNAs may be altered in many different diseases. Furthermore, one mRNA can be affected by several miRNAs. Therefore, circulating miRNAome should be considered an additional tool to improve the accuracy of current diagnostic molecules such as PSA, and other diagnostic tests such as the digital rectal exam, echography and others. Similarly, the tumor miRNAome may help to improve the pathological classification of prostate tumors. Up to date the miRNA profile cannot substitute other clinical tools, but can efficiently supplement them.

2.3.3. Targeting miRNAs as therapeutic strategies

The discovery of miRNAs a decade ago and the subsequent study of their role in the pathogenesis of disease, unveiled a new scenario where miRNA modulators could be used in order to restore the homeostasis of an altered cell or tissue. Recently, a novel class of synthetic inhibitory molecules (antagomirs) that compete with target mRNAs for the binding of miRNAs, allowing mRNA translation, has been introduced as silencers of oncomirs. The antagomirs uncover the way to miRNA-base therapeutic strategies. As the number of *in vivo* studies that analyze the use of miRNAs as therapeutic molecules is restricted to a very small number, further investigations are needed. In spite of all the data being generated, the knowledge and understanding of miRNA in prostate cancer is still at the early stage. Once the normal/pathological role of each alteration is deciphered, and the results validated in a vast cohort of patients, the selected miRNAs might be attractive candidates for prostate cancer diagnosis, patients' management and therapeutic strategy.

2.4. The nuts and volts of prostate cancer survival, mastering the tumoral vasculature: angiogenesis, vasculogenic mimicry or vessel co-option?

2.4.1. Angiogenesis as a hallmark of cancer

The hallmarks of cancer define distinctive and complementary capabilities that allow tumors to grow and disseminate. One of those capacities is the induction of angiogenesis. This process specifically refers to the sprouting of new blood vessels from pre-existing ones, involving proliferation of endothelial cells and migration towards pro-angiogenic molecules. The expansion of the existing vasculature also relies on the accumulation of circulating endothelial progenitor cells. The latter are immature endothelial cells, typically arising in the bone marrow, with the capacity to extravasate in response to pro-angiogenic factors and promote new vessel formation known as vasculogenesis. This process also takes place in the tumor microenvironment; however, it is generally associated with embryogenesis and development and involves the birth of new endothelial cells and their assembly into tubes in addition to the sprouting. Following this morphogenesis, the normal vasculature results in a quiescent action, becoming in the adult only an active process in wound healing events and in female reproductive cycling, but only transiently.

The tumor and its microenvironment display a completely different scenario, allowing pro-inflammatory molecules to switch on the angiogenic process enabling the tumor to grow, persist and disseminate. The tumor-associated angiogenesis was previously considered to be important in growing macroscopic tumors; however, the clinical evidence show that it directly contributes to the microscopic premalignant phase of neoplastic progression, further securing its position as an integral hallmark of cancer. This angiogenic switch is governed by angiogenic regulators that bind to stimulatory or inhibitory cell-surface receptors displayed by vascular endothelial cells. The well-known inducers of angiogenesis include among others: VEGF-A, TGFβ and IL8; while inhibitors include: thrombospondin-1 (TSP-1) and angiostatin, among others. In tumors, these molecules support the rapid division of tumor cells [59]. VEGF signaling occurs via three main subtypes of receptor tyrosine kinases known as VEGFR1, VEGFR2 and VEGFR3. Its expression can be upregulated both by hypoxia and by oncogene signaling [99, 100]. Additionally, VEGF ligands can be sequestered in the ECM in latent forms that can then be activated by ECM-degrading proteases such as MMP9. Also the fibroblast growth factor (FGF) family is capable of activating VEGF and has been implicated in sustaining tumor angiogenesis. TSP-1 emerges as a counterpart of the angiogenic process, that when activated suppresses proangiogenic stimuli [101]. Of note, *Ras* and *Myc*, dominant oncogenes can also upregulate angiogenic factors in the tumoral microenvironment, and these signals can also be produced indirectly by immune inflammatory cells.

It is of particular interest the fact that angiogenesis inhibitors, such as TSP-1, angiostatin and endostatin offer natural barriers to tumor angiogenesis. This was described by Ribatti *et al.* [102], followed by several studies reporting other endogenous inhibitory agents. Most of these molecules appear to derive from proteolytic cleavage of structural proteins that are not angiogenic regulators *per se*, and some can be detected in normal mice and human plasma. These agents serve under normal circumstances as physiologic rheostats modulating angiogenesis during tissue remodeling and wound healing but may also act as intrinsic barriers to the sustained angiogenesis in emerging neoplasias.

How do these counterpart molecules behave in the tumoral process? How can we decipher the cross talk of this aberrant mix of proangiogenic signals? A massive amount of information describes the features of a cancer cell. However, it is wise to acknowledge the differential concepts of causes, oncogenic events, signal transduction programs, and hallmarks to show that there is a complexity under this network of interrelations that dynamically changes in different cells, between cells, and most importantly at different times in any given cell. Cancer is an evolving, heterogeneous system, hence the intricacy of the forming vasculature supporting tumor growth and progression.

2.4.2. Intussusception and vessel co-option

While sprouting angiogenesis requires VEGF for endothelial cells to proliferate, migrate and maturate into new vessels, in the absence of this factor, the blood vessels split into new vessels without the need of endothelial cell proliferation. This phenomena is termed intussusception and has been demonstrated in various tumors [103]. Intussusception cannot be stopped by anti-VEGF strategies.

Intussusceptive microvascular growth refers to vessel network formation by insertion of connective tissue columns, called tissue pillars, into the vessel lumen and to the subsequent growth of these pillars, resulting in the sub-division of the vessel lumen. Intussusception is observed in a variety of normal and malignant tissues. It is faster and more inexpensive than sprouting, occurring within hours or even minutes and besides its autonomy from endothelial cell proliferation, it also becomes independent from basement membrane degradation, or even invasion of the connective tissue. However, intussusceptive microvascular growth displays a limiting factor: it can only work on existing vessel networks. Therefore intussusceptive microvascular growth has the ability to increase the complexity and density of the tumor microvessel mesh already built by sprouting. Although the molecular networks underlying this vascularization mechanism are poorly understood, the role of some local stimuli, such as intravascular shear stress, may induce a cascade of physiological or pathological reactions in endothelial cells, such as new capillary development by tissue pillar formation [104].

The absence of intense endothelial cell proliferation in intussusceptive microvascular growth implies that neovascularization by this mechanism would be resistant to angiosuppressive treatment in itself. Clinically, accumulation of tumor blood vessels by intussusceptive vessel growth is associated with a poor outcome for various types of cancers [105].

Until recently, vascularization of malignant tumors was considered the exclusive result of directed capillary ingrowth (endothelial sprouting). However, recent advances have been made in identifying the processes involved in angiogenesis and vascular remodeling. Consequently, the simplistic model of an invading capillary sprout has been deemed insufficient to describe the entire spectrum of morphogenic and molecular events required to form a neovascular network. Cancer tissue can acquire its vasculature by co-option of pre-existing vessels, intussusceptive microvascular growth, postnatal vasculogenesis, glomeruloid angiogenesis, or vasculogenic mimicry [103, 105].

Before discussing the different ways a tumor is vascularized, we should highlight that these mechanisms may not be mutually exclusive; the literature has shown that in most cases there is a cross-talk between these systems, participating in conjunction in physiological as well as in pathological angiogenesis. Although the various types of cancer vascularization may share similar molecular signaling cascades and may be controlled partly by almost identical regulatory factors, a significant variety of differences also prevail.

It is widely accepted that the primary tumors and metastases have an initial avascular growth stage and then the angiogenic switch is turned on to support the exponential tumor growth. Tumor-induced angiogenesis and tumor cell vessel interactions are one of the most important events during all the stages of tumor development. However, it is not fully understood what is exactly happening before or during the initiation of vascularization of the primary tumor and the micrometastasis. In the beginning malignant cells may associate with and grow preferentially along pre-existing microvessels, prior to building their own vasculature. This process is called vessel co-option and was first proposed by Holash *et al.* [106]. Although at first, it is limited to the early stages of human tumorigenesis, morphological evidence suggests that co-option of pre-existing blood vessels might persist during the entire period of primary or metastatic tumor growth. During solid tumor growth, no signs of directed vessel ingrowth can be appreciated; instead, these tumors decide to develop by co-opting the massive vascular plexus present in the peritumoral connective tissue. Several controversies have been raised regarding how tumors progress, whether microtumors may initiate growth by exploiting pre-existing vessels without inducing angiogenesis or initiating through the induction of angiogenic sprouts from host vessels [107]. These discrepancies may have aroused given the differences in vascular niches in applied experimental models. Although unresolved from a mechanistic point of view, this uncertainty may raise important challenges when outlining a rationale for therapeutic strategies. This implies that, whereas compounds may be efficient inhibitors of angiogenesis and tumor growth in angiogenesis-dependent tumors (such as subcutaneous tumor xenografts), their effects may be limited in tumors growing in tissues with an intrinsic vascular density that allows for co-option by infiltrative tumors or other forms of neo-vasculature.

Based on this knowledge, new ways to inhibit the various vascular modalities have been developed in the past decade. When applying these targeted therapies, there are several aspects to take into consideration: the stage of tumor progression, the type of vascularization of the cancerous tissue and the molecular signaling networks behind the vascularization process.

What are the key aspects in determining the vascularization patterns of tumors? First, the local microenvironment, important during tumor initiation. Second, the cell number, subsidizing microtumors ability of inducing angiogenesis. Moreover, to trigger exponential growth, tumors must depend on vascularization through angiogenesis, which is much more powerful than vessel co-option to increase the tumoral mass and to acquire nutrition and oxygen from the host circulation system. If possible, tumors will prefer this kind of vascularization pattern. Alternatively, another choice is the strategy of co-opting host vessels in order for tumor cells to survive when they cannot acquire enough support from its niche and have no capacity to establish intrinsic vessels through angiogenesis. This is consistent with the observations that anti-angiogenic therapies result in an increase of vascular co-option

http://dx.doi.org/10.5772/52636

[108]. Third, the co-option and migration along host vessels will be inhibited once angiogenic sprouts begin to be induced.

Of note in liver metastases of human colorectal carcinomas, different growth patterns can be observed, depending on the degree of differentiation. These liver metastases represent a truly heterogeneous group and their growth patterns (replacement, pushing and desmoplastic) predict the fraction of immature blood vessels, the fraction of proliferating endothelial cells and the fraction of apoptotic tumor cells. The replacement growth pattern expands mainly by co-opting the stroma with the sinusoidal blood vessels of the liver [109].

The use of anti-vascular endothelial growth factor antibodies have been used for the abrogation of angiogenesis and growth of human prostate carcinoma microtumors and even metastasis in orthotopic prostate cancer xenografts. Although up to date there are no reports suggesting that vessel co-option is also an alternative route for growth and dissemination of prostate tumors, the contribution of this vascular route to prostate tumorigenesis needs further exploration; specifically, the involvement of this survival tool for growth of microtumors [110, 111].

Many studies have reported the close association between host vessels and extravasated cells during the onset of metastases. The co-opting manner makes these tumoral cells cover vessel surface area as much as possible and obtain the necessary support from host, such as nutrients or oxygen, with remarkable vessel-like pseudopodia. As Weinberg articulated for this kind of behaviour "tumor cells require effective interactions with the vasculature in order to acquire nutrients and to shed metabolic waste products and carbon dioxide.... In some normal tissues with an especially high metabolic activity, most cells enjoy direct contact with at least one capillary. This intimate association means that their access to oxygen and critical nutrients not dependent on the diffusion of these molecules over large distances and through densely packed cell layers" [112].

The tumoral vascular picture clearly displays differential contributions of vessel co-option and angiogenesis at the earliest stage of tumor initiation and metastasis. While angiogenesis appears as a key player for tumor exponential growth, the strategy of co-opting host vessels seems indispensable for cancer cell survival. Future anti-vascular therapies should seriously take into consideration the alternative ways in which a tumor disseminate and evades conventional anti-angiogenic treatments.

2.4.3. *Vasculogenic mimicry*

How can we distinguish normal angiogenesis from tumor-associated angiogenesis? Tumor neovasculature is marked by precocious capillary sprouting, convoluted and excessive vessel branching, distorted and enlarged vessels, erratic blood flow, leakiness leading to blood lakes, and distorted levels of endothelial cell proliferation and apoptosis [59]. Also, certain types of cancer cells have the capacity to mimic the activities of endothelial cells and to participate in processes that involve the formation of a fluid-conducting, matrix-rich meshwork, metamorphosing into vessels that either carry blood or connect to the host's blood supply. This new mechanism, by which some aggressive tumors may acquire a blood supply, was first described by Maniotis and coworkers [113] and was termed 'vasculogenic mimicry'. However, it cannot be considered a vasculogenic event as true vasculogenesis involves de novo formation of endothelial cell-lined vessels. Since its discovery, vasculogenic mimicry has been catalogued in several types of tumors. How does vasculogenic mimicry contribute to tumor growth and progression, and can it be targeted by therapeutic agents?

Several interpretations of vasculogenic mimicry have evolved since tumor angiogenesis was recognized as not the only mechanism of blood supply for tumor microcirculation. Vasculogenic mimicry describes the ability of aggressive tumoral cells to express endothelium-associated genes and to form ECM-rich vasculogenic-like networks in three-dimensional (3D) cultures. These new vessels have no endothelial lining and are mainly composed of basement membrane-like material. The formation of these networks, seem to mimic the embryonic development of vasculogenic meshes and they were associated with the distinctly patterned ECM-rich networks that are observed in aggressive tumors. Since its discovery, vasculogenic mimicry has been described in several kinds of tumors, including melanoma, synovial sarcoma, rhabdomyosarcoma, osteosarcoma, breast carcinoma and ovarian carcinoma. Most of these studies correlate the aggressiveness of the tumor with angiogenesis or vasculogenic mimicry proliferation [114]. But how do they form and what is their contribution to tumorigenesis?

In the beginning, researchers observed in xenograft models and human biopsies, patterned loops and arcs that confined spheroidal clusters of tumoral cells. These loops and arcs formed networks that were lined with cancer cells and contained laminin and other components of the ECM yet not explored. Studies of tumor-tissue sections showed that the spheroidal tumor clusters contained either small, channel-like spaces between them, or seemed to be partially or totally juxtaposed by ECM. Some of these channel-like spaces were originally defined as 'vascular channels', because they were found to contain erythrocytes and plasma and were thought to provide a perfusion mechanism and a dissemination path within the tumor that might work independently or together with angiogenesis or vessel co-option.

Blood lakes within the tumor are another physiological phenomena that also draw attention. These are large collections of extravascular erythrocytes lining tumor spaces or channels. As hemorrhage is a manifestation of the defective endothelial barrier function in tumors the reason as why some tumors are bloodier than others, might rely on the balance between erythrocyte extravasation and the vessel wall stability. Rapid endothelial cell proliferation and defective pericyte coverage might contribute to the instability of tumor vessel walls leading to this hemorrhage. Pericytes are supporting cells that are closely apposed to the outer surfaces of the endothelial tubes in normal tissue vasculature, providing mechanical and physiologic support to the endothelial cells and have been associated with the maintenance of a functional neo-vasculature of most if not all tumors [115].

The literature on vasculogenic mimicry in prostate cancer is scarce, although therapeutic implications of it have been described in aggressive prostate cancer *in vitro* [116]. The prognostic value of vasculogenic mimicry remains debatable as there is at least one study showing that there is no significant correlation between vasculogenic mimicry channels and histological grading of prostate cancer [117].

http://dx.doi.org/10.5772/52636

Interestingly, Liu *et al.* [114] looked at this correlation in human tissue samples to determine clinical pathology, prognosis and a possible molecular mechanism. They statistically correlated histological with clinicopathological data from prostate carcinoma cases confirming that vasculogenic mimicry was more often seen in those patients with seminal vesicle invasion, lymph node metastasis, distant metastasis tissues or shorter PSA doubling time (PSADT), all important clinical prognostic factors of prostate cancer. They concluded that vasculogenic mimicry mainly exists in the high-risk prostate cancer patients and is a new independent marker of poor prognosis of the disease. Though more studies with larger sample sizes are needed to further confirm the correlation of vasculogenic mimicry and prostate cancer prognosis, these results might explain why some anti-angiogenesis treatments remain clinically less effective.

2.4.4. Molecular signaling

The identification of molecules that are uniquely expressed on the surface of endothelial cells of tumor vessels has been a holy grail of vascular biology. Such molecules could serve as therapeutical targets. Although there is no molecule truly associated to tumor vessels, several show higher expression in tumors. Among those relevant in prostate cancer we find: endoglin (CD105), VEGF/VEGFR-2 complexes, thrombospondin-1 receptor (CD36), Thy-1 cell surface antigen (Thy-1), phosphatidylserine, prostate-specific membrane antigen (PSMA), MMP, Her2/Neu and multiple tumor endothelial markers. The absence of absolute specificity of these molecules for tumor vessels drives the search for better targets [118]. Of note, Her2/Neu plays an important role in the spreading of prostate carcinomas to the bone and its high expression is associated with a poorer prognosis in patients with bone metastases. The Her2/Neu receptor is part of a molecular signaling cascade that involves Akt and MMP-9 activation, enabling the cancer cell to penetrate the matrix and facilitating angiogenesis.

It is wise to recognize the lead role of MMP in facilitating the invasiveness of prostate cancer. These molecules are important in the degradation of the ECM, allowing tumoral cells to metastasize to distant sites throughout the body. This protease activity, not only allows for cell migration, but also facilitate angiogenesis, providing the tumor with nutrition and further proliferation [119]. Of note, MMP-2 plays an important role in the preliminary stages of the vasculogenic mimicry genesis, degrading collagen IV. Reports showed that human prostate carcinoma samples positive for vasculogenic mimicry had a significantly higher MMP-2 expression levels compared to vasculogenic mimicry-negative patients. Metastat, an inhibitor of MMP, decreased the formation of vasculogenic mimicry networks in aggressive prostate tumors. However, further studies are needed to elucidate the mechanism of formation of vasculogenic mimicry in detail [114].

In bone metastases, the prostate metastatic tissue might allow for angiogenesis via the MMP9 derived from osteoclasts. Interesting, some MMP have a higher expression with higher Gleason's scores. This fact has led to the revamping of the MMP as possible prognostic factors and even more, as valid candidates for therapy. However, the MMP field is at a crossroad; in the last few years, accumulating evidence from experimental models of cancer, knockout mice and proteomics studies has challenged our views on how MMP function in the tumoral process. This challenge has been compounded by the fact that the clinical trials with MMP inhibitors failed to show therapeutic efficacy in cancer patients. MMPs have a vast repertoire of substrates not limited to the ECM components, and multiple proteins can be potentially targeted by MMPs and may be important for the anti-tumor activity of the host. This may partly explain why broad-spectrum synthetic MMP inhibitors failed to show clinical efficacy.

The MMP picture is not simple and reveals a complex contribution to cancer progression, putting aside the long-held view of MMP as a family that promotes cancer metastasis. Today, the evidence shows that members of the MMP family may promote or inhibit cancer development. Moreover, an individual MMP may act positively or negatively on tumor progression depending on other factors, on the tumor stage, tumor site (primary, metastasis), enzyme localization (tumor vs. stromal) and substrate profile [120]. In the *–omics era*, the identification of the substrates targeted by MMP in biological samples, known as degradomics, promises to become an important tool for defining the role of MMP in cancer. Establishing correlations, particularly in advanced prostate carcinomas, may assist in better patient stratification.

2.4.5. Cell plasticity and cancer stem cells

In fact, more questions than answers have been raised about the relevance of the *in vivo* studies on tumor vasculature. Is there a morphological and functional connection between prostate tumor-cell-lined networks and endothelium-lined vasculature? Is it possible for aggressive prostate cancer cells to form functional vessels when placed in an ischaemic, non-tumor microenvironment? What is the potential relevance of a 'plastic' tumor-cell phenotype, and how can we identify and target tumor cells that can masquerade as other cell types? Many of the biological properties that are relevant to embryogenesis are also important for tumor growth. For example, during embryonic development, the formation of primary vascular networks occurs by the process of vasculogenesis (the differentiation of mesodermal progenitor cells (angioblasts and hemangioblasts) to endothelial cells) and their organization into a primitive network [121]. The remodeling of the vasculogenic network into a more refined microvasculature occurs through angiogenesis in the same way as tumors require a blood supply for growth and also use the blood supply for metastatic dissemination [122].

Cells capable of vasculogenic mimicry display a high degree of plasticity, causing them to resemble dedifferentiated cell types. A stem cell is considered the most dedifferentiated cell, holding the capacity to generate various novel cell types. However, a new concept comes into the picture, the cancer stem cells (CSCs). These cells hold the capacity to self-renew, differentiate and proliferate indefinitely, being the latter a key event in tumor growth. Tumoral vasculogenic mimicry is characterized by an undifferentiated molecular signature together with embryonic-like differentiation plasticity implying a link between cancer stem cells and aggressive tumor cells capable of vasculogenic mimicry. Moreover, these two cell types share the potentiality of unlimited proliferation capacity, cellular plasticity and the expression of a gene signature responsible of maintaining pluripotency.

Among the signaling molecules known to influence stem cell renewal and differentiation in aggressive forms of prostate cancer, we find: Wnt, Src, BMP (bone morphogenic proteins) and TGFβ [5]. Other transcription factors are also involved in bone metastasis. HIF1α in tumor cells, inhibits osteoblasts differentiation, induces osteoclasts differentiation and promotes tumor growth. Hypoxia and TGFβ signaling in parallel drive the development of tumor bone metastases and regulate a common set of tumor genes stimulating the production of VEGF and CXCR4 in both tumor cells and bone microenvironment to enhance angiogenesis and tumor homing. VEGF, a target gene of Runx2, facilitates tumor growth and both the osteolytic and the osteoblastic disease [123, 124]. Additionally, prostate cancer cell lines express mediators of tumor growth and bone destruction, among them IL8, IL6 and PTHrP. Runx2 is also a key regulator of metastasis related genes and its presence in the primary tumor could be critical for the diagnosis of prostate cancer bone metastasis [125].

The Notch signaling pathway is now recognized as an important player in tumor angiogenesis. Two key Notch ligands have been implicated in this process, Delta-like 4 (Dll4) and Jagged1. Notch appears to be very attractive because specifically, bone metastases from prostate cancer patients expressed Notch-1 protein in the osteoblastic lesions. Correspondingly, Notch ligand Jagged-1 was found to be highly-expressed in metastatic prostate cancer compared to localized disease or benign prostate tissues, and high Jagged-1 expression in a subset of clinically localized tumors was found to be significantly associated with tumor recurrence [5]. Although the molecular mechanism of Notch signaling is not completely understood, silencing of Notch-1 inhibits MMP9, uPA and VEGF expression, given support to the effect of Notch in invasion [126, 127]. Moreover, Wang et al [126] recently proposed a down-regulated signaling cascade downstream of Notch-1, with reduced Akt and mTOR phosphorylation and inactivated NF-κB signaling. The interplay between these pathways provides a balance between self-renewal and differentiation. Dll4 expression activates Notch resulting in restriction of new sprout development. In agreement with this activity, inhibition of Dll4-mediated Notch signaling in tumors results in hyper sprouting of nonfunctional vasculature [128]. This Dll4 inhibition may paradoxically lead to increased angiogenesis but poor tumor growth because the newly growing vessels are not functional. In contrast, Jagged1 has been described as a Notch ligand expressed in tumor cells that may influence tumor angiogenesis by activating Notch on tumor endothelium. Of note, Notch activation is also critical for the maintenance of stem cell self-renewal potency in several stem cell microenvironments. These results indicate that Notch signaling can have diverse signaling outcomes dependent on the cellular niche, as it is able to induce (endothelial) differentiation in some cases, while promoting self-renewal potency in others [128].

TGFβ signaling also draws our attention given that it is a key molecule in the maintenance of an undifferentiated state in human embryonic stem cells. Various components of the TGFβ signaling cascade are highly expressed in stem cells, including Nodal and its regulators Cripto and LEFTY1/2 [101,102]. However little is known about signaling cascades governing the pluripotent state [129]. Taken together multiple stimuli provided by prostate tumors and their effective microenvironment can trigger differential signaling cascades that in turn will define the fate of the host. Thus a variety of therapeutic venues may have to co-exist in order to be translated into clinical utility.

2.4.6. Clinical significance

Undoubtfully, there are more questions than answers at this time regarding the functional significance of vasculogenic networks and vascular marker expression by prostate cancer cells. If tumor vasculogenesis can be demonstrated in experimental models, does it occur concomitantly with angiogenesis or as a remodeling of angiogenesis in aggressive tumors? Is vessel co-option involved? Is tumor cell vasculogenesis an alternative angiogenic switch in aggressive tumors? Regardless of the terms employed to describe the expression and mimicry of vascular-like gene by aggressive prostate cancer tumor cells, this area of research is worthy of analysis. It is wise to consider that in addition to the current anti-vascular treatments, the novel therapeutic approaches against tumor vasculature must be harmonized with the stage of tumor progression and with the molecular mechanism responsible for the angiogenic phenotype.

In our perspective the challenge relies in combining the anti-vascular strategies with the existing therapeutic regimes. The rational application of antivascular agents must be tagged along with the notion that these therapies must be individually tailored for the different types of cancer cells. The clinical management of prostate cancer would benefit greatly from the better understanding of the diverse vascularization mechanisms helping to fine-tune these novel anti-cancer strategies.

3. Conclusions

It is clear that multiple host and environmental factors contribute to prostate cancer and that inflammation sets the scene for the appearance of a reactive stroma, providing growth factors, chemokines and proteins that stimulate among other things, invasion. In return, this cancer finds a fertile soil to proliferate and disseminate in the bone, which acts as a specialized niche for prostate cancer cells. Moreover, the vascular compartment contributes significantly to prostate cancer growth through provision of oxygen and nutrients. Prostate cancer cells break into the scene co-opting blood vessels, by intussusception or even enhancing angiogenesis, attracting endothelial cells, promoting their growth in the tumor microenvironment and even transdifferentiating through the EMT. The intricacy relies on deciphering the diabolic liaison of all these factors and physiological processes. How can successful therapeutic strategies be designed if there are still so many hidden molecular variables waiting to be unveiled? The path in building promising clinical action plans will depend on unraveling the rheostat molecules that control the metabolic reprogramming of tumoral cells and the tumor microenvironment. Who are the key players controlling all the biochemical reactions producing ROS and RNS within cancer cells? Even more who are their exact targets? Several microRNA signatures are identified and described in the inflammatory milieu associated to

http://dx.doi.org/10.5772/52636

prostate cancer, hence are miRNA-base therapeutic strategies a promising option for the disease? The possibility to target cancer cell malignancy by intervention on both its metabolic reprogramming and its interplay with environmental factors is in truth captivating. The key molecules and pathophysiological process outlined throughout this chapter drive home the concept that the tumor microenvironment enhanced by an inflammatory wand offers interesting homoestatic targets for prostate cancer therapy. In this synopsis, blocking the sustained inflammatory network will offer new promising avenues to achieve significant therapeutic gains in the treatment of prostate cancer.

Abbreviations

AR→androgen receptor

COX-2→cyclooxygenase-2

CXCR4→C-X-C chemokine receptor type 4,bonzo, STRL33 or TYMSTR

CXCR7→C-X-C chemokine receptortype 7, RDC1

ECM→extracellular matrix

ELR→glutamic acid-leucine-arginine motif

EMT→epithelial mesenchymal transition

HIF-1α →hypoxia-inducible factor 1 alpha

HO-1→heme-oxygenase 1

IFNs→interferons

IGF-IR→insulin-like type I growth factor receptor

IL6→interleukin 6

IL8→interleukin 8

miRNAs or miRs→microRNAs

MMP →matrixmetalloproteinase

MnSOD→manganesesuperoxidedismutase

NF-κB→nuclear factor κB

Nrf2→nuclear factor (erythroid-derived 2)-like 2

RNS →reactive nitrogen species

PARs→serine proteases

PI3K →phosphatidylinositol-3 kinase

PIN→prostaticintraepithelial neoplasia→

Prx→peroxiredoxin

PSA →prostate specific antigen

PTEN→phosphatase and tensin homolog

RECIST →Response Evaluation Criteria in Solid Tumors

RNS →reactive nitrogen species

ROS →reactive oxygen species

SDF-1 →stromal derived factor 1

STAT3→signal transducers and activators of transcription-3

TGFβ→transforming growth factor beta

TMPRSS2-ERG →transmembrane protease, serine 2 – ets related gene

TNFα→tumor necrosis factor alpha

TRAIL →tumor necrosis factor-related apoptosis-inducing ligand

VEGF →vascular endothelial growth factor

Acknowledgements

This work was supported by grants from the University of Buenos Aires, Argentina, UBA-CyT (20020100100179) and ANPCYT (PICT RAICES 2010-0431).

Author details

Geraldine Gueron, Javier Cotignola and Elba Vazquez*

*Address all correspondence to: elba@qb.fcen.uba.ar

IQUIBICEN-CONICET, Department of Biological Chemistry, School of Sciences, University of Buenos Aires, Ciudad Universitaria, Buenos Aires, Argentina

References

[1] Mantovani A. Cancer: Inflaming metastasis. Nature, 2009. 457(7225): 36-37.

[2] Vandercappellen J., Van Damme J., and Struyf S. The role of CXC chemokines and their receptors in cancer. Cancer Lett, 2008. 267(2): 226-244.

[3] Thobe M.N., Clark R.J., Bainer R.O., Prasad S.M., and Rinker-Schaeffer C.W. From Prostate to Bone: Key Players in Prostate Cancer Bone Metastasis. Cancers (Basel), 2011. 3(1): 478-493.

[4] Petit I., Jin D., and Rafii S. The SDF-1-CXCR4 signaling pathway: a molecular hub modulating neo-angiogenesis. Trends Immunol, 2007. 28(7): 299-307.

[5] Gueron G., De Siervi A., and Vazquez E. Advanced prostate cancer: reinforcing the strings between inflammation and the metastatic behavior. Prostate Cancer Prostatic Dis, 2011.

[6] Gueron G., De Siervi A., and Vazquez E. Key questions in metastasis: new insights in molecular pathways and therapeutic implications. Curr Pharm Biotechnol, 2011. 12(11): 1867-1880.

[7] Hardy C.L. The homing of hematopoietic stem cells to the bone marrow. Am J Med Sci, 1995. 309(5): 260-266.

[8] Aiuti A., Tavian M., Cipponi A., Ficara F., Zappone E., Hoxie J., Peault B., and Bordignon C. Expression of CXCR4, the receptor for stromal cell-derived factor-1 on fetal and adult human lympho-hematopoietic progenitors. Eur J Immunol, 1999. 29(6): 1823-1831.

[9] Mochizuki H., Matsubara A., Teishima J., Mutaguchi K., Yasumoto H., Dahiya R., Usui T., and Kamiya K. Interaction of ligand-receptor system between stromal-cell-derived factor-1 and CXC chemokine receptor 4 in human prostate cancer: a possible predictor of metastasis. Biochem Biophys Res Commun, 2004. 320(3): 656-663.

[10] Darash-Yahana M., Gillespie J.W., Hewitt S.M., Chen Y.Y., Maeda S., Stein I., Singh S.P., Bedolla R.B., Peled A., Troyer D.A., Pikarsky E., Karin M., and Farber J.M. The chemokine CXCL16 and its receptor, CXCR6, as markers and promoters of inflammation-associated cancers. PLoS One, 2009. 4(8): e6695.

[11] Xing Y., Liu M., Du Y., Qu F., Li Y., Zhang Q., Xiao Y., Zhao J., Zeng F., and Xiao C. Tumor cell-specific blockade of CXCR4/SDF-1 interactions in prostate cancer cells by hTERT promoter induced CXCR4 knockdown: A possible metastasis preventing and minimizing approach. Cancer Biol Ther, 2008. 7(11): 1839-1848.

[12] Frigo D.E., Sherk A.B., Wittmann B.M., Norris J.D., Wang Q., Joseph J.D., Toner A.P., Brown M., and McDonnell D.P. Induction of Kruppel-like factor 5 expression by androgens results in increased CXCR4-dependent migration of prostate cancer cells in vitro. Mol Endocrinol, 2009. 23(9): 1385-1396.

[13] Cai J., Kandagatla P., Singareddy R., Kropinski A., Sheng S., Cher M.L., and Chinni S.R. Androgens Induce Functional CXCR4 through ERG Factor Expression in TMPRSS2-ERG Fusion-Positive Prostate Cancer Cells. Transl Oncol, 2010. 3(3): 195-203.

[14] Akashi T., Koizumi K., Tsuneyama K., Saiki I., Takano Y., and Fuse H. Chemokine receptor CXCR4 expression and prognosis in patients with metastatic prostate cancer. Cancer Sci, 2008. 99(3): 539-542.

[15] Singh R.K. and Lokeshwar B.L. The IL-8-regulated chemokine receptor CXCR7 stimulates EGFR signaling to promote prostate cancer growth. Cancer Res, 2011. 71(9): 3268-3277.

[16] Raggo C., Ruhl R., McAllister S., Koon H., Dezube B.J., Fruh K., and Moses A.V. Novel cellular genes essential for transformation of endothelial cells by Kaposi's sarcoma-associated herpesvirus. Cancer Res, 2005. 65(12): 5084-5095.

[17] Miao Z., Luker K.E., Summers B.C., Berahovich R., Bhojani M.S., Rehemtulla A., Kleer C.G., Essner J.J., Nasevicius A., Luker G.D., Howard M.C., and Schall T.J. CXCR7 (RDC1) promotes breast and lung tumor growth in vivo and is expressed on tumor-associated vasculature. Proc Natl Acad Sci U S A, 2007. 104(40): 15735-15740.

[18] Wang J., Lu Y., Koch A.E., Zhang J., and Taichman R.S. CXCR6 induces prostate cancer progression by the AKT/mammalian target of rapamycin signaling pathway. Cancer Res, 2008. 68(24): 10367-10376.

[19] Ha H.K., Lee W., Park H.J., Lee S.D., Lee J.Z., and Chung M.K. Clinical significance of CXCL16/CXCR6 expression in patients with prostate cancer. Mol Med Report, 2011. 4(3): 419-424.

[20] Unutmaz D., Xiang W., Sunshine M.J., Campbell J., Butcher E., and Littman D.R. The primate lentiviral receptor Bonzo/STRL33 is coordinately regulated with CCR5 and its expression pattern is conserved between human and mouse. J Immunol, 2000. 165(6): 3284-3292.

[21] Chandrasekar B., Bysani S., and Mummidi S. CXCL16 signals via Gi, phosphatidylinositol 3-kinase, Akt, I kappa B kinase, and nuclear factor-kappa B and induces cell-cell adhesion and aortic smooth muscle cell proliferation. J Biol Chem, 2004. 279(5): 3188-3196.

[22] Deng L., Chen N., Li Y., Zheng H., and Lei Q. CXCR6/CXCL16 functions as a regulator in metastasis and progression of cancer. Biochim Biophys Acta, 2010. 1806(1): 42-49.

[23] Nakayama T., Hieshima K., Izawa D., Tatsumi Y., Kanamaru A., and Yoshie O. Cutting edge: profile of chemokine receptor expression on human plasma cells accounts for their efficient recruitment to target tissues. J Immunol, 2003. 170(3): 1136-1140.

[24] Shimaoka T., Nakayama T., Fukumoto N., Kume N., Takahashi S., Yamaguchi J., Minami M., Hayashida K., Kita T., Ohsumi J., Yoshie O., and Yonehara S. Cell surface-anchored SR-PSOX/CXC chemokine ligand 16 mediates firm adhesion of CXC chemokine receptor 6-expressing cells. J Leukoc Biol, 2004. 75(2): 267-274.

[25] Seaton A., Scullin P., Maxwell P.J., Wilson C., Pettigrew J., Gallagher R., O'Sullivan J.M., Johnston P.G., and Waugh D.J. Interleukin-8 signaling promotes androgen-in-

dependent proliferation of prostate cancer cells via induction of androgen receptor expression and activation. Carcinogenesis, 2008. 29(6): 1148-1156.

[26] Inoue K., Slaton J.W., Eve B.Y., Kim S.J., Perrotte P., Balbay M.D., Yano S., Bar-Eli M., Radinsky R., Pettaway C.A., and Dinney C.P. Interleukin 8 expression regulates tumorigenicity and metastases in androgen-independent prostate cancer. Clin Cancer Res, 2000. 6(5): 2104-2119.

[27] Kim S.J., Uehara H., Karashima T., McCarty M., Shih N., and Fidler I.J. Expression of interleukin-8 correlates with angiogenesis, tumorigenicity, and metastasis of human prostate cancer cells implanted orthotopically in nude mice. Neoplasia, 2001. 3(1): 33-42.

[28] Lamont K.R. and Tindall D.J. Minireview: alternative activation pathways for the androgen receptor in prostate cancer. Mol Endocrinol, 2011. 25(6): 897-907.

[29] Mijatovic T., Mahieu T., Bruyere C., De Neve N., Dewelle J., Simon G., Dehoux M.J., van der Aar E., Haibe-Kains B., Bontempi G., Decaestecker C., Van Quaquebeke E., Darro F., and Kiss R. UNBS5162, a novel naphthalimide that decreases CXCL chemokine expression in experimental prostate cancers. Neoplasia, 2008. 10(6): 573-586.

[30] George D.J., Halabi S., Shepard T.F., Sanford B., Vogelzang N.J., Small E.J., and Kantoff P.W. The prognostic significance of plasma interleukin-6 levels in patients with metastatic hormone-refractory prostate cancer: results from cancer and leukemia group B 9480. Clin Cancer Res, 2005. 11(5): 1815-1820.

[31] Alcover J., Filella X., Luque P., Molina R., Izquierdo L., Auge J.M., and Alcaraz A. Prognostic value of IL-6 in localized prostatic cancer. Anticancer Res, 2010. 30(10): 4369-4372.

[32] Fizazi K., De Bono J.S., Flechon A., Heidenreich A., Voog E., Davis N.B., Qi M., Bandekar R., Vermeulen J.T., Cornfeld M., and Hudes G.R. Randomised phase II study of siltuximab (CNTO 328), an anti-IL-6 monoclonal antibody, in combination with mitoxantrone/prednisone versus mitoxantrone/prednisone alone in metastatic castration-resistant prostate cancer. Eur J Cancer, 2012. 48(1): 85-93.

[33] Sottnik J.L., Zhang J., Macoska J.A., and Keller E.T. The PCa Tumor Microenvironment. Cancer Microenviron, 2011. 4(3): 283-297.

[34] Rojas A., Liu G., Coleman I., Nelson P.S., Zhang M., Dash R., Fisher P.B., Plymate S.R., and Wu J.D. IL-6 promotes prostate tumorigenesis and progression through autocrine cross-activation of IGF-IR. Oncogene, 2011. 30(20): 2345-2355.

[35] Blaszczyk N., Masri B.A., Mawji N.R., Ueda T., McAlinden G., Duncan C.P., Bruchovsky N., Schweikert H.U., Schnabel D., Jones E.C., and Sadar M.D. Osteoblast-derived factors induce androgen-independent proliferation and expression of prostate-specific antigen in human prostate cancer cells. Clin Cancer Res, 2004. 10(5): 1860-1869.

[36] Culig Z., Steiner H., Bartsch G., and Hobisch A. Interleukin-6 regulation of prostate cancer cell growth. J Cell Biochem, 2005. 95(3): 497-505.

[37] Carswell E.A., Old L.J., Kassel R.L., Green S., Fiore N., and Williamson B. An endotoxin-induced serum factor that causes necrosis of tumors. Proc Natl Acad Sci U S A, 1975. 72(9): 3666-3670.

[38] Pennica D., Nedwin G.E., Hayflick J.S., Seeburg P.H., Derynck R., Palladino M.A., Kohr W.J., Aggarwal B.B., and Goeddel D.V. Human tumour necrosis factor: precursor structure, expression and homology to lymphotoxin. Nature, 1984. 312(5996): 724-729.

[39] Vandenabeele P., Declercq W., Van Herreweghe F., and Vanden Berghe T. The role of the kinases RIP1 and RIP3 in TNF-induced necrosis. Sci Signal, 2010. 3(115): re4.

[40] Chen G. and Goeddel D.V. TNF-R1 signaling: a beautiful pathway. Science, 2002. 296(5573): 1634-1635.

[41] Hsu H., Xiong J., and Goeddel D.V. The TNF receptor 1-associated protein TRADD signals cell death and NF-kappa B activation. Cell, 1995. 81(4): 495-504.

[42] Malik S.T. Tumour necrosis factor: roles in cancer pathophysiology. Semin Cancer Biol, 1992. 3(1): 27-33.

[43] Wu Y. and Zhou B.P. TNF-alpha/NF-kappaB/Snail pathway in cancer cell migration and invasion. Br J Cancer, 2010. 102(4): 639-644.

[44] Davis J.S., Nastiuk K.L., and Krolewski J.J. TNF is necessary for castration-induced prostate regression, whereas TRAIL and FasL are dispensable. Mol Endocrinol. 25(4): 611-620.

[45] Josson S., Matsuoka Y., Chung L.W., Zhau H.E., and Wang R. Tumor-stroma co-evolution in prostate cancer progression and metastasis. Semin Cell Dev Biol, 2010. 21(1): 26-32.

[46] De Marzo A.M., Platz E.A., Sutcliffe S., Xu J., Gronberg H., Drake C.G., Nakai Y., Isaacs W.B., and Nelson W.G. Inflammation in prostate carcinogenesis. Nat Rev Cancer, 2007. 7(4): 256-269.

[47] Debes J.D. and Tindall D.J. Mechanisms of androgen-refractory prostate cancer. N Engl J Med, 2004. 351(15): 1488-1490.

[48] Sun S., Sprenger C.C., Vessella R.L., Haugk K., Soriano K., Mostaghel E.A., Page S.T., Coleman I.M., Nguyen H.M., Sun H., Nelson P.S., and Plymate S.R. Castration resistance in human prostate cancer is conferred by a frequently occurring androgen receptor splice variant. J Clin Invest, 2010. 120(8): 2715-2730.

[49] Shiota M., Yokomizo A., and Naito S. Oxidative stress and androgen receptor signaling in the development and progression of castration-resistant prostate cancer. Free Radic Biol Med, 2011. 51(7): 1320-1328.

[50] Shiota M., Yokomizo A., Tada Y., Inokuchi J., Kashiwagi E., Masubuchi D., Eto M., Uchiumi T., and Naito S. Castration resistance of prostate cancer cells caused by castration-induced oxidative stress through Twist1 and androgen receptor overexpression. Oncogene, 2010. 29(2): 237-250.

[51] Yang J., Mani S.A., Donaher J.L., Ramaswamy S., Itzykson R.A., Come C., Savagner P., Gitelman I., Richardson A., and Weinberg R.A. Twist, a master regulator of morphogenesis, plays an essential role in tumor metastasis. Cell, 2004. 117(7): 927-939.

[52] Bostwick D.G., Alexander E.E., Singh R., Shan A., Qian J., Santella R.M., Oberley L.W., Yan T., Zhong W., Jiang X., and Oberley T.D. Antioxidant enzyme expression and reactive oxygen species damage in prostatic intraepithelial neoplasia and cancer. Cancer, 2000. 89(1): 123-134.

[53] Sharifi N., Hurt E.M., Thomas S.B., and Farrar W.L. Effects of manganese superoxide dismutase silencing on androgen receptor function and gene regulation: implications for castration-resistant prostate cancer. Clin Cancer Res, 2008. 14(19): 6073-6080.

[54] Pang S.T., Dillner K., Wu X., Pousette A., Norstedt G., and Flores-Morales A. Gene expression profiling of androgen deficiency predicts a pathway of prostate apoptosis that involves genes related to oxidative stress. Endocrinology, 2002. 143(12): 4897-4906.

[55] Shiota M., Yokomizo A., Kashiwagi E., Takeuchi A., Fujimoto N., Uchiumi T., and Naito S. Peroxiredoxin 2 in the nucleus and cytoplasm distinctly regulates androgen receptor activity in prostate cancer cells. Free Radic Biol Med, 2011. 51(1): 78-87.

[56] Paget S. The distribution of secondary growths in cancer of the breast. 1889. Cancer Metastasis Rev, 1989. 8(2): 98-101.

[57] Tuxhorn J.A., Ayala G.E., and Rowley D.R. Reactive stroma in prostate cancer progression. J Urol, 2001. 166(6): 2472-2483.

[58] Zhang X., Wang W., True L.D., Vessella R.L., and Takayama T.K. Protease-activated receptor-1 is upregulated in reactive stroma of primary prostate cancer and bone metastasis. Prostate, 2009. 69(7): 727-736.

[59] Hanahan D. and Weinberg R.A. Hallmarks of cancer: the next generation. Cell, 2011. 144(5): 646-674.

[60] Harfouche R., Malak N.A., Brandes R.P., Karsan A., Irani K., and Hussain S.N. Roles of reactive oxygen species in angiopoietin-1/tie-2 receptor signaling. FASEB J, 2005. 19(12): 1728-1730.

[61] Lander H.M., Milbank A.J., Tauras J.M., Hajjar D.P., Hempstead B.L., Schwartz G.D., Kraemer R.T., Mirza U.A., Chait B.T., Burk S.C., and Quilliam L.A. Redox regulation of cell signalling. Nature, 1996. 381(6581): 380-381.

[62] Chiarugi P. and Fiaschi T. Redox signalling in anchorage-dependent cell growth. Cell Signal, 2007. 19(4): 672-682.

[63] Visconti R. and Grieco D. New insights on oxidative stress in cancer. Curr Opin Drug Discov Devel, 2009. 12(2): 240-245.

[64] Toullec A., Gerald D., Despouy G., Bourachot B., Cardon M., Lefort S., Richardson M., Rigaill G., Parrini M.C., Lucchesi C., Bellanger D., Stern M.H., Dubois T., Sastre-Garau X., Delattre O., Vincent-Salomon A., and Mechta-Grigoriou F. Oxidative stress promotes myofibroblast differentiation and tumour spreading. EMBO Mol Med, 2010. 2(6): 211-230.

[65] Shimojo Y., Akimoto M., Hisanaga T., Tanaka T., Tajima Y., Honma Y., and Takenaga K. Attenuation of reactive oxygen species by antioxidants suppresses hypoxia-induced epithelial-mesenchymal transition and metastasis of pancreatic cancer cells. Clin Exp Metastasis, 2012.

[66] Eliceiri B.P. Integrin and growth factor receptor crosstalk. Circ Res, 2001. 89(12): 1104-1110.

[67] Shukla S., MacLennan G.T., Fu P., Patel J., Marengo S.R., Resnick M.I., and Gupta S. Nuclear factor-kappaB/p65 (Rel A) is constitutively activated in human prostate adenocarcinoma and correlates with disease progression. Neoplasia, 2004. 6(4): 390-400.

[68] Kong D., Li Y., Wang Z., Banerjee S., and Sarkar F.H. Inhibition of angiogenesis and invasion by 3,3'-diindolylmethane is mediated by the nuclear factor-kappaB downstream target genes MMP-9 and uPA that regulated bioavailability of vascular endothelial growth factor in prostate cancer. Cancer Res, 2007. 67(7): 3310-3319.

[69] Ryter S.W. and Choi A.M. Heme oxygenase-1: molecular mechanisms of gene expression in oxygen-related stress. Antioxid Redox Signal, 2002. 4(4): 625-632.

[70] Min K.J., Lee J.T., Joe E.H., and Kwon T.K. An IkappaBalpha phosphorylation inhibitor induces heme oxygenase-1(HO-1) expression through the activation of reactive oxygen species (ROS)-Nrf2-ARE signaling and ROS-PI3K/Akt signaling in an NF-kappaB-independent mechanism. Cell Signal, 2011. 23(9): 1505-1513.

[71] Sacca P., Meiss R., Casas G., Mazza O., Calvo J.C., Navone N., and Vazquez E. Nuclear translocation of haeme oxygenase-1 is associated to prostate cancer. Br J Cancer, 2007. 97(12): 1683-1689.

[72] Lin Q., Weis S., Yang G., Weng Y.H., Helston R., Rish K., Smith A., Bordner J., Polte T., Gaunitz F., and Dennery P.A. Heme oxygenase-1 protein localizes to the nucleus and activates transcription factors important in oxidative stress. J Biol Chem, 2007. 282(28): 20621-20633.

[73] Lin Q.S., Weis S., Yang G., Zhuang T., Abate A., and Dennery P.A. Catalytic inactive heme oxygenase-1 protein regulates its own expression in oxidative stress. Free Radic Biol Med, 2008. 44(5): 847-855.

[74] Gueron G., De Siervi A., Ferrando M., Salierno M., De Luca P., Elguero B., Meiss R., Navone N., and Vazquez E.S. Critical role of endogenous heme oxygenase 1 as a tu-

ner of the invasive potential of prostate cancer cells. Mol Cancer Res, 2009. 7(11): 1745-1755.

[75] Ferrando M., Gueron G., Elguero B., Giudice J., Salles A., Leskow F.C., Jares-Erijman E.A., Colombo L., Meiss R., Navone N., De Siervi A., and Vazquez E. Heme oxygenase 1 (HO-1) challenges the angiogenic switch in prostate cancer. Angiogenesis, 2011. 14(4): 467-479.

[76] Li Y., Su J., DingZhang X., Zhang J., Yoshimoto M., Liu S., Bijian K., Gupta A., Squire J.A., Alaoui Jamali M.A., and Bismar T.A. PTEN deletion and heme oxygenase-1 overexpression cooperate in prostate cancer progression and are associated with adverse clinical outcome. J Pathol, 2011. 224(1): 90-100.

[77] Griffiths-Jones S. The microRNA Registry. Nucleic Acids Res, 2004. 32(Database issue): D109-111.

[78] Friedman R.C., Farh K.K., Burge C.B., and Bartel D.P. Most mammalian mRNAs are conserved targets of microRNAs. Genome Res, 2009. 19(1): 92-105.

[79] Osman A. MicroRNAs in health and disease--basic science and clinical applications. Clin Lab, 2012. 58(5-6): 393-402.

[80] Chen C.Z. MicroRNAs as oncogenes and tumor suppressors. N Engl J Med, 2005. 353(17): 1768-1771.

[81] Calin G.A., Sevignani C., Dumitru C.D., Hyslop T., Noch E., Yendamuri S., Shimizu M., Rattan S., Bullrich F., Negrini M., and Croce C.M. Human microRNA genes are frequently located at fragile sites and genomic regions involved in cancers. Proc Natl Acad Sci U S A, 2004. 101(9): 2999-3004.

[82] Cortez M.A., Bueso-Ramos C., Ferdin J., Lopez-Berestein G., Sood A.K., and Calin G.A. MicroRNAs in body fluids--the mix of hormones and biomarkers. Nat Rev Clin Oncol, 2011. 8(8): 467-477.

[83] Lu J., Getz G., Miska E.A., Alvarez-Saavedra E., Lamb J., Peck D., Sweet-Cordero A., Ebert B.L., Mak R.H., Ferrando A.A., Downing J.R., Jacks T., Horvitz H.R., and Golub T.R. MicroRNA expression profiles classify human cancers. Nature, 2005. 435(7043): 834-838.

[84] Koturbash I., Zemp F.J., Pogribny I., and Kovalchuk O. Small molecules with big effects: the role of the microRNAome in cancer and carcinogenesis. Mutat Res, 2011. 722(2): 94-105.

[85] Coppola V., De Maria R., and Bonci D. MicroRNAs and prostate cancer. Endocr Relat Cancer, 2010. 17(1): F1-17.

[86] Ribas J., Ni X., Haffner M., Wentzel E.A., Salmasi A.H., Chowdhury W.H., Kudrolli T.A., Yegnasubramanian S., Luo J., Rodriguez R., Mendell J.T., and Lupold S.E. miR-21: an androgen receptor-regulated microRNA that promotes hormone-depend-

ent and hormone-independent prostate cancer growth. Cancer Res, 2009. 69(18): 7165-7169.

[87] Mercatelli N., Coppola V., Bonci D., Miele F., Costantini A., Guadagnoli M., Bonanno E., Muto G., Frajese G.V., De Maria R., Spagnoli L.G., Farace M.G., and Ciafre S.A. The inhibition of the highly expressed miR-221 and miR-222 impairs the growth of prostate carcinoma xenografts in mice. PLoS One, 2008. 3(12): e4029.

[88] Scott G.K., Goga A., Bhaumik D., Berger C.E., Sullivan C.S., and Benz C.C. Coordinate suppression of ERBB2 and ERBB3 by enforced expression of micro-RNA miR-125a or miR-125b. J Biol Chem, 2007. 282(2): 1479-1486.

[89] Craft N., Shostak Y., Carey M., and Sawyers C.L. A mechanism for hormone-independent prostate cancer through modulation of androgen receptor signaling by the HER-2/neu tyrosine kinase. Nat Med, 1999. 5(3): 280-285.

[90] Zhao Y., Hao Y., Ji H., Fang Y., Guo Y., Sha W., Zhou Y., Pang X., Southerland W.M., Califano J.A., and Gu X. Combination effects of salvianolic acid B with low-dose celecoxib on inhibition of head and neck squamous cell carcinoma growth in vitro and in vivo. Cancer Prev Res (Phila), 2010. 3(6): 787-796.

[91] Hao Y., Gu X., Zhao Y., Greene S., Sha W., Smoot D.T., Califano J., Wu T.C., and Pang X. Enforced expression of miR-101 inhibits prostate cancer cell growth by modulating the COX-2 pathway in vivo. Cancer Prev Res (Phila), 2011. 4(7): 1073-1083.

[92] Khan A.P., Poisson L.M., Bhat V.B., Fermin D., Zhao R., Kalyana-Sundaram S., Michailidis G., Nesvizhskii A.I., Omenn G.S., Chinnaiyan A.M., and Sreekumar A. Quantitative proteomic profiling of prostate cancer reveals a role for miR-128 in prostate cancer. Mol Cell Proteomics, 2010. 9(2): 298-312.

[93] Lin S.L., Chiang A., Chang D., and Ying S.Y. Loss of mir-146a function in hormone-refractory prostate cancer. RNA, 2008. 14(3): 417-424.

[94] Pang Y., Young C.Y., and Yuan H. MicroRNAs and prostate cancer. Acta Biochim Biophys Sin (Shanghai), 2010. 42(6): 363-369.

[95] Hudson R.S., Yi M., Esposito D., Watkins S.K., Hurwitz A.A., Yfantis H.G., Lee D.H., Borin J.F., Naslund M.J., Alexander R.B., Dorsey T.H., Stephens R.M., Croce C.M., and Ambs S. MicroRNA-1 is a candidate tumor suppressor and prognostic marker in human prostate cancer. Nucleic Acids Res, 2012. 40(8): 3689-3703.

[96] Selth L.A., Tilley W.D., and Butler L.M. Circulating microRNAs: macro-utility as markers of prostate cancer? Endocr Relat Cancer, 2012. 19(4): R99-R113.

[97] Brase J.C., Johannes M., Schlomm T., Falth M., Haese A., Steuber T., Beissbarth T., Kuner R., and Sultmann H. Circulating miRNAs are correlated with tumor progression in prostate cancer. Int J Cancer, 2011. 128(3): 608-616.

[98] Zhang H.L., Yang L.F., Zhu Y., Yao X.D., Zhang S.L., Dai B., Zhu Y.P., Shen Y.J., Shi G.H., and Ye D.W. Serum miRNA-21: elevated levels in patients with metastatic hor-

mone-refractory prostate cancer and potential predictive factor for the efficacy of docetaxel-based chemotherapy. Prostate, 2011. 71(3): 326-331.

[99] Carmeliet P. VEGF as a key mediator of angiogenesis in cancer. Oncology, 2005. 69 Suppl 3: 4-10.

[100] Ferrara N. Pathways mediating VEGF-independent tumor angiogenesis. Cytokine Growth Factor Rev, 2010. 21(1): 21-26.

[101] Kazerounian S., Yee K.O., and Lawler J. Thrombospondins in cancer. Cell Mol Life Sci, 2008. 65(5): 700-712.

[102] Ribatti D. Endogenous inhibitors of angiogenesis: a historical review. Leuk Res, 2009. 33(5): 638-644.

[103] Azam F., Mehta S., and Harris A.L. Mechanisms of resistance to antiangiogenesis therapy. Eur J Cancer, 2010. 46(8): 1323-1332.

[104] Osawa M., Masuda M., Kusano K., and Fujiwara K. Evidence for a role of platelet endothelial cell adhesion molecule-1 in endothelial cell mechanosignal transduction: is it a mechanoresponsive molecule? J Cell Biol, 2002. 158(4): 773-785.

[105] Dome B., Hendrix M.J., Paku S., Tovari J., and Timar J. Alternative vascularization mechanisms in cancer: Pathology and therapeutic implications. Am J Pathol, 2007. 170(1): 1-15.

[106] Holash J., Maisonpierre P.C., Compton D., Boland P., Alexander C.R., Zagzag D., Yancopoulos G.D., and Wiegand S.J. Vessel cooption, regression, and growth in tumors mediated by angiopoietins and VEGF. Science, 1999. 284(5422): 1994-1998.

[107] Vajkoczy P., Farhadi M., Gaumann A., Heidenreich R., Erber R., Wunder A., Tonn J.C., Menger M.D., and Breier G. Microtumor growth initiates angiogenic sprouting with simultaneous expression of VEGF, VEGF receptor-2, and angiopoietin-2. J Clin Invest, 2002. 109(6): 777-785.

[108] Zhao C., Yang H., Shi H., Wang X., Chen X., Yuan Y., Lin S., and Wei Y. Distinct contributions of angiogenesis and vascular co-option during the initiation of primary microtumors and micrometastases. Carcinogenesis, 2011. 32(8): 1143-1150.

[109] Vermeulen P.B., Colpaert C., Salgado R., Royers R., Hellemans H., Van Den Heuvel E., Goovaerts G., Dirix L.Y., and Van Marck E. Liver metastases from colorectal adenocarcinomas grow in three patterns with different angiogenesis and desmoplasia. J Pathol, 2001. 195(3): 336-342.

[110] Borgstrom P., Bourdon M.A., Hillan K.J., Sriramarao P., and Ferrara N. Neutralizing anti-vascular endothelial growth factor antibody completely inhibits angiogenesis and growth of human prostate carcinoma micro tumors in vivo. Prostate, 1998. 35(1): 1-10.

[111] Sweeney P., Karashima T., Kim S.J., Kedar D., Mian B., Huang S., Baker C., Fan Z., Hicklin D.J., Pettaway C.A., and Dinney C.P. Anti-vascular endothelial growth factor

receptor 2 antibody reduces tumorigenicity and metastasis in orthotopic prostate cancer xenografts via induction of endothelial cell apoptosis and reduction of endothelial cell matrix metalloproteinase type 9 production. Clin Cancer Res, 2002. 8(8): 2714-2724.

[112] Weinberg R.A., ed. The Biology of Cancer. ed. Weinberg R.A. 2007, Garland Science: New York.

[113] Maniotis A.J., Folberg R., Hess A., Seftor E.A., Gardner L.M., Pe'er J., Trent J.M., Meltzer P.S., and Hendrix M.J. Vascular channel formation by human melanoma cells in vivo and in vitro: vasculogenic mimicry. Am J Pathol, 1999. 155(3): 739-752.

[114] Liu R., Yang K., Meng C., Zhang Z., and Xu Y. Vasculogenic mimicry is a marker of poor prognosis in prostate cancer. Cancer Biol Ther, 2012. 13(7): 527-533.

[115] Raza A., Franklin M.J., and Dudek A.Z. Pericytes and vessel maturation during tumor angiogenesis and metastasis. Am J Hematol, 2010. 85(8): 593-598.

[116] Sharma N., Seftor R.E., Seftor E.A., Gruman L.M., Heidger P.M., Jr., Cohen M.B., Lubaroff D.M., and Hendrix M.J. Prostatic tumor cell plasticity involves cooperative interactions of distinct phenotypic subpopulations: role in vasculogenic mimicry. Prostate, 2002. 50(3): 189-201.

[117] Ahmadi S.A., Moinfar M., Gohari Moghaddam K., and Bahadori M. Practical application of angiogenesis and vasculogenic mimicry in prostatic adenocarcinoma. Arch Iran Med, 2010. 13(6): 498-503.

[118] Baluk P., Hashizume H., and McDonald D.M. Cellular abnormalities of blood vessels as targets in cancer. Curr Opin Genet Dev, 2005. 15(1): 102-111.

[119] Dasgupta S., Srinidhi S., and Vishwanatha J.K. Oncogenic activation in prostate cancer progression and metastasis: Molecular insights and future challenges. J Carcinog, 2012. 11: 4.

[120] Bonfil R.D., Chinni S., Fridman R., Kim H.R., and Cher M.L. Proteases, growth factors, chemokines, and the microenvironment in prostate cancer bone metastasis. Urol Oncol, 2007. 25(5): 407-411.

[121] Hendrix M.J., Seftor E.A., Hess A.R., and Seftor R.E. Vasculogenic mimicry and tumour-cell plasticity: lessons from melanoma. Nat Rev Cancer, 2003. 3(6): 411-421.

[122] Kerbel R.S. Tumor angiogenesis: past, present and the near future. Carcinogenesis, 2000. 21(3): 505-515.

[123] Yang Q., McHugh K.P., Patntirapong S., Gu X., Wunderlich L., and Hauschka P.V. VEGF enhancement of osteoclast survival and bone resorption involves VEGF receptor-2 signaling and beta3-integrin. Matrix Biol, 2008. 27(7): 589-599.

[124] Dai J., Kitagawa Y., Zhang J., Yao Z., Mizokami A., Cheng S., Nor J., McCauley L.K., Taichman R.S., and Keller E.T. Vascular endothelial growth factor contributes to the

prostate cancer-induced osteoblast differentiation mediated by bone morphogenetic protein. Cancer Res, 2004. 64(3): 994-999.

[125] Akech J., Wixted J.J., Bedard K., van der Deen M., Hussain S., Guise T.A., van Wijnen A.J., Stein J.L., Languino L.R., Altieri D.C., Pratap J., Keller E., Stein G.S., and Lian J.B. Runx2 association with progression of prostate cancer in patients: mechanisms mediating bone osteolysis and osteoblastic metastatic lesions. Oncogene, 2010. 29(6): 811-821.

[126] Wang Z., Li Y., Banerjee S., Kong D., Ahmad A., Nogueira V., Hay N., and Sarkar F.H. Down-regulation of Notch-1 and Jagged-1 inhibits prostate cancer cell growth, migration and invasion, and induces apoptosis via inactivation of Akt, mTOR, and NF-kappaB signaling pathways. J Cell Biochem, 2010. 109(4): 726-736.

[127] Bin Hafeez B., Adhami V.M., Asim M., Siddiqui I.A., Bhat K.M., Zhong W., Saleem M., Din M., Setaluri V., and Mukhtar H. Targeted knockdown of Notch1 inhibits invasion of human prostate cancer cells concomitant with inhibition of matrix metalloproteinase-9 and urokinase plasminogen activator. Clin Cancer Res, 2009. 15(2): 452-459.

[128] Dufraine J., Funahashi Y., and Kitajewski J. Notch signaling regulates tumor angiogenesis by diverse mechanisms. Oncogene, 2008. 27(38): 5132-5137.

[129] Paulis Y.W., Soetekouw P.M., Verheul H.M., Tjan-Heijnen V.C., and Griffioen A.W. Signalling pathways in vasculogenic mimicry. Biochim Biophys Acta, 2010. 1806(1): 18-28.

Section 7

Role of Androgen Receptor

Chapter 19

Expression and Function of Stromal Androgen Receptor in Prostate Cancer

Mandeep Singh, Garrett Daniels, Yirong Li and Peng Lee

Additional information is available at the end of the chapter

http://dx.doi.org/10.5772/52425

1. Introduction

Prostate cancer has the highest incidence in the United States and the second highest in the world among cancers in the male population. It is also one of the leading causes of cancer deaths in males in the United States. Like other glandular organs, benign prostate has an epithelial compartment containing mainly secretory luminal cells outlined with basal cells and a stromal compartment including fibroblasts and smooth muscle cells. The development and function of the prostate is mediated by circulating androgens which act via androgen receptor (AR). Amongst the epithelial cells, AR is expressed only in secretory luminal cells, while in the stroma, AR is expressed primarily by fibroblasts and smooth muscle cells in adulthood. In the past, investigators mainly focused on studying epithelial AR function in prostate cancer, defined the involved mechanisms and developed numerous hypotheses which have been published and are widely accepted. However, limited data is available which can be used to describe the function of stromal AR in prostate cancer. This review of the literature examines the current knowledge and understanding of stromal AR function in prostate cancer and endeavors to illustrate its translational significance.

2. Stromal cells in prostate carcinogenesis

The role of stromal cells on the initiation and promotion of carcinogenesis has been studied over many years. This concept was pioneered from previous studies showing [1-3] that tumor stroma, termed as CAF (cancer associated fibroblast), TAS (tumor associated stroma), or RS (reactive stroma), is often different from the normal stroma [1]. Normal prostate stromal cells play a protective role and maintain growth quiescence within the prostatic tissue. Some investigators have demonstrated in animal studies that when normal prostate stromal cells are associated with malignant epithelial cells, there is a decrease in the proliferation rate [4,5] and an apparent loss of former malignant properties of epithelial cells[6]. Some studies have also shown restriction of growth of epithelial cells and induction into a more differentiated phenotype [7]. Recombination studies using Dunning rat adenocarcinoma revealed that normal stromal environment may override the effects of oncogenic mutations in tumor cells [8]. Normal stromal cells therefore, retain properties of growth control and can prevent the proliferation of cells undergoing neoplastic transformation.

Modification of stromal environment is necessary for carcinogenesis and it is adequately evident on observation of stroma immediately adjacent to carcinoma cells in several tumors [1]. Recombination experiments by viral transfection of oncogenes *myc* and *ras* into urogenital sinus mesenchyme and epithelium have illustrated that changes are required in both epithelium and stroma for prostatic carcinogenesis to occur [9]. The principal stromal cells – smooth muscle cells and fibroblasts undergo a phenotype switching to emerge as myofibroblasts during tumorigenesis. Morphologically and on the basis of cytoskeletal protein expression, myofibroblasts are an intermediate between fibroblasts and smooth muscle cells [10,11]. They are identified by increased expression of vimentin, alpha actin and decreased expression of calponin and smooth muscle myosin. Other phenotypic changes seen in the cancer associated stroma include abnormal migratory behavior *in vitro*, alterations in the cell surface molecules, expression of prostaglandin synthesizing enzymes, alterations in extra cellular matrix (ECM) and altered expression of growth factors – platelet derived growth factor (PDGF), insulin-like growth factor (IGF) 1 & 2, transforming growth factor beta 1(TGF-b1), hepatocyte growth factor (HGF) and keratinocyte growth factor (KGF) [1]. There are several possible factors which promote the modification of normal stromal cells into cancer associated stroma. Some signals from epithelial cancer cells to surrounding stromal cells have been shown to alter the function of stromal cells and ECM production, such as TGF-b1, which induces stromal secretion of 'versican' an extracellular chondroitin sulfate proteoglycan [12]. In a hormone sensitive cell model, variations in ECM have been shown to regulate stromal cell phenotype [13]. There is also evidence that the genetic modifications seen in the cancer associated stroma [14] are a result of epithelial to mesenchymal transitions of previously genetically abnormal epithelial cells. There is a genome-wide change in stromal genes associated with prostate cancer. In an analysis by Rowley et al. [15], when compared with normal stroma, a total of 544 unique genes were significantly higher in the reactive stroma and 606 unique genes were lower. Gene ontology analysis revealed significant alterations in a number of novel processes in prostate cancer reactive stroma, including neurogenesis, axonogenesis, and the DNA damage/repair pathways, as well as an evidence of increased number of stem cells in prostate cancer reactive stroma.

Alternatively, in the 'reactive stroma' hypothesis [11] the stroma of prostate cancer has been correlated with the granulation tissue in wound repair mechanism with reference to similar biological responses. As in any wound repair situation the microenvironment would be expected to be growth promoting which correlates with the promotion of survival and proliferation of carcinoma cells by stroma in prostatic carcinogenesis. Tissue recombination studies have demonstrated that human prostatic tumor associated stroma can promote carcinogenesis in genetically initiated human prostatic epithelial cells [1,16]. The results of this experiment revealed an important inference that the cancer associated stroma, when formed, exhibit a significant role in the epithelial cells promoting prostate carcinogenesis.

In contrast, some investigators [17] have shown that tumor associated stromal cells inhibit epithelial cell growth by production of a specific inhibitory factor termed as prostatic epithelium inhibiting factor (PEIF). The expression of this factor by stromal cells was only in the conditioned media collected from isolated stromal cell subcultures. Later in another experiment [18], stromal cells derived from surgically obtained prostatic carcinoma specimens were co-cultured with PC-3 cells using double layer soft agar system. It was noticed that growth of PC-3 cells was inhibited by the stromal cells.

The diversity in stromal cell function in inhibiting or promoting epithelial cell growth may be explained by the heterogeneity of stromal cells in the stromal compartment. During carcinogenesis, the stromal cells display heterogeneity in their morphology as smooth muscle cells, fibroblasts and myofibroblasts. Also, they are heterogenous in AR expression as AR positive and AR negative cells. It may be possible that the presence and absence of AR in stromal cells can dictate cancer epithelial cell proliferation or growth suppression.

3. Progressive loss of AR expression

Numerous studies have focused on AR expression in the epithelial cells during prostate carcinogenesis and the progression of prostate cancer from primary to metastatic cancer and from hormone sensitive to castration resistant prostate cancer (CRPC). It has been established that epithelial AR is continuously expressed throughout prostate cancer disease progression. Increased AR expression has been associated with aggressive disease and decreased progression free survival (PFS) in patients [19].

The expression and function of stromal AR may be distinct from epithelial AR. As a result of the structural, genetic and genomic [11,15] modifications of the stromal cells, there are behavioral modifications expressed in tumor associated stroma. AR expression in stroma is progressively decreased during the transition from benign tissue to cancer and during progression of prostate cancer from low grade to high grade, primary to metastatic, hormone sensitive to CRPC, as well as aggressive prostate cancer in African Americans.

In immunohistochemistry (IHC) studies, some investigators [20] found that AR expression declines in the peri-epithelial stroma as early as in high grade prostatic intraepithelial neoplasia (HGPIN) compared to normal prostate. In their analysis using tissue samples of HGPIN, expression of AR was found to be absent in 80% and weak in 20% of peri-epithelial stromal cell sections.

Analysis of stromal tissue of prostate cancer showed that loss of AR expression increased linearly with higher histological grades in several studies. AR expression was absent in 67% of peri-epithelial stromal tissue in well differentiated (Gleason score 2-4), 91% in moderately differentiated (Gleason score 5-7) and 94% in poorly differentiated (Gleason score 8-10) prostate cancer [20]. In our study [21], we have shown a statistically significant decrease of stromal AR expression ($p < 0.001$) in the areas of prostate cancer compared with benign prostate with up to a 6% decrease in stromal AR expression. When stratified with Gleason score, we established a trend of greater decrease of AR-positive stromal cells in cancerous areas compared to benign areas with increased tumor grade. Later on, other investigators have also demonstrated that magnitude of loss of stromal AR is directly proportional to advanced pathological stage along with higher Gleason scores [22]. By AR antibody immunostaining of TURP (Trans Urethral Resection of Prostate) specimens obtained from patients with varying Gleason scores and pathological stages, they found lower expression of AR in tumor stroma compared to areas with normal stroma. This difference was notable ($p < 0.05$) in tumor specimens of stage T2 and tumors with Gleason score of 7, while it was more statistically significant ($p < 0.01$) in tumor stage T3 and T4 and in specimens with Gleason score of 8-10.

Decreased stromal AR expression has also been correlated to disease progession including metastasis and androgen-independence. Bergh et al. showed [22] that specimens with metastatic disease displayed significantly lower ($p < 0.01$) stromal AR expression. The AR staining was only 1.6% in metastatic tumor stroma compared to 18 % in normal stroma which was equivalent to a loss of expression by 11 fold. While in the non-metastatic disease specimens, the AR staining was 13% in tumor stroma compared to 48 % in normal stroma, equivalent to a loss of expression by 3.5 fold. Evidence is available [21] that during transition of prostate cancer from hormone sensitive to CRPC, there is a significant decrease in stromal AR expression. AR levels were determined in the prostate stroma of 44 cases of hormone sensitive prostate cancer and in 22 cases of CRPC by IHC analysis using affinity purified polyclonal AR antibodies. Scoring was performed by selecting three areas with 100 cells each in benign and cancerous regions in prostate stromal tissue sections to determine the relative percentages of stromal cells that were AR-positive and AR-negative, respectively. The levels of stromal AR expression were expressed as an average percentage of AR-positive stromal cells. When comparing hormone sensitive and CRPC tumor sections, a statistically significant 3-fold decrease of AR-positive stromal cells was observed, from 4 % in hormone sensitive to 12 % in CRPC tumors. Most importantly, some investigators have also reported an association of loss of stromal AR expression with clinical outcome or prostate cancer specific death in patients [25].

These studies suggest that there is a natural selection of stromal AR negative cells over AR positive cells as the tumor progresses. With these results, we established that stromal AR expression proportionately decreases as tumor grade increases and as cancer advances towards metastatic and androgen independent disease. The mechanism behind the loss of AR expression in the peri-epithelial stroma is not well understood. It has been attributed that during the malignant transformation of epithelial cells, there is a shift in AR axis from stromal cell dependent paracrine pathways to autocrine dependent pathways [23] and is increased during tumor progression. When these cancer cells shift to autocrine mechanism of proliferation, it appears that epithelial AR regulates a new series of genes for survival and proliferation, not normally expressed by prostate epithelial cells [7]. The consequence of this may be that

http://dx.doi.org/10.5772/52425

malignant epithelial cells no longer depend upon stromal-epithelial interactions and stromal AR mediated growth factors for their survival and proliferation.

4. Stromal AR inhibits cancer epithelial cells

We have observed and previously demonstrated by co-culture experiments using well characterized stromal cell lines, both *in vitro* and *in vivo* that, in the presence of androgen, stromal cells expressing AR decrease the growth and invasive ability of prostate cancer epithelial cells. It was hypothesized that this distinct effect of AR in stromal cells is due to the involvement of paracrine factors/mechanisms regulated by both the epithelial and stromal cells.

The analysis was established [21] by using a well characterized prostate stromal cell line morphologically similar to the tumor stroma. We constructed an immortalized stromal cell line from prostate with BPH, termed as PShTert, stably expressing the human telomerase catalytic subunit – hTert. Morphologically and ultra structurally, the cells expressed typical characteristics of myofibroblasts. IHC showed diffuse, strongly positive stain for Vimentin with a strong SMA staining in 25% of cells, and negative staining for Desmin. Together these data support the myofibroblastic phenotype of the PShTert stromal cells. Western blot analysis showed the absence of AR in these cell lines. We transduced this cell line with pBabeAR retroviral vector and selected stable clonal cell lines expressing AR, termed as PShTertAR. Functionality of the ectopic AR was confirmed by *in vivo* dual luciferase assay eliciting ligand dependent transcriptional activation in the presence of androgens.

For *in vitro* analysis, transwell indirect co-culture assays using these two stromal cell lines with PC3 cells were performed. In the presence of androgen, co-culture with PShTertAR resulted in inhibition of PC3 cell proliferation compared to PC3 cell growth when cultured alone ($p = 0.045$). In contrast, co-culture with AR negative PShTert cells resulted in enhancement of growth rate of PC3 cells compared to PC3 cells grown alone ($p = 0.03$). Flow cytometric analysis revealed that PC3 cells co-cultured with PShTertAR showed 20% S-phase cells, decreased from the 27% S-phase cells measured inPC3 cells co-cultured with PShTert cells. We examined the expression of cell cycle genes, including cyclin A, cyclin B, p21 and p27, and the expression of Skp2, and all were decreased in PC3 cells co-cultured with PShTertAR compared with PC3 cells co-cultured with PShTert cells.

However, with co-cultures in androgen free media, both PShTert and PShTertAR cells stimulated the growth of PC3 cells. Similarly *in vivo* analysis by co-injecting PC3 cells with PShTert subcutaneously in the flank region of nude male mice resulted in development of tumors twice as large as when PC3 was injected alone. On the other side, co-injection of PC3 cells and PShTertAR cell line resulted in statistically significant reductions of tumor growth and size.

There were two important observations drawn from the analysis. Firstly, both AR negative and AR positive stromal cells promote growth of prostate cancer epithelial cells in the absence of androgen by secretion of a paracrine factor which is independent of AR. Secondly, AR positive stromal cells secrete another paracrine factor which is growth inhibitory for prostate cancer epithelial cells and is dependent on the presence of androgen and AR.

5. Conclusion

With reference to our hypothesis that AR positive stromal cells inhibit the growth of PC3 cells in the presence of androgen, we also analyzed and found similar results while using LNCaP cells. However, the magnitude of growth inhibition was less significant in LNCaP cells as compared to PC3 cells.

Therefore, there is a need to re-identify the role of continued androgen deprivation therapy (ADT) during progression to CRPC. It may be possible that due to androgen deprivation, the growth promoting stromal effects counteract the apoptotic effects of androgen ablation on epithelial cells. On the contrary, the growth inhibiting effects of the stromal AR are lost during ADT. The permanent methods of androgen ablation such as surgical castration can be replaced by reversible methods of castration such as medical castration with LHRH analogues. Interestingly, some investigators have even observed that using androgen replacement therapy (ART) in metastatic CRPC displayed biochemical improvement in patients [24]. Newer therapies targeting the prostate cancer stromal cells should be evaluated.

Acknowledgements

This study is supported by NIH 1U01CA149556-01, DOD PCRP (PC080010 and PC111624), and NYUSOM Center of Excellence on Urologic Disease Fund to PL.

Author details

Mandeep Singh, Garrett Daniels, Yirong Li and Peng Lee*

*Address all correspondence to: peng.lee@nyumc.org

Department of Pathology and Urology, New York University School of Medicine, New York, NY, USA

References

[1] Cunha, G. R, Hayward, S. W, & Wang, Y. Z. Role of stroma in carcinogenesis of the prostate. Differentiation (2002)., 70, 473-85.

[2] Bosman, F. T, De Bruïne, A, Flohil, C, & Van Der Wurff, A. ten Kate J, Dinjens WW. Epithelial-stromal interactions in colon cancer. International Journal of Developmental Biology. (1993)., 37(1), 203-211.

[3] Seljelid, R, Jozefowski, S, & Sveinbjörnsson, B. Tumor stroma. Anticancer Research. (1999). A):, 4809-22.

[4] Decosse, J. J, Gossens, C. L, Kuzma, J. F, & Unsworth, B. R. Breast cancer: induction of differentiation by embryonic tissue. Science. (1973)., 181(4104), 1057-8.

[5] Decosse, J. J, Gossens, C, Kuzma, J. F, & Unsworth, B. R. Embryonic inductive tissues that cause histologic differentiation of murine mammary carcinoma in vitro. Journal of National Cancer Institute. (1975)., 54(4), 913-22.

[6] Cooper, M, & Pinkus, H. Intrauterine transplantation of rat basal cell carcinoma as a model for reconversion of malignant to benign growth. Cancer Research. (1977)., 37, 2544-52.

[7] Arnold, J. T, & Isaacs, J. T. Mechanisms involved in the progression of androgen-independent prostate cancers: it is not only the cancer cell's fault. Endocrine Related Cancer. (2002). Mar;, 9(1), 61-73.

[8] Hayashi, N, Sugimura, Y, Kawamura, J, Donjacour, A. A, & Cunha, G. R. Morphological and functional heterogeneity in the rat prostatic gland. Biology of Reproduction. (1991). Aug;, 45(2), 308-21.

[9] Thompson, T. C, Timme, T. L, Kadmon, D, Park, S. H, Egawa, S, & Yoshida, K. Genetic predisposition and mesenchymal-epithelial interactions in ras+myc-induced carcinogenesis in reconstituted mouse prostate. Molecular Carcinogenesis. (1993). , 7(3), 165-79.

[10] Gabbiani, G, Hirschel, B. J, Ryan, G. B, Statkov, P. R, & Majno, G. Granulation tissue as a contractile organ. A study of structure and function. Journal of Experimental Medicine. (1972)., 135(4), 719-34.

[11] Tuxhorn, J. A, Ayala, G. E, & Rowley, D. R. Reactive stroma in prostate cancer progression. Journal of Urology. (2001)., 166, 2472-83.

[12] Sakko, A. J, Ricciardelli, C, Mayne, K, & Tilley, W. D. LeBaron RG, Horsfall DJ. Versican accumulation in human prostatic fibroblast cultures is enhanced by prostate cancer cell-derived transforming growth factor beta1. Cancer Research. (2001). , 61(3), 926-930.

[13] Arnold, J. T, Kaufman, D. G, Seppälä, M, & Lessey, B. A. Endometrial stromal cells regulate epithelial cell growth in vitro: a new co-culture model. Human Reproduction. (2001). , 16(5), 836-45.

[14] Macintosh, C. A, Stower, M, Reid, N, & Maitland, N. J. Precise microdissection of human prostate cancers reveals genotypic heterogeneity. Cancer Research. (1998). , 58(1), 23-28.

[15] Dakhova, O, Ozen, M, Creighton, C. J, Li, R, Ayala, G, Rowley, D, & Ittmann, M. Global gene expression analysis of reactive stroma in prostate cancer. Clinical Cancer Research. (2009). , 15(12), 3979-89.

[16] Olumi, A. F, Grossfeld, G. D, Hayward, S. W, Carroll, P. R, Tlsty, T. D, & Cunha, G. R. Carcinoma-associated fibroblasts direct tumor progression of initiated human prostatic epithelium. Cancer Research. (1999). , 59(19), 5002-11.

[17] König, J. J, Romijn, J. C, & Schröder, F. H. Prostatic epithelium inhibiting factor (PEIF): organ specificity and production by prostatic fibroblasts. Urological Research. (1987). , 15(3), 145-149.

[18] Kooistra, A, Romijn, J. C, & Schröder, F. H. Stromal inhibition of epithelial cell growth in the prostate; overview of an experimental study. Urological Research. (1997). Supplement 2): S , 97-105.

[19] Li, R, Wheeler, T, Dai, H, Frolov, A, Thompson, T, & Ayala, G. High level of androgen receptor is associated with aggressive clinicopathologic features and decreased biochemical recurrence-free survival in prostate: cancer patients treated with radical prostatectomy. American Journal of Surgical Pathology. (2004). , 28(7), 928-34.

[20] Olapade-olaopa, E. O. MacKay EH, Taub NA, Sandhu DP, Terry TR, Habib FK. Malignant transformation of human prostatic epithelium is associated with the loss of androgen receptor immunoreactivity in the surrounding stroma. Clinical Cancer Research. (1999). , 5(3), 569-76.

[21] Li, Y, Li, C. X, Ye, H, Chen, F, Melamed, J, Peng, Y, Liu, J, Wang, Z, Tsou, H. C, Wei, J, Walden, P, Garabedian, M. J, & Lee, P. Decrease in stromal androgen receptor associates with androgen-independent disease and promotes prostate cancer cell proliferation and invasion. Journal of Cellular and Molecular Medicine. (2008). B): , 2790-2798.

[22] Wikström, P, Marusic, J, Stattin, P, & Bergh, A. Low stroma androgen receptor level in normal and tumor prostate tissue is related to poor outcome in prostate cancer patients. Prostate. (2009). Jun 1; , 69(8), 799-809.

[23] Gao, J, Arnold, J. T, & Isaacs, J. T. Conversion from a paracrine to an autocrine mechanism of androgen-stimulated growth during malignant transformation of prostatic epithelial cells. Cancer Research. (2001). , 61(13), 5038-44.

[24] Morris, M. J, Huang, D, Kelly, W. K, Slovin, S. F, Stephenson, R. D, Eicher, C, Delacruz, A, Curley, T, Schwartz, L. H, & Scher, H. I. Phase 1 trial of high-dose exogenous

testosterone in patients with castration-resistant metastatic prostate cancer. European Urology. (2009). , 56(2), 237-44.

[25] Grant BuchananFreemasons Foundation Centre for Men's Health, The Bazil Hetzel Institute for Translational Health Research, University of Adelaide, SA, Australia.

Chapter 20

Prostate Cancer Progression to Androgen Independent Disease: The Role of the PI3K/AKT Pathway

Jacqueline R Ha, Yu Hao D Huang, Amit Persad and
Sujata Persad

Additional information is available at the end of the chapter

http://dx.doi.org/10.5772/53483

1. Introduction

1.1. The androgen receptor and CaP progression

The development and progression of prostate cancer (CaP) is largely dependent on the dysregulation of the androgen/androgen receptor (AR) signaling pathway; though, the mechanism of CaP progression remains elusive. Initial treatments for CaP included prostatectomy or radiation to destroy cancerous cells [1]. However, these treatments were not curative and more often than not there were recurrences and metastases of the cancer. Mainstay treatments that target the androgen/AR pathway through anti-androgen and androgen ablation therapies have been promising; yet again, these therapies seem to fail as the tumor progresses. This suggests that the androgen/AR dependence of CaP cells vary over time such that alterations in androgen availability, AR sensitivity and receptor promiscuity fuel a more aggressive CaP.

Approximately 80-90% of CaPs are originally androgen dependent (AD) at diagnosis [2]. Androgens stimulate the proliferation and inhibit the apoptosis of cells, thus implicating that CaP cells require a certain level of androgens to maintain their proliferation and survival [1]. This is primarily the reason why androgen ablation therapy is initially successful—it removes the stimulation these cells require for proliferation, ultimately causing the regression of the tumor. However, over time patients often fail androgen ablation therapy as the tumor becomes a more lethal androgen independent (AI) or castration resistant form. There is no effective therapy for AI-CaP.

The prostate requires androgenic steroids for development and function. Testosterone is the main circulating androgen and is secreted from the testes as well as the adrenal glands (adrenal steroid conversion). Once in the blood stream, the majority of the testosterone binds to albumin and sex-hormone-binding globulin (SHBG) while a small fraction is freely dissolved within serum. Within the prostate, testosterone is converted to a derivative, dihydrotestosterone (DHT), by 5-alpha-reductase. DHT is a more potent and active form of testosterone and has a greater affinity for the AR relative to testosterone. Testosterone and DHT bind to the AR and causes its nuclear localization, transcriptional activation and its interaction with co-regulators/ co-activators to mediate AR-directed gene transcription [2].

The AR is required for the development of prostate carcinogenesis from early prostate intraepithelial neoplasia (PIN) to organ-confined or locally invasive primary tumors [3]. As a member of the steroid-thyroid-retinoid nuclear receptor superfamily of proteins, the AR is in its inactive form within the cytoplasm, bound to heat shock proteins (HSP) [4-7] and components of the cytoskeleton [7,8], preventing AR nuclear localization and transcriptional activation. The binding of DHT or testosterone causes a conformational change leading to the dissociation of the AR from the HSPs and its subsequent phosphorylation [1, 9]. Once ligand bound, the AR is stabilized within the cytoplasm and translocates to the nucleus. The androgen-AR complex is in a conformational state to now homodimerize within the nucleus and bind to androgen response elements (AREs) in the promoter region of target genes [1] such as prostate specific antigen (PSA), a routine biomarker for prostate cancer diagnosis and progression [7, 10] and, probasin, a prostate-specific gene that has been exploited as a marker of prostate differentiation [11]. The AR has both a cytoplasmic and nuclear distribution, and shows a certain degree of trafficking either to or from the nucleus [12]. There are varying reports on the subcellular distribution of the AR in different cell types; however, this two-step model for steroid hormone receptor activation is a clear representation of ligand activated translocation and the observed focal accumulations of the AR within the nucleus [12].

1.2. AR structure and function

The AR gene is located on the X chromosome (q11-12), and contains eight exons that produce a protein of approximately 920 amino acids [7]. Exon 1 codes for the N-terminal domain (NTD), exons 2 and 3 translate into the central DNA binding domain (DBD) which contains two zinc fingers for specific binding of DNA sequences [1], and exon 4 to 8 code for a hinge region and a conserved C-terminal ligand binding domain (LBD).

The NTD (1-558) is a poorly conserved region that houses important sequence motifs for AR conformation and activity [7]. There are three regions of tri-nucleotide repeats, which include poly-glutamine (Q) and poly-glycine tracts [7, 13]. The poly-Q tract is encoded by a polymorphic CAG repeat [14]. The length of the repeats inversely affects the stability of the AR-NTD and C-terminal LBD interaction, and, AR expression and activity [7, 15, 16]. CAG tri-nucleotide repeats can vary between 11 and 31 repeats; less than 18 repeats are thought be an indicator of CaP risk.

The NTD also contains the transcriptional activation function-1 (AF1) comprising two transcriptional activation units (TAU): TAU-1 and TAU-5. The AF1 subdomain of the AR is the predominant site for transactivation, where TAU-1 is required for ligand-dependent transcription of the AR; TAU-5 is responsible for the majority of the constitutive activity associated with the NTD, and the recruitment of the Steroid Receptor Co-activator (SRC)/p160 family of co-activators. For example, TIF2 (Transcriptional Intermediary Factor 2), SRC-1, and GRIP-1 are members of the SRC/p160 family which increase AR transcription through their interactions with the NTD and DBD [4, 5, 7, 17]. These co-activators also recruit other co-regulators such as histone acetyl transferase (HAT) activity containing enzymes such as cAMP response element binding protein (CREB)-binding protein (CBP)/p300 and p300/CBP-associated factor (p/CAF) to initiate chromatin remodeling [7, 18] in preparation for DNA transcription [7, 19].

The LBD folds into 12 helices to form the ligand binding pocket. Interaction of ligands to the LBD promotes AR stability by the formation of the C-terminal transcriptional activation function -2 (AF2) domain and the subsequent interactions between the NTD/LBD [7]. The NTD interacts with the LBD through its sequence motifs ^{23}FQNLF^{27} and ^{433}WHTLF^{437} [5, 7, 20], while co-activators/co-regulators (E.g. SRC/p160 family of co-activators) bind to the LBD by a highly conserved consensus sequence LXXLL (L is Leucine and X is any amino acid) motif (also known as the NR box) [7]. The LBD LXXLL binding region primarily serves to recruit LXXLL motif containing co-activators/co-regulators and structurally enables the NTD FXXLF containing region to interact with the LBD [7]. The LXXLL motifs of such co-regulators form a two-turn amphipathic α-helix which binds to the hydrophobic cleft of the LBD (specifically AF2) [21].

The LBD AF2 domain is comprised of helices 3, 4, 5 and 12 [22]. The ligand binding pocket is formed by helices 3, 5, and 10. Helix 12 is thought to lie across the ligand binding pocket and stabilize the ligand-AR interaction and increase ligand-activated transcription. The AR NTD and C-terminal domain (CTD) interaction in conjunction with Helix 12 serve to stabilize agonist ligand binding and receptor transcriptional activity [23]. Furthermore, the interaction of AR-interacting proteins or co-regulators such as androgen receptor co-activator, ARA70, (which binds to both the AR-DBD and AR-LBD) can increase the receptivity of the AR-LBD to other activating ligands such as hydroxyflutamide (non-steroidal anti-androgen) and estrogens [7, 24-26]. However, it was shown that the AR NTD and CTD interaction was not absolutely required for transcriptional activity. For example, ligands used at high concentrations and peptides that blocked the NTD and CTD interaction did not absolutely inhibit transcriptional activity of the AR [23, 27, 28].

The AR is opposed by co-repressors which inhibit its transcriptional activation. Nuclear receptor co-repressor (NCor) and silencing mediator for retinoid and thyroid hormone receptors (SMRT) disrupts the NTD-LBD interaction and the binding of SRC/p160 co-activators [7]. NCor and SMRT are able to recruit histone deacetylases (HDAC) to promote the repackaging of DNA and prevent the binding of transcriptional machinery, activators, and receptors [7, 29]. However, NCor requires the presence of a ligand (agonist or antagonist) whereas SMRT is able to mediate its effects in the presence or absence of ligands [7, 29-31]. The LBD also houses the nuclear export signal (NES) (amino acids 742-817) and the nuclear localization sequence (NLS), found at the junction between the hinge region and DBD (50 amino acids, 625-676) [7]. Upon ligand binding the NES becomes inactive and the NLS is bound by co-activators such as Filamin-A and importin-α. These interactions direct the nuclear localization of the AR [6, 7, 26, 31, 33, 34, 35]. Upon the loss of ligand interactions, the NES co-ordinates the shuttling of the AR to the cytoplasm where AR can tether to cytoskeletal proteins to again prepare for ligand binding [5,7].

The DBD (559-624) is comprised of two zinc fingers domains created by three α-helices and a 12 amino acid C-terminal extension [1]. The first zinc finger contains a P-Box motif for specific nucleotide interactions and the second, a D-Box motif which functions as a DBD/DBD site for receptor homodimerization [7]. It is thought that Lysine (Lys;K) 580 and Arginine (Arg;R) 585 in the first zinc finger bind respectively to the second and fifth nucleotide pairs in the first ARE repeat: GGTACA [22, 36-39]. The second zinc finger stabilizes the binding complex by making hydrophobic interactions with the first zinc finger and contributes to the specificity of receptor DNA binding [22, 39]. Due to the similarity of the hormone response elements (HREs) of the nuclear receptor family, there is an overlap of nucleic acid sequences in which these receptors can bind. Steroid receptors recognize a palindromic sequence spaced by three nucleotides [40]. The AR, glucocorticoid, mineralcorticoid and progesterone receptors recognize the 5′-TGTTCT-3′ core sequence [40]. However, it has been found that ARs can also recognize specific AREs that consist of two hexameric half-sites separated by 3 base pairs [41-45]. Although ligand specificity brings about hormone specific responses, the specificity of hormone receptors has been questioned as each receptor can bind to similar or the same sequence [45]. It is thought that protein-protein interactions play a role in discriminating AR and other steroid mediated effects [46, 47] to enable ARE dependent gene transcription rather than the activation of other HREs.

1.3. AR and post translational modifications

Despite the AR's role in genomic upregulation of androgen dependent gene transcription, its activation can signal through alternative means at the plasma membrane and cytoplasm (referred to as non-genomic signaling) [1]. For example, the AR can trigger intracellular calcium release and the activation of protein kinases such as the Mitogen Activated Protein Kinases (MAPK), Protein Kinase A (PKA), AKT and PKC [7]. Phosphorylation of the AR by MAPK, JNK, AKT, ERK, p38, increases AR response to low level of androgens, estrogens, and anti-androgens as well as enhances the recruitment of co-activators [7]. Furthermore, the AR itself is a downstream substrate for phosphorylation by receptor-tyrosine kinases and G-protein coupled receptor signaling. The phosphorylation of AR is mediated by the recruitment of kinases in the presence or absence of androgens. Phosphorylation at Serine (Ser) residues, Ser80, Ser93, and Ser641 is thought to protect the AR from proteolytic degradation [7, 48]. Alternatively, AR degradation is regulated by the phosphorylation of specific residues recognized by E3 ubiquitin ligase. For example, MDM2 E3 ubiquitin ligase promotes polyubiquitylation of the AR by recognizing AKT dependent phosphorylated serine [3,49]. Moreover, transactivation of the AR largely relies upon the phosphorylation of Ser213, Ser506, and Ser650 [7]. Phosphorylation of the AR is required for its effects within the nucleus and the AR should remain hyperphosphorylated to mediate its transcriptional role [3]. Studies have also shown constitutive phosphorylation of the AR at Ser94 as well as on other serine residues such as Ser16, 81, 256, 309, and 424. The loss of phosphorylation results in the loss of transcriptional activity and nuclear localization [3, 50-52]. Specifically, Yang et al., (2005) demonstrated that dephosphorylation of AR at the NTD by protein phosphatase 2A (PP2A), resulted in the loss of AR activity.

The AR receptors can also be acetylated, and sumoylated. These types of post translational modifications have also been shown to affect receptor stability and activity. The KXKK motif of the hinge region is a site for acetylation. Mutations of lysine to alanine reduced the transcriptional activity of AR by favoring NCoR interactions [3, 53]. Sumoylation of the AR is hormone dependent and competes with ubiquitination of lysine residues. Sumoylation is thought to repress AR activity. Disruption of sumoylation on Lys386 and Lys520 resulted in an increase in AR transactivation [3, 54].

1.4. AR in CaP progression

The efficacy of many CaP treatments is often temporary, as CaP cells often become refractory to hormone ablation therapies. The current therapeutics are largely targeted towards the inhibition of AR activation, such as anti-androgens, chemical castration (treatment with gonadotropin releasing hormone (GnRH) super agonists to inhibit testosterone secretion from the testes), or surgery (orchidectomy) [7]. AI-CaP or castration resistant CaP is thought to occur due to the androgen deprivation therapies as they may induce altered protein activity and expression in the cancer cells. Despite androgen blockade in AI-CaP patients, expressions of AR target genes such as PSA remain high. Furthermore, hormone refractory CaP continues to rely on AR expression, suggesting that the AR is necessary to maintain proliferative and anti-apoptotic effects. Therefore, CaP acquires the phenotype of oncogenic addiction to the AR for its continued growth and resistance to therapy. The progression of CaP from an hormone sensitive AD to a hormone resistant AI state is likely due to mechanisms involving alterations in AR expression, amplification, mutations, and/or AR activity.

AR mutations in primary CaP are relatively low when compared to metastatic CaP where frequencies are as high as 50% [1, 55-57]. Germline or somatic mutations of the AR leads to AR overexpression and hypersensitivity due to point mutations and promiscuous mutant AR proteins. Germline mutations of the AR are rarely found. Familial inheritance of CaP with at least two first degree relatives account for 20% of cases and transmission compatible with Mendellian inheritance is described to be 50% of the cases observed [3]. Genetic susceptibility seems to be more significant in patients <55 years old [3]. Recently, a R726L mutation was reported in only Finnish patients with sporadic or familial CaP [3, 58, 59]. Genomic alterations to the AR have been found in both non-coding and coding sequences such as polymorphisms of CAG and GGC repeats, single nucleotide polymorphisms, as well as silent and missense mutations [3, 58, 60, 61]. Koochekpour et al., (2010) screened 60 CaP patients of African-American and Caucasian families with a history of familial CaP. Using exon-specific PCR, bi-directional sequencing and restriction enzyme genotyping, they found that one African-American family had a novel germline AR misssense mutation (exon 2 of DBD A1675T; T559S) in three siblings with early onset CaP. This mutation was transmitted in an X-linked pattern and located at the N-terminal region of the DBD. Koochekpour et al., (2010) reason that the location of this particular mutation likely affected AR ligand binding.

Somatic mutations are largely single base substitutions: 49% at the LBD, 37% at the NTD, and 7% at the DBD [3]. For those CaP that harbor gain of function mutations the result is primarily an increase in ligand promiscuity. The AR is activated by testosterone and DHT; however, mutations in the LBD make the AR less stringent of its partners. For example, in LNCaP cells, a Threonine (Thr; T) to Alanine (Ala;A) mutation (T877A) caused the expansion of ligand binding activity [1, 8]. This mutation permitted AR activation by androgens, estrogens, progesterones as well as the non-steroidal antagonist, flutamide. A study by Gaddipati et al., (1994) found that 25% of patient metastatic tumors had a T877A mutation. Patients that were treated with flutamide often experienced a worsening of symptoms over time. Once flutamide was withdrawn, patients tended to do better. Interestingly, some patients also experienced a rise in serum PSA levels upon flutamide treatment. Taplin et al., (1999) studied patients that were on flutamide treatment relative to those that were not given this particular treatment. Tumor cells that had the T877A mutation increased in proliferation while patients who were not treated with flutamide harboured different mutations of the AR that were not activated by flutamide. Therefore, there seems to be a strong selective pressure for AR mutants arising from flutamide treatment such that discontinuation of flutamide resulted in tumor regression before growth resumed again. Other mutations such as the H874Y (Histadine to Tyrosine) mutation in the CWR22 cell line have been found to affect co-activator interactions by altering the conformation of Helix 12 of the LBD. Helix 12 regulates co-activator binding and creates a specific groove with helices 3, 4, and 5 [63-67]. Helix 12 rotates over the ligand binding pocket and assumes favorable or unfavorable positions depending on agonist or antagonist binding, respectively. Helix 12 mutations have also been detected in CaP patients, such as Q902R (Glutamine to Arginine), and M894D (Methionine to Aspartic Acid) (an androgen insensitive mutation) [56, 67, 68]. The importance of Helix 12 and the NTD-LBD interaction for AR activity is underscored by the fact that spontaneous mutations in Helix 12, NTD, and LBD caused either complete or partial androgen insensitivity [67, 68]. Additionally, a L701H mutation was also identified in conjunction with the T877A mutation in MDA CaP 2a cell lines [1, 69]. L701H mutation alone decreased the ability of AR to bind DHT, but increased binding of other non specific adrenal corticosteroids. The presence of the T877A mutation together with L701H potentiated this interaction by more than 300% as both mutations were located within the LBD [1, 70]. Hence, the susceptibility of the AR to minimize its ligand specificity in AI-CaP makes AR dependent disease progression difficult to treat. On the other hand, other anti-androgens such as Casodex (bicalutamide) do not seem to have the same response to T877A AR [1]. Novel truncated AR mutant, mRNA splice variants and mutant AR lacking exon 3 (coding for C-terminal portion of the DBD) tandem duplication have also been found in the 22RV1 cell line (AI-CaP), derived from the CWR22R cell line [3, 71]. Furthermore, an important study by Han et al., (2001) demonstrated that prostate tumors from a genetically engineered mouse model upon androgen ablation resulted in AR gene mutations within AR NTD. Specifically, amino acid substitution A229T and E231G (Glutamic Acid to Glycine) within the AR NTD signature motif: ARNSM (Ala-Arg-Asn-Ser-Met), increased ligand independent basal activity, whereas, E231G increased responsiveness to androgen receptor co-activator ARA160 and ARA70. The ARNSM motif is unique to the AR and the most highly conserved region of the AR NTD.

Another possible mechanism for the progression of AI disease is mediated by AR amplification. Overexpression of the AR causes hypersensitivity of the AR under low levels of androgens. Visakorpi et al., (1995) were the first to show that the AR was amplified in 305 hormone refractory tumors subsequent to androgen ablation therapy. Although these tumors were clinically presenting as AI-CaP, there was increased levels of the AR, and, continued proliferation of the tumor still required androgen. This suggested that some AR amplified tumors may require the presence of residual androgens that remain in the serum after monotherapy [1, 74]. Similarily, mouse models of CaP progression characterized by high expression of AR, increased AR stability, and AR nuclear localization, had hypersensitive tumor growth promoting effects upon DHT administration. DHT concentrations of 4 orders of magnitude lower were able to stimulate growth relative to DHT levels required for AD LnCaP cell proliferation [1, 75].

Although AR gene amplification and hypersensitivity serves to be a sound model for AI-CaP progression, the AR may be activated by alternative means including activation by co-regulators, increased androgen production, and/or intermediary downstream signaling pathways. Greater levels of co-activator expression such as SRC-1, ARA70, and TIF2 were demonstrated to be elevated in CaP and correlated with increased CaP grade, stage, and decreased disease free survival. For example, Cdk-activating phophatase B, an identified co-activator of the AR was overexpressed and also highly amplified in tumors with high Gleason scores [3]. Local production of androgens within the prostate can also increase AR transactivation by compensating for decreased serum testosterone resulting from androgen ablation therapy. Studies have shown that serum testosterone levels can decrease 95%, contrasting the DHT levels within prostate tissue which only reduce by 60% [1, 76]. Locke et al., (2008) demonstrated that there was de novo and organ synthesis of androgens in LNCaP xenograft mouse models, suggesting that CaP cells had steroidogenic properties that enable them to survive in androgen depleted environments. Moreover, this was also indicative of greater levels of intratumoral 5-alpha-reductase activity. It is likely then, that during AI-CaP disease progression, there is a switch in androgen source whereby testicular androgens are replaced by prostatic androgen. Bennett et al., (2010) have deemed this as 'androgen self-sufficient'. There is also a hypothesis that conversion of adrenal steroids can sustain the androgen signal by supplying adrenal androgens such as DHEA and androstenedione [78]. After castration, adrenal androgens could account for as much as 40% of the total DHT in the prostate [76, 78].

Hormone receptors that are activated by ligand independent mechanisms are known as 'outlaw' receptors [1]. Certain growth factors such as Insulin Growth Factor (IGF)-1, Keratinocyte Growth Factor (KGF), and Epidermal Growth Factor (EGF) have been demonstrated to activate AR and induce the expression of AR target genes. Culig et al., (1994) showed that there was a 5-fold increase in PSA levels in LNCaP cells upon IGF-1 stimulation. Moreover, the addition of Casodex abolished the activation of the AR by IGF-1, KGF and EGF, indicating that the LBD was necessary for this activation. Overexpression of these growth factors has been observed in CaP; however, it is unclear whether it is the AR pathway or indirect downstream effects that are mediating tumorigenesis. In fact, patients with AI-CaP can fail Casodex therapy suggesting that other mechanisms are in play for ligand independent activation of the AR.

Furthermore, patients who received androgen ablation therapy have tumor cells that overexpress growth factor receptors, the receptor tyrosine kinases. Craft et al., (1999) demonstrated that an AI-CaP cell line, generated from xenografts implanted in castrated mice, consistently overexpressed Her-2/neu (from the EGF receptor family of receptor tyrosine kinases) [1]. Interestingly, AD-CaP cell lines could also be converted to AI-CaP cells by overexpressing Her-2/neu. This pathway was not blocked by Casodex, which indicated that the LBD of the AR was not necessary to transduce the effects of Her-2/neu. Although Trastuzumab (Herceptin) is used primarily to treat breast cancer, Herceptin had anti-proliferative effects on AD- and AI-CaP xenografts when combined with the chemotherapeutic drug paclitaxel. Yeh et al., (1999) believe that Her-2/neu activated AR via the MAPK pathway, as inhibitors of MAPK decreased HER-2/neu mediated activation of the AR. In effect, a positive feedback loop is created where the AR can activate kinases and in turn, where kinases can activate the AR through its phosphorylation (in the presence or absence of ligand), regardless of the varying levels of androgens [1].

The AR pathway is thought to be in interplay with other signaling pathways. AR activation due to cross regulation by receptor tyrosine kinases and their downstream effectors provides alternative and sustained routes for AR activation despite androgen depletion. Currently, there has been accumulating evidence that the phosphatidylinositol 3-kinase (PI3K)-AKT pathway plays a significant role in CaP tumor progression. The cross-regulatory mechanism by which the PI3K/Akt pathway modulates the expression and activity of AR is a novel area of study. Growing evidence continues to support the increased role of the PI3K/Akt and AR signaling pathways in mediating the progression of CaP to castrate resistant disease.

2. Phosphatidylinositol 3-kinase (PI3K)-AKT pathway: A brief overview

Evidence has largely supported the phosphatidylinositol 3-kinase (PI3K)-AKT signalling pathway as a key regulatory system essential to mammalian cell proliferation, survival, and metabolism. The gain- or loss-of-function of components of this pathway lead to neoplastic transformation in a wide spectrum of human cancers, including CaP. Briefly, the canonical PI3K/AKT pathway is activated by mitogenic growth factor stimulation of receptor tyrosine kinases (RTKs), the most common RTKs include Epidermal Growth Factor Receptor (EGFR, ERBB1), Her2 (EGFR-2, ERBB2), KIT, PDGFRα, and MET. Receptor activation causes RTKs to dimerize and undergo autophosphorylation at tyrosine residues and enables interaction with Src Homology 2 (SH2) domain-containing molecules. The signal then becomes transduced, through the oncogene, RAS, and ultimately leads to the conversion of membrane phosphatidylinositol-bis-phosphate (PI(3,4)P_2; PIP_2) to phosphatidylinositol-tri-phosphate (PI(3,4,5)P_3; PIP_3) by PI3K. The presence of PIP_3 mediates the recruitment of AKT (also known as PKB) to the plasma membrane and its subsequent phosphorylation by 3-Phosphoinositide- Dependent protein Kinase (PDK) 1 and PDK 2 at Threonine 308 (T308) and Serine 473 (S473), respectively. Activated AKT or phosphorylated AKT (P-AKT) is the central effector of many downstream signaling pathways regulating protein synthesis, cell cycle, cell death, cell growth, and cell survival [summarized in Reference 82]. The loss and/or mutation of the tumor suppressor

http://dx.doi.org/10.5772/53483

protein and negative regulator of the PI3K/AKT pathway, Phosphatase and Tensin homolog deleted on chromosome TEN (PTEN), is a common event in various cancers, causing the constitutive activation of PI3K/Akt signalling. PTEN, a dual protein and lipid phosphatase, dephosphorylates PIP_3 to PIP_2, hence, buffering the proliferative and transformative effects of the PI3K. This review will primarily focus on the most studied canonical PI3K/AKT pathway.

2.1. Phosphatidylinositol 3-kinases

The PI3Ks are enzymes that are grouped into three classes (I-III). Most members of this family are bound to regulatory subunits which determine its specificty and function [83-85]. Class I PI3Ks are subdivided into IA and IB and are members to the canonical PI3K/AKT pathway. They are heterodimeric serine and threonine kinases comprising a catalytic subunit, p110, and a regulatory subunit encoded by the PIK3CA and PIK3R1 genes, respectively [83]. The four isoforms of p110 (α-δ) and their regulatory subunits have distinct structure-function domains and specificity. For p110α, β, and δ the most commonly associated regulatory subunit has been identified as p85 [83]. Specific isoforms of the p85 adaptor subunit (p85α, p85β, p50α, p55α, or p55γ) facilitate the interaction with RTKs as well as the p110 catalytic domain isoforms [86]. The p85 subunit directly associates with active RTKs through the physical interaction of its SRC homology 2 (SH2) domain at phosphotyrosine residues of RTKs [87]. The consensus sequence has been identified to be YXXM [87]. In particular, Class IA PI3Ks' p85α subunit encodes an adaptor-like protein that has two SH2 domains and an inter-SH2 domain that binds constitutively to the p110 catalytic subunit [87]. The two splice variants (p55α and p50α) retain such regions but lack an amino terminal SH3 domain (mediates the binding of proline rich sequences) and a breakpoint cluster region (BCR) homology domain (a protein-protein interaction motif) [87]. The p110 isoforms (α, β, δ) have the same basic structure, including a kinase domain and a C2 domain for membrane anchoring [87].

Class I PI3Ks, once activated by RTKs (Class IA) or G-protein-coupled receptors (GPCRs, [Class IB]), have preferred substrates, in particular, the non-phosphorylated phosphatidylinositol (PI), inositol monophosphate (PI(4)P), and phosphatidyl-bis-phosphate ($PI(4,5)P_2$), and mediate the addition of a phosphate group in the D-3 position of the inositol ring to generate PI(3)P, PIP_2, and PIP_3, respectively [83, 88]. PIP_3 is a potent second messenger in the cell and the predominant arbitrator of PI3K signalling. Class IA PI3K p110α domain isoform is the most mutated amongst cancers, causing the kinase to be more active [86, 89, 90] and perpetuating a constitutively active PI3K pathway. Class II and III PI3Ks, on the other hand, are less studied and are recognized for their involvement in membrane trafficking and receptor internalization, and, vesicle trafficking, respectively [91-93]. PI3Ks within Class II generate $PI(3,4)P_2$ from PI(3)P and can also produce PI(3)P from PI. However, they cannot recognize $PIP(4,5)P_2$ as substrate to produce PIP and PIP_2. Class II PI3Ks use only PI to convert it to PIP [83, 94]. Furthermore, unlike Class I PI3Ks, Class II PI3Ks do not require a regulatory subunit but comprise three distinct isoforms to mediate their functions. Class IA PI3K will be discussed in this review and will be referred to as PI3K unless otherwise stated.

PI3K activity is normally strictly regulated within the cell by growth factor-receptor interactions [95]. As such, the majority of the PI3K is inactive in the cytosplasm and remains removed from its plasma membrane substrates. Moreover, only a small fraction of these PI3Ks become activated upon growth factor stimulation [95]. Currently, it is thought that there are preformed inactive p85-p110 complex present in the cytoplasm, whereby ligand mediated activation of kinase activity and transphosphorylation of RTK's cytoplasmic tail recruits p85-p110 complexes to the receptor by the SH2 domain of p85 [87]. This brings PI3K in close proximity to its lipid substrates; moreover, it is reasoned that the RTK-p85 interaction may remove an inhibitory effect of p85 on p110 kinase activity [87, 96]. This is thought to involve conformational changes in the p85-p110 complex through the SH3 and BCR domains.

Mutations have now been identified in the genes coding for the p110 and p85 subunits which have shed light on the pathology of metabolic diseases and cancer [83, 93]. These mutations occur at a frequency of 5-25% in common cancers such as breast, endometrium and large intestine [83]. Activating mutations or 'hot spots' of PIK3CA occur at a frequency of 80% and are located in the PI3K catalytic kinase domain, H1074 and the helical domain, E542 and E545 [93]. Both mutations have been demonstrated to drive transformation *in vitro* [93, 97]. As a result, the lipid kinase activity is increased [83, 89, 98-102], downstream signalling no long requires upstream growth factor stimulation, and increased oncogenic potency. Expression of these hot spot mutants induced oncogenic transformation in avian and mammalian cell culture and transgenic expression of H1047R p110α in mouse models induced adenocarcinoma of the lung [83, 103]. As such, hot spot mutations then can be suggested to function as drivers of cellular transformation to a more oncogenic phenotype. Conversely, mutational inactivation of the ability of p110α to interact with RAS has the opposite effect by decreasing the oncogenicity of helical domain mutants and minimizing downstream signaling [83]. On the other hand, kinase domain mutants become independent of RAS binding, and its oncogenicity is preserved [83]. PIK3R1 mutations occur within a stretch of six residues (560-565) located in the inter-SH2 domain of p85 [83]. This area is the contact point for p85 with the C2 domain of p110α whereby mutation leads to improper binding to p110α and relieve the inhibitory interaction of p85 [83]. Enhanced AKT signalling, stimulation of cell replication, and oncogenic transformation were some of the observed effects [83, 104, 105]. As such, p85 mutations in the inter-SH2 domain can be thought to be equivalent to activation mutations of the p110α C2 domain.

2.2. Phosphatase and tensin homolog deleted on chromosome TEN (PTEN)

The tumor suppressor, PTEN, is a dual phosphatase that has activity for both lipid and protein substrates. It is a gene that is lost in both heritable and spontaneous cancers where germline mutations cause autosomal dominant hamartoma tumor syndromes and where spontaneous missense mutations occur frequently in the central nervous system (20%), endometrial (39%), colorectal (9%), skin (17%), prostate (14%), and breast (6%) cancers [95]. Its role within the PI3K pathway serves to negatively regulate PI3K signalling. PTEN functions to remove phosphates in position 3' from phosphoinositides [93, 106, 107], therefore, returning PIP_3 to PIP_2 and terminating the PI3K signal. Monoallelic loss (loss of heterozygosity) and/or mutation of PTEN thus, leads to a hyperactive PI3K pathway to drastically impact tumor growth and disease severity. PTEN mutants that retain protein tyrosine phosphatase activity but lose the ability to dephosphorylate PIP_3 are found in many tumours indicating that PTEN lipid phosphatase activity is required for tumour suppression.

PTEN is tightly regulated at the transcriptional level as well as by post translational modification, primarily through ubiquitylation. Incidentally, the levels of PTEN are controlled by PI3K itself, through the regulation of the transcription factor NF-κB, while, PPARβ/δ agonists and TNFα repress PTEN expression [93, 108]. Furthermore, the activity of PTEN is also controlled by the PI3K pathway. In p85 conditional knockout mice, the loss of p85 resulted in PTEN activity, while loss of p110δ isoform regulated PTEN activity through a RhoA-ROCK-depedent signaling [93, 109]. Currently, NEDD4-1 is the first and only identified E3 ligase for PTEN [93, 110]. Similar to PTEN, NEDD4-1 is also regulated by the PI3K pathway, thus representing a positive feedback for PTEN degradation and PI3K activation [93, 111]. More often than not, heterozygous alterations of PTEN are most common in the initial steps of tumorigenesis. Surprisingly, complete PTEN deletion does not have pro-tumorigenic effect. For example actute PTEN loss within prostate cells leads to a strong p53 dependent senescence response that opposes cancer progression. Hence, it can be suggested that tumors may not select for a complete loss of function of PTEN during the initial states of tumorigenesis. For example, in CaP patients, approximately 70% of tumors have heterozygous alteration in PTEN at presentaiton and then lose the other allele at later stages [93].

The co-existence of both PIK3CA mutations and PTEN loss has been observed in various cancers. This suggests that these two genetic aberrations are not completely redundant and may have additional selective advantage [95]. Yuan and Cantley, (2008) postulate that PTEN and p110α exist in a negative feedback loop to regulate pathway activity, such that any alterations to these enzymes results in heightened oncogenic potency of the PI3K pathway.

2.3. AKT/PKB

The formation of PIP_3 is the central initiating event which functions to recruit plekstrin homology (PH) domain containing proteins to the plasma membrane. Of relevance here, is AKT/PKB, as it is the critical mediator of signal tranduction events downstream the PI3K cascade. There are three members of the AKT family (AKT1, AKT2, and AKT3) and they are broadly expressed to have some isoform specific features [87]. AKT1 is the major isoform implicated in cancers, whereas AKT2 is more so involved in insulin signaling and glucose transport. AKT3 on the other hand has well known features and functions, however is thought to play a specific role in brain tissue [86, 112].

The AKT gene encodes a serine/threonine kinase with an amino-terminal PH domain, a central catalytic domain, and a carboxyl-terminal regulatory domain. The regulation of AKT function is two- fold, requiring its translocation to the plasma membrane and its sequential phosphorylation at Threonine 308 (T308) and Serine 473 (S473). Within unstimulated cells, AKT is constitutively phosphorylated at S124 and T450. Upon PIP_3 formation, there is direct interaction of AKT to PIP_3 via is PH domain. Here, PDK1 phosphorylates AKT on T308. The phosphorylation of T308 is a priming event to mediate the phosphorylation of S473 by PDK2, now thought to be the mammalian target of rapamycin complex 2 (mTORC2). This secondary event is necessary for maximal activation of the kinase, increasing AKT activity 10-fold [86, 113,

114]. Once activated AKT has many substrates within the cytoplasm and nucleus, including those that regulate apoptosis, proliferation, and protein translation. Although the activation of AKT has been well established, there is little known regarding the dephosphorylation of AKT as no AKT specific phosphatase has been identified. However heat-shock protein 90 (HSP90) has been demonstrated to protect AKT from dephosphorylation by the ubiquitous phosphatase, PP2A.

The activation of AKT regulates many cellular processes including cell proliferation and survival, cell size and glucose homeostasis, metabolism, angiogenesis, and tissue invasion [86, 93]. Amplification and mutations of AKT have been reported for pancreas, ovarian, head and neck and breast cancers. This includes a recently identified missense mutation to the PH domain of AKT1 (E17K) [95]. Such a mutation resulted in constitutive association of AKT with the plasma membrane and its prolonged activation. The biological effects of AKT activation relevant to cancer is primarily associated with cell survival, proliferation and growth. First, AKT functions as an anti-apoptotic response to various stimuli. This is through a series of phosphorylation and inhibition events of key pro-apoptotic proteins including, BAD, MDM2 and members of the Forkhead family of proteins.

BAD is a member Bcl-2 family of pro-apoptotic protein where these members form non-function hetero-dimer complexes with the survival factor BCL-X_L [87]. Once AKT phosphorylates BAD on S136, it prevents the interaction of BAD with BLC-X_L to restore the anti-apoptotic function of BCL-X_L [86, 115]. AKT also phosphorylates the pro-death enzyme, caspase 9, and inhibits its catalytic activity; this is in addition to preventing the nuclear localization of the Forkhead family of transcription factor, FKHR which transcriptionally inhibits the expression of pro-apoptotic proteins, BIM and FAS ligand. Alternatively, an indirect mechanism of AKT regulation of apoptosis is mediated by the NF-κB pathway and p53. Specifically, phosphorylation of and hence, the activation of IκB kinase (IκK) results in the degradation of NF-κB inhibitor, IκB, causing the nuclear translocation of NF-κB and the expression of anti-apoptotic genes. The pro-apoptotic effects of p53 tumour suppressor protein are mediated by AKT phosphorylation of the p53 binding protein MDM2. MDM2 is a negative regulator of p53 function as it targets p53 for ubiquitin mediated proteosomal degradation through its E3 ubiquitin ligase activity. The phosphorylation of MDM2 increases the efficiency by which MDM2 translocates to the nucleus thereby enhancing p53 degradation.

The proliferative effects of AKT activation can be attributed to its role by inactivating the cell cycle inhibitor p27 and p21, and, by inhibiting the enzyme, glycogen synthase kinase (GSK) 3β at its Serine 9 phosphoryaltion site. The regulation of cell cycle progression is through cyclin-cyclin-dependent kinase (CDK) complexes and CDK inhibitors (CKI). p27and p21 are CKIs that become phosphorylated by AKT and through indirect mechanisms, AKT phosphorylation can modulate the expression of CKIs as well as their activities. Phosphorylation of p27 renders it inactive and promotes cell cycle entry. Additionally, phosphorylation of the transcription factor, FOXO3A, by AKT causes the nuclear expulsion of the transcription factor, and therefore decreases the expression of p27 [116]. Alongside CKIs, cyclin D1 levels are important for G1/S phase transition through the cell cycle. AKT has an important role in preventing cyclin D1 degradation by inhibiting the cyclin D1 kinase, GSK3β. This prevents the phosphorylation

http://dx.doi.org/10.5772/53483

of cyclin D1 thereby increasing its levels to enable cell cycle progression. Interestingly, cyclin D1 expression is also tightly controlled by FOXO3A. Upon AKT phosphorylation of FOXO, its exclusion from the nucleus increases cyclin D1 expression. In effect, FOXO3A is considered a transcriptional repressor for this gene.

The significance of AKT in cancer progression is further heightened by its role in cell growth and metabolism. In highly proliferating tumor cells, there is rapid synthesis of macromolecules to meet the biosynthetic demands required by the cell. Incidently, AKT is one of the main regulators of protein translation and ribosome biogenesis [93], facilitating the means for cell growth. This is primarily achieved through the serine/threonine kinase, mammalian target of rapamycin (mTOR or FRAP1) Complex 1, which is composed of the protein kinase mTOR and a series of interactors. This complex serves as a molecular sensor of nutrient availability and in effect, modulates protein synthesis. It is unlikely that the PI3K/AKT pathway is the sole simulator of mTOR activity. Nonetheless, AKT's phosphorylation of two independent substrates of this complex contributes to the oncogenic phenotype. Specifically, AKT phosphorylates and inactivates the GTPase-activating protein (GAP) Tuberous Sclerosis Complex (TSC) 2 which forms a complex with TSC1 to inhibit the GTPase, Ras-homolog enriched in brain (Rheb). Rheb then directly interacts with mTOR and activates mTORC1 through the inhibition of FKBP38, the negative regulator of mTORC1. Alternatively, the phosphorylation and inhibition of another negative regulator of mTORC1, PRAS40 (proline-rich AKT substrate of 40kDa), enhances the activity of mTORC1 through its competition with GTPase Rheb. Altogether then, AKT promotes the activation of mTORC1 which initiates the translational machinery to produce ribosomes and increase the rate of protein synthesis. REFS

2.4. Mammalian Target of Rapamycin (mTOR)

mTOR is a member of two distinct complexes, mTOR Complex 1 (mTORC1) and mTOR Complex 2 (mTORC2) [83, 117]. It is thought that the mTORC1 complex plays a more dominant role in tumor progression while the mTORC2 complex is more significant to mediating signals to the cytoskeleton [116] and now identified as the factor responsible for the phosphorylation of AKT at S473. This phosphorylation event maximizes the activity of AKT and opens its targets to include PRAS40 and FOXO [83]. Moreover, it is another mechanism through which to provide positive feedback on the PI3K pathway [86,113].

The mTORC1 pathway is a central point of signal integration for growth factor signalling, energy state (AMP levels), and, nutrient and oxygen availability [118] which are fundamental for regulating tumor cell growth. The particular interest for this pathway has been largely determined by the discovery of the specific inhibitor, rapamycin, which blocks mTORC1 activity through yet unknown mechanisms. mTORC1 is comprised of Regulatory Associated Protein of TOR (RAPTOR), LST8 and PRAS40 [83]. The complex itself has many substrates, which upon its activation phosphorylates and activates S6 kinases (S6K) 1 and 2 (activation of protein translation and ribosome biogenesis), as well as inactivates 4E binding protein (4EBP) 1, 4EBP2, 4EBP3, which releases the inhibition of eukaryotic intiation factor 4E (eIF4E). mTOR dependent protein synthesis affects 5' untranslated polypyrimidine tracts of complex secondary mRNA structures. Such mRNA structures require eIF4A helicase activity together with eukaryotic initiation factors eIF4E and eIF4G to from the EIF4F initation complex. Altogether, the main effect is to upregulated protein synthesis.

Although the PI3K/AKT pathway serves to activate the mTORC1 pathway, mTORC1 itself negatively regulated the PI3K pathway. Over the years, studies have shown that mTORC1 inhibition can lead to PI3K activation. Moreover, mTOR activity can be suppressed by PI3K inhibitors such as wortmannin and LY294002 [87]. However, it is unclear whether the mechanism of activation of mTOR by AKT can completely drive tumorigenesis. As rapamycin can inhibit AKT dependent cancers, it is presumed that in some part mTORC1 does have tumorigenic effects. Although there is correlation between increased translation and tumorigeneisis, whether this is sufficient for increased cancer susceptibility is yet to be determined.

3. The PI3K/Akt signaling pathway and prostate cancer

In the recent years, emerging evidence has strongly linked the deregulation of the PI3K pathway to prostate carcinogenesis and castrate resistance, although its precise role remains elusive. Two components of this pathway, PTEN and PI3K, are currently the focus of intense investigation and this section aims to address their role in the pathology of prostate cancer.

3.1. The incidence of genetic *PTEN* alteration

The deletions involving the chromosome 10q, which hosts the *PTEN* locus, 10q23, in CaP is a frequently observed phenomenon. Modifications to *PTEN* in various stages of CaP have been characterized to include both homozygous and hemizygous deletions, as well as inactivating mutations. Although the incidence and the modes of these alterations have been inconsistent across studies, the severity of *PTEN* loss seems to correlate with disease progression [119]. Whereas locally confined CaP presents homozygous deletions of *PTEN* ranging from 0% to 15%, the incidence within metastases can increase up to 30%. Likewise, heterozygosity loss occurs in 13% of the locally confined cases and up to 39% in metastatic phenotypes [120]. Further support has comefrom interphase fluorescence in situ hybridization (FISH) analysis of histologic sections, which reported genomic deletion of *PTEN* in 23% of high-grade intraepithelial neoplasia (HGPIN) and 68% of prostate tumors [121]. Recently, Han et al., (2009) demonstrated that *PTEN* deletion occurs in 9% of premalignant prostate, a proportion which increases to 17% in localized CaP and to 54% when metastasized. Functional loss of *PTEN* can also be generated through point mutations, which are seen in upwards of 16% of primary tumor and 20% to 30% in advanced stages [120]. Taken together, these studies suggest the deletion of *PTEN* is likely a late genetic occurrence in CaP progression.

3.1.1. Mechanism of PTEN loss

Although the incidence *PTEN* alterations in CaP have been extensively characterized in the past ten years, the mechanism by which genomic *PTEN* deletions occur remains to be elucidated. The high frequency of large-scale chromosomal events leading to the loss of *PTEN* locus suggests unique features that may enhance DNA rearrangements at 10q23. Yoshimoto et al.,

(2012) identified recombination hotspots known as segmental duplications (SD) 17 and 18 to be located between *PTEN* and *BMPR1A*. The SDs are typically part of a 1-400 kB genomic region exhibiting over 90% homology [123, 124] responsible for improving the likelihood of constitutional microdeletion events [125]. Utilizing meta-analysis of published prostate cancer genomes to map 10q23 deletion sites and FISH for confirmation, Yoshimoto et al., (2012) demonstrates SD17-SD18 colocalizes with a deletion breakpoint hotspot occurring in 69% of PTEN losses, which suggests SD17 and SD18 facilitate homology-dependent rearrangements of DNA that lead to a *PTEN* deletion breakpoint. The presence of these SDs thus destabilizes the genome, predisposing CaP progenitors to genomic microdeletions that ultimately result in *PTEN* loss. Subsequent attenuated *PTEN* expression has been shown to further diminish genomic stability [126], leading to the acquirement of other chromosomal abnormalities [127]. Cells bearing homozygous *PTEN* deletion would have significant stronger growth advantage and predominate due a constitutively activation of the PI3K pathway. This sequence of events may explain the progressive loss of *PTEN* as prostate turmorigenesis continues.

3.1.2. The clinical and cellular impact of PTEN loss

The functional loss of *PTEN* in CaP has been shown by numerous studies to confer poor clinical prognosis and predict disease progression. Genomic *PTEN* deletions studied through either immunohistochemistry or FISH have been correlated with increased Akt phosphorylation, higher Gleason grade, biochemical relapse, angiogenesis, and larger tumor sizes [123, 128-132]. Specifically, Yoshimoto et al., (2007) demonstrated that haploinsufficiency of *PTEN* is associated with an earlier onset of biochemical relapse after prostatectomy while bi-allelic deletion of *PTEN* is associated with an even shorter time to relapse. Additionally, loss of *PTEN* near the time of prostatectomy correlated strongly with extraprostatic extension and seminal vesicle invasion.

Decreased expression of PTEN profiled by high-density tissue microarray was shown to also increase the risk of tumor recurrence after radical prostatectomy [129]. Similar findings were reached in immunohistochemical evaluation of PTEN expression in CaP glands. Using a nested case-control study, the group Chaux et al., (2012) found patients with reduced PTEN expression was at a higher risk of relapse, independent of identified clinicopathological covariates. Their previous study also linked attenuated PTEN levels to faster onset of metastasis in CaP patients [134]. Additionally, the use of transgenic mouse models have served to recapitulate features of PTEN loss in humans and concomitantly fostered a greater understanding of the PI3K pathway alongside clinical studies. Prostate specific PTEN$^{-/-}$ null knockout mice proceeds linearly from acquiring prostatic intraepithelial neoplasia (PIN) to adenocarcinoma to metastasis, mimicking the disease progression in human CaP [135]. The prostate tumors also exhibited temporary regression following androgen ablation, but eventually proliferated androgen independently. Further, mice with one deactivated *PTEN* allele combined with *p27KIP1* loss exhibit accelerated spontaneous neoplastic transformation and tumorigenesis [136]. These studies of mouse and human prostate cancers combine to emphasize haploinsufficiency of *PTEN* as a key predictor of disease states in prostate cancer.

3.2. The role of PI3K isoforms

The catalytic isoform p110β and its regulatory complex p85α have been shown to mediate AR transactivation in the presence of androgens [137]. Overexpression of wild type p110β led to androgen-independent AR transactivation while the overexpression of p110α gene showed no effects. Interestingly, short interference RNA (siRNA) disruption of p110β gene in prostate cancer cells abrogated tumor progression *in vivo*. Moreover, clinical analysis of tumor samples linked high p110β and p85α expression at the mRNA and protein level to malignant prostate tumors, metastasis and poor differentiation.

Conditional knockout mouse models of p110β have further provided insight into the oncogenic potential of the catalytic subunit. Prostate epithelium remained normal in the absence p110β alone while PTEN loss alone resulted in tumor growth in the anterior lobe by 12 weeks; subsequent ablation of the *p110β* gene rescued PTEN null anterior prostate from tumorigenesis [138]. Increased phosphorylation of Akt on Ser473 was achieved through PTEN loss while additional ablation of *p110β* attenuated Akt activation. These results are not attributable to changes in the p110α subunit as minimal changes in tumor growth and Akt phosphorylation were observed upon *p110α* ablation. One study ascribed the differential functions of the p110α and p110β catalytic subunits to the distinct pools of PIP3 they generate [139]. The p110α, in response to growth factor stimuli, will cause an immediate flux of PIP3 coupled with efficient Akt phosphorylation, whereas p110β will maintain a basal level of PIP3 with minimal effects on Akt phosphorylation. Together with the observation that p110β-specific inhibitors effectively reduce Akt phosphorylation in the absence of *PTEN in vitro* [139], oncogenic transformation of prostate cancer cells upon PTEN loss is likely derived from the p110β-catalyzed pool of PIP3 [138]. These data collectively support distinct functionalities of the p110α and p110β catalytic subunits in PI3K/AKT signaling.

Recent studies have also shed light onto the third isoform of PI3K catalytic subunit, p110δ. Tzenaki et al., (2012) reported CaP cells that contain high levels of p110δ activity have dampened PTEN functionality. Treatment with p110δ -specific inhibitor in DU145 cells promoted PTEN activation, reduced Akt phosphorylation and inhibited cell proliferation. In another cell line (22Rv1) with wild-type PTEN and low p110δ expression, measured basal PTEN activity was comparatively higher than that in DU145 cells. Inhibition of p110δ in 22Rv1 likewise did not affect Akt phosphorylation status or cell proliferative abilities. Hence, the development of p110δ -selective inhibitors may hold promise since blocking p110δ activity will also indirectly inhibit other catalytic isoforms through PTEN activation.

4. PI3K/AKT and AR Signalling axis

The role of the PI3K/AKT pathway in CaP cell proliferation, survival and progression from AD to AI disease has been linked to androgen receptor (AR) transcriptional activity, stability and expression. This section of the review will discuss the various modes of crosstalk between the PI3K-Akt and AR axis.

4.1. PI3K/PTEN and AR

The activation of Akt has provided a mechanistic link between PI3K and AR transactivation. However, other modes of interaction have been shown. AR can directly interact with the p85 regulatory subunit of PI3K. Upon their binding, the AR enhances PI3K enzyme activity to ultimately upregulate Akt phosphorylation [141]. Conversely, EGFR stimulated PI3K activity was decreased in PC-3 cells transfected with wildtype AR relative to AR null PC-3 cell line [141-142]. PI3K activity was further reduced upon R1881 treatment, suggesting AR activation as a negative regulator of PI3K stimulation. The role of androgens within the AR-PI3K axis has also shown their significance in modulating cell proliferation and growth. Multiple reports have demonstrated that androgens enhance PI3K activity and increase downstream Akt phosphorylation. In NIH3T3 fibroblasts, there was rapid activation of the PI3K/AKT pathway upon androgen stimulation. While this required the presence of the AR, AR transactivation was not essential [141, 143]. Low concentration of androgen further stimulated the association of the AR with Src and PI3K, which triggered the cells into S-phase entry [141, 143].

The negative regulator of the PI3K pathway, the PTEN tumor suppressor gene, as discussed previous is frequently inactivated in CaP as well as in CaP cell lines which include PC-3 and LNCaP. Functional loss of PTEN is associated with increased AKT phosphorylation, higher Gleason score, and poor prognosis [120, 144]. The development of conditional mouse models of PTEN -/- has shown that PTEN alone can drive the progression of CaP through invasion, metastasis and AI proliferation [82]. Although there was heightened PI3K activity, there was continued evidence of AR gain-of-function despite reduced steroid ligand levels [45, 82]. For example, prostatic epithelium in PTEN-/- mice was still sensitive to androgen withdrawal. As such, Mullholland et al., (2006) suggest that while the AR remains functional and sensitive to androgens, the PI3K/AKT and AR oncogenic signaling may complement and compensate for one another during the time of androgen ablation therapy. This is supported by studies demonstrating cells lacking PTEN had elevated PI3K/AKT axis activity upon androgen withdrawal [45, 46, 82]. Hence, PTEN loss may allow for epithelium with sufficient PI3K/AKT signaling to maintain cell proliferation and promote AR gain of function [82].

Currently, there is no direct method that supports PTEN loss for promoting AR-specific gene activation. However, CaP xenograft studies have shown that amplification of AR does occur [82, 147] under a PTEN null background, which can be correlated to increased AR stabilization [82]. Li et al, (2001) demonstrated that PTEN itself can negatively regulate AR gene targets such as PSA, reduce the nuclear localization of the AR and promote receptor degradation through caspase 3 or the proteosome [82]. Alternative to AR amplification and stabilization, the loss of PTEN may also contribute to AR activation through the various coregulators of the AR, this includes ARA70 [149] and ARA54 [150]. Such regulation by PTEN would allow for heightened AR response to low androgen concentrations or responsiveness to non-androgen ligands. On the other hand, at low androgen levels, AR expression alone can also stimulate cell proliferation (Denmeade et al., 1996) while PTEN restoration induced apoptosis and growth arrest [151]. However, in the presence of androgens, PTEN expression was sufficient to reduce cell proliferation but not induce apoptotic response [82, 148, 152]. PTEN loss then, results in an indirect AR gain-of-function phenotype by establishing an environment that may increase AR oncogenicity and CaP metastatic potential.

4.2. AKT and AR cross-talk

The regulation of the AR by Akt through direct and indirect modes of interactions has been demonstrated in literature. These include, but not limited to 1) direct phosphorylation of the AR by AKT, 2) AKT/mTOR dependent regulation of the AR, 3) AR interaction with FOXO family of transcription factors downstream AKT, and 4) AR regulation by AKT via the Wnt/GSK3β/β-catenin cross-talk.

4.2.1. AKT and direct AR phosphorylation

AKT binds to the AR to directly phosphorylate at AR consensus sites, S213 and S791. Upon phosphorylation by AKT, the AR becomes transcriptionally active under physiological androgen concentrations. However, a study Xin et al, (2006) demonstrated that AR phosphorylations at S213 and S791 were not critical for tumor progression, which indicated that AR phosphorylation may not be the sole regulatory event inducing AR transcriptional activity [153, 141]. Alternatively, at high androgen concentrations, AKT can protect CaP cells from apoptosis and suppress AR transcriptional activity by phosphorylation at S210 and S790 [49]. Lin et al, (2002) also demonstrated that AR phosphorylation by AKT resulted in MDM2 mediated ubiquitlyation of the AR, leading to its proteosomal degradation. Taken together, these data indicate AKT-mediated regulation of AR activity is dependent on the external environment.

4.2.2. PI-3K/AKT/mTOR and AR

A potent nutrient and growth/survival pathway kinase, mTOR has been implicated in the progression of several types of cancer. Interestingly, it has been identified as a regulator of AI-CaP growth, but not CaP growth, by Ghosh et al. (2005). Further, it has been implicated in regulating the progression to androgen-independent disease [155-156] alongside AR signaling. There are three key routes through which mTOR could potentially interact with AR signaling: through its kinase activity as mTORC1 or mTORC2, post-transcriptional regulation via regulation of translation factors, or indirectly through a signaling cascade. Several broad studies have implicated a connection between the two molecules. Sircar et al. (2009) showed that AKT activation, mTOR activity and AR nuclear expression concurrently occur in several PTEN-null patient samples. Additionally, Müller et al. (2012) demonstrated that loss of phosphorylation of Ser2448 of mTOR, an inhibitory alteration, resulted in decreased levels of cellular AR in ERG-fusion-positive prostate cancer cells. Kaarbø et al. (2010) also show a reduction of AR by mTOR in LNCaP cells. Furthermore, they demonstrate that mTOR inhibtion increases ligand-dependent AR activity.

Work by Wang et al. (2008) further demonstrated evidence of a connection between mTORC1 signaling and AR by demonstrating an induction of AR activity by rapamycin. The application of rapamycin to LNCaP and C4-2 cells resulted in inhibition of the mTORC1 pathway, but an increase in AR transcriptional activity. They further determined that this relationship was through AKT. Inhibition of mTORC1 by rapamycin was shown to activate a parallel AR-mediated survival pathway putatively downstream of mTORC2. This potentially matches results by Müller et al. (2012), who showed that loss of mTOR deactivation resulted in AR reduction, suggesting an inverse relationship between the two molecules. Upon dual inhibition using rapamycin and bicalutamide, apoptosis occurred [159], signifying that there is a parallel compensatory effect for mTORC1 signaling through AR. This relationship was expanded on by Wu et al., (2010) who determined that the relationship between AR and mTORC1 is dependent upon testosterone availability, and generates a self perpetuating cycle that promotes cell survival. In low testosterone conditions, application of bicalutamide repressed mTOR activity, as did siRNA against AR in both low and high testosterone conditions. This was shown to be through AR repression of TSC2, a negative regulator of mTORC1. Conversely, rapamycin treatment induced AR activity, as was previously shown by Wang et al. (2008). Furthermore, in low testosterone conditions, where AR activity is low and thus TSC2 is not repressed, bicalutamide leads to apoptosis [160].

These data support the compensatory AR-mediated growth pathway found by Wang et al. (2008), as the lack of TSC2 repression would inhibit mTOR signaling while bicalutimide inhibits AR, leading to a similar dual inhibition of mTORC1 and AR which Wang et al. (2008) reported to induce apoptosis. The interactions between mTOR and AR have been shown to play a key role in progression to AICaP. The mechanism elucidated by Wu et al. (2010) demonstrated that LNCaP cells can become attuned to low testoterone by mTOR/AR crosstalk. When testosterone is low, AR activity drops, but so then does AR-mediated inhibition of TSC2. This represses mTOR activity, leading to induction of AR activity once more. If this cycle is perpetuated, the cells will become able to self-induce AR signaling, and thus also reestablish mTORC1 activity, leading to the development of an androgen-resistant and highly proliferative tumor. Additionally, LNCaP cells acclimatized to low-testosterone conditions showed resistance to glucose deprivation, another way of repressing mTOR. The mTORC1 repression leads to higher levels of AR transactivity, activating a postulated second survival pathway that can compensate for the canonical PI-3K/AKT/mTOR axis. Thus, inhibition of one pathway would sensitize to inhibition of the other. Only by inhibition of both mTOR and AR was apoptosis achieved in both studies [159, 160]. Squillace et al. (2012) show similar results using bicalutamide and ridaforolimus, an mTOR inhibitor. In their study, they [161] also demonstrate that the combination therapy does not induce apoptosis in healthy RWPE-1 PTEN-expressing prostate cells. This is important, as it indicates that the targeted AR/mTOR system is an aberrancy in the tumour.

AR/mTOR dual inhibition was shown to be key to regulation of CaP progression by Schayowitz et al. (2010), who demonstrated that usage thereof can prolong androgen sensitivity of a tumour. Using mouse models, Schayowitz et al. (2010) showed that combination therapy had significant effect on both xenografted androgen-dependent (LNCaP) and androgen-independent (HP-LNCaP) tumours. In both LNCaP and HP-LNCaP xenografts, treatment with a single inhibitor caused no significant decrease in tumour volume, while combination therapy reduced tumour volume significantly. Bicalutamide or everolimus (an mTOR inhibitor) did not decrease tumour volume in LNCaP xenografts, while combination treatment offered significant reduction after 15 days [162]. Likewise, in HP-LNCaP xenografts bicalutamide, everolimus or VN124-1 (a novel androgen/AR inhibitor) did not significantly decrease tumour volume, while dual inhibition did. Interestingly, combination everolimus/VN124-1 treatment reduced tumour volume far more than did everolimus/bicalutamide treatment. Everolimus/VN124-1 treatment also resulted in significant decreases in AR, p-mTOR, p-S6K and p-S6 levels as visualized by western blotting [162], signifying an inhibition of the AR/mTOR pathways. Single inhibition often led to increased pathway activation, further evidencing compensatory crosstalk. This study is notable because treatment of xenografts with the combination treatment was not overcome, nor was its efficacy as compared to tumour volume decreased over a 45-day period. This indicates that sensitivity to the dual inhibition was maintained, and compensatory crosstalk did not rescue the xenograft. Suppression of CaP progression to AI disease in this manner was also shown by Friedrichs et al. (2011), albeit through a different treatment. Omega-3 polyunsaturated fatty acids (PUFAs) were shown to inhibit CaP progression through suppression of mTOR and AR signalling. Application of DHA, an omega-3 PUFA, inhibited AKT signaling and decreased cell growth in AI clones of LNCaP. Friedrichs et al. (2011) also observed the effect of omega-3 PUFAs on suppression of CaP progression using an assay that mimics progression to androgen-independent disease with androgen ablation. In the control group, ~35% of the cells initally underwent growth arrest and then recovered, while ~42.5% stayed arrested. In the omega-3 PUFA groups (+DHA, +EPA), a majority of cells stayed arrested, as did cells treated with an AKT inhibitor. Treatment with DHA was also accompanied by suppression of AR and p-mTOR expression, along with downregulation of p-S6 and of p-TSC2, an AKT target. This data taken together with data by Wang et al. (2008), Wu et al. (2010), Schayowitz et al. (2011) and Squillace et al. (2012) suggest that suppression of both mTOR and AR signaling is key to inhibition of CaP progression, and that single inhibition leads to activation of the other in a compensatory mechanism.

Such a mechanism was postulated by Wang et al. (2008) to be downstream of mTORC2. Facompre et al., (2012) report that that mTORC2 is involved in an AR-mediated growth pathway. Addition of 5μM p-XSC, or 1,4-phenylenebis(methylene)selenocyanate, a known AKT and AR inhibitor, was shown by Facompre et al. (2012) to inhibit mTORC2 kinase activity *in vitro*, supporting Wang et al. (2008) in proposing that mTORC2 plays a role in AR-mediated crosstalk. This dual inhibition of AR and mTORC2 could indicate that either p-XSC is an mTORC2 inhibitor and inhibits AR downstream of TORC2, or that AR is upstream of mTORC2 and thus suppression of AR inhibits mTORC2 signaling. Treatment with p-XSC resulted in decreased growth of both androgen-dependent LNCaP and androgen-independent C4-2 CaP cell lines by ~25%, with rapamycin showing similar results [163]. As indicated by several other sources, dual inhibition had a far more marked effect. Addition of 1nM rapamycin in combination with the mTORC2/AR inhibitor p-XSC heavily decreased cell viability by ~50% in LNCaP calls, and by ~60% in C4-2 cells. The dual inhibitor treatment resulted in extremely efficient repression of phosphorylation downstream of both mTOR complexes, further supporting the postulation that an AR survival pathway is related to mTORC2. The role of mTORC2 in AR signaling has been investigated by Fang et al. (2011), who report that an mTORC2-mediated growth pathway is downstream of AR. Treatment of CWR22R3 cells with

DHT led to proteosome-mediated degradation of p27, a protein that induces cell cycle arrest through CDK inhibition. Such an action would contribute to the inhibited growth noted in CaP progression. This degradation was shown to be through mTORC2-mediated phosphorylation of AKT at Ser473, but not Thr308. AKT has previously been shown to be phosphorylated at Thr308 by PDK1 [165], so the modification of AKT in this context seems to be purely mediated by mTORC2 without influence from PDK1 molecules, leading to selective activation of only certain downstream substrates, such as SGK and PKCa. Fang et al. (2011) went on to demonstrate that DHT stimulation of AR is inducing nuclear accumulation of SIN1, a factor required for complexing of mTORC2, which signals for the assembly of mTORC2 and subsequent partial phophorylation of AKT. The actual phosphorylation of p27, required for its degradation, could be mediated by AKT or one of its selectively activated substrates. Growth pathways downstream of AKT, such as the SGK pathway, would also lead to increased viability and proliferation of CaP. Xu et al. (2006) implicated mTOR in a similar manner, showing that AR induces cyclin proteins, especially cyclin D1, D2 and D3. RT-PCR results did not indicate a similar increase at an mRNA level. This was because AR regulation of cyclin D was at a post-transcriptional level, through mTOR. Co-activation of cyclin proteins together with degradation of p27, a CDK inhibitor, could lead to potent activation of a CDK-Cyclin growth pathway.

AR has also been shown to be post-transcriptionally modified by mTOR [167] in an EGF/PI-3K/AKT-dependent manner. This study elucidates the manner in which mTORC1 regulates and rapamycin induces AR. Through modulation of the interactions between translation initiation factor eIF4E and scaffolding protein eIF4G, mTOR putatively regulates the rate of translation of AR. Thus, rapamycin inhibition of mTORC1 would lead to an increased rate of translation of AR, leading to increased expression and revitalization of mTORC1 signaling. This combined pathway contains a failsafe in the form of the mTOR-mediated repression of AR and the AR regulation of TSC2, leading to cyclic and self-perpetuating support of two growth pathways. This pathway has consistently been implicated as important to CaP survival, growth and progression to AICaP. The data suggests that this crosstalk leads to maintainance of parallel mTORC1 and mTORC2 survival pathways. The pathway is protected from itself: induction of mTOR signaling decreases AR activity, which would enhance TSC2 and thus return mTORC1 to normal levels, rescuing AR. Repression of mTORC1 induces AR through attenuation of its post-transcriptional inhibition, leading to downstream mTORC2/CDK-Cyclin signaling. Additionally, AR represses TSC2, revitalizing the mTORC1 pathway. Repression of AR increases TSC2 activity, leading to inhibited mTORC1 and thus increased AR, hypersensitizing the cell and possibly leading to progression towards AI disease.

4.2.3. PI-3K/AKT/FOXO and AR

FOXO, a family of apoptosis-promtoing transcription factor, has shown relevance to AR and prostate cancer progression. AR has previously been shown to be a positive regulator of the PI-3K pathway, which represses FOXO family transactivity. Additionally, tissue microarray data from TM3-AR CaP cells treated with testosterone display marked downregulation of 65 FOXO-family proteins [168]. Sixteen of these have been shown to be important in development, including FOXO1. These data suggest that AR and FOXO are antagonistic towards one another. Li et al. (2001) first indicated an antagonistic nature of AR and PTEN/FOXO.

Ma et al. (2008) characterized one side of this antagonism, showing that FOXO1 mediates PTEN inhibition of AR. By expressing fragments of FOXO1 and determining their ability to repress AR activity, they discerned that the FOXO1 inhibition of AR required its AD and forkhead box. Further, the inhibition of AR was found to be through disruption of its NTD/CTD interaction. This disruption was found to be mediated by FOXO1 binding the AR NTD and repressing interaction with SRC1, a promoter of AR activity [169]. Completing the dichotomy, Li et al. (2003) showed that AR can also disrupt the activity of FOXO-family transcription factors, including FKHR. Androgen treatment and subsequent AR activation in PTEN-null cells was shown to repress FKHR and related FOXO-family protein activity in a manner independent of transcriptional coactivators. This repression was found to be by complexing of activated AR and FKHR, leading to an inability of FKHR to bind DNA. Two points of interaction were found for each molecule: AR binds to the FKHR C-terminus and binds weakly to the forkhead domain, while FKHR binds to the AR NTD and weakly to the LBD. Through flow cytometry, Li et al. (2003) demonstrated that FKHR when bound by AR can no longer induce cell cycle arrest, thereby leading to an attenuation of its role in growth control. This suggests that androgen ablation therapy might reintroduce FKHR and related FOXO activity, leading to arrest of cell growth. Thus, the progression to androgen independence would require compensation for androgen deprivation, such as those discussed earlier. In particular, mTOR and FOXO seem to have related roles. AR inhibition of FOXO combined with mTOR-mediated growth signaling could lead to potent CaP proliferation. Additionally, mTOR-related crosstalk could rescue FOXO-mediated AR inhibition.

Another similarity between FOXO and mTOR crosstalk with AR is the role of p27. Unlike FOXO1 and FKHR, FOXO3a has been shown to transcriptionally upregulate AR by binding its promoter [171], while AR deactivates FOXO3a [172]. FOXO3a also promotes transcription of p27 via its promoter [173]. These interactions lead to a system where AR deactivates FOXO3a, leading to inhibition of p27. If AR were reduced, FOXO3a would become active, promote AR expression and thus reinstate the same state. Disruption of this cycle was shown by Li et al. (2007), using a DIM compound called B-DIM. Treatment with B-DIM repressed FOXO3a binding to the AR promoter while maintaining its binding to the p27 promoter, leading to cell cycle arrest. In CaP, redundant repression by mTOR might prevent this method of rescue. Additionally, AR disruption of FOXO proteins in conjunction with AR/mTOR crosstalk would lead to a deadly regulatory loop whereby cell cycle regulation is suppressed and growth is promoted. Zhang et al. (2010) also showed potential for FOXO-based therapy in response to AR signaling. Methylseleninic acid (MSA) can be metabolized to methylselenol, which has been shown to have anticancer effects and to induce apoptosis [175]. Zhang et al (2010) found that treatment of LNCaP cells with MSA leads to induction of FOXO1 expression and transactivity. Additionally, knock down of FOXO1 after MSA treatment was found to nullify its apoptotic effects. The critical role of FOXO1 in this context was found to be repression of AR activity, though the mechanism for this inhibition remains unknown. Based on results from Ma et al. (2008), FOXO1 could be attenuating NTD/CTD interactions of AR. Results from treatments with FOXO-associated drugs such as B-DIM and MSA implicate it as an important molecule in AR-mediated CaP growth and its role as an antagonist of AR could potentially implicate it in CaP progression. Since AR/FOXO crosstalk is seemingly similar but opposite to AR/mTOR crosstalk, investigation of both AKT-dependent and AKT-independent crosstalk between the two pathways could elucidate important mechanisms of CaP progression.

4.2.4. PI-3K/AKT/GSK3β and AR

The evidence thus far clearly shows that increased activation of the PI-3K/AKT signaling pathway and transcriptional activity of AR are closely intertwined. The role that AKT plays in modulating AR activity, however, remains obscure. One of the many downstream substrates of AKT, GSK3β has also been shown to play a role in AR regulation [176-179], and is ubiquitously expressed in CaP cell lines, including COS-1, PC-3, LNCaP and DU145 (Wang et al., 2004). It has increased expression in AICaP cell lines [176, 179], and appears to be a key player in the progression of CaP to androgen-independent disease. However, the nature of this role is at present ambiguous. In varied contexts, GSK3β has been shown to both promote and antagonize AR transactivaton independently of its interactors and other substrates in both a ligand-dependent and ligand-independent manner.

A repressor of several EMT pathways, GSK3β has been shown by Salas et al. (2004) to be capable of repressing ligand-dependent AR activity by phosphorylation. Transfection of wild type GSK3β or constitutively active GSK-3B$^{\Delta 9}$, a mutant of GSK3β devoid of its first 9 amino acids, into AR-expressing LNCaP, A103 and V28 cells significantly increased phosphorylated AR compared to transfection of empty pCMV$_4$ or inactivated tyrosine 216 mutated GSK3β (GSK3β^{Y216F}). Furthermore, treatment of cells with LiCl, a GSK3β inhibitor, significantly decreased phosphorylation of AR (Salas et al., 2004), indicating that altered modification of AR is indeed due to the activity of GSK3β. In AR- COS-1 prostate cancer cells, co-transfection of wtGSK3β or GSK3β$^{\Delta 9}$ with AR lead to increased phosphorylation of AR, as opposed to cotransfection of AR with empty pCMV$_4$ or GSK3β^{Y216F} which did not elevate phosphorylation of AR. This suggests that the activity of GSK3β is essential to the phosphorylation of AR, as the active forms of GSK3β were the only ones to display an effect. Upon treatment of AR-expressing COS-1 cells with LY294002, phosphorylation of AR increased [176]. This is due to reduced deactivation of endogenous GSK3β through indirect inhibition of AKT via the PI3K pathway. When these cells were treated with LiCl, AR phosphorylation decreased in a dose-dependent manner, indicating that these results are related to increased GSK3β activity. In following with the increased phosphorylation of AR, Salas et al. (2004) also reported that AR-mediated transactivation in the presence of R1881 (metribolone), a synthetic nonmetabolizable androgen, was decreased with increased GSK3β activity. This was shown through luciferase reporter assays both with an ARE-driven ARE$_2$LUC construct as well as with a PB-LUC (a promoter from an endogenous AR target). By using C-terminal and N-terminal domain mutants of AR, Salas et al. (2004) were able to determine that GSK3β preferentially phosphorylates AR on its CTD. Furthermore, usage of a GST-tagged ARLBD revealed that GSK3β could phosphorylate AR on its LBD. This may provide a mechanism by which AR-driven transcription is decreased by GSK-3β. The effect of GSK3β being through the AR LBD is further evidenced by the fact that Salas et al. (2004) did not note any suppression of the ligand-independent, constitutively active AR5 and AR104 constructs.

Wang et al. (2004) also showed a reductive effect of GSK3β on AR transcription. Co-transfection of AR, wtGSK3β and two reporter constructs in a dual luciferase system with an ARE-driven promoter (ARE_4) revealed that increased GSK3β decreased AR transactivation. Further, usage of a constitutively active GSK3β mutant ($GSK3\beta^{S9A}$) further restricted AR-driven transcription. These data taken together suggest that GSK3β kinase activity regulates the level of AR transactivation. GSK3β was also shown to decrease AR transcription in LNCaP cells, which express endogenous AR. These effects were shown to be reversible by LiCl treatment. However, in contrast to the work by Salas et al. (2004), Wang et al. (2004) demonstrated that GSK3β phosphorylates AR on its NTD more significantly than its LBD or a DBD-LBD fragment by using GST-tagged fragments. Moreover, they showed that GSK3β repressed transcription by GAL4-AR-N-terminal in the presence of a pG5-Luc reporter, which contains the ligand-independent AF-1 domain, while failing to repress activity of the AF-2 domain-containing GAL4-AR-LBD. These data suggest that GSK3β inhibits ligand-independent activity of AR. Wang et al. (2004) also demonstrated that GSK3β binds to the CTD and NTD of AR in both transfected and endogenously expressing CaP cell lines, leading to the postulation that GSK3β-mediated suppression of AR transcription may be due to attenuated AR CTD-NTD interactions, which are required for transactivation. Supporting the interaction of the two molecules, Salas et al. (2004) noted that there was a physical co-distribution of the two molecules in CaP cell lines and in CaP tissue. Salas et al, (2004) reported that inhibition of GSK3β by Ser9 phosphorylation is elevated in the androgen-dependent LNCaP in comparison to the androgen-independent PC3 and DU145 CaP lines, which may signify an increased role for GSK3β in androgen-dependent tumours. Liao et al (2004) also show that GSK3β Tyr216 phosphorylation is elevated in AICaP cells, especially 22-RV1. Aberrant activity of the PI-3KAKT signaling system has been demonstrated in AI 22-RV1 CaP cells, and has been associated with an increased Gleason grade [82], which in turn has been shown to be an accurate predictor of progression to AICaP [182]. These data taken together suggest that the increased activity of PI-3K/AKT in AICaP, usually due to PTEN deficiency, may have the effect of disabling GSK3β and thus increasing activity of AR in a ligand-independent manner.

Work by Liao et al. (2004), Mazor et al. (2004) and Schütz et al. (2011) contradicts Salas et al. (2004) and Wang et al. (2004), reporting that inhibition of GSK3β actually represses AR-mediated transcription. Mazor et al. (2004) reported that GSK3β sequestration or knockdown inhibits AR signaling, while transfection of a constitutively active form ($GSK3\beta^{S9A}$) into LNCaP cells with majority Ser9-phosphorylated GSK3β increased AR transcriptional activity. Moreover, this effect was independent of its downstream substrate, the oncogenic β-catenin. Liao et al. (2004) demonstrate that GSK3β is necessary for ligand-dependent transcriptional activity to occur. In the presence of LiCl, two other GSK3β inhibitors RO318220 and GF109203X and siRNA against GSK3β, R1881-stimulated AR transcriptional activity as measured by a PSA-SEAP reporter was significantly reduced. This was not due to reduced nuclear translocation, as no inhibitors blocked AR nuclear localization with R1881 treatment. Knockdown of AKT and β-catenin, another substrate of GSK3β, did not yield any similar results, implicating that

http://dx.doi.org/10.5772/53483

GSK3β activity is directly inducing the observed effect. Interestingly, in the presence of R1881 GSK3β Tyr216 phosphorylation was also increased, signifying a synergistic relationship between GSK3β and the androgen-dependent AR signaling cascade.

Schütz et al. (2011) further complicate the story, reporting that GSK3β is necessary for androgen-independent AR activity, though not by directly affecting the AF-1 or AF-2 activity domains. Instead, this inhibition is in a CRM1-dependent manner, as discerned in an earlier study [179]. CRM1 is an export receptor for substrates containing an L-rich NES, likely acting in a RanGTP-dependent manner [182]. CRM1 activity is inhibited by leptomycin B (LMB). Upon treatment of 22-RV1 cells with SB216763, a GSK3β inhibitor, AR was increasingly localized in the cytoplasm and experienced a two-fold drop in the nucleus. When LMB was added, the effects were reversed. AR transcriptional activity was also shown to drop with the inhibitor, and was rescued by LMB. Furthermore, AR association with CRM1 was shown to increase with SB216763, and a putative binding site was reported to be located within the C-terminal LBD. This was found using a mutant deleted of its LBD (Schütz et al., 2010). In their future work, Schütz et al. (2011) showed that unliganded AR in AI LNCaP lines, which was localized to the nucleus, is exported upon application of SB216763 in a CRM1-dependent manner, rescued by LMB. Decreased AR signaling with GSK3β was also shown in vivo using a tumor-engrafted chick choriallantoic membrane model. Of note, knockdown (shRNA) or long-term inhibition (SB216763) reduced the nuclear and cellular levels of AR respectively. Mazor et al (2004) showed similar data, suggesting that GSK3β may also play a role in maintaining stability of the AR protein.

The evidence clearly indicates that GSK3β plays a crucial role in regulation of AR; however the nature of that role is highly controversial. Upregulation of GSK3β has been shown to be associated with an elevated Gleason grade [180], which would suggest that support of AR signaling would be likely. Moreover, as Gleason grade often indicates increased risk for AICaP progression [182], however, GSK3β is also a target of AKT for Ser9 phsophorylation, which deactivates its kinase activity. Thus it would seem detrimental that GSK3β induction and reduced inhibition of the PI-3K pathway occur concurrently, as is the situation in several AICaP lines such as 22-RV1. It may be important to note that while Salas et al. (2004) and Wang et al. (2004) made liberal usage of overexpression models, while Liao et al. (2004), Schütz et al (2010) and Schütz et al. (2011) used mainly endogenous protein. This is largely due to the nature of the work, using GSK3β as a suppressant as opposed to studying the effects of repressed GSK3β activity, however ectopic expression can alter a system from the *in situ* function. From the presented results, it becomes apparent that endogenous GSK3β-AR interactions seem to be AR-promoting. Mullholland et al. (2006) suggests that a baseline level of GSK3β may be necessary for AR activity, and ectopic expression may alter the nature of the system, causing an inhibition and suggesting that GSK3β Tyr216 phosphorylation may ultimately be AR-inhibitory. However, the recent results by Schütz et al. (2011) contradict this, while results by Mazor et al. (2004) indicate that overexpression of GSK3β in a system with active endogenous GSK3β, such as 22-RV1 cells, has little effect. The mechanism outlined by Schütz et al. (2010) may be key to note: GSK3β could have a higher affinity for CRM1, thereby preferentially preventing AR export and thus promoting AR transactivation. Further, it would seem that these interaction play a different role in ligand-dependent and AI disease, which may suggest a role in promoting the progression of CaP to an AI state. Alteration of GSK3β or alteration of its interactions *in situ* may play an important role in regulating GSK3β function with respect to CaP, as it has been shown to play a wide variety of tumour-suppressing and oncogenic roles when in different environments. Thus, a change in cellular context may be key to its role in CaP progression.

4.3. PI-3K/Wnt/AR Axis

The Wnt pathway and the PI-3K have both been implicated in CaP progression. Additionally, crosstalk has been evidenced between the two systems, usually downstream of AKT. In particular, GSK3β is a common intermediary between the Wnt and PI-3K pathways through which crosstalk is often implicated. In the Wnt pathway, GSK3β phosphorylates β-catenin, the central effector of the pathway, to mark it for ubiquitination and subsequent proteosomal degradation [184]. β -catenin is a multifunctional protein that both aids in the stabilization of the adherens junction with E-cadherin and activates transcription of Wnt target genes. Wnt ligands activate the Wnt pathway by binding to their seven-pass transmembrane receptor frizzled (Fzd) and its co-receptors LDL receptor related proteins 5 and 6 (LRP5/6). The Wnt pathway is divided into the canonical Wnt pathway, which signals through β-catenin, and the non-canonical Wnt pathway. The non-canonical Wnt pathway includes the calcium dependent pathway and the planar cell polarity pathway, both of which play vital roles in development. [185,186]. The canonical Wnt pathway is stimulated when a member of a subset of Wnt ligands binds Fzd. This transduces a signal through dishevelled (Dvl) to disrupt the β-catenin destruction complex, made up of adenomatous polyposis coli (APC), casein kinase 1 (CK1) and GSK3 β unified by the scaffolding protein Axin. By sequential phosphorylation, ubiquitination and degradation in the presence of an active destruction complex, β-catenin is maintained at reasonable levels. Upon stimulation by a Wnt ligand, GSK3βis deactivated by Dvl and Axin is seuestered to the membrane by the now-phosphorylated LRP5/6. This allows β-catenin to accumulate unchecked, and translocate to the nucleus. The mechanism for β-catenin translocation remains unclear. In order to play its role as a transcativator, β-catenin must bind its nuclear interactor T-cell factor (TCF). In a cell unstimulated by Wnt activation, TCF is bound to its repressor, Groucho. With Wnt activation, β-catenin displaces Groucho, and the β-catenin/TCF complex transcribes a plethora of Wnt target genes, many of which play oncogenic roles. In this way, β-catenin itself is a potent oncogene.

Wang et al. (2008) used castration resistant mouse models to demonstrate that AR expression seems to be concurrently expressed with increased levels of cytoplasmic β-catenin that is unattached to the adherens junction. This is significant because free β-catenin has the potential to shuttle to the nucleus and activate transcription of Wnt target genes. Trucia et al. (2000) establish a direct significance for this co-expression: β-catenin and AR can directly interact, leading to enhanced AR signaling and hypersensitivity to androgens. In LNCaP cells β-catenin and AR were shown to complex both in the presence and absence of androgen, but binding was markedly enhanced in the presence of DHT. However, using a stabilized mutant of β-catenin (β-catenin S33F) it was shown that AR activity is only enhanced in the presence of androgen, signifying a ligand-dependent activation. This was measured using a luciferase reporter assay. Trucia et al. (2000) went on to show that β-catenin binds AR on its LBD, and reduces the effects of bicalutamide on AR. This was shown to be through alteration of the AR LBD, broadening the scope of AR-ligand interactions to include other ligands. In this way β-catenin was show by Trucia et al. (2000) to be a co-activator of AR, providing it with increased significance beyond its role as a coactivator of Wnt target genes with TCF. β-catenin's interaction with AR were shown to be increasingly important by Mullholland et al. (2002), who showed that the AR/β-catenin complex can serve as a vehicle for β-catenin translocation in a ligand-dependent manner. Treatment with androgen in LNCaP cells led to colocalization of AR and β-catenin to the nucleus. Mullholland et al. (2002) went on to show that there are several points of overlap between β-catenin-driven and AR-driven transcription by noting several common targets, including cell cycle proteins such as cyclin D1. Others since have showed interaction between the two molecules, both in support [67] and in contention [47, 189]. In fact, data by Chesire et al. (2002) indicates that ligand-dependent AR/ β-catenin interactions inhibit β-catenn/TCF activity.

The most obvious point of crosstalk between PI-3K and Wnt is their common intermediary, GSK3. Sharma et al. (2002) investigated the crosstalk between these two molecules and AR. Treatment of LNCaP cells with LY294002 resulted in inhibition of AR-driven PSA expression, demonstrating a regulation of AR activity similar to that seen by Li et al. (2001). Upon application of LY294002, phosphorylation of AKT decreased, as did inhibitory phosphorylation of GSK3 β. In conjunction with the lack of deactivation of GSK3 β, nuclear accumulation of β-catenin was significantly reduced. Usage of a mutant β-catenin mutated at its GSK3 βphosphorylation site attenuated the results, showing that the modulation of AR transactivation by the PI-3K pathway occurs through β-catenin. This finding is contradicted by Liao et al. (2004) and Mazor et al. (2003), who demonstrate that GSK3 βis required for AR transactivation. Liao et al (2004) showed that knockdown of β-catenin by pooled siRNA does not affect the levels of R1881-stimulated AR transactivation as measured using a PSA-SEAP reporter construct. Mazor et al. (2003) also show that depletion of β-catenin levels by siRNA treatment does not inhibit transactivation by endogenous AR in 22-RV1, LNCaP and CWR-R1 cells. In fact, they demonstrate that knockdown of β-catenin leads to increased levels of AR activity. It is worthy to note that both Liao et al. (2004) and Mazor et al. (2003) worked with primarily endogenous proteins, using knockdown models, and demonstrating that endogenous β-catenin is not a co-activator of AR. Mazor et al. (2003) notes the importance of confirming results obtained using ectopic expression with studies of endogenous protein.

For the most part, this section focuses on crosstalk through GSK3β. However, it is important to note that AKT modulates a variety of substrates downstream of PI-3K, and a number of these could be means for crosstalk. Hoogeboom et al. (2008) noted that FOXO interrupts β-catenin/TCF transcription by binding and sequestering β-catenin. This type of interference could play a role in inhibiting β-catenin/AR transcription as well, should that interaction take place. If β-catenin Is truly a coactivator of AR, or if AR does act as a shuttle for β-catenin, a great depth of understanding could be arrived at. In order to understand CaP progression and the roles of the Wnt, PI-3K and AR pathways therein, these interactions must be studied and understood. Should β-catenin coactivate with AR, the question arises as to whether it might do the same with FOXO. Many other proteins adapt functions based on their interactors and β-catenin is no different, being responsible for maintaining anchorage dependence when interacting with E-cadherin at the adherens junction. Mazor et al. (2003) had justification in commenting that the endogenous interactions of a protein should be understood. Until the relationships underlying β-catenin and its interactors are characterized, its role in CaP progression will remain elusive.

5. Current therapy, implications and future directions

The reciprocal interactions and interplay between the AR and PI3K/AKT axis suggests that the underlying mechanism potentiating CaP progression is complex and impacts the very balance of these prosurvival pathways. Current literature shows that there is indeed crosstalk between the AR and PI3K/AKT pathway occuring at various levels. The integration of these oncogenic pathways potentiates CaP tumorigenesis and this is further complicated by the levels of androgens and stage of CaP progression. In effect, the transition from AD-CaP to AI-CaP in prostate carcinogenesis provides major clinical challenges. Androgen ablation and/or anti-androgen therapies are only temporarily effective. Such therapies yield a hormone refractory tumor that is essentially untreatable with the most effective standard chemotherapeutic regimens which only increase patient survival for 2 months [191]. In this case, the pharmacological challenge then, will be to consider the contributions from both PI3K/AKT and AR signalling pathways throughout CaP progression [82].

The mTORC1 pathway has been a primary focus for drug development due to the discovery of rapamycin [93]. However, selective inhibitors from this family of compounds have not proven to be effective. Although, it seems promising to use drug combinations for the inhibition of the main survival pathways (mTORC1, PI3K, AKT) this may incidently result in high toxicity. The concept of intercepting signaling cross-talk with drug combinations to target multiple nodes of integration and/or multiple kinases may be useful in controlling upstream and downstream the PI3K pathway. In addition, the ability of the PI3K/AKT pathway to synergistically heighten AR signaling together with non-genomic cross talk between other pro-survival factors make targetable areas for therapy difficult. Now, with the integration of the Wnt/β-catenin signalling pathway in AR regulation the interplay between PI3K, Wnt and AR signaling becomes further complicated. As such, putative chemotherapeutic agents that inhibit upstream the Wnt or PI3K signaling may pose a viable option [194].

The oncogenic role of the PI3K/AKT pathway in CaP progression is clearly evident. However, the mechanisms underlying the interplay between PI3K and AR signaling still remains unclear. Therefore, understanding how crosstalks are regulated in CaP progression will provide a means by which to elucidate the complexities and contexts of AI disease that are necessary for successful therapeutic intervention.

http://dx.doi.org/10.5772/53483

Author details

Jacqueline R Ha, Yu Hao D Huang, Amit Persad and Sujata Persad

University of Alberta, Department of Pediatrics, Canada

References

[1] Feldman, BJ., & Feldman, D. (2001). The development of androgen-independent prostate cancer. Nat Rev Cancer, Vol.1, pp. 34-45, ISSN 1474-175X

[2] Niu, Y., Chang, TM., Yeh, S., Ma, WL., Wang, YZ., & Chang, C. (2010). Differential androgen receptor signals in different cells explain why androgen-deprivation therapy of prostate cancer fails. Oncogene, Vol.29, pp. 3593-3604, ISSN 0950-9232

[3] Koochekpour, S. (2010). Androgen receptor signaling and mutations in prostate cancer. Asian J Androl, Vol.12, pp.639-657, ISSN 1008-682X

[4] He, B., Kemppainen, JA., Voegel, JJ., Gronemeyer, H., Wilson, EM. (1999). Activation function 2 in the human androgen receptor ligand binding domain mediates interdomain communication with the NH(2)-terminal domain. J Biol Chem, Vol. 274 (52), pp. 37219-37225

[5] He, B., Lee, LW., Minges, JT., Wilson, EM.(2000). Dependence of selective gene activation on the androgen receptor NH2- and COOH-terminal interaction. J Biol Chem, Vol. 275 (30), pp. 22986-22994

[6] Loy, CJ., Sim, KS., Yong, EL. (2003). Filamin-A fragment localizes to the nucleus to regulate androgen receptor and coactivator functions. Proc Natl Acad Scie USA, Vol. 100(8), pp. 4562-4567

[7] Bennett, NC., Gardiner, RA., Hooper, JD., Johnson, DW., & Gobe, GC. (2010). Molecular cell biology of androgen receptor signalling. Int J Biochem Cell Biol, Viol.42, pp. 813-827, ISSN 1357-2725

[8] Veldscholte, J., Berrevoets, CA., Zegers, ND., van der Kwast, TH., Grootegoed, J.S., Mulder, E. (1992). Hormone-induced dissociation of the androgen receptor-heat-shock protein complexes: use of a new monoclonal antibody to distinguish transformed from nontransformed receptors. Biochemistry, Vol. 31(32), pp. 7422-7430

[9] Nazareth, LV., & Weigel, NL. (1996). Activation of the human androgen receptor through a protein kinase A signaling pathway. J Biol Chem, Vol. 271, pp. 19900-19907

[10] Whitaker, H.C., Girling, J., Warren, A.Y., Leung, H., Mills, I.G., Neal, D.E. (2008). Alterations in β-Catenin expression and localization in prostate cancer. The Prostate, 68, 1196-1205

[11] Johnson, MA., Hernandez, I., Wei, Y., & Greenberg, N. (2000). Isolation and characterization of mouse probasin: An androgen-regulated protein specifically expressed in the differentiated prostate. Prostate, Vol.43, pp. 255-262, ISSN 0270-4137

[12] Mulholland, DJ., Cheng, H., Reid, K., Rennie, PS., Nelson, CC. (2002). The androgen receptor can promote beta-catenin nuclear translocation independently of adenomatous polyposis coli. J Biol Chem, Vol.277, pp. 17933-17943, ISSN 0021-9258

[13] Choong, CS., & Wilson, EM. (1998). Trinucleotide repeats in the human androgen receptor: a molecular basis for disease, J Mol Endocrinol, Vol. 21(3), pp. 235-257

[14] Southwell, J., Chowdhury, SF., Gottlieb, B., Beitel, LK., Lumbroso, R., Purisima, EO., & Trifiro, M. (2008). An investigation into CAG repeat length variation and N/C terminal interactions in the T877A mutant androgen receptor found in prostate cancer. J Steroid Biochem Mol Biol, Vol.111, pp. 138-146, ISSN 0960-0760

[15] Chamberlain, ML., Driver, ED., Miesfeld, RL. (1994). The length and location of CAG trinucleotide repeats in the androgen receptor N-terminal domain affect transactivation function. Nucleic Acids Res, Vol. 22(15), pp. 3181-3186

[16] Ding, D., Xu, L., Mennon, M., Reddy, GP., Barrack, ER. (2004). Effect of a short CAG (glutamine) repeat on human androgen receptor function. Prostate,Vol. 58(1), pp. 23-32

[17] Hong, H., Darimont, BD., Tang, L., Tamamoto, KR., Stallcup, MR. (1999). An additional region of coactivator GRIP1 required for interaction with the hormone-binding domains of a subset of nuclear receptors. J Biol Chem, Vol. 274(6), pp. 3496-3502

[18] Lemon, B., & Tjian, R. (2000). Orchestrated response: a symphony of transcription factors for gene control. Genes Dev, Vol. 14(20), pp. 2551-2569

[19] Shen, HC., Buchanan, G., Butler, LM., Prescott, J., Henderson, M., Tilley, WD., Coetzee, GA. (2005). GRIP1 mediates the interaction between the amino- and carboxyl-termini of the

[20] Simental, JA., Sar., M., Lane, MV., French, RS., Wilson, EM. (1991). Transcriptional activation and nuclear targeting signals of the human androgen receptor. J BiolChem, Vol. 266(1), pp. 510-518

[21] Yang, F., Li, X., Sharma, M., Sasaki, CY., Longo, DL., Lim, B., & Sun, Z. (2002). Linking beta-catenin to androgen-signaling pathway. J Biol Chem, Vol.277, pp. 11336-11344, ISSN 0021-9258

[22] Gelmann, EP. (2002). Molecular biology of the androgen receptor. J Clin Oncol, Vol. 20, pp. 3001-3015, ISSN 0732-183X

[23] Masiello, D., Chen, SY., Xu, Y., Verhoeven, MC., Choi, E., Hollenberg, AN., & Balk, SP. (2004). Recruitment of beta-catenin by wild-type or mutant androgen receptors

correlates with ligand-stimulated growth of prostate cancer cells. Mol Endocrinol, Vol.18, pp. 2388-2401, ISSN 0888-8809

[24] Miyamoto, H., & Chang, C. (2000). Antiandrogens fail to block androstenedione-mediated mutated androgen receptor transactivation in human prostate cancer cells. Int, J Urol, Vol. 7(1), pp. 32-34

[25] Miyamoto, H., Yeh, S., Wilding, G., Chang, C. (1998). Promotion of agonist activity of antiandrogens by the androgen receptor coactivator, ARA70, in human prostate cancer DU145 cells. Proc Natl Acad Sci USA, Vol. 95(13), pp. 7370-7384

[26] Rahmann, M., Miyamoto, H., Chang, C. (2004). Androgen receptor coregulators in prostate cancer: mechanisms and clinical implications. Clin Cancer Res, Vol. 10(7), pp. 2208-2219

[27] Kemppainen, J.S., Langley, E., Wong, C.I., Bobseine, K., Kelce, W.R., Wilson, E.M. (1999). Mol. Endocrinol, Vol. 13, pp. 440-454.

[28] Chang, CY., & McDonnell, DP. (2002). Evaluation of ligand-dependent changes in AR structure using peptide probes.Mol Endocrinol, Vol. 16, pp. 440-454

[29] Liao, G., Chen, LY., Zhang, A., Godavarthy, A., Xia F., Ghosh, JC., Li, H., Chen, JD. (2003). Regulation of androgen receptor activity by the nuclear receptor corepressor SMRT. J Biol Chem, Vol. 278(7), pp. 5052-5061

[30] Cheng, S., Brzostek, S., Lee, SR., Hollenberg, AN., Balk, SP. (2002). Inhibition of the dihydrotestosterone-activated androgen receptor by nuclear receptor corepressor. Mol Endocrinol, Vol. 16(7), pp. 1492-1501

[31] Heinlein, CA., & Chang, C. (2002). Androgen receptor (AR) coregulators: an overview. Endocr Rev, Vol. 23(2), pp. 175-200

[32] Liao, X., Thrasher, JB., Holzbeierlein, J., Stanley, S., & Li, B. (2004). Glycogen synthase kinase-3beta activity is required for androgen-stimulated gene expression in prostate cancer. Endocrinology, Vol.145, pp. 2941-2949, ISSN 0013-7227

[33] Cutress, ML., Whitaker, HC., Mills, IG, Stewart, M., Neal, DE. (2008). Structural basis for the nuclear import of the human androgen receptor. J Cell Sci, Vol. 121 (Part 7), pp.957-968

[34] Ozanne DM., Brady, ME., Cook, S., Gaughan, L., Neal, DE., Robson, CN. (2000). Androgen receptor nuclear translocation is facilitated by the f-actin cross-linking protein filamin, Mol Endocrinol, Vol. 14(10), pp. 1618-1626

[35] Schaufele, Fl, Carbonell, X., Guerbadot, M., Borngraeber, S., Chapman, MS., Ma, AA., Miner, JN., Diamond, MI. (2005). The structural basis of androgen receptor activation: intramolecular and intermolecular amino-carboxy interactions. Proc Natl Acad Sci USA, Vol. 102 (28), pp. 9802-9807

[36] Gewirth, DT., & Sigler, PB. (1995). The basis for half-site specificity explored through a non-cognate steroid receptor-DNA complex. Nat Struc Biol, Vol. 2, pp. 386-394

[37] Luisi, BF., Xu, WX., Otwinoswski, Z., Freedman, LP., Yamamoto, KR>, Sigler, PB. (1991). Crystallographic analysis of the interaction of the glucocorticoid receptor with DNA. Nature, Vol. 352(6335), pp. 497-505

[38] Schwabe, JW., Chapman, L., Finch, JT., Rhodes, D. (1993). The crystal structure of the estrogen receptor DNA-binding domain bound to DNA: How receptors discriminate between their response elements. Cell, Vol. 75, pp. 567-578

[39] Rastinejad, F., Perlmann, T., Evans, RM., Sigler, PB. Structural determinants of nuclear receptor assembly on DNA direct repeats. Nature, Vol. 375(6528), pp. 203-211

[40] Haelens, A., Verrijdt. G,, Callewaert. L., Christiaens, V., Schauwaers, K., Peeters, B., Rombauts, W., & Claessens, F. (2003). DNA recognition by the androgen receptor: evidence for an alternative DNA-dependent dimerization, and an active role of sequences flanking the response element on transactivation. Biochem J, Vol.369, pp. 141-151, ISSN 0264-6021

[41] Claessens, F., Alen, P., Devos, A., Peeters, B., Verhoeven, G., Rombauts, W. the androgen-specific probasin response element 2 interacts differentially with androgen and glucocorticoid receptors. J Biol Chem, Vol. 271(32), pp. 19013-19016

[42] Rennie, PS., Bruchovsky, M., Leco, KJ., Sheppard, PC., McQueen, SA., Cheng, H., Snoek, R., Hamel, A., Bock, ME., MacDonald, BS., et al. (1993). Characterization of two cis-acting DNA elements involved in the androgen regulation of the probasin gene. Mol Endocrinol, Vol. 7(1), pp. 23-26

[43] Verrijdt, G., Schoenmakers, E.., Alen, P., Haelens, A., Peeters, B., Rombauts, W., Claessens, F. (1999). Androgen specificity of a response unit upstream of the human secretory component gene is mediated by differential receptor binding to an essential androgen response element. Mol Endocrinol, Vol. 13(9), pp. 1558-1570

[44] Verrijdt, G., Schoenmakers, E., Haelens, A., Peeters, B., Verhoeven, G., Rombauts, W., Claessens, F. (2000). Change of specificity mutations in androgen-selective enhances. Evidence for a role of differential DNA binding by the androgen receptor. J Biol Chem, Vol. 275(16), pp. 12298-12305

[45] Shaffer, PL., Jivan, A., Dollins, DE., Claessens, F., & Gewirth, DT. (2004). Structural basis of androgen receptor binding to selective androgen response elements. Proc Natl Acad Sci U S A, Vol.101, pp. 4758-4763, ISSN 0027-8424

[46] Adler, AJ., Scheller, A., Robins, DM. (1993). The stringency and magnitude of androgen-specific gene activation are combinatorial functions of receptor and nonreceptor binding site sequences. Mol Cell Biol, Vol 13(10), pp. 6326-6335

[47] Pawlowski, JE., Ertel, JR., Allen, MP., Xu, M., Butler, C., Wilson, EM., & Wierman, ME. (2002). Liganded androgen receptor interaction with beta-catenin: nuclear co-lo-

calization and modulation of transcriptional activity in neuronal cells. J Biol Chem, Vol.277, pp. 20702-20710, ISSN 0021-9258

[48] Blok, LJ., de Ruiter, PE., Brinkmann, AO. (1998). Forskolin-induced dephosphorylation of the androgen receptor impairs ligand binding. Biochemistry, Vol. 37(11), pp. 3850-3857

[49] Lin, HK., Wang, L., Hu, YC., Altuwaijri, S., Chang, C. (2002). Phosphorylation dependent ubiquitylation and degradation of androgen receptor by Akt require Mdm2 E3 ligase. EMBO J, Vol. 21, pp. 4037-4048

[50] Grossmann, ME., Huang, H., Tindall, DJ. (2001). Androgen receptor signaling in androgen-refractory prostate cancer. J Natl Cancer Inst, Vol 93, pp.1687-1697

[51] Gioeli, D., Ficarro, SB., Kwiek, JJ., Aaronson, D., Hancock, M., Catling, AD., White, FM., Christian, RE., Settlage, RE., Shabanowitz, J., Hunt, DF., Weber, MJ. (2002). Androgen receptor phosphorylation. Regulation and identification of the phosphorylation sites. J Biol Chem, Vol. 277(32), pp. 29304-29314

[52] O'Malley, BW., Tsai, SY., Bagchi, M., Weigel, NL., Schrader, WT., Tsai MJ. (1991). Molecular mechanism of action of a steroid hormone receptor. Recent Prog Horm Res, Vol. 47, pp. 1-24

[53] Fu, M., Rao, M., Wu, K., Wang, C., Zhang, S., Hessien, M., Yeung, YG., Gioeli, D., Weber,,MJ., Pestell, RG. (2004). The androgen receptor acetylation site regulates cAMP and AKT but not ERK-induced activity. J Biol Chem, Vol. 279(28), pp. 29436-29449

[54] Poukka, J., Karvonen, U., Janne, OA., Palvimo, JJ. (2000). Covalent modification of the androgen receptor by small ubiquitin-like modifier 1 (SUMO-1). Proc Natl Acad Sci USA, Vol. 97, pp.14145-14150

[55] Koivisto, P., Kononen, J., Palmberg, C., Tammela, T., Hyytinen, E., Isola, J., Trapman, J., Cleutjens, K., Noordzij, A., Visakorpi, T., Kallioniemi, OP. (1997). Androgen receptor gene amplification: a possible molecular mechanism for androgen deprivation therapy failure in prostate cancer. Cancer Res, Vol. 57(2), pp. 314-319

[56] Taplin, ME., Bubley, GJ., Shuster, TD., Frantz, ME., Spooner, AE., Ogata, GK., Keer, HN., Balk, SP. (1995). Mutation of the androgen-receptor gene in metastatic androgen-independent prostate cancer. N Engl J Med, Vol. 332(21), pp. 1393-1398

[57] Tilley, WD., Buchanan, G., Hickey, TE., Bentel, JM. (1996). Mutations in the androgen receptor gene are associated with progression of human prostate cancer to androgen independence. Clin Cancer Res, Vol. 2(2), pp. 277-285

[58] Gruber, SB., Chen, H., Tomsho, LP., Lee, M., Perrone, EE., Cooney, KA. (2003). R726L androgen receptor mutation is uncommon in prostate cancer families in the united states. Prostate, Vol. 54(4), pp. 306-309

[59] Mononen, N., Syrjakoski, K., Matikainen, M., Tammela, TL., Schleutker J., Kallioniemi, OP, Trapman, J., Koivisto, PA. (2000). Two percent of Finnish prostate cancer patients have a germ-line mutation in the hormone-binding domain of the androgen receptor gene. Cancer Res, Vol. 60(22), pp. 6479-6481

[60] Ingles, SA., Ross, RK., Yu, MC., Irvine, RA., La Pera, G., Haile, RW, Coetzee, GA. (1997). Association of prostate cancer risk with genetic polymorphisms in vitamin D receptor and androgen receptor. J Natl Cancer Inst, Vol. 89(2), pp. 166-170

[61] Crocitto, LE., Henderson, BE., Coetzee, GA. (1997). Identification of two germline point mutations in the 5'UTR of the androgen receptor gene in men with prostate cancer. J Urol, Vol. 158, pp.1599-1601

[62] Crocitto, LE., Henderson, BE., Coetzee, GA. (1997). Identification of two germline point mutations in the 5'UTR of the androgen receptor gene in men with prostate cancer. J Urol, Vol. 158, pp.1599-1601

[63] Darimont, BD., Wagner, RL., Apriletti, JW, Stallcup, MR., Kushner, PJ., Baxter, JD., Fletterick, RJ., Yamamoto, KR. (1998). Structure and specificity of nuclear receptor-coactivator interactions. Genes Dev, Vol. 12, pp. 3343-3356

[64] McInerney, EM., Rose, DW., Flynn, SE., Westin, S., Mullen, TM., Krones, A., Inostroza, J., Torchia, J., Nolte, RT., Assa-Munt, N., Milburn, MV., Glass, CK., Rosenfeld, MG. (1998). Determinants of coactivator LXXLL motif specificity in nuclear receptor transcriptional activation. Genes Dev, Vol. 12, pp. 3357-3368

[65] Shiau, AK., Barstad, D., Loria, PM., Cheng, L., Kushner, PJ., Agard DA., Greene, GL. (1998). The structural basis of estrogen receptor/coactivator recognition and the antagonism of this interaction by tamoxifen. Cell, Vol. 95, 927-937

[66] Westin, SR., Kurokawa, R., Nolte, RT., Wisely, GB., McInerney, EM., Rose, DW., Milburn, MV., Rosenfeld, MG., Glass, CK. (1998). Iinteractions controlling the assembly of nuclear-receptor heterodimers and co-activators. Nature, Vol. 395, pp. 199-202

[67] Song, DH., Dominguez, I., Mizuno, J., Kaut, M., Mohr, SC., & Seldin, DC. (2003) CK2 phosphorylation of the armadillo repeat region of beta-catenin potentiates Wnt signaling. J Biol Chem, Vol.278, pp. 24018-24025, ISSN 0021-9258

[68] Thompson, J., Saatciogl, F., Janne, O.S., Palvimo, J.J. (2001). Disruped amino-and carboxyl-terminal interactions of the androgen receptor are linked to androgen insensitivity. Molecular Endocrinology, Vol. 15 (6), pp. 923-935.

[69] Zhao, XY., Boyle, B., Krishnan, AV., Navone, NM., Peehl, DM, Feldman, D. (1999). Two mutations identified in the androgen receptor of the new human prostate cancer cell line MDA PCa. J Urol, Vol. 162(6), pp. 2192-2199

[70] Zhao, XY., Malloy, PJ., Krishnan, AV., Swami, S., Navone, NM., Peehl, DM., Feldman, D. (2000). Glucocorticoids can promote androgen-independent growth of pros-

tate cancer cells through a mutated androgen receptor. Nat Med, Vol 6(6), pp. 703-706

[71] Marcias, G., Erdmann, El, Lapouge, G., Siebert, C., Barthelemy, P., Duclos, B., Bergerat, JP., Ceraline, J., Kurtz, JE. (2010). Identification of novel truncated androgen receptor (AR) mutants including unreported pre-mRNA splicing variants in the 22Rv1 hormone-refractory prostate cancer (PCa) cell line. Hum Mutat, Vol. 31(1), pp. 74-80

[72] Han, G., Foster, B.A., Mistry, S., Buchanan, G., Harris., J.M., Tilley, W.D., Greenberg, N.M. (2001). Hormone statis selects for spontaneous somatic androgen receptor variant that demonstrate specific ligand and cofactor dependent activities in autochthonous prostate cancer. The Journal of Biological Chemistry Vol.276 (14), pp. 11204-11213

[73] Visakorpi, T., Hyytinen,E., Koivisto, P., Tanner, M., Keinanen, R., Palmberg., C., Palotie, A., Tammela, T., Isola, J., Kallioniemi, O.P. (1995). In vivo amplification of the androgen receptor gene and progression of human prostate cancer. Nat. Genet, Vol. 9, pp.401-406.

[74] Palmberg, C., Koivisto, P., Kakkola., L., Tammela, TL., Kallioniemi, OP., Visakorpi, T. (2000). Androgen receptor gene amplification at primary progression predicts response to combined androgen blockade as second line therapy for advanced prostate cancer. J Urol, Vol 164(6), pp. 1992-1995

[75] Gregory, CW., Johnson, RT Jr., Mohler,,JL., French, FS., Wilson, EM. (2001). Androgen receptor stabilization in recurrent prostate cancer is associated with hypersensitivity to low androgen. Cancer Res, Vol. 61(7), pp. 2892-2898

[76] Labrie, F., Belanger, A., Simard, J., Labrie, C., Dupont A. (1993). Combination therapy for prostate cancer. Endocrine and biologic basis o(2003).f its choice as new standard first-line therapy. Cancer (Phila.), Vol. 71, pp. 1059-1067

[77] Locke, JA., Guns, ES., Lubik, AA., Adomat, HH., Hendy, SC., Wood CA., Ettinger, SL., Gleave, ME., Nelson, CC. (2008). Androgen levels increase by intratumoral de novo steroidogenesis during progression of castration-resistant prostate cancer. Cancer Res, Vol. 68(15), pp. 6407-6415

[78] Truica, CI., Byers, S., & Gelmann, EP. (2000). Beta-catenin affects androgen receptor transcriptional activity and ligand specificity. Cancer Res, Vol.60, pp. 4709-4713, ISSN 0008-5472

[79] Culig, Z., Hobisch, A., Cronauer, MV., Radmayr, C., Trapman, J., Hittmair, A., Bartssch, G., Klocker, H. (1994). Androgen receptor activation in prostatic tumor cell lines by insulin-like growth factor-1, keratinocyte growth factor, and epidermal growth factor. Cancer Res, Vol. 54(20), pp. 5474-5478

[80] Craft, N., Shostak,., Carey, M., Sawyer, C. (1999). A mechanism for hormone independent prostate cancer through modulation of androgen receptor signaling by HER-2/neu tyrosine kinase. Nature Me Vol. 5, pp. 280-285.

[81] Yeh, S., et al. (1999). From Her2.Neu signal cascade to androgen receptor and its coactivators: a novel pathway by induction of androgen targen genes through MAK kinase in prostate cancer cell. Proc. Natl Acad. Sci, Vol. 95, pp. 5458-5463.

[82] Mulholland, D.J., Dedhar, S., Wu, H., Nelson, C.C. (2006). PTEN and GSK3β: key regulators of progression to androgen-independent prostate cancer. Oncogene, 25, 329-337.

[83] Vogt, P.K., Hart, J.R., Gymnopoulos, M., Jiang, H., Kang, Sohye, Bader, A.G., Zhao, L., Denley, A. (2010). Phosphatidylinositol 3-Kinase: The oncoprotein. Phosphoinositide 3-kinase in Health and Disease Vol 2, Current Topics in Microbiology and Immunology, 347, 79-104

[84] Fruman D.A., Meyers, R.E., Cantley, L. (1998). Phosphoinositide kinases. Annu Rev Biochem, 67, 481-507

[85] Vanhaesebroeck, B., Waterfield, M.D. (1999). Signaling by distinct classes of phosphoinositide 3-kinases. Exp Cell Res, 253, 239-254

[86] McCall, P. The interaction between the PI3K/Akt cascade and the androgen receptor in the development and progression of castrate resistant prostate cancer. PhD thesis. University of Glasgow; 2010

[87] Vivanco, I., Sawyers, C.L. (2002). The phosphatidylinositol 3-kinase-akt pathway in human cancer. Nature Review, 2, 489-501

[88] Carpenter, C.L., Duckworth, B.C., Auger, K.R., Cohen, B., Schaffhausen, B.S., Cantley, L.C. (1990). Purification and characterization of phosphoinositide 3-kinase from rat liver. J Biol Chem, 265, 19704-19711

[89] Ikenoue, T., Kanai, F., Hikiba, Y., Obata, T., Tanaka, Y., Imamura, J., et al. (2005). Functional analysis of PIK3CA gene mutations in human colorectal cancer. Cancer Res, 65(11), 4562-4567

[90] Samuels, Y., Ericson, K. (2006). Oncogenic PI3K and its role in cancer. Curr Opin Oncol, 18(1), 77-82

[91] Engelman, J.A., Luo, J., Cantley, L.C. (2006). The evolution of phosphatidylinositol 3-kinases as regulators of growth and metabolism. Nat Rev Genet, 7, 606-619

[92] Backer, J.M. (2008). The regulation and function of class II PI3Ks: novel roles for Vps34. Biochem J, 410, 1-17

[93] Carracedo A., Pandolfi, P.P. (2008). The PTEN-PI3K pathway: of feedbacks and cross-talks. Oncogene, 27, 5527-5541

[94] Pirola, L., Zvelevil, M.J., Bulgarelli-Leva, G., Van Obberghen, E., Waterfield, M.D., Wymann, M.P. (2001). Activation loop sequences confer substrate specificity to phosphoinositide 3-kinase alpha (PI3Kalpha). Functions of lipid kinase-deficient PI3Kalpha in signaling. J Biol Chem, 276, 21544-21554

[95] Yuan, T.L., Cantley, L.C. (2008). PI3K pathway alterations in cancer: variations on a theme. Oncogene, 27, 5497-5510

[96] Yu, J., et al. (1998). Regulation of the p85/p110 phosphatidylinositol 3-kinase: stabilization and inhibition of the p110α catalytic subunit by the p85 α regulatory subunit. Mol. Cell. Biol. 20, 8035-8046

[97] Zhao, L., Vogt, P.K. (2008). Class I PI3K in oncogenic cellular transformation. Oncogene, 5486-96

[98] Carson, J.D., van Aller, G., Lehr, R., Sinnamon, R.H., Kirkpatrick, R.B., Auger, K.R., Dhanak, D., Copeland, R.A., Gontarek, R.R., Tummino, P.J., Luo, L. (2008). Effects of oncogenic p110alpha subunit mutations on the lipid kinase activity of phosphoinositide 3-kinase. Biochem J, 409, 519-524

[99] Kang, S., Bader, A.G., Vogt, P.K. (2005). Phosphatidylinositol 3-kinase mutations identified in human cancer are oncogenic. Proc Natl Acad Sci USA, 102, 802-807

[100] Sugita, H., Dan, S., Kong, D., Tomida, A., Tamori, T. (2008). A new evaluation method for quantifying PI3K activity by HTRF assay. Biochem Biophys Res Commun, 377, 941-945

[101] Zhao, J.J., Roberts, T.M. (2006). PI3 kinases in cancer: from oncogene artifact to leading cancer target. Sci STKE, pe52

[102] Chaussade, C., Cho, K., Mawson,C., Rewcastle, G.W., Sheperd, P.R. (2009). Functional differences between two classes of oncogenic mutation in the PIK3CA gene. Biochem Biophys Res Commun, 381, 577-581

[103] Engelman, J.A., Chen, L., Tan, X., Crosby, K., Guimaraes, A.R., Upadhyay, R., Maira, M., McNamara, K., Perera, S.A., et al. (2008). Effective use of PI3K and MEK inhibitors to treat mutant Kras G12D and PIK3CA H1047R murine lunch cancers. Nat Med, 14, 1351-1356

[104] Jaiswal, B.S., Janakiraman, V., Kljavin, N.M., Chaudhuri, S., Stern H.M., et al. (2009). Somatic mutations in p85alpha promote tumorigenesis through class IA PI3K activation. Cancer Cell, 16, 463-474

[105] Wu, H., Shekar, S.C., Flinn, R.J., El-Sibai, M., Jaiswal, B.S., et al. (2009). Regulation of Class IA PI 3-kinases. C2 domain-iSH2 domain contacts inhibit p85/p110alpha and are disrupted in oncogenic p85 mutants. Proc Natl Acad Sci USA, 106, 20258-20263

[106] Maehama, T., Dixon, J.E. (1998). The tumor suppressor, PTEN/MMAC1, dephosphorylates the lipid second messenger, phosphatidylinositol 3,4,5-trisphosphate. J Biol Chem, 273, 13375-13378

[107] Stambolic, V., Suzuki, A., de la Pompa, J.L., brothers, G.M., Mirtsos, C., Sasaki, T. et al. (1998). Negative regulation of PKB/Akt-dependent cell survival by the tumor suppressor PTEN. Cell, 95, 29-39

[108] Vasudvan, K.M., Guruurthy, S., Rangnekar, V.M. (2007). Suppression of PTEN expression by NF-kappa B prevents apoptosis. Mol Cell Biol, 24, 1007-1021

[109] Papakonstanti, E.A., Ridley, A.J., Vanhaesebroeck, B. (2007). The p110delta isoform of PI 3-kinase negatively controls RhoA and PTEN. EMBO J, 26, 3050-3061

[110] Wang, W., Trotman, L.C., Koppie, T., Alimonti, A., Chen, Z., Gao, Z., et al. (2007). NEDD4-1 is a proto-oncogenic ubiquitin ligase for PTEN. Cell, 128, 129-139

[111] Ahn, Y., Hwang, C.Y., Lee, S.R., Kwon, K.S., Lee, C. (2008). Tumor suppressor PTEN mediates a negative regulation of E3 ubiquitin-protein ligase Nedd4. Biochem J, 412, 331-338

[112] Yang, Z.Z., Tschopp, O., Baudry, A., Dummler, B., Hynx, D., Hemmings, B.A. (2004). Physiological functions of protein kinase B/Akt. Biochem Soc Trans, 32(Pt 2), 350-354

[113] Sarbassov, D.D., Guertin, D.A., Ali, S.M., Sabtini, D.M. Phosphorylation and regulation of Akt/PKB by the Rictor-mTOR complex. Science, 307 (5712), 1098-1101

[114] Stephens, L., Anderson, K., Stokoe, D., Erdjument-Bromage, H., Painter, G.F., Holmes A.B., et al. (1998). Protein Kinase B kinases that mediate phosphatidylinositol 3,4,5-trisphosphate-dependent activation of protein kinase B. Science, 279 (5351), 710-714

[115] Chang, F., Lee, J.T., Navolanic, P.M., Stellman, L.S., Shelton, J.G., Blalock, W.L. (2003). Involvement of PI3K/Akt pathway in cell cycle progression, apoptosis, and neoplastic transformation: a target for cancer chemotherapy. Leukemia, 17(3), 590-603

[116] Cully, M., You, H., Levine, A.J., Mak, T.W. (2006). Beyond PTEN mutations: the PI3K pathway as an integrator of multiple inputs during tumorigenesis. Nature Reviews, 6, 184-192

[117] Jacinto, E., Loewith, R., Schmidt, A., Lin S., Ruegg, M.A., Hall, A., Hall, M.N. (2004). Mammalian TOR complex 2 controls the actin cytoskeleton and is rapamycin insensitive. Nat Cell Biol, 6, 1122-1128

[118] Engelman, J.A. (2009). Targeting PI3K signalling in cancer: opportunities, challenges, and limitations. Nature Reviews, 9, 550-562

[119] Weigui, S., Yiping, G., Zhangqun, Y., Qiangguo, Y., Zhenguo, M., et al. (2009). A comparative study on different characteristics between prostate cancer model and BPH model of BALB/c Mice. Gene Ther Biol, 13, 205-213

[120] Sarker, D., Reid, A.H.M., Yap, T.A., et al. (2009). Targeting the PI3K/AKT pathway for the treatment of prostate cancer. Clin Cancer Res, 4799-4805

[121] Yoshimoto M, Cunha IW, Coudry RA, Fonseca FP, Torres CH, Soares FA, Squire JA (2007) FISH analysis of 107 prostate cancers shows that PTEN genomic deletion is associated with poor clinical outcome. Br J Cancer 97: 678-685

[122] Han B, Mehra R, Lonigro RJ, Wang L, Suleman K, Menon A, Palanisamy N, Tomlins SA, Chinnaiyan AM, Shah RB (2009) Fluorescence in situ hybridization study shows association of PTEN deletion with ERG rearrangement during prostate cancer progression. Mod Pathol 22, 1083-1093

[123] Yoshimoto M, Ludkovski O, DeGrace D, Williams JL, Evans A, Sircar K, Bismar TA, Nuin P, Squire JA (2012) PTEN genomic deletions that characterize aggressive prostate cancer originate close to segmental duplications. Genes Chromosomes Cancer 51,149-160

[124] Khurana E, Lam HY, Cheng C, Carriero N, Cayting P, Gerstein MB (2010) Segmental duplications in the human genome reveal details of pseudogene formation. Nucleic Acids Res 38, 6997-7007

[125] Bengesser K, Cooper DN, Steinmann K, Kluwe L, Chuzhanova NA, Wimmer K, Tatagiba M, Tinschert S, Mautner VF, Kehrer-Sawatzki H (2010) A novel third type of recurrent NF1 microdeletion mediated by nonallelic homologous recombination between LRRC37B-containing low-copy repeats in 17q11.2. Hum Mutat 31, 742-751

[126] Alimonti A, Carracedo A, Clohessy JG, Trotman LC, Nardella C, Egia A, Salmena L, Sampieri K, Haveman WJ, Brogi E, Richardson AL, Zhang J, Pandolfi PP (2010) Subtle variations in Pten dose determine cancer susceptibility. Nat Genet 42, 454-458

[127] Bismar TA, Yoshimoto M, Vollmer RT, Duan Q, Firszt M, Corcos J, Squire JA (2011) PTEN genomic deletion is an early event associated with ERG gene rearrangements in prostate cancer. BJU Int 107, 477-485

[128] Sircar K, Yoshimoto M, Monzon FA, Koumakpayi IH, Katz RL, Khanna A, Alvarez K, Chen G, Darnel AD, Aprikian AG, Saad F, Bismar TA, Squire JA (2009) PTEN genomic deletion is associated with p-Akt and AR signalling in poorer outcome, hormone refractory prostate cancer. J Pathol 218, 505-513

[129] Halvorsen OJ, Haukaas SA, Akslen LA (2003) Combined loss of PTEN and p27 expression is associated with tumor cell proliferation by Ki-67 and increased risk of recurrent disease in localized prostate cancer. Clin Cancer Res, 9, 1474-1479

[130] McMenamin ME, Soung P, Perera S, Kaplan I, Loda M, Sellers WR (1999) Loss of PTEN expression in paraffin-embedded primary prostate cancer correlates with high Gleason score and advanced stage. Cancer Res 59, 4291-4296

[131] Koksal IT, Dirice E, Yasar D, Sanlioglu AD, Ciftcioglu A, Gulkesen KH, Ozes NO, Baykara M, Luleci G, Sanlioglu S (2004) The assessment of PTEN tumor suppressor gene in combination with Gleason scoring and serum PSA to evaluate progression of prostate carcinoma. Urol Oncol 22, 307-312

[132] Dreher T, Zentgraf H, Abel U, Kappeler A, Michel MS, Bleyl U, Grobholz R (2004) Reduction of PTEN and p27kip1 expression correlates with tumor grade in prostate cancer. Analysis in radical prostatectomy specimens and needle biopsies. Virchows Arch 444, 509-517

[133] Chaux A, Peskoe SB, Gonzalez-Roibon N, Schultz L, Albadine R, Hicks J, De Marzo AM, Platz EA, Netto GJ (2012) Loss of PTEN expression is associated with increased risk of recurrence after prostatectomy for clinically localized prostate cancer. Mod Pathol, [Epub ahead of print]

[134] Lotan TL, Gurel B, Sutcliffe S, Esopi D, Liu W, Xu J, Hicks JL, Park BH, Humphreys E, Partin AW, Han M, Netto GJ, Isaacs WB, De Marzo AM (2011) PTEN protein loss by immunostaining: analytic validation and prognostic indicator for a high risk surgical cohort of prostate cancer patients. Clin Cancer Res 17, 6563-6573

[135] Wang S, Gao J, Lei Q, Rozengurt N, Pritchard C, Jiao J, Thomas GV, Li G, Roy-Burman P, Nelson PS, Liu X, Wu H (2003) Prostate-specific deletion of the murine Pten tumor suppressor gene leads to metastatic prostate cancer. Cancer Cell 4, 209-221

[136] Di Cristofano A, De Acetis M, Koff A, Cordon-Cardo C, Pandolfi PP (2001) Pten and p27KIP1 cooperate in prostate cancer tumor suppression in the mouse. Nat Genet 27, 222-224

[137] Zhu Q, Youn H, Tang J, Tawfik O, Dennis K, Terranova PF, Du J, Raynal P, Thrasher JB, Li B (2008) Phosphoinositide 3-OH kinase p85alpha and p110beta are essential for androgen receptor transactivation and tumor progression in prostate cancers. Oncogene 27, 4569-4579

[138] Jia S, Liu Z, Zhang S, Liu P, Zhang L, Lee SH, Zhang J, Signoretti S, Loda M, Roberts TM, Zhao JJ (2008) Essential roles of PI(3)K-p110beta in cell growth, metabolism and tumorigenesis. Nature 454: 776-779

[139] Knight ZA, Gonzalez B, Feldman ME, Zunder ER, Goldenberg DD, Williams O, Loewith R, Stokoe D, Balla A, Toth B, Balla T, Weiss WA, Williams RL, Shokat KM (2006) A pharmacological map of the PI3-K family defines a role for p110alpha in insulin signaling. Cell 125, 733-747

[140] Tzenaki N, Andreou M, Stratigi K, Vergetaki A, Makrigiannakis A, Vanhaesebroeck B, Papakonstanti EA (2012) High levels of p110delta PI3K expression in solid tumor

cells suppress PTEN activity, generating cellular sensitivity to p110delta inhibitors through PTEN activation. FASEB J 26, 2498-2508

[141] Wang., Y., Krisberg, J.R., Ghosh, P.M. (2007). Cross-talk between the androgen receptor and the phosphatidylinositol 3-kinase/Akt pathway in prostate cancer. Current Cancer Drug Targets, 7, 591-604.

[142] Bonaccorsi, L., Marchiani, S., Muratori, M., Carloni, V., Forti, G., Baldi, E. (2004). Signaling mechanisms that mediate invasion in prostate cancer cells. Ann. N Y Acad Sci, 1028, 283-288

[143] Castoria, G., Lombardi, M., Barone, M.V., Bilancio, A., Di Domenico, M., De Auricchio, F. (2004). Rapid signalling pathway activation by androgens in epithelial and stromal cells. Steroids, 69, 517-522

[144] Ayala, G., Thompson, T., Yang G., et al. (2004). High levels of phosphorylated form of Akt-1 in prostate cancer and non-neoplastic prostate tissues are strong predictors of biochemical recurrence. Clin Cancer Res, 10, 6572-6578

[145] Wang, S., Gao, J., Lei, Q., Rozengurt H., Pritchard, C., Jiao, J., et al. (2003). Prostate-specific deletion of the murine Pten tumor suppressor gene leads to metastatic prostate cancer. Cancer Cell, 4, 209-221

[146] Murillo, H., Huang, H., Schmidt, L.J., Smith, D.I., Tindall, D.J. (2001). Role of PI3K signaling in survival and progression of LNCaP prostate cancer cells to the androgen refractory state. Endocrinol, 142, 4795-4805

[147] Chen, G., Shukeir, N., Potti, A., Sircar, K., Aprikian, A., Goltzman, D., et al. (2004). Up-regulation of Wnt-1 and beta-catenin production in patients with advanced metastatic prostate carcinoma: potential pathogenetic and prognostic implications. Cancer, 101, 1345-1356

[148] Li, P., Nicosia, S.V., Bai, W. (2001). Antagonism between PTEN/MMAC1/TEP-1 and androgen receptor in growth and apoptosis of prostatic cancer cells. J Biol Chem, 276 (23), 20444-20450

[149] Yeh, S., Chang, C. (1996). Cloning and characterization of a specific coactivator, ARA_{70} for the androgen receptor in human prostate cells. Proc Natl Acad Sci USA, 93, 5517-5521

[150] Kang, H.Y., Yeh, S., Fujimoto, N., Chang, C. (1999). C loning and characterization of human prostate coactivator ARA54, a novel protein that associates with the androgen receptor. J Biol Chem, 274, 8570-8576

[151] Yuan, S., Trachtenberg, J., Mills, G.B., Brown, T.J., Xu, F., Keating, A. (1993). Androgen-induced inhibition of cell proliferation in an androgen-insensitive prostate cancer cell line (PC-3) transfected with a human androgen receptor complementary DNA. Cancer Res, 62, 1008-1013

[152] Lin, H.K., Hu, Y.C., Lee, D.K., Chang, C. (2004). Regulation of androgen receptor signaling by PTEN (phosphatase and tensin homolog deleted on chromosome 10) tumor suppressor through distinct mechanisms in prostate cancer cells. Mol Endocrinol, 10, 2409-2423

[153] Sharma M., Chuang, W.W., Sun, Z. (2002)Phospatidylinositol 3-kinase/Akt stimulates androgen pathway through GSK3beta inhibition and nuclear beta-catenin accumulation. J Biol Chem, 277, 30935-3094

[154] Ghosh P.M., Malik S.N, Bedolla RG, Wang Y, Mikhailova M, Prihoda TJ, Troyer DA, Kreisberg JI. (2005). Signal transduction pathways in androgen-dependent and -independent prostate cancer cell proliferation. Endocr Relat Cancer, 119-134

[155] Friedrichs W., Ruparel S.B., Marciniak R.A., de Graffenried L. (2011). Omega-3 fatty acid inhibition of prostate cancer progression to hormone independence is associated with suppression of mTOR signaling and androgen receptor expression. Nutr Cancer, 771-777

[156] Schayowitz A., Sabnis G., Goloubeva O., Njar V.C., Brodie A.M. (2010). Prolonging hormone sensitivity in prostate cancer xenografts through dual inhibition of AR and mTOR. Br J Cancer, 1001-1007

[157] Sircar K., Yoshimoto M., Monzon F.A., Koumakpayi I.H., Katz R.L., Khanna A., Alvarez K., Chen G., Darnel A.D., Aprikian A.G., Saad F., Bismar T.A., Squire J.A. (2009). PTEN genomic deletion is associated with p-Akt and AR signalling in poorer outcome, hormone refractory prostate cancer. J Pathol, 505-513

[158] Müller J., Ehlers A., Burkhardt L., Sirma H., Steuber T., Graefen M., Sauter G., Minner S., Simon R., Schlomm T., Michl U. (2012). Loss of p(Ser2448) -mTOR expression is linked to adverse prognosis and tumor progression in ERG-fusion-positive cancers. Int J Cancer, Epub ahead of print

[159] Kaarbø M., Mikkelsen O.L., Malerød L., Qu S., Lobert V.H., Akgul G., Halvorsen T., Maelandsmo G.M., Saatcioglu F. (2010). PI3K-AKT-mTOR pathway is dominant over androgen receptor signaling in prostate cancer cells. Cell Oncol, 11-27

[160] Wang Y., Mikhailova M., Bose S., Pan C.X., de Vere White R.W., Ghosh P.M. (2008). Regulation of androgen receptor transcriptional activity by rapamycin in prostate cancer cell proliferation and survival. Oncogene, 7106-7117

[161] Wu Y., Chhipa R.R., Cheng J., Zhang H., Mohler J.L., Ip C. (2010). Androgen receptor-mTOR crosstalk is regulated by testosterone availability: implication for prostate cancer cell survival. Anticancer Res, 3895-3901

[162] Squillace R.M., Miller D., Wardwell S.D., Wang F., Clackson T., Rivera V.M. (2012). Synergistic activity of the mTOR inhibitor ridaforolimus and the antiandrogen bicalutamide in prostate cancer models. Int J Oncol, 425-432

[163] Facompre N.D., Sinha I., El-Bayoumy K., Pinto J.T., Sinha R. (2012). Remarkable inhibition of mTOR signaling by the combination of rapamycin and 1,4-phenylenebis(methylene)selenocyanate in human prostate cancer cells. Int J Cancer, 2134-2142

[164] Fang Z., Zhang T., Dizeyi N., Chen S., Wang H., Swanson K.D., Cai C., Balk S.P., Yuan X. (2012). Androgen Receptor Enhances p27 Degradation in Prostate Cancer Cells through Rapid and Selective TORC2 Activation. J Biol Chem, 2090-2098

[165] Alessi D.R., James S.R., Downes C.P., Holmes A.B., Gaffney P.R., Reese C.B., Cohen P. (1997). Characterization of a 3-phosphoinositide-dependent protein kinase which phosphorylates and activates protein kinase Balpha. Curr Biol, 261-269

[166] Xu Y., Chen S.Y., Ross K.N., Balk S.P. (2006). Androgens induce prostate cancer cell proliferation through mammalian target of rapamycin activation and post-transcriptional increases in cyclin D proteins. Cancer Res, 7783-7792

[167] Cinar B., De Benedetti A., Freeman M.R. (2005). Post-transcriptional regulation of the androgen receptor by Mammalian target of rapamycin. Cancer Res, 2547-2553

[168] Bagchi G., Zhang Y., Stanley K.A., Waxman D.J. (2011). Complex modulation of androgen responsive gene expression by methoxyacetic acid. Reprod Biol Endocrinol

[169] Li P., Nicosia S.V., Bai W. (2001). Antagonism between PTEN/MMAC1/TEP-1 and androgen receptor in growth and apoptosis of prostatic cancer cells. J Biol Chem, 20444-20450

[170] Ma Q., Fu W., Li P., Nicosia S.V., Jenster G., Zhang X., Bai W. (2009). FoxO1 mediates PTEN suppression of androgen receptor N- and C-terminal interactions and coactivator recruitment. Mol Endocrinol, 213-225

[171] Li P., Lee H., Guo S., Unterman T.G., Jenster G., Bai W. (2003). AKT- independent protection of prostate cancer cells from apoptosis mediated through complex formation between the androgen receptor and FKHR. Mol Cell Biol 104-118

[172] Yang L., Xie S., Jamaluddin M. S., Altuwaijri S., Ni J., Kim E., Chen Y. T., Hu Y. C., Wang L., Chuang K. H., Wu C. T., Chang C. (2005). Induction of androgen receptor expression by phosphatidylinositol 3-kinase/Akt downstream substrate, FOXO3a, and their roles in apoptosis of LNCaP prostate cancer cells. J Biol Chem, 33558-33565

[173] Hu Y., Wang X., Zeng L., Cai D. Y., Sabapathy K., Goff S. P., Firpo E. J., Li B. (2005). ERK phosphorylates p66shcA on Ser36 and subsequently regulates p27kip1 expression via the Akt-FOXO3a pathway: implication of p27kip1 in cell response to oxidative stress. Mol Biol Cell, 3705-3718

[174] Li Y., Wang Z., Kong D., Murthy S., Dou Q.P., Sheng S., Reddy G.P., Sarkar F.H. (2007). Regulation of FOXO3a/beta-catenin/GSK-3beta signaling by 3,3'-diindolylmethane contributes to inhibition of cell proliferation and induction of apoptosis in prostate cancer cells. J Biol Chem, 21542-21550

[175] Zhang H., Fang J., Yao D., Wu Y., Ip C., Dong Y. (2010). Activation of FOXO1 is critical for the anticancer effect of methylseleninic acid in prostate cancer cells. Prostate, 1265-1273

[176] Ip C., Ganther H.E. (1990). Activity of methylated forms of selenium in cancer prevention. Cancer Res, 1206-1211

[177] Salas T.R., Kim J., Vakar-Lopez F., Sabichi A.L., Troncoso P., Jenster G., Kikuchi A., Chen S.Y., Shemshedini L., Suraokar M., Logothetis C.J., DiGiovanni J., Lippman S.M., Menter D.G. (2004). Glycogen synthase kinase-3 beta is involved in the phosphorylation and suppression of androgen receptor activity. J Biol Chem, 19191-19200

[178] Wang L., Lin H.K., Hu Y.C., Xie S., Yang L., Chang C. (2004). Suppression of androgen receptor-mediated transactivation and cell growth by the glycogen synthase kinase 3 beta in prostate cells. J Biol Chem, 32444-32452

[179] Mazor M., Kawano Y., Zhu H., Waxman J., Kypta R.M. (2004). Inhibition of glycogen synthase kinase-3 represses androgen receptor activity and prostate cancer cell growth. Oncogene, 7882-7892

[180] Schütz S.V., Schrader A.J., Zengerling F., Genze F., Cronauer M.V., Schrader M. (2011). Inhibition of glycogen synthase kinase-3β counteracts ligand-independent activity of the androgen receptor in castration resistant prostate cancer. PloS One, e25341

[181] Liao X., Thrasher J.B., Holzbeierlein J., Stanley S., Li B. (2004). Glycogen synthase kinase-3beta activity is required for androgen-stimulated gene expression in prostate cancer. Endocrinology, 2941-2949

[182] Mulholland D.J., Dedhar S., Wu H., Nelson C.C. (2006). PTEN and GSK3beta: key regulators of progression to androgen-independent prostate cancer. Oncogene, 329-337

[183] Benaim E.A., Pace C.M., Roehrborn C.G. (2002). Gleason score predicts androgen independent progression after androgen deprivation therapy. Eur Urol, 12-17

[184] Schütz S.V., Cronauer M.V., Rinnab L. (2010). Inhibition of glycogen synthase kinase-3beta promotes nuclear export of the androgen receptor through a CRM1-dependent mechanism in prostate cancer cell lines. J Cell Biochem, 1192-1200

[185] Fornerod M., Ohno M., Yoshida M., Mattaj I.W. (1997). CRM1 is an export receptor for leucine-rich nuclear export signals. Cell, 1051-1060

[186] Li R., Erdamar S., Dai H., Sayeeduddin M., Frolov A., Wheeler T.M., Ayala G.E. (2009). Cytoplasmic accumulation of glycogen synthase kinase-3beta is associated with aggressive clinicopathological features in human prostate cancer. Anticancer Res, 2077-2081

[187] Wang G., Wang J., Sadar M.D. (2008). Crosstalk between the androgen receptor and beta- catenin in castrate-resistant prostate cancer. Cancer Res, 9918-9927

[188] Trucia C.I., Byers S., Gelmann E.P. (2000). Beta-catenin affects androgen receptor transcriptional activity and ligand specificity. Cancer Res, 4709-4712

[189] Mulholland D.J., Cheng H., Reid K., Rennie P.S., Nelson C.C. (2002). The androgen receptor can promote beta-catenin nuclear translocation independently of adenomatous polyposis coli. J Biol Chem, 17933-17943

[190] Song L.N., Herrell R., Byers S., Shah S., Wilson E.M., Gelmann E.P. (2003). Beta-catenin binds to the activation function 2 region of the androgen receptor and modulates the effects of the N-terminal domain and TIF2 on ligand-dependent transcription. Mol Cell Biol, 1674-1687

[191] Chesire D.R., Isaacs W.B. (2002). Ligand-dependent inhibition of beta-catenin/TCF signaling by androgen receptor. Oncogene, 8453-8469

[192] Hoogeboom D., Essers M.A., Polderman P.E., Voets E., Smits L.M., Burgering B.M. (2008). Interaction of FOXO with beta-catenin inhibits beta-catenin/T cell factor activity. J Biol Chem, 9224-9230

[193] Shen, MM., & Abate-Shen, C. (2011). Molecular genetics of prostate cancer: new prospects for old challenges. Gene Dev, Vol.24, pp. 1967-2000

[194] Mulholland, DJ., Dedhar, S., Coetzee, GA., & Nelson, CC. (2005). Interaction of nuclear receptors with the Wnt/beta-catenin/Tcf signaling axis: Wnt you like to know? Endocr Rev, Vol.26, pp. 898-915, ISSN 0163-769X

Section 8

Non-Androgen Gene Transcripts in Prostate Cancer

Chapter 21

Non-Androgen Regulated Transcription Factors as Novel Potential Targets for Prostate Cancer Therapy

J. Nathan Davis, Adam H. Greer, Thomas Yong and
Shari Meyers

Additional information is available at the end of the chapter

http://dx.doi.org/10.5772/53090

1. Introduction

1.1. Overview of prostate cancer and standard treatments

The estimated number of new prostate cancer cases for 2011 was 240,890. The majority of diagnosed prostate cancers (PCa) is found early due to the widespread use of the screening test for prostate specific antigen (PSA) and are considered low risk [1]. The prognosis for men diagnosed with low-risk prostate cancer is good and the NIH is recommending active surveillance [1]. Active surveillance has the benefit of reducing treatment side effects, including erectile dysfunction and incontinence, for men that are unlikely to die from their cancer [2]. Locally advanced prostate cancers are higher risk, and a substantial fraction of these patients will eventually die of the disease, though median survival may be as long as 5 years. If prostate cancer has spread to distant organs, current therapy will inevitably fail [3]. Because the androgen receptor (AR) is important for prostate cancer development and progression, androgen deprivation therapy (ADT), which either reduces the production of androgens by surgical or medical castration, or interferes with AR function via the use of antiandrogens, is increasingly becoming a central component in the management of metastatic prostate cancer [3]. ADT initially leads to improved clinical outcomes in about 90% of the cases. However, most tumors become androgen independent (AI) and no longer respond to standard hormonal therapies, chemotherapeutics or radiotherapy [3]. Thus, improved therapeutic strategies that target key pathways and molecules are essential to improve the outcome for patients with AI prostate cancer (AIPC). Interestingly, recent data shows that the AR pathway is often still engaged in AIPC, possibly due to receptor promiscuity or hypersensitivity. Therefore, some scientists believe that a strategy of targeting AR expression, either directly or indirectly, may be helpful in these cases [4]. Indeed, elegant methods employing genome wide analysis are being used to identify small molecule antagonists of AR function [5]. Other ideas for targeted therapies include small molecule inhibition of metabolic enzymes such as fatty acid synthase (FASN) because cancer cells, unlike their normal counterparts, synthesize de novo large quantities of fatty acids and cholesterol [6] and inhibitors of vascular endothelial growth factor receptor (VEGFR) to suppress vascularization [7].

2. Non-androgen regulated transcription factors in prostate cancer; rationale for targeting

Most targeted small molecule therapies under development interfere with the function of receptors on the cell surface or kinases located in the cytoplasm. Transcription factors have been underutilized as targets of cancer therapeutics, the exceptions being the steroid hormone receptors, such as the AR, and nuclear factor kappa B (NF- ▪ B) [8, 9]. However, it is imperative to identify novel targets for the design of molecular treatments for cancers, including AIPC. Advances in drug delivery systems and a better understanding of how transcription factors act should overcome issues with targeting this important group of proteins. Thus, we believe that effective therapeutics for AIPC can be developed by identifying and targeting key transcriptional regulators, other than the AR, that are required for prostate cancer proliferation and survival. To identify potential targets that are master transcriptional regulators, one looks for DNA binding proteins whose activity is required for cell fate decisions, stem cell homeostasis, proliferation, and development. The regulatory roles played by Core Binding Factor (CBF) [10] and CBF1, Suppressor of Hairless, Lag-1 (CSL), the downstream effector of Notch receptors, place these transcription factors at the pinnacle of signaling cascades required for malignancy [11, 12]. Perhaps not surprisingly, these two pathways are genetically linked and exhibit cross talk. For example, enforced expression of RUNX1 rescues the Notch1-null phenotype in zebrafish [13] and in Notch1-null mice RUNX1 expression is greatly reduced [14]. Moreover, Notch and RUNX1 cooperate during T-cell specification in mammals and CBF is required for pre-thymic cells response to Notch signaling [15]. Thus, these two important transcriptional pathways are linked and, together, present a number of novel targets for the development of cancer therapies.

3. Core binding factor

More than twenty years ago, Nancy Speck and David Baltimore identified a DNA binding activity that bound to the core site (TGTGGTAA) in the enhancer of Moloney Murine Leukemia Virus that, when mutated, altered disease specificity to produce thymic leukemia instead of erythroleukemia [16, 17]. This DNA binding activity, which was named Core Binding Factor, was identified in a variety of cell lines [16]. Dr. Speck's laboratory purified several peptides that had core- binding activity from calf thymus nuclei [18]. The Speck laboratory then went on to sequence 5 peptides and used these sequences to isolate 3 cDNA

http://dx.doi.org/10.5772/53090

clones from a murine thymus library that encoded the three mammalian isoforms of CBFβ (CBFβ p22.0, CBFβ p21.5, and CBFβ p17.6). [19]. The Speck study demonstrated that CBFβ did not bind to DNA itself but, instead, partnered with a DNA binding protein, at that time termed acute myeloid leukemia-1 (AML-1), since one of their peptides appeared to be contained in the bovine homologue of the human AML-1. AML-1 had been identified by virtue of its involvement in the t(8;21) chromosomal translocation in 1991 [20]. A similar DNA binding activity was also isolated via interaction with the polyomavirus enhancer and was called polyomavirus enhancer binding protein 2 (PEBP2) [21]. CBF also binds to the Type B leukemogenic virus enhancer [22]. In 1993, Scott Hiebert's laboratory demonstrated that AML-1 selected a site related to the enhancer core motif (TGT/cGGT) and identified the DNA binding domain [23]. Later, Dr. Hiebert's group identified a larger isoform of AML-1 (termed AML-1B) produced from the *AML-1* gene using a homology screen of a human B-cell library [24]. Two other AML-1 family members expressed from independent genes were identified; AML-2 and AML-3 [25]. Following these studies, the AML-1 family of proteins underwent a revision in nomenclature with guidance from the Human Genome Organization [26]. AML-1 is now termed RUNX1, AML-2 is now termed RUNX3, and AML-3 is now termed RUNX2. The murine nomenclature is written in small case. This nomenclature will be used for the remainder of the chapter.

Mammalian CBF is a heterodimeric complex consisting of RUNX1, RUNX2, or RUNX3. As the Speck laboratory suggested, these three proteins bind to promoters and enhancers of target genes (or viral LTRs) as a heterodimer with CBFβ [10, 27]. DNA binding is achieved with a central domain (runt domain), consisting of an S-type immunoglobulin fold resembling the DNA binding domains of p53 and NF-kB [23, 28]. Although CBFβ does not contact DNA it regulates and enhances RUNX protein DNA binding via interactions with the Runt domain [28]. Complexity in CBF-regulated transcription comes about not only through co-expression in many tissues and a highly conserved DNA binding domain and recognition sequence, but also through the existence of multiple isoforms. For example, the *RUNX1* gene produces three main isoforms, all of which contain the DNA binding domain. These isoforms are thought to have both overlapping and unique functions. For example, RUNX1 isoforms are differentially expressed during hematopoietic differentiation of human embryonic stem cells (ESCs) and the RUNX1c isoform is expressed at the time of emergence of definitive HSCs [29]. Such complexity makes it difficult to assign function to each RUNX isoform and clearly, we are just at the beginning of understanding the distinct roles played by each protein. CBFβ is encoded on one gene in mammals but, as noted above, multiple isoforms are produced that may have distinct functions [19].

CBF is conserved in all multicellular organisms examined but is not present in yeast or any nonmetazoan studied to date. RUNX and CBFβ genes were identified in the nematode *C. elegans*, the fruit fly *Drosophila melanogaster*, which contains two CBFβ genes and four RUNX genes, the sea urchin (*Strongylocentrotus purpuratus*), sponges, puffer fish (*Takifugu rubripes)*, and the zebrafish (*Danio rerio*) [30-32]. In *Drosophila, RUNT*, the first RUNX gene identified in that organism, is required for segmentation [33]. *RUNT* gene mutations produce fly embryos with segmentation defects while *Lozenge*, a second RUNX gene in fruit flies, is required for eye development (Coffman 2009). In sea urchin, the *spRunt-1* gene is required throughout development for cellular proliferation, cell survival, and tissue-specific gene expression [30]. Unlike mammals, two CBFβ homologs exist in *Drosophila. Big brother* and *Brother (Bgb* and *Bro)* display high homology to human CBFβ and are required for RUNX gene function in flies [34]. Studies in these model organisms have clearly demonstrated that CBF coordinates cellular proliferation, stem cell fate and terminal differentiation [30, 35].

Mouse genetics further demonstrate specific requirements for CBF in development and stem cell function. For example, RUNX1 is required for hematopoietic development and *Runx1* null animals die *in utero* by day E12.5 due to a complete absence of fetal-liver derived hematopoiesis [36]. Runx2 is critical for skeletal morphogenesis and *Runx2* null mice survive until birth but die shortly thereafter due to a complete lack of bone formation [37]. Interestingly, Runx1 and Runx3 are also expressed in bone cells and support skeletal development [27, 38]. *Runx3* null mice were reported to display gut hyperplasia due to an increase in cell proliferation and a reduced rate of apoptosis [39]. However, a second study showed that Runx3-deficient mice develop severe limb ataxia due to a defect in the dorsal root ganglion (DRG) proprioceptive neurons [40]. Runx3 is also important for hematopoiesis [27, 41]. Similar genetic studies demonstrated that CBFβ is required for RUNX protein function. For example, CBFβ knockdown mice recapitulate the *Runx1* null phenotype and hematopoietic-specific rescue of CBFβ null animals has demonstrated that CBFβ, like Runx2, is required for skeletal development [42, 43]. Thus, CBF functions as a master regulator of genes required for development, differentiation and stem cell maintenance [44, 45]. The requirement for CBFβ is likely due to it's ability to enhance RUNX DNA binding and, therefore, to augment the transcriptional strength of the RUNX factors [46].

4. Cancers associated with alterations to CBF

Alterations to CBF activity result in human disease. For example, human RUNX1 was first identified as the target of the t(8;21) chromosomal translocation associated with acute myelogenous leukemia (AML) [20, 47]. The t(8;21) is associated with approximately 12% of AML cases [48]. The t(8;21) results in the production of a chimeric transcription factor that retains the RUNX1 (chromosome 21) DNA binding domain but replaces the entire C-terminus with MTG8 (also called ETO), a transcriptional co-repressor [24, 49, 50]. RUNX1 is also the target of the rarer t(16;21) found in both de novo and therapy-related AML [51] and the t(12;21) identified in pre-B-cell acute lymphoblastic leukemia (ALL) [52]. These translocations fuse the RUNX1 DNA binding domain to an ETO-related protein termed MTG16 (CBFA2T3) and to an ETS-related transcription factor, respectively, to create chimeric gene regulatory factors [51, 52]. CBFβ is also targeted by genomic abnormalities that lead to AML. For example, the pericentric inversion of chromosome 16 produces a chimeric CBFβ/smooth muscle myosin heavy chain (SMMHC) protein termed CBFβ–SMMHC [53]. These chimeric transcription factors are thought to contribute to leukemogenesis by interfering with CBF-regulated transcription [54]. Moreover, these chromosomal abnormalities demonstrate that CBF alterations can result in both lymphoid and myeloid leukemias.

http://dx.doi.org/10.5772/53090

CBF's role in blood development and in leukemia was brought into sharp focus by animal studies and by the identification of the molecular defects associated with AML. For many years, RUNX1 was considered blood specific, in part because of the strong phenotype obtained in *Runx1*-null mice. More recently, the expression, composition and function of CBF was studied in a wide variety of normal and cancerous cell lines and tissues. For example, RUNX protein expression was identified in the hair follicle stem cells (HFSCs) of the skin, and CBF is required to regulate HFSC proliferation [55]. Moreover, RUNX1 expression is activated in a chemical-induced model of rodent skin squamous cell carcinoma [55].

The expression of RUNX factors in prostate epithelial cell lines and normal prostate tissue was identified by real-time RT-PCR [56]. RUNX1, RUNX2, and RUNX3 were variously expressed in normal prostate tissue, an immortalized, non-transformed cell line, prostate cancer cell lines and primary prostate cancers [56]. To confirm that mRNA expression led to active DNA binding activity, CBF presence was confirmed using electrophoretic mobility shift assay (EMSA) [56]. While RUNX1 and RUNX2 were always expressed in prostate cancer cell lines, RUNX3 expression was not observed in most prostate cancer cell lines [56]. This correlates well with other studies that have identified RUNX2 expression in prostate cancer cell lines and showed that decreasing RUNX2 expression inhibits cell growth [57]. RUNX2 may play a role in tumor spread since RUNX2 triggers expression of bone-specific genes in prostate cancers, which may be involved in bone metastasis [58, 59]. Moreover, in a PTEN-deleted mouse model of prostate cancer, developing tumors increased Runx2 expression [60]. Thus, there is evidence that Runx2 expression is increased in malignant versus benign prostate tissue and is associated with tumor metastasis [61]. Interestingly, in a study of 314 patients with clinically localized prostate cancer that were treated with radical prostatectomy, the allelic variant RUNX1 rs2253319 was associated with metastasis to lymph nodes [62]. These data illustrate both the complexity of CBF expression in prostate and the involvement of CBF in cancer growth and metastasis. CBF is also highly expressed or altered in lung, endometrioid, and breast cancers [63-65].

CBF interacts with steroid hormones in various tissues. For example, the vitamin D receptor (VDR) associates with RUNX2 to regulate osteocalcin gene expression [66] and inappropriate expression of osteocalcin in prostate cancer cells depends upon RUNX2 [38]. CBF also interacts with the androgen receptor. RUNX1 and RUNX2 have both been shown to activate transcription from the prostate specific antigen (PSA) promoter and RUNX1 and RUNX2 physically associate with the AR [56] [57]. In prostate cancer cell lines, RUNX2 enhances TGF-β and androgen response [57]. Thus, the CBF and AR transcriptional pathways intersect in a way that enhances AR signaling. These data suggest that targeting CBF in prostate tumors should negatively impact AR signaling as well.

5. CBF inhibitors

Given that CBF and the AR pathways intersect and that CBF has been shown to regulate gene expression changes associated with tumorigenesis and metastasis in prostate cancer cell lines, it seems reasonable to identify small molecules that can inhibit CBF function. Small molecules that interfere with the interaction between the RUNX proteins and CBFβ were recently described. In the first of these studies, the 3D structure of CBFβ was solved using NMR and the RUNX1 binding interface was determined [67]. This information was then used to perform a virtual chemical screen and using that information, allosteric inhibitors of CBFβ were identified. The most potent inhibitor, "17", inhibited proliferation of the ME-1 cell line, a line derived from a patient with acute myelomonocytic leukemia containing the inv(16), by about 40% and showed very little cytotoxicity [67]. Treatment of cells with 100 μm concentrations of Inhibitor 17 reduced RUNX1 DNA binding by about 30%. Thus, compound 17 binds to a site removed from the heterodimerization interface and produces moderate changes in CBF DNA binding and cellular proliferation. These data suggest that allosteric inhibitors of protein complex formation could be useful for probing CBF's role in cancer.

A recent approach to identify a role for CBF in prostate and ovarian cancer provides compelling evidence that CBF is a druggable target. Davis and co-workers showed that CBFβ - specific shRNAs inhibited the malignant phenotype of prostate and ovarian cancer cell lines [68]. Cell lines displaying 70% reduction in CBFβ were unable to grow in an anchorage independent manner and did not form xenograft tumors in mice. Gene array data (Agilent whole genome array) gathered during this study suggested that CBF-mediated gene expression was inhibited. Bioinformatic searches for RUNX DNA binding sites in the promoter regions of the differentially expressed genes revealed that of the 200 genes that exhibited altered expression, over 20% contained multiple putative RUNX binding sites (analyzed using the consensus TGT/CGGT) within their upstream regulatory regions [68]. EMSA was used to confirm a loss in CBF DNA binding activity [68]. These data clearly demonstrate that inhibition of CBFβ expression leads to a reduction in CBF activity and that CBF activity is required for the transformed phenotype.

The DNA binding activity of recombinant CBF is amenable to high throughput screening (HTS) assays and a recent screen of the NIH Clinical Collection Library has identified compounds that inhibit CBF (Davis and Meyers, unpublished data). The CBFβ siRNAs and compounds identified via HTS or virtual screens show promise as tools for discovery and as molecules that can be further developed into small molecule therapeutics in prostate cancer.

6. The Notch pathway

Notch gene mutations were first discovered in *Drosophila* via malformations of the wing [69]. This ligand-activated signaling pathway is a highly conserved mechanism for maintaining stem cell function and regulating apoptosis, proliferation and cell fate specification [69]. Mammals express four Notch receptor family members, termed Notch 1-4 and five ligands; two Jagged family ligands (jagged-1 and jagged-2) and three delta-like ligands (Dll1, Dll3 and Dll4) [69]. The Notch receptors are highly similar in structure and the extracellular domains contain epidermal growth factor-like repeats. The Notch ligands are also transmembrane proteins. Thus, the Notch receptors regulate cell behavior via juxatacrine signaling that requires direct contact between the ligand-expressing cells and those cells expressing the receptor. Ligand binding activates two consecutive proteolytic cleavages to free the intracellular portion of the receptor, which is referred to as the Notch intracellular domain (NICD) [70]. The first cleavage is carried out by an A Disintegrin And Metalloprotease (ADAM)-family of transmembrane metalloproteases. The second cleavage is carried out by γ-secretase, an integral membrane enzyme complex, that is perhaps best known for its role in generating the amyloid-beta peptide found in brains of Alzheimer's disease patients [70, 71]. The NICD is a transcriptional co-activator. Once released, it travels to the nucleus via a nuclear transport signal where it binds to DNA-bound CSL. NICD binding to CSL displaces repressor complexes and recruits the mastermind family (MAML, mastermind like) of transcriptional coactivators, thereby activating the transcription of Notch-responsive genes [69]. In the absence of Notch receptor activation, CSL nucleates transcriptional repressive complexes via recruitment of histone deacetylase activities through interaction with SHARP (SMART and HDAC associated repressor) and corepressors like SMART/NcoR, CtIP/CtBP or ETO family members [72]. Interestingly, ETO (also called MTG8) is the target of the t(8;21) that produces a RUNX1/ETO fusion gene. Thus, the t(8;21) targets components of both the CBF and Notch pathways, highlighting yet another way in which these pathways intersect.

To date, a limited number of Notch-responsive genes have been identified. Some of the first gene targets identified include the transcription factors Hairy and enhancer of split-1 (Hes1) and Hairy and enhancer-of-split related with YRPW motif 1 (Hey1). Both Hes1 and Hey1 can be activated by a constitutively activated Notch1 receptor suggesting that these genes are bona fide targets [69]. Other CSL target genes are important mediators of signaling, including Akt and NF-κB, and important cell cycle regulators such as c-myc, D-type cyclins, $p21^{Waf1/Cip1}$ and p53 [69]. CSL is the only down-stream transcription factor directly responsive to Notch activation and, therefore, is crucial to Notch function.

The Notch pathway is deregulated in a variety of leukemias and solid cancers. For example, the mammalian orthologue of Notch was identified as TAN1 the target of the t(7;9)(q34;q34.4) in T-cell acute lymphocytic leukemia (T-ALL). While the t(7;9) is relatively rare (1% of all T-ALL) [73], the Notch1 receptor is constitutively activated by point mutations in the majority of T-ALL (almost 60%) [74]. Subsequent to the identification of Notch alterations in T-cell leukemia, the Notch pathway has been implicated in a variety of other human malignancies including cancers of the breast, ovarian, prostate, colorectal, and pancreas, as well as other leukemias [75-78]. In breast cancer, the Notch pathway components are commonly over-expressed and increased expression of Notch or Jag1 correlates with poor prognosis [76]. More recently, some studies suggest that breast cancer stem cell fate is regulated through the Notch pathway [79]. The Notch pathway is required for normal development of the murine prostate, and like breast cancers, prostate cancers also utilize the Notch pathway [80]. For example, Notch-1 and Jagged-1 expression constitute part of a gene expression signature for prostate cancer [81]. Other evidence indicating a role for Notch signaling in prostate cancer includes studies showing that Jagged-1 expression correlates with prostate cancer recurrence and proliferation of prostate cancer cell lines [82, 83]. Moreover, down-regulation of both Notch-1 and Jagged-1 expression in the androgen insensitive prostate cancer cell line, PC3, was associated with a loss of malignancy and a reduction in Akt, mTOR and NF-κB activation [84].

As discussed above, the constitutive activation of Notch receptor signaling in diverse cancers is well documented, but the contribution of CSL to Notch-dependent oncogenesis has not been well studied. Our recent publication was the first to demonstrate that CSL was essential for the growth of prostate and breast cancer derived cell lines [85]. In these cancer cells, where Notch signaling is constitutive, CSL is required for growth *in vitro*. Thus, CSL is not only the focal point of Notch-dependent transcriptional control but appears to be central to the oncogenic Notch pathway as well [85].

In addition to the oncogenic functions associated with Notch signaling, the Notch pathway can also be tumor suppressive in cells or tissues where Notch predominately promotes differentiation [86]. Notch associated tumor suppressor activity is best illustrated in carcinoma of the skin, where keratinocyte specific inactivation of Notch1, Delta-like 1 (Dl1) or γ-secretase treatment accentuates tumor formation in chemical carcinogenesis models [87]. Increasingly, tumor suppressive activities of the Notch pathway are being reported, as interest in Notch signaling and the use of γ-secretase inhibitors to block Notch receptor activation has expanded. Inactivating mutations of Notch1 have been identified in head and neck squamous cell carcinoma [88] and haploinsufficiency of Notch1 or inhibition of Notch signaling with monoclonal antibodies to the Notch ligand Delta-like 4 induces vascular tumors in model systems [89]. As if to highlight the context dependent nature of Notch signaling, one report provided evidence that activated Notch1 alleles cooperated with oncogenic Ras to induce pancreatic cancer while a second report indicated that inactivation of Notch1 cooperated with Ras pathways in pancreatic cancers [90, 91]. This duality of function associated with Notch signaling has led to serious concerns regarding Notch receptor activation as a target of therapeutic intervention [86].

In prostate cancer, like in other cancers discussed above, Notch pathway signaling can be tumor suppressive. For example, NICD activity and Hes1 expression have been observed to be high in benign prostatic hyperplasia but low in prostate cancer indicating that Notch pathway activation can be lost during malignant transformation. Additionally, activation of the Notch pathway in the androgen independent prostate cancer cell line, DU145, inhibited cell growth and resulted in the activation of the PTEN tumor suppressor. Interestingly, knockdown of CSL in the DU145 cell line results in loss of cell growth (Yong and Davis, unpublished data). These data demonstrate that CSL (in a repressed complex) is required in cells where the Notch pathway can display tumor-suppressing activity. Clearly, the activity of the Notch pathway in prostate cancer is context dependent and complex.

7. Notch pathway inhibitors

Regardless of the data implicating the Notch pathway in tumor suppression as well as oncogenesis, chemotherapeutic targeting of the Notch pathway employing γ-secretase inhibitors (GSI) to block release of the NICD has generated much interest [92]. GSIs, which were designed primarily for Alzheimer's disease, developed by Merck, Novartis, Pfizer and Roche are currently in clinical trials for a number of malignancies including T-ALL, lymphoma, breast, colorectal, brain, pancreatic, and non-small cell lung carcinoma. However, targeting the Notch pathway through the use of GSIs is problematic. Preclinical studies examining GSI function *in vitro* are difficult because, with the notable exception of GSI-1, these drugs do not display strong inhibitory effects on cell growth or survival *in vitro*. Also, while these drugs do inhibit Notch signaling, they display poor specificity. As an example, the inhibition of survival of breast carcinoma cell lines by GSI-1 was associated with inhibition of the proteosome and not effects on Notch signaling [93]. In addition to off-target effects, Notch inhibition by GSI has adverse effects on the intestinal system and immune function [94]. Lastly, as discussed above, the cell context determines whether the Notch pathway is oncogenic or tumor suppressive even within cancers of the same organ [86]. Thus, the consequence of inhibition of Notch receptor activation by GSI or inhibitory antibodies to Notch receptors/ligands is difficult to predict.

Inhibition of Notch activation by GSIs, inhibitory antibodies that bind DSL ligands, or other inhibitors of receptor activation target only the Notch activated state and they are less than ideal. However, the Notch pathway is central to oncogenesis, and this idea fuels the search for novel ways to inhibit the Notch signaling pathway [11]. Recently, the Bradner laboratory developed a stabilized peptide that mimics MAML and binds to the NICD-CSL complex to block interaction with endogenous MAML [95]. SAHM1, a 16 amino acid peptide which blocks MAML binding to the NICD-CSL complex is cell-permeable and lowers NOTCH-target gene expression when added to cells in culture [95]. SAHM1 lowers proliferation of T-ALL cell lines suggesting that these small molecules will be useful as probes to dissect the requirement for MAML in Notch signaling and as building blocks for a new generation of Notch inhibitors.

Davis and co-workers tested the idea that direct inhibition of CSL would not only abrogate Notch pathways in the activated oncogenic state, but also disrupt the transcriptional regulation of Notch pathway genes that are repressed in the Notch quiescent state [85]. According to this argument, in cells or tissues where Notch activation is tumor suppressive, inhibition of CSL would release the strong transcriptional repressive complexes positioned on Notch targets. Removal of CSL-dependent repressive complexes could mimic the tumor suppressive activity of the Notch pathway. Indeed, Davis and co-workers addressed the role of CSL in Notch-dependent signaling in prostate cancer cell lines, using lentiviral mediated transfer of shRNA specific for CSL to knockdown expression of CSL. CSL knockdown was tracked by EMSA and expression of the Notch pathway genes was documented using RT-PCR array profiling. Knockdown of CSL expression produced gene expression changes distinct from those induced by GSI inhibition of Notch signaling [85]. For example, inhibition of Notch receptor activation by DAPT resulted in repression of Hes1, a well-characterized CSL target in prostate and breast cancer cell lines. In contrast, Hes1 mRNA levels were unaffected by CSL ablation in prostate cancer cell lines, indicating that Hes1 expression does not require the activating function of CSL [85]. Thus, Notch pathway-dependent transcriptional regulation of Hes1 is primarily through repression and ablation of CSL partially mimics Notch receptor activation. While HES1 expression was not significantly altered by CSL knockdown, the expression of other Notch pathway genes did change. One such gene, DTX1 is thought to regulate Notch signaling either by targeting the NICD for ubiquitination and degradation or by altering NICD transcriptional functions, possibly by competing for co-activators [96]. Davis and coworkers failed to generate stable cell lines after infection with the CSL-specific shRNA but not with the control non-target (NT) shRNA. CSL knockdown cells were poorly attached and growth inhibited as compared to the NT infected cells [96]. These data provide strong evidence that CSL, the major Notch pathway effector, is required for cell growth in prostate cancer cells lines, and suggest that CSL is an important candidate for small molecule therapies in AIPC.

8. Summary and future directions

Although the AR is an important target of therapeutics in the struggle against prostate cancer, it remains imperative to develop effective strategies to target other important transcirption pathways, especially in AIPC. To alter gene transcription, some scientists, for example, are developing histone acetyl transferase inhibitors [97]. However, any such therapeutic would be expected to lack specificity for particular oncogenic pathways. DNA binding transcription factors represent druggable targets that should produce a more specific outcome, and are under appreciated as targets of small molecule inhibitors. Master transcriptional regulatory factors such as CBF and CSL clearly play important roles in cancer cell biology. Numerous studies show that inhibiting their function results in cancer cell death or loss of malignancy. These may be particularly useful targets in prostate cancers as the pathways intersect and CBF enhances AR function. In the case of CBF, it may make sense to target CBFβ to inhibit CBF activity in cancers since the activity of CBF is clearly oncogenic, while individual RUNX proteins can act either as oncogenes or tumor suppressors [10]. Developing inhibitors against these key transcriptional regulators will allow their use not only for therapy but also as probes to understand specific transcriptional pathways that support cancer growth, proliferation and metastasis.

Acknowledgements

Drs. Davis and Meyers are supported by the Department of Defense award W81XWH-09-1-0277. Funding was also provided by the Feist-Weiller Cancer Center. Dr. Meyers would like to thank Ellie Shaina Davis and Dr. Arrigo De Benedetti for editorial assistance. T.S., rest in peace.

http://dx.doi.org/10.5772/53090

Abbreviations

ADT: androgen deprivation therapy

AI: androgen independent

AIPC: androgen independent prostate cancer

ALL: acute lymphoblastic leukemia

AR: androgen receptor

CBF: Core Binding Factor

DRG: dorsal root ganglion

ECS: embryonic stem cells

GSI: γ-secretase inhibitors

NT: non-target

PCa: prostate cancer

PSA: prostate specific antigen

VEGFR: vascular endothelial growth factor receptor

Author details

J. Nathan Davis[3], Adam H. Greer[1], Thomas Yong[2] and Shari Meyers[1]

*Address all correspondence to: smeyer@lsuhsc.edu

1 Department of Biochemistry and Molecular Biology, LSUHSC-S and Feist-Weiller Cancer Center, USA

2 Department of Medicine, LSUHSC-S and Feist-Weiller Cancer Center, USA

3 Department of Medical Sciences, Frank H. Netter School of Medicine at Quinnipiac University, USA

References

[1] Brawley, O.W., Prostate cancer epidemiology in the United States. World J Urol, 2012. 30(2): p. 195-200.

[2] Singer, E.A., et al., Active surveillance for prostate cancer: past, present and future. Curr Opin Oncol, 2012. 24(3): p. 243-50.

[3] Bluemn, E.G. and P.S. Nelson, The androgen/androgen receptor axis in prostate cancer. Curr Opin Oncol, 2012. 24(3): p. 251-7.

[4] Shiota, M., A. Yokomizo, and S. Naito, Increased androgen receptor transcription: a cause of castration-resistant prostate cancer and a possible therapeutic target. J Mol Endocrinol, 2011. 47(1): p. R25-41.

[5] Zhu, Z., et al., Dose-dependent effects of small-molecule antagonists on the genomic landscape of androgen receptor binding. BMC Genomics, 2012. 13(1): p. 355.

[6] Flavin, R., G. Zadra, and M. Loda, Metabolic alterations and targeted therapies in prostate cancer. J Pathol, 2011. 223(2): p. 283-94.

[7] Kluetz, P.G., W.D. Figg, and W.L. Dahut, Angiogenesis inhibitors in the treatment of prostate cancer. Expert Opin Pharmacother, 2010. 11(2): p. 233-47.

[8] Moretti, M., et al., Cancer: NF-kappaB regulates energy metabolism. Int J Biochem Cell Biol, 2012.

[9] Haddad, H. and J.A. Garcia, Novel agents for the management of castration-resistant prostate cancer. Curr Opin Urol, 2012. 22(3): p. 175-82.

[10] Cameron, E.R. and J.C. Neil, The Runx genes: lineage-specific oncogenes and tumor suppressors. Oncogene, 2004. 23(24): p. 4308-14.

[11] Groth, C. and M.E. Fortini, Therapeutic approaches to modulating Notch signaling: current challenges and future prospects. Semin Cell Dev Biol, 2012. 23(4): p. 465-72.

[12] Martinez Arias, A., V. Zecchini, and K. Brennan, CSL-independent Notch signalling: a checkpoint in cell fate decisions during development? Curr Opin Genet Dev, 2002. 12(5): p. 524-33.

[13] Nakagawa, M., et al., AML1/Runx1 rescues Notch1-null mutation-induced deficiency of para-aortic splanchnopleural hematopoiesis. Blood, 2006. 108(10): p. 3329-34.

[14] Kumano, K., et al., Notch1 but not Notch2 is essential for generating hematopoietic stem cells from endothelial cells. Immunity, 2003. 18(5): p. 699-711.

[15] Guo, Y., et al., Core binding factors are necessary for natural killer cell development and cooperate with Notch signaling during T-cell specification. Blood, 2008. 112(3): p. 480-92.

[16] Speck, N.A. and D. Baltimore, Six distinct nuclear factors interact with the 75-base-pair repeat of the Moloney murine leukemia virus enhancer. Mol Cell Biol, 1987. 7(3): p. 1101-10.

[17] Speck, N.A., B. Renjifo, and N. Hopkins, Point mutations in the Moloney murine leukemia virus enhancer identify a lymphoid-specific viral core motif and 1,3-phorbol myristate acetate-inducible element. J Virol, 1990. 64(2): p. 543-50.

[18] Wang, S.W. and N.A. Speck, Purification of core-binding factor, a protein that binds the conserved core site in murine leukemia virus enhancers. Mol Cell Biol, 1992. 12(1): p. 89-102.

[19] Wang, S., et al., Cloning and characterization of subunits of the T-cell receptor and murine leukemia virus enhancer core-binding factor. Mol Cell Biol, 1993. 13(6): p. 3324-39.

[20] Miyoshi, H., et al., t(8;21) breakpoints on chromosome 21 in acute myeloid leukemia are clustered within a limited region of a single gene, AML1. Proc Natl Acad Sci U S A, 1991. 88(23): p. 10431-4.

[21] Bae, S.C., et al., Isolation of PEBP2 alpha B cDNA representing the mouse homolog of human acute myeloid leukemia gene, AML1. Oncogene, 1993. 8(3): p. 809-14.

[22] Mertz, J.A., et al., Type B leukemogenic virus has a T-cell-specific enhancer that binds AML-1. J Virol, 2001. 75(5): p. 2174-84.

[23] Meyers, S., J.R. Downing, and S.W. Hiebert, Identification of AML-1 and the (8;21) translocation protein (AML-1/ETO) as sequence-specific DNA-binding proteins: the runt homology domain is required for DNA binding and protein-protein interactions. Mol Cell Biol, 1993. 13(10): p. 6336-45.

[24] Meyers, S., N. Lenny, and S.W. Hiebert, The t(8;21) fusion protein interferes with AML-1B-dependent transcriptional activation. Mol Cell Biol, 1995. 15(4): p. 1974-82.

[25] Levanon, D., et al., AML1, AML2, and AML3, the human members of the runt domain gene-family: cDNA structure, expression, and chromosomal localization. Genomics, 1994. 23(2): p. 425-32.

[26] van Wijnen, A.J., et al., Nomenclature for Runt-related (RUNX) proteins. Oncogene, 2004. 23(24): p. 4209-10.

[27] Cohen, M.M., Jr., Perspectives on RUNX genes: an update. Am J Med Genet A, 2009. 149A(12): p. 2629-46.

[28] Zhang, L., et al., Structural and functional characterization of Runx1, CBF beta, and CBF beta-SMMHC. Blood Cells Mol Dis, 2003. 30(2): p. 147-56.

[29] Challen, G.A. and M.A. Goodell, Runx1 isoforms show differential expression patterns during hematopoietic development but have similar functional effects in adult hematopoietic stem cells. Exp Hematol, 2010. 38(5): p. 403-16.

[30] Coffman, J.A., Is Runx a linchpin for developmental signaling in metazoans? J Cell Biochem, 2009. 107(2): p. 194-202.

[31] Rennert, J., et al., The evolution of Runx genes I. A comparative study of sequences from phylogenetically diverse model organisms. BMC Evol Biol, 2003. 3: p. 4.

[32] Robertson, A.J., et al., The evolution of Runx genes II. The C-terminal Groucho recruitment motif is present in both eumetazoans and homoscleromorphs but absent in a haplosclerid demosponge. BMC Res Notes, 2009. 2: p. 59.

[33] Kania, M.A., et al., The Drosophila segmentation gene runt encodes a novel nuclear regulatory protein that is also expressed in the developing nervous system. Genes Dev, 1990. 4(10): p. 1701-13.

[34] Golling, G., et al., Drosophila homologs of the proto-oncogene product PEBP2/CBF beta regulate the DNA-binding properties of Runt. Mol Cell Biol, 1996. 16(3): p. 932-42.

[35] Wang, C.Q., et al., Runx family genes, niche, and stem cell quiescence. Blood Cells Mol Dis, 2010. 44(4): p. 275-86.

[36] Okuda, T., et al., AML1, the target of multiple chromosomal translocations in human leukemia, is essential for normal fetal liver hematopoiesis. Cell, 1996. 84(2): p. 321-30.

[37] Komori, T., et al., Targeted disruption of Cbfa1 results in a complete lack of bone formation owing to maturational arrest of osteoblasts. Cell, 1997. 89(5): p. 755-64.

[38] Lian, J.B., et al., Regulatory controls for osteoblast growth and differentiation: role of Runx/Cbfa/AML factors. Crit Rev Eukaryot Gene Expr, 2004. 14(1-2): p. 1-41.

[39] Li, Q.L., et al., Causal relationship between the loss of RUNX3 expression and gastric cancer. Cell, 2002. 109(1): p. 113-24.

[40] Levanon, D., et al., The Runx3 transcription factor regulates development and survival of TrkC dorsal root ganglia neurons. EMBO J, 2002. 21(13): p. 3454-63.

[41] Inoue, K., T. Shiga, and Y. Ito, Runx transcription factors in neuronal development. Neural Dev, 2008. 3: p. 20.

[42] Wang, Q., et al., The CBFbeta subunit is essential for CBFalpha2 (AML1) function in vivo. Cell, 1996. 87(4): p. 697-708.

[43] Kundu, M., et al., Cbfbeta interacts with Runx2 and has a critical role in bone development. Nat Genet, 2002. 32(4): p. 639-44.

[44] Coffman, J.A., Runx transcription factors and the developmental balance between cell proliferation and differentiation. Cell Biol Int, 2003. 27(4): p. 315-24.

[45] Kurosaka, H., et al., Core binding factor beta functions in the maintenance of stem cells and orchestrates continuous proliferation and differentiation in mouse incisors. Stem Cells, 2011. 29(11): p. 1792-803.

[46] Tang, Y.Y., et al., Energetic and functional contribution of residues in the core binding factor beta (CBFbeta) subunit to heterodimerization with CBFalpha. J Biol Chem, 2000. 275(50): p. 39579-88.

[47] Erickson, P., et al., Identification of breakpoints in t(8;21) acute myelogenous leukemia and isolation of a fusion transcript, AML1/ETO, with similarity to Drosophila segmentation gene, runt. Blood, 1992. 80(7): p. 1825-31.

[48] Lam, K. and D.E. Zhang, RUNX1 and RUNX1-ETO: roles in hematopoiesis and leukemogenesis. Front Biosci, 2012. 17: p. 1120-39.

[49] Davis, J.N., L. McGhee, and S. Meyers, The ETO (MTG8) gene family. Gene, 2003. 303: p. 1-10.

[50] Miyoshi, H., et al., The t(8;21) translocation in acute myeloid leukemia results in production of an AML1-MTG8 fusion transcript. EMBO J, 1993. 12(7): p. 2715-21.

[51] Gamou, T., et al., The partner gene of AML1 in t(16;21) myeloid malignancies is a novel member of the MTG8(ETO) family. Blood, 1998. 91(11): p. 4028-37.

[52] Golub, T.R., et al., Fusion of the TEL gene on 12p13 to the AML1 gene on 21q22 in acute lymphoblastic leukemia. Proc Natl Acad Sci U S A, 1995. 92(11): p. 4917-21.

[53] Liu, P., et al., Fusion between transcription factor CBF beta/PEBP2 beta and a myosin heavy chain in acute myeloid leukemia. Science, 1993. 261(5124): p. 1041-4.

[54] Hart, S.M. and L. Foroni, Core binding factor genes and human leukemia. Haematologica, 2002. 87(12): p. 1307-23.

[55] Hoi, C.S., et al., Runx1 directly promotes proliferation of hair follicle stem cells and epithelial tumor formation in mouse skin. Mol Cell Biol, 2010. 30(10): p. 2518-36.

[56] Fowler, M., et al., RUNX1 (AML-1) and RUNX2 (AML-3) cooperate with prostate-derived Ets factor to activate transcription from the PSA upstream regulatory region. J Cell Biochem, 2006. 97(1): p. 1-17.

[57] van der Deen, M., et al., The cancer-related Runx2 protein enhances cell growth and responses to androgen and TGFbeta in prostate cancer cells. J Cell Biochem, 2010. 109(4): p. 828-37.

[58] Stein, G.S., et al., Runx2 control of organization, assembly and activity of the regulatory machinery for skeletal gene expression. Oncogene, 2004. 23(24): p. 4315-29.

[59] Pratap, J., J.B. Lian, and G.S. Stein, Metastatic bone disease: role of transcription factors and future targets. Bone, 2011. 48(1): p. 30-6.

[60] Lim, M., et al., Runx2 regulates survivin expression in prostate cancer cells. Lab Invest, 2010. 90(2): p. 222-33.

[61] Akech, J., et al., Runx2 association with progression of prostate cancer in patients: mechanisms mediating bone osteolysis and osteoblastic metastatic lesions. Oncogene, 2010. 29(6): p. 811-21.

[62] Huang, S.P., et al., Clinical significance of runt-related transcription factor 1 polymorphism in prostate cancer. BJU Int, 2011. 107(3): p. 486-92.

[63] Tandon, M., et al., Runx2 mediates epigenetic silencing of the bone morphogenetic protein-3B (BMP-3B/GDF10) in lung cancer cells. Mol Cancer, 2012. 11: p. 27.

[64] CBFB Mutations and MAGI3-AKT3 Fusions Recur In Breast Cancer. Cancer Discov, 2012. 2(8): p. OF10.

[65] Planaguma, J., et al., A differential gene expression profile reveals overexpression of RUNX1/AML1 in invasive endometrioid carcinoma. Cancer Res, 2004. 64(24): p. 8846-53.

[66] Paredes, R., et al., Bone-specific transcription factor Runx2 interacts with the 1alpha, 25-dihydroxyvitamin D3 receptor to up-regulate rat osteocalcin gene expression in osteoblastic cells. Mol Cell Biol, 2004. 24(20): p. 8847-61.

[67] Gorczynski, M.J., et al., Allosteric inhibition of the protein-protein interaction between the leukemia-associated proteins Runx1 and CBFbeta. Chem Biol, 2007. 14(10): p. 1186-97.

[68] Davis, J.N., et al., Association of core-binding factor beta with the malignant phenotype of prostate and ovarian cancer cells. J Cell Physiol, 2010. 225(3): p. 875-87.

[69] Borggrefe, T. and F. Oswald, The Notch signaling pathway: transcriptional regulation at Notch target genes. Cell Mol Life Sci, 2009. 66(10): p. 1631-46.

[70] Kaether, C., C. Haass, and H. Steiner, Assembly, trafficking and function of gamma-secretase. Neurodegener Dis, 2006. 3(4-5): p. 275-83.

[71] van Tetering, G. and M. Vooijs, Proteolytic cleavage of Notch: "HIT and RUN". Curr Mol Med, 2011. 11(4): p. 255-69.

[72] Oswald, F., et al., SHARP is a novel component of the Notch/RBP-Jkappa signalling pathway. EMBO J, 2002. 21(20): p. 5417-26.

[73] Ellisen, L.W., et al., TAN-1, the human homolog of the Drosophila notch gene, is broken by chromosomal translocations in T lymphoblastic neoplasms. Cell, 1991. 66(4): p. 649-61.

[74] Weng, A.P., et al., Activating mutations of NOTCH1 in human T cell acute lymphoblastic leukemia. Science, 2004. 306(5694): p. 269-71.

[75] Pece, S., et al., Loss of negative regulation by Numb over Notch is relevant to human breast carcinogenesis. J Cell Biol, 2004. 167(2): p. 215-21.

[76] Reedijk, M., et al., High-level coexpression of JAG1 and NOTCH1 is observed in human breast cancer and is associated with poor overall survival. Cancer Res, 2005. 65(18): p. 8530-7.

[77] Park, J.T., et al., Notch3 gene amplification in ovarian cancer. Cancer Res, 2006. 66(12): p. 6312-8.

[78] Reedijk, M., et al., Activation of Notch signaling in human colon adenocarcinoma. Int J Oncol, 2008. 33(6): p. 1223-9.

[79] Sharma, A., et al., A monoclonal antibody against human Notch1 ligand-binding domain depletes subpopulation of putative breast cancer stem-like cells. Mol Cancer Ther, 2012. 11(1): p. 77-86.

[80] Whelan, J.T., et al., Notch-1 signaling is lost in prostate adenocarcinoma and promotes PTEN gene expression. J Cell Biochem, 2009. 107(5): p. 992-1001.

[81] Kong, D., et al., Cancer Stem Cells and Epithelial-to-Mesenchymal Transition (EMT)-Phenotypic Cells: Are They Cousins or Twins? Cancers (Basel), 2011. 3(1): p. 716-729.

[82] Zhang, Y., et al., Down-regulation of Jagged-1 induces cell growth inhibition and S phase arrest in prostate cancer cells. Int J Cancer, 2006. 119(9): p. 2071-7.

[83] Santagata, S., et al., JAGGED1 expression is associated with prostate cancer metastasis and recurrence. Cancer Res, 2004. 64(19): p. 6854-7.

[84] Wang, Z., et al., Down-regulation of Notch-1 and Jagged-1 inhibits prostate cancer cell growth, migration and invasion, and induces apoptosis via inactivation of Akt, mTOR, and NF-kappaB signaling pathways. J Cell Biochem, 2010. 109(4): p. 726-36.

[85] Yong, T., et al., Down regulation of CSL activity inhibits cell proliferation in prostate and breast cancer cells. J Cell Biochem, 2011. 112(9): p. 2340-51.

[86] Lobry, C., P. Oh, and I. Aifantis, Oncogenic and tumor suppressor functions of Notch in cancer: it's NOTCH what you think. J Exp Med, 2011. 208(10): p. 1931-5.

[87] Nicolas, M., et al., Notch1 functions as a tumor suppressor in mouse skin. Nat Genet, 2003. 33(3): p. 416-21.

[88] Stransky, N., et al., The mutational landscape of head and neck squamous cell carcinoma. Science, 2011. 333(6046): p. 1157-60.

[89] Ryeom, S.W., The cautionary tale of side effects of chronic Notch1 inhibition. J Clin Invest, 2011. 121(2): p. 508-9.

[90] Hanlon, L., et al., Notch1 functions as a tumor suppressor in a model of K-ras-induced pancreatic ductal adenocarcinoma. Cancer Res, 2010. 70(11): p. 4280-6.

[91] De La, O.J., et al., Notch and Kras reprogram pancreatic acinar cells to ductal intraepithelial neoplasia. Proc Natl Acad Sci U S A, 2008. 105(48): p. 18907-12.

[92] Takebe, N., et al., Targeting cancer stem cells by inhibiting Wnt, Notch, and Hedgehog pathways. Nat Rev Clin Oncol, 2011. 8(2): p. 97-106.

[93] Han, J., et al., The cytotoxicity of gamma-secretase inhibitor I to breast cancer cells is mediated by proteasome inhibition, not by gamma-secretase inhibition. Breast Cancer Res, 2009. 11(4): p. R57.

[94] Imbimbo, B.P., et al., Therapeutic intervention for Alzheimer's disease with gamma-secretase inhibitors: still a viable option? Expert Opin Investig Drugs, 2011. 20(3): p. 325-41.

[95] Moellering, R.E., et al., Direct inhibition of the NOTCH transcription factor complex. Nature, 2009. 462(7270): p. 182-8.

[96] Yamamoto, N., et al., Role of Deltex-1 as a transcriptional regulator downstream of the Notch receptor. J Biol Chem, 2001. 276(48): p. 45031-40.

[97] Perry, A.S., et al., The epigenome as a therapeutic target in prostate cancer. Nat Rev Urol, 2010. 7(12): p. 668-80.

Chapter 22

Trithorax Genes in Prostate Cancer

Pier-Luc Clermont, Francesco Crea and
Cheryl D. Helgason

Additional information is available at the end of the chapter

http://dx.doi.org/10.5772/52905

1. Introduction

For several years, prostate cancer (PCa) has been considered a genetic disease, driven by somatic mutations occurring at critical oncogenic or tumor suppressive *loci* [1]. This view has changed over the last decades, thanks to mounting evidence on the role of epigenetics in PCa initiation and progression [2]. The term "epigenetics" derives from a Greek word, and literally means "above the gene". In molecular biology, this definition includes all heritable gene expression patterns, which are not derived from an alteration of DNA primary sequence [3]. The first epigenetic alteration to be linked with cancer was DNA methylation, which occurs at 5-cytosine residues in specific genomic regions, called CpG islands [2, 4]. Cytosine methylation results in gene silencing, especially when occurring at the promoter region of a targeted *locus*. This process is mediated by enzymes called DNA methyltransferases (DNMTs) [5]. Functional studies demonstrated that, along with inactivating mutations, DNA methylation is an alternative way of tumor suppressor silencing, and that this event might even anticipate the occurrence of a genetic mutation. For example, the *PTEN* (Phosphatase and tensin homolog) gene encodes for a phosphatase which acts as a potent tumor suppressor in PCa [6]. Indeed, PTEN protein is able to inhibit AKT (protein kinase B), which in turn activates several anti-apoptotic and proliferative signals in PCa cells. In keeping with these observations, PTEN- knockout mice display an early onset of PCa [7]. *PTEN* inactivating mutations are found in approximately 20% of PCa samples, and are associated with hormone refractory disease and higher tumor stage [8]. However, *PTEN* mutation is rarely homozygous, and approximately 50% of PCa patients are PTEN-negative, even if they do not display any genetic alteration [9]. Subsequent studies found that DNA methylation is the main mechanism of *PTEN* silencing in PCa, as well as in other neoplasms [10]. This event may occur in association with mutation on the other allele [11]. DNA methylation in the *PTEN* promoter region acts as a docking site for MeCP2 (methyl-CpG-binding protein 2), which in turn recruits several chromatin remodelling factors. Those complexes are able to turn transcriptionally active chromatin (euchromatin) into an inactive form (heterochromatin) [12]. Since then, several tumor suppressor genes were shown to be methylated in a significant fraction of PCa patients [13]. DNA methylation patterns are useful biomarkers for early diagnosis and patient stratification. Unlike genetic alterations, epigenetic changes are reversible, and thus can be targeted by specific drugs [2]. DNMT inhibition is able to reactivate silenced oncogenes, thereby inducing apoptosis and reducing treatment resistance [14]. Pharmacological inhibitors of DNMTs have been developed and tested in clinical trials, and some of them are approved for the treatment of haematological malignancies [15]. In PCa, as well as in other solid tumors, DNMT inhibitors displayed encouraging effects in pre-clinical models [14], but often failed to demonstrate clinically relevant activity [16]. One possible explanation for this discrepancy is that DNA methylation is not the key epigenetic mechanism in PCa.

As basic research on epigenetic gene regulation proceeds, it is becoming increasingly clear that gene expression regulation in human cells is finely tuned by the concurrent activity of different protein complexes. To understand the foundation of this intricate process, it is necessary to consider the tridimensional structure of chromatin [17]. The nucleosome is the basic chromatin unit. It is composed by approximately 150 bp of DNA, which are wrapped around a cylindrical protein complex (histone core) [18]. The core is an octamer composed of two copies of histone H2a, H2b, H3 and H4. Histone H1 acts as a linker between two nucleosomes. Nucleosomes can restrict the access of RNA polymerases to the DNA; thus, their local interaction with DNA is critical for gene expression control. Histones are characterized by long N-terminal tails, which mainly interact with the DNA phosphate backbone [19]. For this reason, post-translational modifications at histone tails can shape the local tridimensional structure of chromatin, thereby affecting RNA polymerase (and transcription factor) accessibility, and eventually modifying gene expression. Seminal studies revealed that the range of possible histone post-translational modifications (HPTMs) is wide, including acetylation, methylation, phosphorylation, ubiquitination, sumoylation and ADP-ribosylation [20]. Another layer of complexity is represented by the variable number of amino-acidic residues that can be modified. In addition, some modifications may be repeated on the same residue. For example, histone H3 Lys 27 (H3K27) can be mono-, di- or tri-methylated (me) [19]. Each single modification affects gene activity, and likely interacts with others [20]. As it is easy to understand, the combinatorial complexity of those modifications is immense, and we still lack appropriate technologic tools to comprehensively investigate this phenomenon [21]. Some authors proposed the systematic discovery of the histone code, i.e. the hidden language by which HPTMs cooperate to determine local gene activity [22].

Despite this discouraging complexity, some research sheds light on the functional role of specific HPTMs. For example, it is well known that histone lysine acetylation loosens DNA-histone binding, thereby providing transcriptionally active chromatin [23]. Accordingly, histone acetylases (HATs) are a class of activating epigenetic modifiers [24]. For the same reason, histone deacetylases (HDACs) are enzymes that repress gene expression [25]. To the contrary, histone methylation is multifaceted, since it can be associated with gene repression or activation depending on the targeted amino acid residue. For example, H3K9me and H3K27me are repressive marks, while H3K4me and H3K36me activate gene expression [26]. Interestingly, most of those HPTMs are mediated by two classes of histone modifiers, which appear to act as counteracting forces during embryonic development, and are emerging as novel oncogenes and tumor suppressor genes. The first class to be discovered was the Polycomb group (PcG) genes, which are mainly organized in multimeric Polycomb repressive complexes 1 and 2 (PRC1 and PRC2; Table 1) [27]. PRC2 catalyzes H3K27 trimethylation (me3), which acts as a docking site for PRC1. The latter complex then catalyzes histone H2aK119 ubiquitination (ub). Both modifications are repressive marks, and can be associated with DNA methylation [28]. In addition, it has been shown that PRC1 can act independently of PRC2 [29]. The function of PRCs was revealed by mutational analyses conducted on *Drosophila.* PRCs are essential for HOX (homeobox) gene silencing and tissue specification [30]. *Drosophila* PRC homologs are also expressed in human cells, where they regulate stem cell function and differentiation. Studies on human cells also revealed that PRCs can target a wider set of genes, and that they are involved in physiologic and pathologic phenomena, including cancer [31]. In PCa, both PRC1 and PRC2 display oncogenic functions, through the repression of key tumor suppressor genes. For example, PRC1 member BMI1 (B-cell-specific Moloney murine leukemia virus integration site 1) induces resistance to conventional chemotherapy (docetaxel) [32], while PRC2 member EZH2 (enhancer of zeste homolog 2) is essential for PCa cell invasion and metastatic spreading [33].

As anticipated, trithorax group genes (TrxGs) were first discovered as PRC-counteracting forces in *Drosophila,* where their role in switching on and maintaining the activation of HOX genes is well known [30]. TrxG complex organization is more variable than what has been found for PRCs. First, TrxGs include both histone modifiers and ATP-dependent chromatin remodelling factors [34]. The first class acts by decorating histone tails with activating marks, while the latter "reads" those modifications and actively induces a tridimensional change in chromatin structure, which then becomes available for RNA polymerases and transcription factors. Since this chapter is focused on strictly epigenetic mechanisms of gene expression control, we will not discuss chromatin remodelling factors. In mammals, histone modifier TrxGs are grouped in 3 major complexes (refer to Table 1): COMPASS (complex protein associated with SET domain), COMPASS-like and ASH (absent small and homeotic discs). COMPASS contains a histone methyltransferase domain (SET), which is shared with PRC2 [35]. Unlike PRC2, COMPASS mediates H3K4me, a broad activating mark found throughout the genome. COMPASS-like complexes also display the SET domain, which is used to silence a more restricted group of genes [36]. COMPASS-like can also activate gene expression through H4K16 acetylation [34]. Depending on subunit composition, this complex is also able to demethylate H3K27me, thereby directly counteracting PRC2 [37]. Finally, ASH1 is able to catalyze H3K36me, a further activating mark. In mammals, this function is mediated by a single protein rather than a complex [34].

Along with their function in embryonic development, TrxG histone modifiers are emerging as a novel class of cancer-related genes [43]. Due to their multifaceted interaction with PcGs, and due to the role of PcGs in PCa, it is likely that TrxGs also play a role in this neoplasm. For this reason, we decided to summarize current knowledge on the role of TrxGs in cancer initiation and progression, and to query a publically available gene expression database, to get insights into the role of those genes in PCa metastasis, which is the major determinant of death induced by this neoplasm. Based on our literature search and our results, we will propose a model to explain putative mechanisms of TrxG-dependent oncogenic, or tumor suppressive, functions.

Type	Complex	Subunits	HPTMs Catalyzed	Transcriptional Effect	References
PcG	PRC1	BMI1; RING1; RING1B; CBX	H2AK119Ub	Repression	[38-40]
	PRC2	EZH2; SUZ12; EED	H3K27me3	Repression	[38-40]
TrxG	COMPASS	SET1A,B; CXXC1; WDR82; ASH2L*; DPY30; HCF1; RBBP5; WDR5	H3K4me3	Activation	[34, 41, 42]
	COMPASS-like (A)	MLL1,2; MOF; MENIN; ASH2L; DPY30; HCF1; RBBP5; WDR5	H3K4me3; H4K16ac	Activation	[34, 41, 42]
	COMPASS-like (B)	MLL3,4; UTX; NCOA6; PA1; PTIP; ASH2L; DPY30; HCF1; RBBP5; WDR5	H3K4me3; H3K27 demethylation	Activation	[34, 41, 42]
	ASH1	ASH1L	H3K36me3; H3K27ac	Activation	[34, 41, 42]

Note : Red indicates core COMPASS subunits

Table 1. Composition and Activity of TrxG Complexes

2. Body

2.1. Overview of trithorax group activity in prostate cancer

It is now well established that TrxG counteracts PcG HPTMs to promote a transcriptionally competent chromatin state [34, 44]. An intricate regulatory network controls whether the repressive effect of PcG activity or the activating role of TrxG dominates at specific *loci* [45]. The best characterized interplay between these two families of epigenetic modifiers occurs during embryonic development. In undifferentiated cells, PcG is highly expressed and maintains lineage-specific genes in a transcriptionally incompetent state while TrxG activity is minimal [46]. In response to external differentiation cues, PcG activity is reduced while TrxG becomes functionally active. As a result, lineage-specific genes are expressed and drive the cell towards a differentiated state [46]. The classic example of TrxG and PcG interplay

http://dx.doi.org/10.5772/52905

involves the regulation of the HOX *locus*(See Figure 1). First silenced by PcG in embryonic stem cells (ESCs), HOX genes are subsequently induced upon TrxG activation during differentiation [47].

The functional relationship between PcG and TrxG is not limited to development. Incorrect regulation of PcG and TrxG also plays an inherent role in cancer initiation and progression [48-51]. In cancer, many embryonic transcriptional programs are orchestrated and push tumor cells towards a more undifferentiated state [43]. This directly implicates PcG and TrxG as they regulate many common target tumor suppressor genes that inhibit differentiation, invasion, and cell cycle progression [41]. These tumor suppressor genes are turned off in cancer, correlating with increased PcG expression and H3K27 trimethylation [52]. This indicates that, in cancer cells, PcG somehow undergoes a gain of function while TrxG activity is lost at key metastasis-inhibitory *loci*. In this classical model, PcG therefore act as oncogenes while TrxG operate as tumor suppressors (See Figure 1).

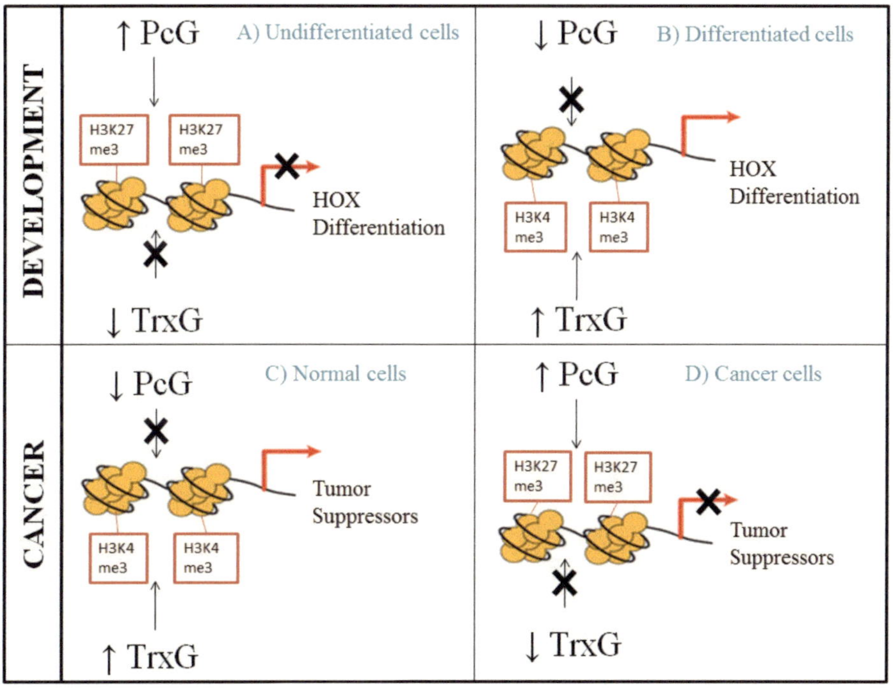

Figure 1. Classical Model of the PcG-TrxG Interplay in Development and Cancer

However, this model does not explain all the data regarding TrxG in cancer as the expression of individual TrxG subunits is highly heterogeneous across, and within, different tumor types. According to the classical model, TrxG genes act as tumor suppressors and should therefore be consistently downregulated in malignant cells. In fact, the expression of some TrxG genes increases in cancerous tissues, suggesting an oncogenic role for these particular TrxG genes [52, 53]. This indicates that there must exist an additional level of complexity which regulates not only the expression of individual TrxG genes, but also the activity and sequence specificity of TrxG complexes. Since TrxG proteins function as multimeric structures, their activity is highly context-dependent [54]. Many factors need to be taken into consideration when trying to assess the molecular function of TrxG complexes in a given temporal and spatial context. First of all, what is the relative expression of the individual subunits present within the TrxG complex? If many subunits are overexpressed or underexpressed, the composition of the complex changes, which might lead to functional differences. Second, which coregulators of these complexes are present? For example, a corepressor could bind to a given TrxG complex and inhibit its H3K4 methyltransferase ability. Another possibility is that a transcription factor expressed specifically in cancer cells binds to a TrxG complex and recruits it to a normally untargeted loci. Finally, how is TrxG activity regulated by PTMs of its individual subunits? Every TrxG complex is composed of multiple proteins, all of them able to be chemically modified at multiple residues. Each PTM potentially affects the activity of the complex and the additive effect of all these possible PTMs accounts for an astronomical number of possible transcriptional outcomes [21]. In summary, although the traditional model by which TrxG simply opposes PcG functions in cancer still represents a good approximation, it remains incomplete as additional factors regulate TrxG activity.

Even though the epigenetic landscape of PCa remains quite complex, interesting links can be found between histone modifiers and the metastatic process. PcG members EZH2 and BMI1 are both overexpressed in PCa and their elevated expression correlates with metastasis and poor prognosis [55-57]. Their importance in PCa progression is reflected by the numerous studies that explored the possibility of targeting them pharmacologically [58-61]. While the role of PcG has been extensively investigated, few studies directly assessed the role of TrxG in PCa. Our analysis revealed that although no individual TrxG genes shows consistently significant up- or downregulation, a very high proportion of metastatic prostate tumors contain at least one TrxG gene whose expression is deregulated. The accumulated evidence suggests that TrxG does not act only as traditional tumor suppressors which counteract PcG activity. In fact, individual TrxG genes can interact with other complexes to either promote or repress progression to metastasis. To account for this functional heterogeneity, we will review the current literature for individual TrxG gene previously associated with cancer and then discuss expression data from a publicly available PCa database. We will finish by proposing putative mechanisms of TrxG misregulation in PCa, with a focus on the metastatic process.

3. Literature review – Individual TrxG genes

3.1. ASH2L

ASH2L is the human homologue of *Drosophila* ASH2 (absent small homeotic 2) and represents a core member of the COMPASS and COMPASS-like complexes. Through interactions with WDR5 (WD-repeat protein 5) and RBBP5 (retinoblastoma binding protein 5), ASH2L activates SET1 domain-containing proteins (SET1A, SET1B and mixed lineage leukemia

(MLL)1-4) which subsequently catalyze H3K4 trimethylation [54]. The presence of ASH2L is essential for optimal H3K4 trimethylation as knockdown of ASH2L led to a genome-wide decrease in H3K4me3 [62]. Since COMPASS and COMPASS-like complexes are required for the transcriptional activation of numerous differentiation genes such as the HOX family, defects in ASH2L activity result in developmental defects [42, 63]. In mice, homozygous knockdown of ASH2L with gene-trap technology resulted in early embryonic lethality [64]. ASH2L also promotes differentiation in muscle during later developmental stages. Through an interaction with ASH2L, PAX7 (paired box 7) recruits the WDR5-ASH2L-MLL2 complex to myogenic gene promoters and promotes trimethylation of H3K4 at these sites [65]. MEF2D (myocyte enhancer factor 2D) is a transcription factor downstream of the p38 MAPK (mitogen-activated protein kinase) that also directs ASH2L-containing complexes to MyoD (myoblast determination protein)-bound genes in myoblasts [66]. At specific *loci*, MyoD, PAX7, and ASH2L cooperate to induce a transcriptional program that leads to myogenic differentiation [67].

In addition to its role in development, ASH2L is also involved in tumor initiation. While ASH2L mRNA levels remain normal in human cancers, ASH2L protein levels increase dramatically in malignant cells, suggesting an oncogenic function for ASH2L [68]. Supporting this hypothesis, ASH2L was also identified in complexes containing MYC (myelocytomatosis viral oncogene homolog) oncogene [68]. Since MYC activity increases in many types of cancers, the interaction between ASH2L and MYC suggests that ASH2L potentially adopts an oncogenic function [69]. Indeed, ASH2L transforms primary rat embryo fibroblasts (REFs) through cooperation with H-Ras (Harvey rat sarcoma viral oncogene homolog) [68]. As expected from an oncogene, knockdown of ASH2L reduces cell proliferation and inhibits transformation of REFs by MYC and H-RAS [68]. A recent study revealed that ASH2L might affect PCa progression by acting as a co-activator of the androgen receptor (AR) [70]. Co-immunoprecipitation experiments showed that AR interacts with ASH2L [70]. Importantly, TrxG genes MLL1 and MLL2 also interact with AR [70], suggesting that ASH2L function in PCa results from association with complexes having H3K4 methyltransferase activity (See Figure 2A). Furthermore, siRNA (small interfering RNA) silencing of MLL or ASH2L significantly repressed AR signalling [70]. However, pathways underlying the oncogenic nature of ASH2L remain poorly characterized. An important question that needs to be addressed is whether ASH2L promotes tumorigenesis through the same pathways in all tumor types or if its activity depends on the availability of other context-specific coregulators.

3.2. MENIN

MENIN (protein encoded by multiple endocrine neoplasia 1 gene – *MEN1*) represents an integral subunit of the COMPASS-like complex that contains MLL1-2, MOF (MYST family histone acetyltransferases), and core COMPASS proteins that trimethylate H3K4 [42]. In contrast to ASH2L, whether MENIN acts as an oncogene or a tumor suppressor highly depends on the specific tissue. Inherited mutations inactivating the *MEN1* gene lead to a condition called multiple endocrine neoplasia type 1, in which the patients develop neoplasias in endocrine organs such as the parathyroid gland, the pituitary gland, and the pancreas [71,

72]. In endocrine organs, MENIN functions as a tumor suppressor and its role has been well characterized [73]. MENIN induces the transcription of cyclin-dependent kinase inhibitors p18 and p27 [74]. A mutated *MEN1* gene therefore leads to a decrease in p18 and p27 expression, which accelerates cell-cycle progression. Loss of MENIN also promotes tumorigenesis by releasing the inhibition of the oncogenic transcription factor JUN D (jun sarcoma virus 17 oncogene homolog) [75], which subsequently induces the expression of genes responsible for proliferation [76]. In summary, mutation of the *MEN1* gene leads to neoplasm formation in endocrine organs, which signifies that MENIN acts as a tumor suppressor in these tissues. However, studies in hematopoietic malignancies containing MLL fusion proteins suggest an oncogenic role for MENIN [77]. In this context, MENIN binds to the MLL fusion protein and the complex activates the expression of key oncogenes which drive leukemogenesis [78]. Since MLL fusion proteins do not possess a SET domain, it is important to note that the oncogenic function of MENIN does not implicate H3K4 methylation [78]. Misregulation of MENIN activity also induces the formation of some solid tumors, although its mechanism of action varies considerably with the tumor type. For example, MENIN has been described as a tumor suppressor in non-small cell lung carcinomas (NSCLC) [79]. MENIN function can also be observed in other solid tumors. In breast cancer, MENIN represents a transcriptional coactivator of ERα (estrogen receptor alpha). [80]. In MCF7 breast cancer cells, MENIN co-localizes with ERα and activates ERα transactivation in a ligand-dependent manner [81]. Interestingly, MLL2 was also independently shown to associate with ERα, suggesting that MENIN's oncogenic function requires the methyltransferase activity of its associated TrxG proteins [82]. Furthermore, ER-positive breast cancer samples highly expressing MENIN had a worse outcome than those with low levels of MENIN after tamoxifen treatment [80]. These findings support the idea that MENIN overexpression promotes the progression to a malignant phenotype in mammary tumors. As in breast cancer, MENIN seems to function as an oncoprotein in PCa [53]. Significant upregulation of MENIN has been described in metastatic prostate tumors in comparison with their non-metastatic counterparts [83]. Copy number gains for *MEN1* represent frequent events in PCa and correlate with an increase in MENIN levels [83]. Depletion of MENIN also significantly suppresses proliferation of DU145 PCa cells, in addition to increasing the levels of Integrin-β1, CASPASE8, and p53 tumor suppressor [53]. Interestingly, MLL and MLL2 interact with AR. Since MENIN associates with MLL and MLL2, it is possible that its oncogenic function stems from cooperation with AR [70]. Given these findings, we propose that MENIN promotes tumorigenesis in PCa.

3.3. MLL

MLL is a H3K4 methyltransferase and its role has been well characterized in certain types of leukemia where it is frequently involved in translocations [84]. Five MLL family members, MLL1-5 are encoded in the mammalian genome [42]. MLL and MLL2 can associate with MENIN, MOF and core TrxG subunits to form a complex with H3K4 and H4K16 methyltransferase activity [54]. MLL3 and MLL4, on the other hand, can only be constituents of TrxG complexes that contain UTX and therefore possess H3K27 demethylase activity [45]. MLL5 does not directly associate with core TrxG members and there is still no evidence that

http://dx.doi.org/10.5772/52905

it has H3K4 methyltransferase activity [85]. The oncogenic role of MLL in leukemia arises through a translocation that removes its SET domain responsible for H3K4 methylation [84]. However, the role of MLL in PCa tumors has not been fully studied yet. Recent reports indicate that MLL enhances androgen signalling by directly interacting with AR and trimethylating H3K4 at AR target genes [70]. In accordance with an activating role of MLL on AR signalling, RNAi-mediated depletion of MLL significantly decreases Prostate-Specific Antigen (PSA) levels [70]. MLL expression is induced by SOX4 (Sex-determining region Y-box 4), a transcription factor that also activates epidermal growth factor receptor (EGFR), Integrin αv, Ras-related C3 botulinum toxin substrate 1 (Rac1), and ADAM metallopeptidase domain 10 (ADAM10) [86]. The pathways influenced by MLL activity suggest that MLL plays a role in promoting tumorigenesis. As is the case with MLL, MLL2 has also been shown to interact with AR. Although the role of MLL2 remains unclear in PCa, it seems to function as an oncoprotein in breast cancer [87]. By acting as a coactivator, MLL2 stimulates the transcription of estrogen receptor (ER) target genes in ER+ breast tumors [88]. Amplification of MLL2 has also been recorded in many solid malignancies including breast, pancreatic, brain, and ovarian tumors [89]. In summary, it seems that the H3K4 methyltransferase activity of MLL1 and MLL2 mediates an oncogenic function in solid tumors.

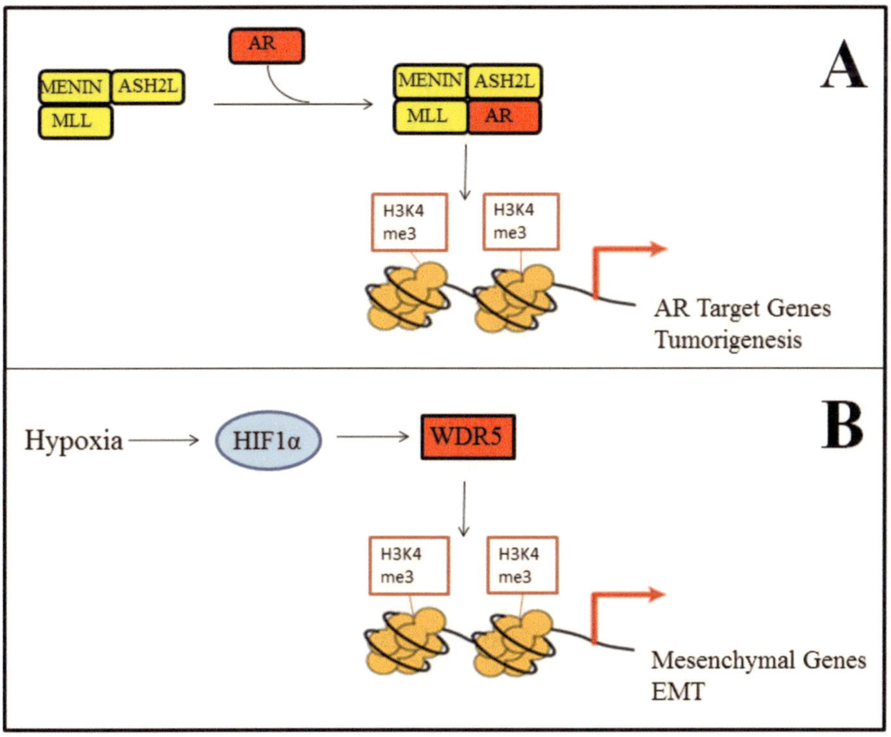

Figure 2. Putative Mechanisms of Oncogenic TrxG Genes in PCa

3.4. MOF

The acetyltransferase MOF (males absent on the first) associates with MENIN, MLL or MLL2, and the core COMPASS proteins (ASH2L, DPY30, HCF1, RBBP5, and WDR5) to form a distinct TrxG complex [90]. MOF specifically acetylates H4K16, a HPTM linked to transcriptional activation [91]. In cancer cells, loss of H4K16ac represents a common event and correlates with general hypomethylation of repetitive DNA sequences [92]. This suggests that MOF activity is inhibited in cancer cells and that MOF therefore functions as an oncosuppressor. Many important growth-regulatory pathways are regulated by MOF, some of which do not require the H3K4 methyltransferase ability of COMPASS-like complexes. First of all, MOF inhibits cancer progression by cooperating with forkhead box protein P3 (FOXP3) [93]. FOXP3 recruits MOF and the H3K4 methyltrasferase complex close to the transcription start site of tumor suppressors [93]. The synergistic effect of H3K4 trimethylation by MLL1-2 and of H4K16 acetylation by MOF results in transcriptional activation of target *loci*. In addition to its regulatory function in transcription, MOF also plays an important role in the DNA damage response (DDR), more specifically in the repair of double-stranded breaks (DSBs) [94]. In response to ATM (ataxia telangiectasia mutated) pathway activation, MOF gets recruited to chromatin where it acetylates H4K16 near DSBs [95]. At sites of DSBs, MOF stimulates the activity of DNA-dependent protein kinases (DNA-PKcs), a critical component of non-homologous end-joining (NHEJ) [96]. Interestingly, studies demonstrated that MOF inhibition also affects homologous recombination (HR) in addition to NHEJ [96]. In short, depletion of MOF leads to a reduction in H4K16 acetylation and is associated with defective DNA repair and chromosomal aberrations following ionizing radiation [97]. MOF also plays another critical role in DDR and apoptosis induction by acetylating the DNA-binding domain of p53 at lysine 120 [98]. This modification leads to increased p53 stability and triggers p53-mediated apoptosis through the upregulation of pro-apoptotic genes [99]. In summary, MOF acts as an important tumor suppressor in PCa through three distinct mechanisms: 1) cooperating with FOXP3 to induce the expression of oncosuppressors 2) recruiting DDR proteins at DSBs by acetylating H4K16 and 3) acetylating p53 on lys120, leading to the expression of pro-apoptotic genes (See Figure 3A).

3.5. UTX

UTX, also called KDM6 (histone lysine demethylase 6), associates with complexes containing the H3K4 methyltransferases MLL3 or MLL4 [42]. UTX possesses H3K27 demethylase activity and therefore plays a prominent role in the balance between PcG-mediated repression and TrxG-mediated activation [100]. The role of UTX has been well characterized in HOX gene regulation during embryonic development [101]. When a cell receives a differentiation signal, UTX promotes HOX gene expression in two ways: 1) It interacts with MLL3 or MLL4, which catalyze the trimethylation of H3K4 at HOX loci and 2) It demethylates H3K27me3, a chemical modification associated with transcriptional repression [101]. Aside from its role in development, UTX has also been linked to cancer where it functions as a tumor suppressor [102]. The demethylase activity of UTX seems particularly relevant to PCa as PRC2 gain of function and H3K27 trimethylation represent common hallmarks of aggressive solid tumors [103].This global increase in H3K27me3 implies a loss of function for UTX in PCa progression. UTX also counteracts PcG-mediated silencing by stimulating the ubiquitination of H2A, a HPTM associated with transcriptional activation [104]. Moreover, UTX further antagonizes PcG function by interacting with BRM (ATP-dependent helicase brahma) and subsequently recruiting CBP (CREB-binding protein), which catalyzes H3K27 acetylation. The added acetyl group restricts the access to PRC2 at the modified sites and therefore inhibits PcG-induced silencing [37]. UTX also plays an important role in repressing cellular proliferation through the regulation of RB levels [105]. It promotes cell cycle arrest by upregulating RB, a commonly altered tumor suppressor that inhibits the transcription of genes responsible for G1/S transition [106]. In summary, UTX represses many molecular processes associated with PCa initiation and progression (See Figure 3B). The tumor suppressive role of UTX has been validated in other tumor types. Systematic sequencing of renal carcinomas, multiple myelomas, medulloblastoma, and different types of leukemias all revealed inactivating mutations in a significant number of patients [107-111] Furthermore, UTX downregulation correlates with poor clinical outcome in breast cancer [112]. Given the prominence of PcG in PCa, inactivation of UTX most likely represents a critical event in the progression to metastasis.

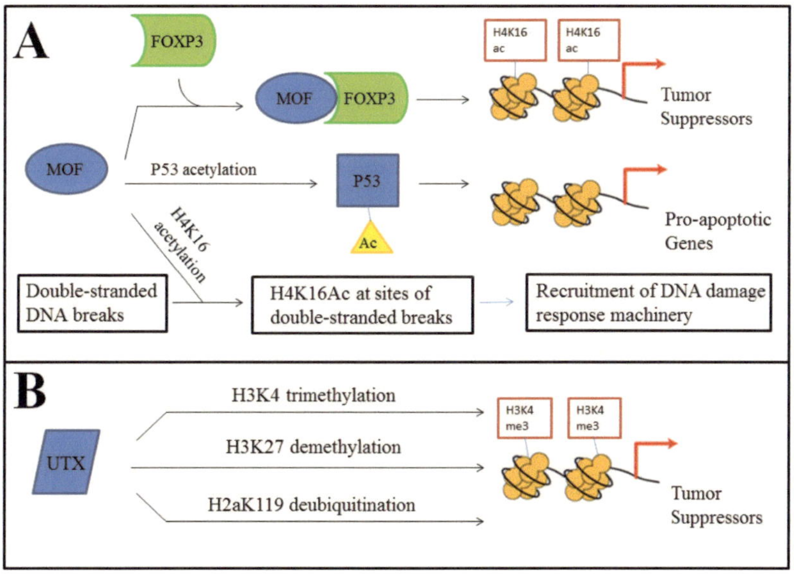

Figure 3. Putative Mechanisms of Oncosuppressive TrxG Genes in PCa

3.6. WDR5

WDR5 represents a core member of the COMPASS and COMPASS-like complexes whose functional role in cancer remains unclear [113]. To date, very few studies have focused solely on the link between WDR5 and oncogenesis. However, WDR5 appears to have a prominent role in embryogenesis. In ESCs, WDR5 interacts with the transcription factors OCT4 (octamer-binding transcription factor-4), SOX2, and NANOG to induce the expression of genes necessary for pluripotency and self-renewal [114]. This transactivational ability correlates with H3K4 trimethylation at the target *loci*. Furthermore, somatic cell reprogramming and formation of induced pluripotent stem cells (iPSCs) also requires the presence of WDR5 [114]. WDR5 has been shown to be essential for proper HOX gene activation as *Xenopus Laevis* tadpoles exhibit a wide range of developmental defects upon WDR5 depletion [115]. Moreover, WDR5 cooperates with the canonical Wnt pathway to induce osteoblast and chondrocyte differentiation [116]. WDR5 is expressed upon bone morphogenetic protein (BMP) signalling, another pathway associated with differentiation [117]. In fact, WDR5 was initially called "BMP-2-induced gene 3 kb" and subsequently changed to its current name [118].

Recently, a study demonstrated that WDR5 is induced under hypoxic conditions and is required for epithelial-mesenchymal transition (EMT) [119]. Hypoxia activates the expression of WDR5 and HDAC3. WDR5 and H3K4 methyltransferase complexes are then recruited to promoters of mesenchymal genes to activate their transcription [119]. In parallel, HDAC3 removes pre-existing acetyl groups from H3K4 to potentiate WDR5 action. HDAC3 also removes histone acetylation marks from promoters of epithelial genes, further pushing the cell towards a mesenchymal phenotype [119]. EMT represents an essential step for tumor metastasis [120-122]. Since WDR5 is required for EMT, WDR5 could potentially act as an oncogene by promoting metastasis of primary prostate tumors (Figure 2B). Although the oncogenic role of WDR5 has not been tested in PCa, studies in head and neck squamous cell carcinoma showed that coexpression of HIF-1α, WDR5, and HDAC3 is associated with metastasis and poor prognosis [119]. These results suggest that WDR5 functions as an oncoprotein by triggering EMT. However, further studies are needed to assess the consequences of WDR5 expression in PCa.

4. Expression data analysis and putative mechanisms of TrxG function in malignant progression

As summarized in previous sections, epigenetic gene regulation plays a crucial role in PCa. In particular, HPTMs mediated by TrxG genes are emerging as novel drivers of tumor progression, or as mediators of tumor suppressive functions. Although these genes have been extensively investigated in hematological neoplasms, their roles in solid tumors such as PCa have not been completely elucidated. As demonstrated for other epigenetic players, it is likely that The functioin of TrxG members is dependent on tissue type, tumor stage, as well as on overlooked or uncharacterized determinants [123]. To gain insights into the possible role of TrxG genes in PCa progression, we conducted an analysis of their expression in primary *vs.* metastatic samples. To this aim, we exploited a publically available database (http://www.cbioportal.org/public-portal/) [124]. Our results are summarized in Table 2. At first glance, it is evident that each TrxG member represented in the table shows up- or down-regulation in a relevant fraction (16-53%) of metastatic PCa cases. This indicates that aberrations in TrxG activity are likely to play an important role in the progression to metastasis.

TrxG	Non-metastatic: 71/131 = 54%	Metastatic: 18/19 Cases = 95%
ASH1L	↓ in 12/131 and ↑ in 1/131 = 10%	↓ in 5/19 = 26%
ASH2L	↓ in 13/131 and ↑ in 3/131 = 12%	↓ in 7/19 = 37%
WDR5	↓ in 3/131 and ↑ in 5/131 = 6%	↓ in 9/19 and ↑ in 1/19 = 53%
MEN1	↓ in 5/131 and ↑ in 19/131 = 19%	↓ in 10/19 = 53%
HCFC1	↓ in 11/131 and ↑ in 14/131 = 19%	↓ in 4/19 and ↑ in 1/19 = 26%
MLL	↓ in 18/131 = 14%	↑ in 6/19 = 32%
MLL2	↓ in 8/131 and ↑ in 12/131 = 15%	↓ in 4/19 and ↑ in 2/19 = 32%
MLL3	↓ in 6/131 and ↑ in 3/131 = 7%	↓ in 2/19 and ↑ in 1/19 = 16%
MLL4	↓ in 10/131 and ↑ in 10/131 = 15%	↓ in 6/19 = 26%
MLL5	↓ in 6/131 = 5%	↓ in 1/19 and ↑ in 2/19 = 16%
UTX	↓ in 2/131 and ↑ in 6/131 = 6%	↑ in 5/19 = 26%

Table 2. CBio portal-derived gene expression data in primary *vs.* metastatic PCa. Arrows pointing up or down indicate increased or decreased expression, respectively. The percentage indicates the fraction of alterted (up- or down-regulated) genes.

In the following paragraphs, we will briefly discuss our findings and conciliate them with published data on each TrxG memember.

1. **ASHL:** although ASH2L has been described as an oncoprotein [68], we found that ASH-1L and -2L expression is reduced in metastatic PCa samples. This discrepancy might be explained by the evidence that ASH2L protein levels rise in cancer, but mRNA level does not increase [68]. This implies additional regulation at the translational level, most likely relating to a defect in proteasomal degradation.

2. **MEN1:** MENIN can function as an oncogene [53, 78] and as a tumor suppressor [73] depending on tissue specificity. MENIN interacts with nuclear proteins like estrogen- and vitamin D-receptor [80, 125], thereby stimulating their transactivation. Since other members of the COMPASS-like complex interact with AR [70], we propose that the oncogenic function of MENIN might result from its association with, and subsequent stimulation of, AR transactivation ability through H3K4 trimethylation (See Figure 2). Since most metastatic PCas are androgen-independent, while almost all primary tumors display an active AR signaling [126], MENIN action is likely required in early tumor stages. This explains the preferential up-regulation of MEN1 in non-metastatic (likely androgen dependent) PCa samples (Table 2).

3. **MLL:** There is no documented role for MLL in PCa. Data from the cBio database shows that MLL expression is increased in metastatic *vs.* primary PCa samples. Therefore we

propose that MLL acts as a metastasis-driving oncogene in PCa. MLL is known to interact with AR [70]. Since metastatic PCa cells are usually AR-independent, the mechanism of MLL action in the metastatic process is likely androgen-independent too. Interestingly, MLL homologs are often down-regulated in metastatic PCa (Table 2), suggesting that they might counteract its oncogenic function.

4. **MOF:** MOF was not included in the cBIO database, but based on its regulation of growth suppressive pathways (See Figure 3), we propose that MOF acts as a tumor suppressor and therefore we expect to see its expression downregulated in PCa. However, since MOF is required for optimal DNA damage response to double-stranded breaks [96], reduced MOF expression could be a predictor of good response to radiotherapy or to chemotherapy agents that induce dsDNA breaks.

5. **UTX:** The protein encoded by this gene possesses H3K27 demethylase activity, which counteracts the repressive effect of PRC2-catalyzed H3K27me3. Due to the preponderance of PRC2 activity in PCa, UTX loss of function appears to be a critical event in the progression to metastasis. UTX also interacts with other histone-modifying complexes that catalyze HPTMs associated with transcriptional activation (See Figure 3). Despite this evidence, we found an increased rate of UTX upregulation in metastatic *vs.* non metastatic PCa samples (Table 2). Those data counteract the common view that UTX acts as a tumor suppressor, at least in PCa. A possible explanation derives from the recent finding that *UTX* is frequently mutated in metastatic PCa [70]. It is worth noting that all experiments on the oncosuppressive role of UTX have been performed on the wild-type gene. We do not know whether the mutated protein simply loses its tumor-suppressive activity, or if it acquires oncogenic features. In the latter case, the upregulation reported in metastatic PCa might even drive tumor progression.

6. **WDR5:** Although no studies have directly assessed the role of WDR5 in PCa, data from ESC suggest that WDR5 might promote metastasis due to its implication in EMT. During EMT, WDR5 promotes the expression of mesenchymal genes by stimulating H3K4 methylation at target *loci* [119]. Since WDR5 triggers EMT, we would expect its expression to increase in metastatic samples. However, in the MSKCC database, WDR5 expression is reduced in metastatic tumors. This could be explained by the fact that only a subset of PCa cells acquires epigenetic alterations in response to cues from the extracellular environment (niche) which predisposes them to metastasis. Since only a minority of the tumor bulk acquire invasive and migratory potential, the elevated expression of WDR5 in those cells would not be detected by micro-array as the levels of WDR5 in non-invasive cells would dominate.

The reader is cautioned that it is necessary to consider that studies comparing metastatic and primary tumors might oversimplify the complex nature of the metastatic process. First, those studies show expression levels of target genes at 2 specific time points, while the metastatic process occurs over several years in the clinical setting [58]. Second, molecular mechanisms of regulating metastasis are complex: if EMT is required as an early step, the opposite (mesenchymal-to-epithelial transition) is needed during metastatic cell homing [127]. Thus, a gene required during early metastatic steps might even be silenced at later stages. These considerations underscore the fact that our conclusions are limited, and need to be complemented by functional and clinical studies. However, results shown in Table 2 indicate that at least some TrxG genes are likely involved in PCa metastasis and thus are candidate therapeutic targets or prognostic factors.

5. Conclusion

While for many years cancers were thought to arise as a result of genetic alterations, an increasing number of studies report that in fact epigenetic misregulation primarily drives PCa progression and metastasis [13, 128]. PcG proteins EZH2 and BMI1 are overexpressed in PCa, an event that correlates with increased metastatic spreading and poor prognosis [57]. Since TrxG antagonizes PcG action, we explored the possibility that aberrant TrxG signalling could also represent a key factor in PCa metastasis. Since PcG is overactive in PCa and TrxG counteracts PcG activity, TrxG were historically thought to be oncosuppressive [41]. Analysis of expression databases revealed that almost all metastatic prostate tumors show deregulated expression of at least one TrxG gene. Interestingly, an in-depth literature review combined with an analysis of expression data indicated that aberration in TrxG complexes impacts PCa progression in a way that goes beyond their anticipated roles as classical tumor suppressors. In fact, some TrxG genes show elevated expression in metastatic PCas and have been shown to interact with, and enhance the activity of, known oncogenes such as AR, c-MYC, h-RAS [68, 70]. The finding that TrxG genes can act as either oncogenes or tumor suppressors implies that the regulation of TrxG activity highly depends on the cellular context [68, 129]. Changes in individual TrxG gene expression, availability of coregulators, as well as post-translational modifications on both individual TrxG subunits and coregulators all regulate the functional output of TrxG complexes. These multiple levels of regulation account for the highly diversified spectrum of molecular processes affected by TrxG activity, and explain why some TrxG genes can act as oncogenes and others as tumor suppressors.

Since it is becoming increasingly clear that misregulated TrxG activity represents a key driver of PCa progression, an important question arises: How can TrxG complexes be targeted clinically? Inhibiting core TrxG subunits like MLL, ASH2L, and WDR5 does not represent a suitable strategy. TrxG complexes play many important physiological roles [130] and therefore disrupting these core TrxG proteins would result in high toxicity. In fact, it is important to recognize that TrxG activity is highly context-dependent and is controlled by many coregulators. This context-dependency can be exploited in the search for new drug targets. An interesting strategy to adopt would be to identify TrxG coregulators that are overexpressed in PCa only. Inhibiting these coregulators would impair TrxG function in PCa cells specifically while leaving normal cells unaffected. Since TrxG complexes can be oncogenic or tumor suppressive, two types of coregulators should be targeted clinically. The first represents coactivators of oncogenic complexes and second, corepressors of oncosuppressive complexes. Pharmacologic disruption of both of these proteins would in theory limit the tumorigenic potential of aberrant TrxG signalling. To date, no such coregulators have been described in PCa. The link between TrxG and PCa remains poorly characterized and many more studies are required to understand the impact of dysregulated TrxG on PCa progression. Nonetheless, the implication of TrxG in PCa supports the idea that epigenetic alterations represent key drivers in the progression to metastatic disease.

Acknowledgements

We thank Stephen Choi for his generous help in the analysis of online databases. This work was partially funded by grants to CDH from Prostate Cancer Canada (Grant #2010-556) and the Canadian Cancer Society (Grant #701097).

Author details

Pier-Luc Clermont, Francesco Crea and Cheryl D. Helgason

*Address all correspondence to: chelgaso@bccrc.ca

Experimental Therapeutics, British Columbia Cancer Research Centre, Vancouver, BC, Canada

References

[1] Baca, S.C. and L.A. Garraway, The genomic landscape of prostate cancer. Front Endocrinol (Lausanne), 2012. 3: p. 69.

[2] You, J.S. and P.A. Jones, Cancer genetics and epigenetics: two sides of the same coin? Cancer Cell, 2012. 22(1): p. 9-20.

[3] Feil, R., Epigenetics, an emerging discipline with broad implications. C R Biol, 2008. 331(11): p. 837-43.

[4] Wilson, V.L., P.A. Jones, and R.L. Momparler, Inhibition of DNA methylation in L1210 leukemic cells by 5-aza-2'-deoxycytidine as a possible mechanism of chemotherapeutic action. Cancer Res, 1983. 43(8): p. 3493-6.

[5] Prokhortchouk, E. and P.A. Defossez, The cell biology of DNA methylation in mammals. Biochim Biophys Acta, 2008. 1783(11): p. 2167-73.

[6] Song, M.S., L. Salmena, and P.P. Pandolfi, The functions and regulation of the PTEN tumour suppressor. Nat Rev Mol Cell Biol, 2012. 13(5): p. 283-96.

[7] Backman, S.A., et al., Early onset of neoplasia in the prostate and skin of mice with tissue-specific deletion of Pten. Proc Natl Acad Sci U S A, 2004. 101(6): p. 1725-30.

[8] Krohn, A., et al., Genomic Deletion of PTEN Is Associated with Tumor Progression and Early PSA Recurrence in ERG Fusion-Positive and Fusion-Negative Prostate Cancer. Am J Pathol, 2012. 181(2): p. 401-12.

[9] Whang, Y.E., et al., Inactivation of the tumor suppressor PTEN/MMAC1 in advanced human prostate cancer through loss of expression. Proc Natl Acad Sci U S A, 1998. 95(9): p. 5246-50.

[10] Carracedo, A., A. Alimonti, and P.P. Pandolfi, PTEN level in tumor suppression: how much is too little? Cancer Res, 2011. 71(3): p. 629-33.

[11] Goel, A., et al., Frequent inactivation of PTEN by promoter hypermethylation in microsatellite instability-high sporadic colorectal cancers. Cancer Res, 2004. 64(9): p. 3014-21.

[12] Bienvenu, T. and J. Chelly, Molecular genetics of Rett syndrome: when DNA methylation goes unrecognized. Nat Rev Genet, 2006. 7(6): p. 415-26.

[13] Jeronimo, C., et al., Epigenetics in prostate cancer: biologic and clinical relevance. Eur Urol, 2011. 60(4): p. 753-66.

[14] Gravina, G.L., et al., Hormonal therapy promotes hormone-resistant phenotype by increasing DNMT activity and expression in prostate cancer models. Endocrinology, 2011. 152(12): p. 4550-61.

[15] Kuendgen, A. and M. Lubbert, Current status of epigenetic treatment in myelodysplastic syndromes. Ann Hematol, 2008. 87(8): p. 601-11.

[16] Schwartsmann, G., et al., A phase I trial of cisplatin plus decitabine, a new DNA-hypomethylating agent, in patients with advanced solid tumors and a follow-up early phase II evaluation in patients with inoperable non-small cell lung cancer. Invest New Drugs, 2000. 18(1): p. 83-91.

[17] Travers, A.A., G. Muskhelishvili, and J.M. Thompson, DNA information: from digital code to analogue structure. Philos Transact A Math Phys Eng Sci, 2012. 370(1969): p. 2960-86.

[18] Travers, A.A., et al., DNA structure, nucleosome placement and chromatin remodelling: a perspective. Biochem Soc Trans, 2012. 40(2): p. 335-40.

[19] Yost, J.M., et al., Targets in epigenetics: inhibiting the methyl writers of the histone code. Curr Chem Genomics, 2011. 5(Suppl 1): p. 72-84.

[20] Oliver, S.S. and J.M. Denu, Dynamic interplay between histone H3 modifications and protein interpreters: emerging evidence for a "histone language". Chembiochem, 2011. 12(2): p. 299-307.

[21] Donzella, V. and F. Crea, Optical biosensors to analyze novel biomarkers in oncology. J Biophotonics, 2011. 4(6): p. 442-52.

[22] Britton, L.M., et al., Breaking the histone code with quantitative mass spectrometry. Expert Rev Proteomics, 2011. 8(5): p. 631-43.

[23] Georghiou, S. and A.M. Ababneh, Maintenance of open DNA base pairs through histone acetylated lysine-purine interaction leading to transcriptional activation: a proposed mechanism. Int J Mol Med, 2005. 16(5): p. 911-7.

[24] Dekker, F.J. and H.J. Haisma, Histone acetyl transferases as emerging drug targets. Drug Discov Today, 2009. 14(19-20): p. 942-8.

[25] Mottet, D. and V. Castronovo, Histone deacetylases: target enzymes for cancer therapy. Clin Exp Metastasis, 2008. 25(2): p. 183-9.

[26] Mathews, L.A., F. Crea, and W.L. Farrar, Epigenetic gene regulation in stem cells and correlation to cancer. Differentiation, 2009. 78(1): p. 1-17.

[27] Crea, F., et al., Polycomb genes and cancer: Time for clinical application? Crit Rev Oncol Hematol, 2012. 83(2): p. 184-93.

[28] Jin, B., et al., DNMT1 and DNMT3B modulate distinct polycomb-mediated histone modifications in colon cancer. Cancer Res, 2009. 69(18): p. 7412-21.

[29] Yu, M., et al., Direct recruitment of polycomb repressive complex 1 to chromatin by core binding transcription factors. Mol Cell, 2012. 45(3): p. 330-43.

[30] Soshnikova, N. and D. Duboule, Epigenetic regulation of vertebrate Hox genes: a dynamic equilibrium. Epigenetics, 2009. 4(8): p. 537-40.

[31] Orlando, D.A., et al., CpG island structure and trithorax/polycomb chromatin domains in human cells. Genomics, 2012.

[32] Crea, F., et al., BMI1 silencing enhances docetaxel activity and impairs antioxidant response in prostate cancer. Int J Cancer, 2011. 128(8): p. 1946-54.

[33] Ren, G., et al., Polycomb Protein EZH2 Regulates Tumor Invasion via the Transcriptional Repression of the Metastasis Suppressor RKIP in Breast and Prostate Cancer. Cancer Res, 2012. 72(12): p. 3091-3104.

[34] Schuettengruber, B., et al., Trithorax group proteins: switching genes on and keeping them active. Nat Rev Mol Cell Biol, 2011. 12(12): p. 799-814.

[35] Takahashi, Y.H., et al., Structural analysis of the core COMPASS family of histone H3K4 methylases from yeast to human. Proc Natl Acad Sci U S A, 2011. 108(51): p. 20526-31.

[36] Wu, M., et al., Molecular regulation of H3K4 trimethylation by Wdr82, a component of human Set1/COMPASS. Mol Cell Biol, 2008. 28(24): p. 7337-44.

[37] Tie, F., et al., Histone demethylase UTX and chromatin remodeler BRM bind directly to CBP and modulate acetylation of histone H3 lysine 27. Mol Cell Biol, 2012. 32(12): p. 2323-34.

[38] Schwartz, Y.B. and V. Pirrotta, Polycomb complexes and epigenetic states. Curr Opin Cell Biol, 2008. 20(3): p. 266-73.

[39] Morey, L. and K. Helin, Polycomb group protein-mediated repression of transcription. Trends Biochem Sci, 2010. 35(6): p. 323-32.

[40] Sauvageau, M. and G. Sauvageau, Polycomb group proteins: multi-faceted regulators of somatic stem cells and cancer. Cell Stem Cell, 2010. 7(3): p. 299-313.

[41] Mills, A.A., Throwing the cancer switch: reciprocal roles of polycomb and trithorax proteins. Nat Rev Cancer, 2010. 10(10): p. 669-82.

[42] Shilatifard, A., The COMPASS family of histone H3K4 methylases: mechanisms of regulation in development and disease pathogenesis. Annu Rev Biochem, 2012. 81: p. 65-95.

[43] Geissler, K. and O. Zach, Pathways involved in Drosophila and human cancer development: the Notch, Hedgehog, Wingless, Runt, and Trithorax pathway. Ann Hematol, 2012. 91(5): p. 645-69.

[44] Ringrose, L. and R. Paro, Epigenetic regulation of cellular memory by the Polycomb and Trithorax group proteins. Annu Rev Genet, 2004. 38: p. 413-43.

[45] Schuettengruber, B., et al., Genome regulation by polycomb and trithorax proteins. Cell, 2007. 128(4): p. 735-45.

[46] Soshnikova, N., Dynamics of Polycomb and Trithorax activities during development. Birth Defects Res A Clin Mol Teratol, 2011. 91(8): p. 781-7.

[47] Hanson, R.D., et al., Mammalian Trithorax and polycomb-group homologues are antagonistic regulators of homeotic development. Proc Natl Acad Sci U S A, 1999. 96(25): p. 14372-7.

[48] Richly, H., et al., Setting and resetting of epigenetic marks in malignant transformation and development. Bioessays, 2010. 32(8): p. 669-79.

[49] Richly, H., L. Aloia, and L. Di Croce, Roles of the Polycomb group proteins in stem cells and cancer. Cell Death Dis, 2011. 2: p. e204.

[50] Marschalek, R., Mechanisms of leukemogenesis by MLL fusion proteins. Br J Haematol, 2011. 152(2): p. 141-54.

[51] Chang, C.J. and M.C. Hung, The role of EZH2 in tumour progression. Br J Cancer, 2012. 106(2): p. 243-7.

[52] Lin, Y.W., H.M. Chen, and J.Y. Fang, Gene silencing by the Polycomb group proteins and associations with cancer. Cancer Invest, 2011. 29(3): p. 187-95.

[53] Paris, P.L., et al., An oncogenic role for the multiple endocrine neoplasia type 1 gene in prostate cancer. Prostate Cancer Prostatic Dis, 2009. 12(2): p. 184-91.

[54] Dou, Y., et al., Regulation of MLL1 H3K4 methyltransferase activity by its core components. Nat Struct Mol Biol, 2006. 13(8): p. 713-9.

[55] Yu, J., et al., A polycomb repression signature in metastatic prostate cancer predicts cancer outcome. Cancer Res, 2007. 67(22): p. 10657-63.

[56] Laitinen, S., et al., EZH2, Ki-67 and MCM7 are prognostic markers in prostatectomy treated patients. Int J Cancer, 2008. 122(3): p. 595-602.

[57] van Leenders, G.J., et al., Polycomb-group oncogenes EZH2, BMI1, and RING1 are overexpressed in prostate cancer with adverse pathologic and clinical features. Eur Urol, 2007. 52(2): p. 455-63.

[58] Crea, F., et al., EZH2 inhibition: targeting the crossroad of tumor invasion and angiogenesis. Cancer Metastasis Rev, 2012.

[59] Crea, F., et al., Pharmacologic disruption of Polycomb Repressive Complex 2 inhibits tumorigenicity and tumor progression in prostate cancer. Mol Cancer, 2011. 10: p. 40.

[60] Avan, A., et al., Molecular Mechanisms Involved in the Synergistic Interaction of the EZH2 Inhibitor 3-Deazaneplanocin A with Gemcitabine in Pancreatic Cancer Cells. Mol Cancer Ther, 2012. 11(8): p. 1735-46.

[61] Cao, L., et al., BMI1 as a novel target for drug discovery in cancer. J Cell Biochem, 2011. 112(10): p. 2729-41.

[62] Steward, M.M., et al., Molecular regulation of H3K4 trimethylation by ASH2L, a shared subunit of MLL complexes. Nat Struct Mol Biol, 2006. 13(9): p. 852-4.

[63] Eissenberg, J.C. and A. Shilatifard, Histone H3 lysine 4 (H3K4) methylation in development and differentiation. Dev Biol, 2010. 339(2): p. 240-9.

[64] Stoller, J.Z., et al., Ash2l interacts with Tbx1 and is required during early embryogenesis. Exp Biol Med (Maywood), 2010. 235(5): p. 569-76.

[65] McKinnell, I.W., et al., Pax7 activates myogenic genes by recruitment of a histone methyltransferase complex. Nat Cell Biol, 2008. 10(1): p. 77-84.

[66] Rampalli, S., et al., p38 MAPK signaling regulates recruitment of Ash2L-containing methyltransferase complexes to specific genes during differentiation. Nat Struct Mol Biol, 2007. 14(12): p. 1150-6.

[67] Aziz, A., Q.C. Liu, and F.J. Dilworth, Regulating a master regulator: establishing tissue-specific gene expression in skeletal muscle. Epigenetics, 2010. 5(8): p. 691-5.

[68] Luscher-Firzlaff, J., et al., The human trithorax protein hASH2 functions as an oncoprotein. Cancer Res, 2008. 68(3): p. 749-58.

[69] Dang, C.V., MYC on the path to cancer. Cell, 2012. 149(1): p. 22-35.

[70] Grasso, C.S., et al., The mutational landscape of lethal castration-resistant prostate cancer. Nature, 2012. 487(7406): p. 239-43.

[71] Larsson, C., et al., Multiple endocrine neoplasia type 1 gene maps to chromosome 11 and is lost in insulinoma. Nature, 1988. 332(6159): p. 85-7.

[72] Thakker, R.V., Multiple endocrine neoplasia type 1 (MEN1). Best Pract Res Clin Endocrinol Metab, 2010. 24(3): p. 355-70.

[73] Lairmore, T.C. and H. Chen, Role of menin in neuroendocrine tumorigenesis. Adv Exp Med Biol, 2009. 668: p. 87-95.

[74] Karnik, S.K., et al., Menin regulates pancreatic islet growth by promoting histone methylation and expression of genes encoding p27Kip1 and p18INK4c. Proc Natl Acad Sci U S A, 2005. 102(41): p. 14659-64.

[75] Agarwal, S.K., et al., Menin interacts with the AP1 transcription factor JunD and represses JunD-activated transcription. Cell, 1999. 96(1): p. 143-52.

[76] Ikeo, Y., et al., JunD-menin interaction regulates c-Jun-mediated AP-1 transactivation. Endocr J, 2004. 51(3): p. 333-42.

[77] Yokoyama, A., et al., The menin tumor suppressor protein is an essential oncogenic cofactor for MLL-associated leukemogenesis. Cell, 2005. 123(2): p. 207-18.

[78] Yokoyama, A. and M.L. Cleary, Menin critically links MLL proteins with LEDGF on cancer-associated target genes. Cancer Cell, 2008. 14(1): p. 36-46.

[79] Pei, X.H., et al., p18Ink4c collaborates with Men1 to constrain lung stem cell expansion and suppress non-small-cell lung cancers. Cancer Res, 2007. 67(7): p. 3162-70.

[80] Dreijerink, K.M., et al., Menin links estrogen receptor activation to histone H3K4 trimethylation. Cancer Res, 2006. 66(9): p. 4929-35.

[81] Imachi, H., et al., Menin, a product of the MENI gene, binds to estrogen receptor to enhance its activity in breast cancer cells: possibility of a novel predictive factor for tamoxifen resistance. Breast Cancer Res Treat, 2010. 122(2): p. 395-407.

[82] Mo, R., S.M. Rao, and Y.J. Zhu, Identification of the MLL2 complex as a coactivator for estrogen receptor alpha. J Biol Chem, 2006. 281(23): p. 15714-20.

[83] Paris, P.L., et al., Whole genome scanning identifies genotypes associated with recurrence and metastasis in prostate tumors. Hum Mol Genet, 2004. 13(13): p. 1303-13.

[84] Marschalek, R., Mixed lineage leukemia: roles in human malignancies and potential therapy. FEBS J, 2010. 277(8): p. 1822-31.

[85] Varier, R.A. and H.T. Timmers, Histone lysine methylation and demethylation pathways in cancer. Biochim Biophys Acta, 2011. 1815(1): p. 75-89.

[86] Moreno, C.S., The Sex-determining region Y-box 4 and homeobox C6 transcriptional networks in prostate cancer progression: crosstalk with the Wnt, Notch, and PI3K pathways. Am J Pathol, 2010. 176(2): p. 518-27.

[87] Natarajan, T.G., et al., Epigenetic regulator MLL2 shows altered expression in cancer cell lines and tumors from human breast and colon. Cancer Cell Int, 2010. 10: p. 13.

[88] Shi, L., et al., Histone demethylase JMJD2B coordinates H3K4/H3K9 methylation and promotes hormonally responsive breast carcinogenesis. Proc Natl Acad Sci U S A, 2011. 108(18): p. 7541-6.

[89] Huntsman, D.G., et al., MLL2, the second human homolog of the Drosophila trithorax gene, maps to 19q13.1 and is amplified in solid tumor cell lines. Oncogene, 1999. 18(56): p. 7975-84.

[90] Dou, Y., et al., Physical association and coordinate function of the H3 K4 methyltransferase MLL1 and the H4 K16 acetyltransferase MOF. Cell, 2005. 121(6): p. 873-85.

[91] Taipale, M., et al., hMOF histone acetyltransferase is required for histone H4 lysine 16 acetylation in mammalian cells. Mol Cell Biol, 2005. 25(15): p. 6798-810.

[92] Fraga, M.F., et al., Loss of acetylation at Lys16 and trimethylation at Lys20 of histone H4 is a common hallmark of human cancer. Nat Genet, 2005. 37(4): p. 391-400.

[93] Katoh, H., et al., FOXP3 orchestrates H4K16 acetylation and H3K4 trimethylation for activation of multiple genes by recruiting MOF and causing displacement of PLU-1. Mol Cell, 2011. 44(5): p. 770-84.

[94] Bhadra, M.P., et al., The role of MOF in the ionizing radiation response is conserved in Drosophila melanogaster. Chromosoma, 2012. 121(1): p. 79-90.

[95] Gupta, A., et al., Involvement of human MOF in ATM function. Mol Cell Biol, 2005. 25(12): p. 5292-305.

[96] Sharma, G.G., et al., MOF and histone H4 acetylation at lysine 16 are critical for DNA damage response and double-strand break repair. Mol Cell Biol, 2010. 30(14): p. 3582-95.

[97] Li, X., et al., MOF and H4 K16 acetylation play important roles in DNA damage repair by modulating recruitment of DNA damage repair protein Mdc1. Mol Cell Biol, 2010. 30(22): p. 5335-47.

[98] Tang, Y., et al., Tip60-dependent acetylation of p53 modulates the decision between cell-cycle arrest and apoptosis. Mol Cell, 2006. 24(6): p. 827-39.

[99] Sykes, S.M., et al., Acetylation of the p53 DNA-binding domain regulates apoptosis induction. Mol Cell, 2006. 24(6): p. 841-51.

[100] Hong, S., et al., Identification of JmjC domain-containing UTX and JMJD3 as histone H3 lysine 27 demethylases. Proc Natl Acad Sci U S A, 2007. 104(47): p. 18439-44.

[101] Agger, K., et al., UTX and JMJD3 are histone H3K27 demethylases involved in HOX gene regulation and development. Nature, 2007. 449(7163): p. 731-4.

[102] Tsai, M.C., J.K. Wang, and H.Y. Chang, Tumor suppression by the histone demethylase UTX. Cell Cycle, 2010. 9(11): p. 2043-4.

[103] Ellinger, J., et al., Global histone H3K27 methylation levels are different in localized and metastatic prostate cancer. Cancer Invest, 2012. 30(2): p. 92-7.

[104] Lee, M.G., et al., Demethylation of H3K27 regulates polycomb recruitment and H2A ubiquitination. Science, 2007. 318(5849): p. 447-50.

[105] Terashima, M., et al., The tumor suppressor Rb and its related Rbl2 genes are regulated by Utx histone demethylase. Biochem Biophys Res Commun, 2010. 399(2): p. 238-44.

[106] Wang, J.K., et al., The histone demethylase UTX enables RB-dependent cell fate control. Genes Dev, 2010. 24(4): p. 327-32.

[107] Dalgliesh, G.L., et al., Systematic sequencing of renal carcinoma reveals inactivation of histone modifying genes. Nature, 2010. 463(7279): p. 360-3.

[108] van Haaften, G., et al., Somatic mutations of the histone H3K27 demethylase gene UTX in human cancer. Nat Genet, 2009. 41(5): p. 521-3.

[109] Robinson, G., et al., Novel mutations target distinct subgroups of medulloblastoma. Nature, 2012. 488(7409): p. 43-8.

[110] Mar, B.G., et al., Sequencing histone-modifying enzymes identifies UTX mutations in acute lymphoblastic leukemia. Leukemia, 2012. 26(8): p. 1881-3.

[111] Jankowska, A.M., et al., Mutational spectrum analysis of chronic myelomonocytic leukemia includes genes associated with epigenetic regulation: UTX, EZH2, and DNMT3A. Blood, 2011. 118(14): p. 3932-41.

[112] Patani, N., et al., Histone-modifier gene expression profiles are associated with pathological and clinical outcomes in human breast cancer. Anticancer Res, 2011. 31(12): p. 4115-25.

[113] Odho, Z., S.M. Southall, and J.R. Wilson, Characterization of a novel WDR5-binding site that recruits RbBP5 through a conserved motif to enhance methylation of histone H3 lysine 4 by mixed lineage leukemia protein-1. J Biol Chem, 2010. 285(43): p. 32967-76.

[114] Ang, Y.S., et al., Wdr5 mediates self-renewal and reprogramming via the embryonic stem cell core transcriptional network. Cell, 2011. 145(2): p. 183-97.

[115] Wysocka, J., et al., WDR5 associates with histone H3 methylated at K4 and is essential for H3 K4 methylation and vertebrate development. Cell, 2005. 121(6): p. 859-72.

[116] Gori, F., L.G. Friedman, and M.B. Demay, Wdr5, a WD-40 protein, regulates osteoblast differentiation during embryonic bone development. Dev Biol, 2006. 295(2): p. 498-506.

[117] Gori, F., P. Divieti, and M.B. Demay, Cloning and characterization of a novel WD-40 repeat protein that dramatically accelerates osteoblastic differentiation. J Biol Chem, 2001. 276(49): p. 46515-22.

[118] Gori, F. and M.B. Demay, BIG-3, a novel WD-40 repeat protein, is expressed in the developing growth plate and accelerates chondrocyte differentiation in vitro. Endocrinology, 2004. 145(3): p. 1050-4.

[119] Wu, M.Z., et al., Interplay between HDAC3 and WDR5 is essential for hypoxia-induced epithelial-mesenchymal transition. Mol Cell, 2011. 43(5): p. 811-22.

[120] Tsuji, T., S. Ibaragi, and G.F. Hu, Epithelial-mesenchymal transition and cell cooperativity in metastasis. Cancer Res, 2009. 69(18): p. 7135-9.

[121] Yao, D., C. Dai, and S. Peng, Mechanism of the mesenchymal-epithelial transition and its relationship with metastatic tumor formation. Mol Cancer Res, 2011. 9(12): p. 1608-20.

[122] Gomes, L.R., et al., Epithelial-mesenchymal transition: implications in cancer progression and metastasis. Curr Pharm Biotechnol, 2011. 12(11): p. 1881-90.

[123] Scacheri, P.C., et al., Homozygous loss of menin is well tolerated in liver, a tissue not affected in MEN1. Mamm Genome, 2004. 15(11): p. 872-7.

[124] Cerami, E., et al., The cBio cancer genomics portal: an open platform for exploring multidimensional cancer genomics data. Cancer Discov, 2012. 2(5): p. 401-4.

[125] Dreijerink, K.M., et al., Regulation of vitamin D receptor function in MEN1-related parathyroid adenomas. Mol Cell Endocrinol, 2009. 313(1-2): p. 1-8.

[126] Attar, R.M., C.H. Takimoto, and M.M. Gottardis, Castration-resistant prostate cancer: locking up the molecular escape routes. Clin Cancer Res, 2009. 15(10): p. 3251-5.

[127] Gunasinghe, N.P., et al., Mesenchymal-epithelial transition (MET) as a mechanism for metastatic colonisation in breast cancer. Cancer Metastasis Rev, 2012.

[128] Perry, A.S., et al., The epigenome as a therapeutic target in prostate cancer. Nat Rev Urol, 2010. 7(12): p. 668-80.

[129] Herz, H.M., et al., The H3K27me3 demethylase dUTX is a suppressor of Notch- and Rb-dependent tumors in Drosophila. Mol Cell Biol, 2010. 30(10): p. 2485-97.

[130] Yap, D.B., et al., Mll5 is required for normal spermatogenesis. PLoS One, 2011. 6(11): p. e27127.

Chapter 23

The Function of YY1 and Its Oncogenic Role in Prostate Cancer

Daniel B. Stovall and Guangchao Sui

Additional information is available at the end of the chapter

http://dx.doi.org/10.5772/53091

1. Introduction

Transcription factors regulate gene expression by interacting with specific DNA elements and other proteins to either activate or repress gene transcription. Aberrant expression and function of transcription factors are commonly observed in human cancers and play a pivotal role in oncogenic transformation. Ultimately, these affect downstream signaling pathways, resulting in acquisition of some or all of the hallmarks of cancer, such as insensitivity to antigrowth or apoptotic signals, production of self-sufficient growth signals, limitless replicative potential and invasive or metastatic capability [1].

Yin Yang 1 (YY1) is a highly conserved transcription factor across species and ubiquitously expressed in human tissues. YY1 has the ability to act as either an activator or repressor of its target genes, depending on the compositional difference of its recruited complexes. Through these complexes YY1 regulates epigenetic modifications, such as DNA methylation and histone acetylation, of its targeted promoters. Originally, YY1 was discovered as a transcription factor capable of binding to the P5 promoter of adeno-associated virus [2]. YY1 executed an inhibitory effect on this promoter, but this inhibition was reversed to activation by its association with a viral protein, E1A. Indeed, the name "Yin Yang" symbolizes these two opposing abilities. "Yin Yang" also represents the ongoing debate over what role YY1 plays in human cancers, although its oncogenic role is clearly more predominant than its tumor suppressive potential based on the current literature.

As discussed below, the evidence supporting the oncogenic role of YY1 has been obtained through its study in various human cancers. In this chapter, we will first describe the studies that suggest a proliferative role for YY1 in cancers, and then specifically discuss what is known to date about the function of YY1 in prostate cancer.

2. YY1 as a transcription factor

The YY1 protein consists of 414 amino acids and multiple functional domains (Figure 1). As a transcription factor, YY1 is capable of directly binding to DNA through the zing-finger domains at its C-terminus. YY1 recognizes and binds its DNA consensus sites with a core sequence of either CCAT or ACAT, and these consensus elements have been identified in over 7% of vertebrate genes, underscoring the importance of YY1 in gene regulation [3].

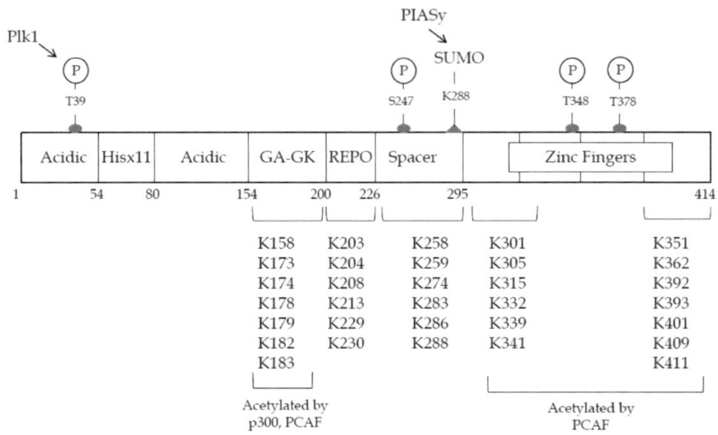

Figure 1. The Domain Structure of the YY1 Protein; YY1 is post-translationally modified at multiple sites. Polo-like kinase 1 (Plk1) phosphorylates T39, while protein inhibitor of activated STAT Y (PIASy) stimulates sumoylation of K288. PCAF and p300 mediate acetylation of residues 171-200, while p300/CBP associated factor (PCAF) also acetylates the C-terminus. All 32 lysine (K) residues are indicated in their respective domains of YY1. Phosphorylation of residues Thr348 and Thr378, but not Ser247, reduces DNA affinity of YY1. The REPO motif (201-226) is both necessary and sufficient for the recruitment of PcG proteins for the initiation and maintenance of gene silencing.

Most YY1 target genes are cancer-related, and can be either transcriptionally activated or repressed by YY1 and its associated factors. YY1-recruited proteins play a large role in determining whether YY1 will execute inhibitory or activating functions on a particular target gene. YY1 can recruit a variety of coactivators, including p300, cyclic adenosine monophosphate response element binding (CREB) protein (CBP), p300/CBP-associated factor (PCAF), and protein arginine methyltransferase (PRMT) 4 as well as corepressors such as histone deacetylases (HDACs), enhancer of zeste (Ezh) 2, and DNA methyltransferases (DNMTs) [4-11]. We will discuss these interaction partners and their effect on YY1-mediated gene regulation in detail below.

2.1. YY1-activated gene expression

We have listed cancer-relevant genes that are activated by YY1 in Table 1. In support of the predominance of YY1's oncogenic effects over its tumor suppressive potential, we note that the majority of its activated targets are oncogenes, which promote either proliferative or invasive phenotypes when overexpressed.

http://dx.doi.org/10.5772/53091

Gene/Promoter	Gene Product Function	Mechanism/Observation	Reference
A. Oncogenic, proliferative and/or overexpressed genes in cancer			
B23/nucleophosmin	Regulates nucleosome formation and inhibits tumor suppressors	HCV core, p300 and B23 itself are involved	[12, 13]
c-Myc	Oncogenic transcription factor in multiple cancers	E1A converts YY1 from a repressor to an activator; p300 and HDAC3 are also involved	[14, 15]
HER2/ERBB2/neu	Proto-oncogene in breast cancer	AP-2 transcriptional activity on the HER2 promoter is enhanced by YY1	[16, 17]
Cyclooxygenase-2 (COX-2]	Oncogene of various cancers	Proposed a model with YY1-mediated recruitment of p300 and HDAC1,2	[18]
c-Fos	Proto-oncogene	E1A converts YY1 from a repressor to an activator in this regulation	[19]
Glucose regulating protein 78/ binding immunoglobulin protein	Promotes tumor proliferation, survival, metastasis and therapeutic resistance	p300 and PRMT1 are recruited	[20-23]
Snail	Enhances cell survival, movement and/or EMT	YY1 binds a distal Snail 3' enhancer	[24, 25]
Msx2	EMT and tumorigenesis	Three YY1-binding sites are involved	[26, 27]
DR-α	Overexpressed in cancers	YY1 binding directly to the promoter	[28, 29]
TGF-β	Overexpressed in tumors; promotes invasiveness and metastasis	A polymorphism mutation in the TGF-β promoter creates a binding site of YY1 that activates the TGF-β gene	[30, 31]
B. Tumor suppression genes			
p53	Tumor suppressor	E1A and p300 can further induce p53 expression	[32]
p73	A member of the p53 family of proteins	YY1 and E2F1 cooperate to promote p73 transcription	[33]
RIZ1	A histone methyltransferase; altered expression in cancers; a potential tumor suppressor	Correlated with reduced H3-K9 dimethylation	[34]
C. Other regulatory proteins in tumorigenesis			
Epidermal growth factor receptor (EGFR)	Cell signaling molecule involved in diverse cellular functions, including cell proliferation, differentiation, motility, and survival	Sp1 and YY1 synergistically induce the EGFR promoter; p53 suppresses this activation	[35]
Histone H2a and H3	Aberrantly modified in cancers	Regulated by the cell cycle	[36]
Histone H4	Aberrantly modified in cancers	Multiple YY1 binding sites are involved	[37]
Poly(ADP-ribose) polymerase 1 (PARP1]	Promoting poly(ADP-ribosyl)ation; related to DNA damage repair	YY1 directly binds the promoter	[38]
Proliferating cellular nuclear antigen (PCNA)	Involved in DNA synthesis and repair; cooperates with nucleophosmin/B23	B23 is involved; accompanied by histone H4 deacetylation	[39, 40]

Table 1. YY1-Activated Genes and Promoters.

The first oncogene shown to be activated by YY1 is c-myc that drives cellular proliferation and leads to oncogenic transformation when constitutively activated [14]. Specifically, YY1 was found to increase levels of two c-myc mRNA transcript variants. It was later discovered that the viral protein E1A dissociates the YY1-p300-HDAC3 complex that normally inhibits c-myc transcription. Thus, with the presence of E1A and the dissociation of HDAC3, the c-myc promoter becomes more accessible due to regional histone hyperacetylation. YY1 acts similarly in regulating expression of c-Fos, another well characterized proto-oncogene driving cellular proliferation [41, 42]. Through interacting with the ATF-CREB transcription complex, YY1 inhibits c-Fos expression; however, this interaction is also disrupted by E1A, which changes the effect of YY1 from repressive to activating on c-Fos gene expression.

Another example of YY1-activated oncogene expression is its regulation of the protein B23. B23 is involved in nuclear export of ribosomes and chaperone activity and stimulates repression of multiple tumor suppressors. YY1 activates B23 in the presence of a viral gene product, the hepatitis C virus (HCV) core, which plays a pivotal role in liver oncogenesis [12]. The HCV core leads to YY1-mediated recruitment of p300 and B23 to the B23 promoter, activating its gene expression. In the absence of the HCV core, YY1 recruits HDAC1 to the B23 promoter to act as a transcriptional repressor. Thus, B23, like E1A, switches YY1 from a transcriptional repressor to an activator [43]. Other YY1-activated oncogenes include proliferating cell nuclear antigen (PCNA) and HER2 [17, 40, 44].

Several genes that directly promote cancer invasion and metastasis are regulated by YY1. Angiogenesis is important to cancer progression and tumor cell invasion. Vascular endothelial growth factor (VEGF) is a key mediator of angiogenesis in cancer. YY1 forms a complex with hypoxia-inducible factor (HIF) 1α to activate VEGF expression and consequently promotes angiogenesis [45]. YY1 also induces expression of cyclooxygenase (COX) -2, an inflammation-associated enzyme that mediates tumor cell bone metastasis [18].

Epithelial-to-mesenchymal transition (EMT) is one of the early and critical steps of the tumor metastatic cascade and characterized by tumor cells losing their epithelial architecture and adopting that of a mesenchymal cell. This morphological transition typically enhances the motile, migratory and invasive abilities of tumor cells [46]. The transcription factor Snail inhibits expression of the epithelial marker and EMT-inhibitor E-cadherin. YY1 binds the 3′ enhancer of Snail to upregulate its expression. Consequently, YY1 overexpression downregulates E-cadherin expression through activating Snail, leading to enhanced EMT and tumor progression [24].

The above studies, among others, demonstrate an oncogenic role of YY1 in human cancers through its transcriptional activation of a number of oncogenes. It is important to mention that YY1 has also been reported to activate several genes with tumor suppressive potential. The negative regulation of p53 activity by YY1 at the posttranslational level is well established [47-49]. However, ectopically overexpressed YY1 activated a p53 promoter driving expression of a reporter, and this activation was reversed in the presence of E1A [32]. Since YY1-mediated histone modifications are essential to its transcriptional activity and this modulation unlikely occurs on extrachromosomal DNA, such as transfected reporter plasmids, the results of this study may not truly reflect YY1's effect on the endogenous p53 promoter.

http://dx.doi.org/10.5772/53091

2.2. YY1-repressed gene expression

Cancer-related genes that are repressed by YY1 are listed in Table 2. Many of them encode gene products with tumor suppressive functions, a phenomenon consistent with YY1's predominantly oncogenic role in human cancers.

Gene/Promoter	Gene Product Function	Mechanism/Observation	Reference
A. Oncogenic and/or overexpressed genes			
Interferon β (IFN-β)	Potential target in cancer therapy	YY2 antagonizes the YY1-mediated repression, Sin3A/NCoR/HDACs complex is recruited by YY1	[50, 51]
Hypoxia-Inducible Factor 2α (HIF-2α)	Oncogenic role	PTEN released this repression	[52]
Matrix Metalloproteinase-9 (MMP-9]	Increasingly expressed in various cancers	Monoubiquitinated YY1 binds CtBP; HDAC3 is recruited	[53]
PVT1	Oncogenic role	A mutation leading to reduced YY1 causes PVT1 overexpression.	[54]
B. Tumor suppression genes			
CCAAT/enhancer-binding protein delta (CEBPD)	Tumor suppressor	Recruits Ezh2, DNMT1, DNMT3A, DNMT3B	[6]
Chondromodulin-I	Inhibitor of angiogenesis	YY1 recruits HDAC2	[55]
Death Receptor 5 (DR5]	A receptor in the extrinsic apoptosis pathway	Rituximab inhibits DNA binding of YY1 and relieves its repression of DR5	[56, 57]
KISS1	Metastasis suppressor	Sp1 is not involved.	[58]
microRNA-29	Tumor suppressor	Through binding to a conserved regulatory region	[59]
microRNA-206	Promotes cell apoptosis	YY1 regulation is antagonized by c-Jun and c-Fos	[60]
p21	Leads to cell cycle arrest	YY1 antagonizes p53-mediated transcription	[49, 61]
p16(INK4a)	Tumor suppressor	HDAC3 and HDAC4 are recruited	[62]
Retinoblastoma (Rb)	Tumor suppressor	GABP and HCF-1 are involved in this regulation	[63]
HOXB13	Inhibits prostate cancer cell growth by suppressing AR and TCF-4 signaling	YY1 recruits HDAC4 to promoter and inhibits transcription	[8]
PTEN	Tumor Suppressor and Antagonist of PI3K/Akt Signaling	MTA1 recruits HDAC4 and YY1 to PTEN promoter	[64]
C. Other regulatory proteins related to cancers			
CD30	A member of the TNF receptor family; related to lymphoma.	Directly binds the promoter	[65]
PPAR-δ	Nuclear receptor proteins regulating gene expression	Directly binds the promoter	[66]
Cyclin D1	Regulates Cdk4 function	HDAC1 is recruited	[61, 67]

Table 2. Y1-Repressed Genes and Promoters.

The tumor suppressor retinoblastoma (Rb) is transcriptionally inhibited by YY1 upon its binding to the Rb promoter [63]. YY1 also recruits HDAC3 and HDAC4 to repress the expression of tumor suppressor p16 that inhibits CDK4 to reduce cell proliferation [62]. YY1-mediated transcriptional repression of the cell cycle-regulator p21 is one of many examples of YY1's role in antagonizing p53 function [49]. Additionally, YY1 represses PTEN through associating with HDAC4 and the chromatin modifier MTA1 [64].

YY1 has been shown to inhibit genes encoding microRNA (miRNA) products with tumor suppressive potential. MiRNAs are critical players in a number of human diseases, including cancers. MiRNAs bind the 5′ UTRs of partially complementary mRNA transcripts, blocking their translation; they may also lead to mRNA degradation. MiR-29 exhibits tumor suppressive potential based on its activation of p53 through targeting its inhibitory proteins p85α and CDC42 [68]. YY1, in cooperation with NF-κB, can inhibit miR-29 transcription [59]. Ring1- and YY1-binding protein (RYBP) enhances YY1-mediated miR-29 silencing and enriches YY1-recruited Ezh2 at target loci [69]. YY1 has also been shown to negatively regulate miR-206, a known promoter of apoptosis [60].

YY1 binding elements are present in over a thousand vertebrate gene promoters. The effect of YY1 on the expression of a given target gene will depend on the extracellular stimuli available to the cell and the presence or absence of YY1-interaction partners that serve as coactivators or corepressors. The transcriptional activity of YY1 on its myriad of cancer-related target genes convolutes the task of determining its role in human cancers. However, the current evidence suggests that YY1 activity is primarily oncogenic, and these effects clearly override any YY1 tumor suppressive function.

2.3. YY1 as a transcription cofactor

Although most studies to date demonstrate the regulation of YY1 as a transcription factor directly binding to target promoters, recent reports have begun to reveal the role of YY1 as a transcription cofactor that is independent of its DNA binding ability.

In prostate cancer cells, YY1 interacts with androgen receptor (AR) and serves as its coactivator in mediating PSA expression. Thus, the putative binding site of YY1 is dispensable in YY1-promoted prostate specific antigen (PSA) expression [70]. YY1 represses RNA methyltransferase-like 1 gene expression, yet there is no YY1 binding site in its gene promoter [71]. In this instance, YY1 regulation depends on transcription factor ATF/CREB. Hypoxia-Inducible Factor (HIF) -2α is stabilized upon inactivation of tumor suppressor von Hippel Lindau (VHL). As a transcription factor, HIF-2α regulates the expression of genes responsible for angiogenesis and metastasis. YY1 acts as a corepressor of HIF-2α, but this repression is abolished by phosphatase and tensin homolog (PTEN) [52].

The recently appreciated function of YY1 as a transcription cofactor expands its role in mediating gene expression. As a cofactor, more or different YY1 functional domains are exposed and available to other proteins for binding or recruitment. This diversifies the interaction partners available to YY1 on its target promoters and extends its role in regulating gene expression [72].

http://dx.doi.org/10.5772/53091

3. YY1 as a regulator of post-translational modifications

YY1 was first identified as a transcription factor and has been shown to regulate the expression of many genes. However, our understanding of YY1 function has evolved with an increasing appreciation for its DNA-binding independent activities, many of which contribute to YY1-mediated gene expression.

Proteins undergo different types of post-translational modifications, including acetylation, methylation, ubiquitination and sumoylation that contribute to the complexity of protein stability, function and interactions. Many YY1-interaction partners mediate YY1-regulated gene expression through instigating post-translational modifications.

3.1. Acetylation

Acetylation is the addition of an acetyl group (CH_3CO) to a lysine residue and mediated by a class of proteins called histone acetyltransferases (HATs). These enzymes catalyze acetylation of both histone and non-histone proteins, and for this reason are more commonly referred to as lysine acetyltransferases (KATs) [73]. Acetylation of non-histone proteins modulates their activity and stablity, while histone acetylation is associated with a relatively loose or open chromatin conformation that is more accessible to transcriptional regulatory proteins, leading to active gene expression.

As we discussed above, YY1 interacts with the KAT p300 and this complex is disrupted in the presence of the viral protein E1A. Notably, YY1 and E1A bind to different domains of p300, and the binding sites of p300 and E1A on YY1 are also well separate [74]. Thus, it is very likely that these three proteins form a ternary complex. Such a complex would promote histone acetylation on promoters, such as P5, c-myc and c-Fos. This explains the role of E1A in converting YY1 from a transcriptional repressor to an activator to promote the expression of these target genes [2, 41, 75].

Acetylation of p53 by p300 both prevents its ubiquitination and subsequent degradation and enhances the p53-DNA interaction, thus promoting p53 transcriptional activity [76, 77]. YY1 inhibits p300-mediated p53 acetylation, thereby antagonizing the tumor suppressive function of p53 [47].

While histone acetylation is associated with active gene expression, histone deacetylation is a mark of gene repression and mediated by a family of proteins called histone deacetylases (HDACs). YY1 has been demonstrated to interact with a number of HDACs and recruit them to target promoters for gene repression. Indeed, YY1 recruitment of HDACs to tumor suppressor gene promoters is important for its role in prostate cancer, and will be discussed below.

3.2. Methylation

Like other modifications, methylation also modulates protein function. In this regard, the most studied activity is the contribution of histone methylation to gene expression. Although DNA methylation usually inhibits gene expression, histone methylation can either activate or repress a target gene, depending on the methylated residues.

Protein arginine methyltransferase (PRMT) 1 catalyzes methylation of histone H4 at arginine 3 (H4-R3). YY1 recruits PRMT1 to the c-myc promoter to activate c-myc gene expression [9]. Similarly, YY1 has also been shown to activate the promoter of a pro-survival chaperone protein, GRP78, through recruiting PRMT1 [22]. YY1-mediated expression of these cell survival genes suggests its proliferative role in oncogenesis.

The proteins enhancer of zeste (Ezh) 1 and 2 are lysine-specific histone methyltransferases mediating methylation of lysine 27 on histone 3 (H3-K27), a hallmark of gene silencing in many cancer-related genes [78]. They are both members of the Polycomb group (PcG) of proteins and core components of the Polycomb repressive complex (PRC) 2, responsible for gene silencing in a number of tumor suppressor genes.

YY1 was first demonstrated to recruit Ezh2 in mouse skeletal muscle cells [4]. The Recruitment of Polycomb (REPO) domain of YY1 is both necessary and sufficient to recruit Ezh2 and other PcG proteins for the establishment of target gene silencing [79].

In addition to histone methylation, YY1 can also mediate DNA methylation. This multi-layered regulation by YY1 has been demonstrated on the promoter of CCAAT/enhancer binding protein delta (CEBPD). YY1 associates with both DNA methyltransferases and PcG proteins to execute gene silencing through modifications of both DNA and histones [80].

3.3. Ubiquitination

Ubiquitination is a modification executed cooperatively by a set of three ubiquitin enzymes (E1, E2, and E3). Protein monoubiquitination typically alters subcellular localization of a protein or modulates its function and additional types of modification, while polyubiquitination usually results in its proteasomal degradation.

In addition to the negative regulatory effects of YY1 on p53 discussed above, YY1 also promotes p53 polyubiquitination and degradation [47, 48]. YY1 directly interacts with both p53 and its E3 ligase Mdm2 and enhances the p53-Mdm2 interaction through the formation of a ternary complex. Both wild-type YY1 and its DNA-binding deficient mutant promote p53 polyubiquitination, indicating that this function of YY1 is independent of its transcriptional activity [48]. Consistently, YY1 depletion in cells leads to an increase in p53 stability and results in cell cycle arrest and apoptosis.

We recently identified negative regulation of the tumor suppressor p27 by YY1 through YY1-promoted ubiquitination [81]. YY1 overexpression enhanced both mono- and polyubiquitination of p27, while YY1 silencing markedly reduced p27 polyubiquitination, but not monoubiquitination.

In summary, the large number of YY1's interaction partners increases the complexity of its biological functions. Many of these proteins (e.g. p300, PRMT1, Ezh2, etc.) contribute to YY1-mediated gene expression and modulate its Yin Yang effects on target genes. This transcriptional modulation is typically executed through YY1-recruited complexes initiating the addition or removal of different modifying groups on histone proteins. Other YY1-binding proteins contribute to the transcription-independent functions of YY1, such as Mdm2-mediated p53 ubiquitination and degradation.

4. Regulation of YY1 expression and activity

In addition to transcriptional regulation, YY1-mediated gene transcription and protein modifications, YY1 expression and function are also modulated at multiple levels.

4.1. YY1 is regulated by gene regulatory proteins

As a transcription factor, YY1 regulates the expression of itself through binding to consensus sequences in the first intron of the YY1 gene [82]. These YY1 binding sites are necessary for YY1 gene transcription. Interestingly, overexpressed exogenous YY1 inhibits the transcription of the endogenous YY1 gene, but the reduction of YY1 to normal levels restores this transcription, suggesting a negative feedback loop. Several other transcription factors regulate YY1 expression, including NF-κB, whose regulation of YY1 in prostate cancer will be discussed below.

Raf kinase inhibitor protein (RKIP) is a potential tumor suppressor gene based on its activity in suppressing metastasis and reduced expression in cancers. RKIP overexpression inhibits YY1 transcription and sensitizes cells to TRAIL-mediated apoptosis [83, 84].

In addition to transcription factors, other gene regulatory proteins also modulate YY1 expression. One example is G-quadruplex resolvase (G4R) 1 (also known as RHAU or DHX36], which upregulates YY1 expression by resolving secondary structures in the YY1 promoter. The G-quadruplex (G4) structure is a 4-stranded secondary DNA or RNA structure that is stabilized by non-canonical Hoogsteen hydrogen bonding of planar guanine quartets and their subsequent stacking [85]. G4 structures in gene promoters inhibit gene transcription, which can be relieved by G4 structure resolving helicases.

Both human and murine YY1 promoters have high contents of cytosine (C) and guanine (G) nucleotides that confer these promoters with the potential to form G4 structures [86, 87]. We recently demonstrated that the presence of G4 structures in the YY1 promoter inhibits YY1 expression [86]. High G/C content is a common feature of many proto-oncogenes, such as c-myc and Bcl-2, whereas the promoters of most tumor suppressor genes have reduced numbers of closely-linked guanosine runs [88]. The high G/C content of YY1 and the presence of G4 structures in its promoter and 5′ UTR are strong indicators of the oncogenic nature of YY1.

4.2. YY1 is regulated by post-translational modifications

Lysine residues are one of the major targets of post-translational modifications, acting as a substrate for the addition of acetyl, methyl, ubiquitin or small ubiquitin modifier (SUMO) groups. YY1 contains 32 lysines, equivalent to 8% of its total amino acids, making YY1 a vulnerable target of multiple modifications. Of the 414 amino acids that compose YY1, all lysine residues are located within the 257 amino acids comprising the middle and C-terminal regions, but not in the first 157 residues (Figure 1).

YY1 recruits p300 and PCAF to mediate histone acetylation of target promoters. Meanwhile, both p300 and PCAF acetylate YY1 in the central region (residues 171-200), augmenting YY1-mediated gene repression [11]. PCAF also acetylates YY1 in the C-terminus and thereby interferes with YY1's ability to bind its DNA consensus sequence [11]. On the other hand, HDACs deacetylate YY1 residues in its central region but not at the C-terminus [11].

YY1 is modified by ubiquitin and SUMO groups. Treatment with a proteasome inhibitor led to an accumulation of YY1 protein, suggesting that YY1 degradation is likely regulated by ubiquitination [48]. However, YY1 mono-ubiquitination enhances its interaction with C-terminal binidng protein (CtBP) and HDAC3 to establish a repressive complex that inhibits the expression of matrix metalloprotease (MMP) -9, a protein promoting cell invasion [53].

PIASy, a SUMO-E3 ligase, promotes the conjugation of SUMO proteins to YY1. We reported that sumoylation exerts an inhibitory effect on YY1-mediated gene expression [89].

YY1 is also subject to other modifications that do not rely on lysine residues. Phosphorylation of YY1 at three particular sites modulates a number of YY1 activities [90]. Among them, serine 247 (Ser247) is located in the spacer region of YY1 while two other sites, threonines 348 and 378, are in YY1's DNA-binding domain (Figure 1). Phosphorylation of the two threonines, but not Ser247, abolishes the DNA binding ability of YY1. Threonine 39 of YY1 was recently identified to be phosphorylated by Polo-like kinase 1; however, its role in modulating YY1 activity remains undetermined [91].

Akt is a well-established oncogene and acts as a critical upstream signaling protein for cell proliferation and survival. YY1 was shown to interact with Akt and is likely a substrate of Akt-mediated phosphorylation. Specifically, YY1 phosphorylation decreased upon treatment with an inhibitor of phosphoinositide 3 kinase (PI3K) that mediates Akt activation [45].

4.3. YY1 is regulated by growth factors & other biomolecules

Oncogenesis involves the upregulation of multiple growth factors, some of which promote YY1 expression. Insulin-like growth factor-1 increases YY1 expression while its depletion significantly decreases YY1 levels [92-94]. Fibroblast growth factor (FGF) -2 also upregulates YY1 expression in vascular cells upon injury [95]. YY1 expression in prostate cancer cells is particularly sensitive to growth factors, which will be discussed below.

Other biomolecules, such as lipopolysaccharide and myeloid nuclear differentiation antigen (MNDA) can promote YY1 expression and modulate its activity through enhancing YY1-DNA association [18, 96]. Conversely, YY1 is negatively regulated by molecules that have anti-growth effects. For example, aphidicolin, the DNA synthesis inhibitor and apoptosis inducer, facilitiates YY1 translocation and cleavage [97, 98].

While YY1 negatively regulates miR-29, this miRNA also binds the 3′ UTR of YY1 mRNA and inhibits its translation [59, 99]. The tumor suppressor miR-34a has also been shown to target YY1 and block its expression [100, 101].

Yin Yang (YY) 2 has 65% similarity to YY1 in the protein coding regions while their amino acid sequences share 56% similarity, which is mostly in their DNA binding regions [102]. Thus, YY2 binds the same consensus sequence as YY1, but with a much lower affinity [103]. Interestingly, YY2 exhibits opposing effects on shared YY1 transcriptional targets [104]. YY2 silencing reversed the antiproliferative effects of YY1 depletion [104]. Nonetheless, more studies are needed to delineate the mechanisms and interaction of YY1 and YY2.

Overall, YY1 is activated by different growth factors, whereas antiproliferative signals tend to antagonize YY1 activity. These data support an oncogenic role of YY1 in tumor development and progression.

5. Evidence of YY1's oncogenic regulation in prostate cancer

Many lines of evidence support an oncogenic role of YY1. Most functions of YY1 discussed above contribute to this role in prostate cancer. Importantly, the overexpression of YY1 in prostate cancer augments the oncogenic effects caused by its regulated pathways. We allocate the role of YY1 in prostate oncogenesis into two categories based on the different regulatory mechanisms.

5.1. Transcriptional regulation

As a transcription factor, YY1 generally activates the expression of oncogenic or proliferative genes and inhibits those with tumor suppressive functions [105].

The Rex1 protein is a marker of both mouse and human embryonic stem cells and exhibits reduced expression in prostate cancer cells compared to normal prostate epithelial cells [106]. YY1 positively regulates Rex1 expression in normal human prostate epithelial cells, but this regulation is not observed in prostate cancer cells, suggesting that YY1 transcriptional activity may be altered during transformation [106].

Prostate stem cell antigen (PSCA) is differentially regulated during prostate oncogenesis and its expression is correlated with the development of malignant human prostate cancer. YY1 cooperates with androgen receptor (AR) to regulate PSCA expression [107]. Two YY1 consensus sites have been identified in the PSCA promoter and YY1 is overall essential to androgen-mediated PSCA upregulation in prostate epithelial cell lines. This suggests that YY1 contributes to prostate cancer progression by modulating genes such as PSCA (Figure 2) [107].

YY1 can act as a transcription coactivator to promote gene expression. We demonstrated that the expression of prostate-specific antigen (PSA) in prostate cancer cells is dependent on YY1 [70]. This effect is unaltered when the YY1 binding site in the PSA promoter is mutated, but lost when the direct YY1-AR interaction is disrupted. Since YY1-DNA association is unnecessary for YY1-mediated PSA transcription, YY1 acts as a coactivator in promoting PSA gene expression. We mapped the AR binding domain to the C-terminus of YY1 where its DNA binding site resides, suggesting that YY1 unlikely interacts simultaneously with the

PSA promoter and AR [70]. Elevated PSA levels serve as a diagnostic marker of prostate cancer development, and androgen hormones, which bind to AR and stimulate its activity, are known to facilitate prostate cancer progression [108]. The positive regulation of PSA expression by YY1 suggests its diagnostic and prognostic value in prostate cancer therapies (Figure 2).

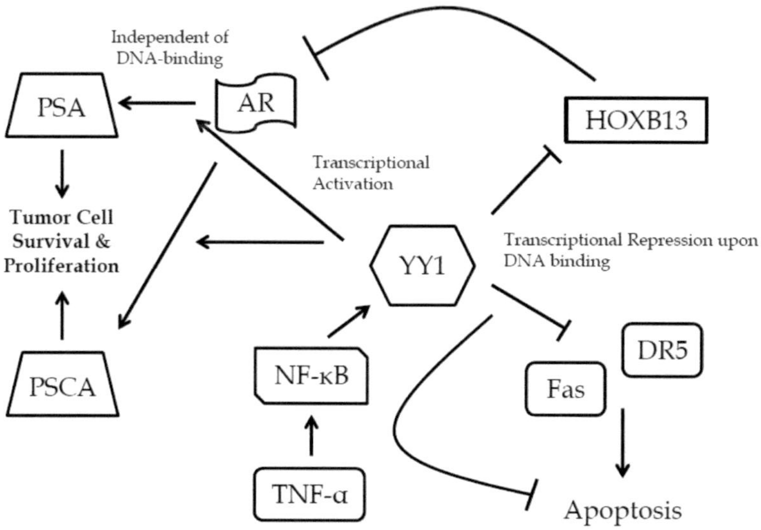

Figure 2. An Overview of Several YY1-Involved Signaling Pathways in Prostate Cancer; YY1 inhibits apoptosis by repressing DR5 and Fas receptors. YY1 and androgen receptor (AR) cooperate to activate expression of prostate specific antigen (PSA) and prostate stem cell antigen (PSCA), both of which contribute to prostate oncogenesis. HOXB13 inhibits prostate cancer cell growth by antagonizing AR signaling. YY1 represses HOXB13 transcription, thereby relieving growth suppression. The growth hormone tumor necrosis factor (TNF)-α enhances NF-κB-mediated YY1 expression and AR activity, promoting cell survival and growth. Overall, YY1 function and regulation support its oncogenic role in prostate cancer development and progression.

More evidence has been demonstrated to show how YY1-mediated transcriptional repression contributes to the oncogenic progression and therapeutic response of prostate cancer.

The homeobox gene HOXB13 suppresses prostate cancer cell growth by negatively regulating AR and T-cell factor (TCF) -4 signaling (Figure 2) [109, 110]. YY1 binds to the HOXB13 promoter and represses its expression through recruiting HDAC4, suggesting that YY1 releases HOXB13-mediated growth arrest of prostate cancer cells [8].

Fas receptor and DR5 are two death receptors regulating extrinsic apoptotic pathways. YY1 negatively regulates the expression of these two receptors (Figure 2) [111, 112]. Nitric oxide (NO) acts as an intracellular second messenger to modify gene expression, including upregulating Fas receptor. The underlying mechanism of this regulation is through NO-induced S-nitrosylation of YY1 and the consequently reduced YY1 DNA binding affinity. This abolishes YY1 mediated Fas receptor gene repression and sensitizes

http://dx.doi.org/10.5772/53091

prostate cancer cells to apoptotic stimuli [111]. A similar mechanism has also been reported in the regulation of YY1 by Rituximab, a synthetic antibody used in the treatment of multiple cancers, including prostate cancer [112]. YY1 inhibits DR5 expression; thus elevated YY1 levels in prostate cancer confer therapeutic resistance to tumor cells through downregulating DR5. Rituximab inhibits both DNA binding and expression of YY1, which consequently activates DR5 gene expression and sensitizes TRAIL-induced apoptosis.

5.2. The regulation of YY1 in prostate cancer-related mechanisms

In addition to the growth stimuli indicated above, YY1 expression is regulated by signaling pathways directly involved in prostate oncogenesis.

NF-κB contributes to prostate cancer development through its constitutive activation of AR expression and therefore serves as a prognostic marker of prostate cancer [113-115]. NF-κB directly binds to the YY1 promoter to enhance YY1 expression (Figure 2) [116]. Thus, genetic deletion of the p65 subunit of NF-κB was associated with decreased YY1 mRNA and protein levels [117]. Consistently, the growth hormone tumor necrosis factor (TNF) -α, an activator of NF-κB transcriptional activity, stimulates NF-κB-mediated YY1 expression in prostate cancer PC-3 cells (Figure 2) [117].

Transforming growth factor (TGF) -β3 is a commonly upregulated growth factor in cancers. A recent study revealed differential regulatory effects of TGF-β3 on YY1 expression in various prostate cell lines [118]. While TGF-β3 promotes YY1 expression in benign prostatic hyperplasia cells, this effect is diminished in LNCaP cells and reversed in DU145 cells. Consistent with other studies, these altered YY1 expression levels inversely correlated to p53 levels [47-49].

The contribution of Akt-mediated signaling pathways to prostate cancer development is well documented. Akt was reported to mediate YY1 phosphorylation and its cytoplasmic translocation, although the target residue(s) and whether the effect is direct or not remain unclear [45]. Tumor suppressor PTEN inhibits the proliferative regulation of Akt through antagonizing its phosphorylation [119-121]. Recent studies demonstrated PTEN-mediated YY1 downregulation through inhibiting PI3K/Akt signaling [52, 122].

Consistent with these mechanistic studies, YY1 was suggested as a biomarker of prostate cancer. A study using a prostate cancer tissue microarray consisting of 1364 representative tissues from 246 hormone-naive prostate cancer patients demonstrated that YY1 levels were increased in tumors of intermediate to high morphologic grades, indicating its upregulation throughout the progression of prostate cancer [3]. Interestingly, YY1 immunohistochemical staining was observed in both nucleus and cytoplasm in tissues of prostate cancer and prostatic intraepithelial neoplasia, consistent with the cytoplasmic localization of YY1 demonstrated in other cells [98]. In another study, YY1 was one of several differentially expressed proteins in prostate cancer in comparison to benign prostatic hyperplasia and contributed to upregulated transcriptional networks [76].

6. YY1 studies in the clinical applications of prostate cancer

Many biological functions of YY1 implicate its oncogenic role in human cancers. Further corroborating these observations is the frequent overexpression of YY1 in cancer cells, including prostate tumors [123]. These oncogenic properties confer YY1 with great potential as a therapeutic target in prostate cancer treatment.

YY1 antagonizes p53 function through multiple mechanisms, including facilitating Mdm2-mediated p53 ubiquitination and degradation, inhibiting p53-mediated transcription, blocking p53 acetylation, and attenuating p14ARF-mediated p53 stablization [47-49]. These suggest that p53 is a primary target of overexpressed YY1's role during prostate oncogenesis. Although p53 is most commonly deleted or mutated in prostate cancers, some tumors retain functional p53, especially at their early stages [124-126]. As a result, many tumors need to overcome p53 tumor suppression early in their cell transformation process, and it is reasonable to hypothesize that YY1 plays a role in overcoming this barrier to tumorigenesis in these developing prostate neoplasms.

YY1 is also implicated as a therapeutic target through its promotion of multiple oncogenes' function and expression. The bona fide oncogene Ezh2 has been used as a marker for aggressive prostate cancers and its overexpression is associated with decreased therapeutic efficacy [127]. Since YY1 is essential to Ezh2-mediated histone H3-K27 methylation, it is possible that YY1 augments the aberrant epigenetics in prostate cancer and contributes to tumor progression by recruiting Ezh2 to its target promoters.

The role of YY1 in prostate cancer therapies has been investigated in multiple studies. As indicated above, YY1 transcriptional activity and expression are negatively regulated by NO and rituximab. Thus, the treatment of the two anticancer drugs DETA/NONOate and rituximab releases YY1-mediated repression of the death receptors Fas and DR5, and sensitizes the ligand-induced apoptosis of prostate cancer cells [111, 112].

7. Summary

YY1 is a multifunctional transcription factor capable of either repressing or activating its target genes, depending on the cellular signals and composition of its recruited complexes. Additionally, YY1 modulates the activity and stability of its interaction proteins by mediating the post-translational modifications of these proteins. Several lines of evidence exist to suggest that YY1 acts as an oncogene in prostate cancer. First, YY1 activates the expression and function of oncogenes, while inhibiting tumor suppressor activity. Secondly, the activity of YY1 itself is promoted by oncogenes and growth factors, and inhibited by tumor suppressors. Third, YY1 is overexpressed in prostate cancers.

Epigenetics implicates reversible processes that do not involve any change of DNA sequence. In theory, simultaneously targeting several epigenetic, cancer-driving pathways should result in more efficient therapies than individually targeting each of them. Thus, if a singular regulatory protein involved in the abnormality of multiple processes contributing to malignancy is identified, therapeutic targeting of this key regulator will display a substantial impact on disease progression or reversal. To date, no YY1 gene or protein mutation has been reported in any disease. YY1's regulatory role in multiple epigenetic processes coupled with its overexpression in prostate cancer lends YY1 therapeutic potential.

Many questions remain about the role of YY1 in prostate cancer-related biological pathways, and it is likely that such a promiscuous protein has more roles in prostate oncogenesis than what are currently known. Nonetheless, present evidence suggests that YY1 exerts a predominantly oncogenic function and therapeutic targeting of YY1 may result in substantial advances in prostate cancer treatment.

Acknowledgements

This work was supported in part by the Research Scholar Grants (116403-RSG-09-082-01-MGO) from the American Cancer Society and the National Institutes of Health R01 Grant (5R01CA106314-09) to GS. DBS was supported by the National Cancer Institute Training Grant 5T32CA079448.

Author details

Daniel B. Stovall and Guangchao Sui

Department of Cancer Biology and Comprehensive Cancer Center, Wake Forest University School of Medicine, Winston-Salem, NC, U.S.A.

References

[1] Hanahan D, Weinberg RA. Hallmarks of cancer: the next generation. Cell. 2011 Mar 4;144(5]:646-74.

[2] Shi Y, Seto E, Chang LS, Shenk T. Transcriptional repression by YY1, a human GLI-Kruppel-related protein, and relief of repression by adenovirus E1A protein. Cell. 1991 Oct 18;67(2]:377-88.

[3] Hyde-DeRuyscher RP, Jennings E, Shenk T. DNA binding sites for the transcriptional activator/repressor YY1. Nucleic Acids Res. 1995 Nov 11;23(21]:4457-65.

[4] Caretti G, Di Padova M, Micales B, Lyons GE, Sartorelli V. The Polycomb Ezh2 methyltransferase regulates muscle gene expression and skeletal muscle differentiation. Genes Dev. 2004 Nov 1;18(21]:2627-38.

[5] Hu HM, Kanda K, Zhang L, Boxer LM. Activation of the c-myc p1 promoter in Burkitt's lymphoma by the hs3 immunoglobulin heavy-chain gene enhancer. Leukemia. 2007 Apr;21(4]:747-53.

[6] Ko CY, Hsu HC, Shen MR, Chang WC, Wang JM. Epigenetic silencing of CCAAT/enhancer-binding protein delta activity by YY1/polycomb group/DNA methyltransferase complex. J Biol Chem. 2008 Nov 7;283(45]:30919-32.

[7] Miao J, Wang Z, Provencher H, Muir B, Dahiya S, Carney E, et al. HOXB13 promotes ovarian cancer progression. Proc Natl Acad Sci U S A. 2007 Oct 23;104(43]:17093-8.

[8] Ren G, Zhang G, Dong Z, Liu Z, Li L, Feng Y, et al. Recruitment of HDAC4 by transcription factor YY1 represses HOXB13 to affect cell growth in AR-negative prostate cancers. Int J Biochem Cell Biol. 2009 May;41(5]:1094-101.

[9] Rezai-Zadeh N, Zhang X, Namour F, Fejer G, Wen YD, Yao YL, et al. Targeted recruitment of a histone H4-specific methyltransferase by the transcription factor YY1. Genes Dev. 2003 Apr 15;17(8]:1019-29.

[10] Sankar N, Baluchamy S, Kadeppagari RK, Singhal G, Weitzman S, Thimmapaya B. p300 provides a corepressor function by cooperating with YY1 and HDAC3 to repress c-Myc. Oncogene. 2008 Sep 25;27(43]:5717-28.

[11] Yao YL, Yang WM, Seto E. Regulation of transcription factor YY1 by acetylation and deacetylation. Mol Cell Biol. 2001 Sep;21(17]:5979-91.

[12] Mai RT, Yeh TS, Kao CF, Sun SK, Huang HH, Wu Lee YH. Hepatitis C virus core protein recruits nucleolar phosphoprotein B23 and coactivator p300 to relieve the repression effect of transcriptional factor YY1 on B23 gene expression. Oncogene. 2006 Jan 19;25(3]:448-62.

[13] Ye K. Nucleophosmin/B23, a multifunctional protein that can regulate apoptosis. Cancer Biol Ther. 2005 Sep;4(9]:918-23.

[14] Riggs KJ, Saleque S, Wong KK, Merrell KT, Lee JS, Shi Y, et al. Yin-yang 1 activates the c-myc promoter. Mol Cell Biol. 1993 Dec;13(12]:7487-95.

[15] Hsu KW, Hsieh RH, Lee YH, Chao CH, Wu KJ, Tseng MJ, et al. The activated Notch1 receptor cooperates with alpha-enolase and MBP-1 in modulating c-myc activity. Mol Cell Biol. 2008 Aug;28(15]:4829-42.

[16] Begon DY, Delacroix L, Vernimmen D, Jackers P, Winkler R. Yin Yang 1 cooperates with activator protein 2 to stimulate ERBB2 gene expression in mammary cancer cells. J Biol Chem. 2005 Jul 1;280(26]:24428-34.

[17] Allouche A, Nolens G, Tancredi A, Delacroix L, Mardaga J, Fridman V, et al. The combined immunodetection of AP-2alpha and YY1 transcription factors is associated with ERBB2 gene overexpression in primary breast tumors. Breast Cancer Res. 2008;10(1]:R9.

[18] Joo M, Wright JG, Hu NN, Sadikot RT, Park GY, Blackwell TS, et al. Yin Yang 1 enhances cyclooxygenase-2 gene expression in macrophages. Am J Physiol Lung Cell Mol Physiol. 2007 May;292(5]:L1219-26.

[19] Natesan S, Gilman MZ. DNA bending and orientation-dependent function of YY1 in the c-fos promoter. Genes Dev. 1993 Dec;7(12B):2497-509.

[20] Li WW, Hsiung Y, Zhou Y, Roy B, Lee AS. Induction of the mammalian GRP78/BiP gene by Ca2+ depletion and formation of aberrant proteins: activation of the conserved stress-inducible grp core promoter element by the human nuclear factor YY1. Mol Cell Biol. 1997 Jan;17(1]:54-60.

[21] Mao C, Tai WC, Bai Y, Poizat C, Lee AS. In vivo regulation of Grp78/BiP transcription in the embryonic heart: role of the endoplasmic reticulum stress response element and GATA-4. J Biol Chem. 2006 Mar 31;281(13]:8877-87.

[22] Baumeister P, Luo S, Skarnes WC, Sui G, Seto E, Shi Y, et al. Endoplasmic reticulum stress induction of the Grp78/BiP promoter: activating mechanisms mediated by YY1 and its interactive chromatin modifiers. Mol Cell Biol. 2005 Jun;25(11]:4529-40.

[23] Lee AS. GRP78 induction in cancer: therapeutic and prognostic implications. Cancer Res. 2007 Apr 15;67(8]:3496-9.

[24] Palmer MB, Majumder P, Cooper JC, Yoon H, Wade PA, Boss JM. Yin yang 1 regulates the expression of snail through a distal enhancer. Mol Cancer Res. 2009 Feb;7(2]: 221-9.

[25] Bonavida B, Baritaki S. Dual role of NO donors in the reversal of tumor cell resistance and EMT: Downregulation of the NF-kappaB/Snail/YY1/RKIP circuitry. Nitric Oxide. 2011 Jan 1;24(1]:1-7.

[26] Tan DP, Nonaka K, Nuckolls GH, Liu YH, Maxson RE, Slavkin HC, et al. YY1 activates Msx2 gene independent of bone morphogenetic protein signaling. Nucleic Acids Res. 2002 Mar 1;30(5]:1213-23.

[27] Satoh K, Ginsburg E, Vonderhaar BK. Msx-1 and Msx-2 in mammary gland development. J Mammary Gland Biol Neoplasia. 2004 Apr;9(2]:195-205.

[28] Hehlgans T, Strominger JL. Activation of transcription by binding of NF-E1 (YY1) to a newly identified element in the first exon of the human DR alpha gene. J Immunol. 1995 May 15;154(10]:5181-7.

[29] Rangel LB, Agarwal R, Sherman-Baust CA, Mello-Coelho V, Pizer ES, Ji H, et al. Anomalous expression of the HLA-DR alpha and beta chains in ovarian and other cancers. Cancer Biol Ther. 2004 Oct;3(10]:1021-7.

[30] Hobbs K, Negri J, Klinnert M, Rosenwasser LJ, Borish L. Interleukin-10 and transforming growth factor-beta promoter polymorphisms in allergies and asthma. Am J Respir Crit Care Med. 1998 Dec;158(6]:1958-62.

[31] de Souza AP, Trevilatto PC, Scarel-Caminaga RM, de Brito RB, Line SR. Analysis of the TGF-beta1 promoter polymorphism (C-509T) in patients with chronic periodontitis. J Clin Periodontol. 2003 Jun;30(6]:519-23.

[32] Furlong EE, Rein T, Martin F. YY1 and NF1 both activate the human p53 promoter by alternatively binding to a composite element, and YY1 and E1A cooperate to amplify p53 promoter activity. Mol Cell Biol. 1996 Oct;16(10]:5933-45.

[33] Wu S, Murai S, Kataoka K, Miyagishi M. Yin Yang 1 induces transcriptional activity of p73 through cooperation with E2F1. Biochem Biophys Res Commun. 2008 Jan 4;365(1]:75-81.

[34] Abbondanza C, de Nigris F, De Rosa C, Rossiello R, Puca GA, Napoli C. Silencing of YY1 downregulates RIZ1 promoter in human osteosarcoma. Oncol Res. 2008;17(1]: 33-41.

[35] Bheda A, Creek KE, Pirisi L. Loss of p53 induces epidermal growth factor receptor promoter activity in normal human keratinocytes. Oncogene. 2008 Jul 17;27(31]: 4315-23.

[36] Eliassen KA, Baldwin A, Sikorski EM, Hurt MM. Role for a YY1-binding element in replication-dependent mouse histone gene expression. Mol Cell Biol. 1998 Dec;18(12]: 7106-18.

[37] Last TJ, van Wijnen AJ, Birnbaum MJ, Stein GS, Stein JL. Multiple interactions of the transcription factor YY1 with human histone H4 gene regulatory elements. J Cell Biochem. 1999 Mar 15;72(4]:507-16.

[38] Oei SL, Shi Y. Transcription factor Yin Yang 1 stimulates poly(ADP-ribosyl)ation and DNA repair. Biochem Biophys Res Commun. 2001 Jun 8;284(2]:450-4.

[39] Labrie C, Lee BH, Mathews MB. Transcription factors RFX1/EF-C and ATF-1 associate with the adenovirus E1A-responsive element of the human proliferating cell nuclear antigen promoter. Nucleic Acids Res. 1995 Sep 25;23(18]:3732-41.

[40] Weng JJ, Yung BY. Nucleophosmin/B23 regulates PCNA promoter through YY1. Biochem Biophys Res Commun. 2005 Sep 30;335(3]:826-31.

[41] Zhou Q, Engel DA. Adenovirus E1A243 disrupts the ATF/CREB-YY1 complex at the mouse c-fos promoter. J Virol. 1995 Dec;69(12]:7402-9.

[42] Zhou Q, Gedrich RW, Engel DA. Transcriptional repression of the c-fos gene by YY1 is mediated by a direct interaction with ATF/CREB. J Virol. 1995 Jul;69(7]:4323-30.

[43] Inouye CJ, Seto E. Relief of YY1-induced transcriptional repression by protein-protein interaction with the nucleolar phosphoprotein B23. J Biol Chem. 1994 Mar 4;269(9]:6506-10.

[44] Harari D, Yarden Y. Molecular mechanisms underlying ErbB2/HER2 action in breast cancer. Oncogene. 2000 Dec 11;19(53]:6102-14.

[45] de Nigris F, Crudele V, Giovane A, Casamassimi A, Giordano A, Garban HJ, et al. CXCR4/YY1 inhibition impairs VEGF network and angiogenesis during malignancy. Proc Natl Acad Sci U S A. 2010 Aug 10;107(32]:14484-9.

[46] Nauseef JT, Henry MD. Epithelial-to-mesenchymal transition in prostate cancer: paradigm or puzzle? Nat Rev Urol. 2011 Aug;8(8]:428-39.

[47] Gronroos E, Terentiev AA, Punga T, Ericsson J. YY1 inhibits the activation of the p53 tumor suppressor in response to genotoxic stress. Proc Natl Acad Sci U S A. 2004 Aug 17;101(33]:12165-70.

[48] Sui G, Affar el B, Shi Y, Brignone C, Wall NR, Yin P, et al. Yin Yang 1 is a negative regulator of p53. Cell. 2004 Jun 25;117(7]:859-72.

[49] Yakovleva T, Kolesnikova L, Vukojevic V, Gileva I, Tan-No K, Austen M, et al. YY1 binding to a subset of p53 DNA-target sites regulates p53-dependent transcription. Biochem Biophys Res Commun. 2004 May 28;318(2]:615-24.

[50] Klar M, Bode J. Enhanceosome formation over the beta interferon promoter underlies a remote-control mechanism mediated by YY1 and YY2. Mol Cell Biol. 2005 Nov; 25(22]:10159-70.

[51] Le May N, Mansuroglu Z, Leger P, Josse T, Blot G, Billecocq A, et al. A SAP30 complex inhibits IFN-beta expression in Rift Valley fever virus infected cells. PLoS Pathog. 2008 Jan;4(1]:e13.

[52] Petrella BL, Brinckerhoff CE. PTEN suppression of YY1 induces HIF-2 activity in von-Hippel-Lindau-null renal-cell carcinoma. Cancer Biol Ther. 2009 Jul;8(14]: 1389-401.

[53] Rylski M, Amborska R, Zybura K, Mioduszewska B, Michaluk P, Jaworski J, et al. Yin Yang 1 is a critical repressor of matrix metalloproteinase-9 expression in brain neurons. J Biol Chem. 2008 Dec 12;283(50]:35140-53.

[54] Meyer KB, Maia AT, O'Reilly M, Ghoussaini M, Prathalingam R, Porter-Gill P, et al. A functional variant at a prostate cancer predisposition locus at 8q24 is associated with PVT1 expression. PLoS Genet. 2011 Jul;7(7]:e1002165.

[55] Aoyama T, Okamoto T, Fukiage K, Otsuka S, Furu M, Ito K, et al. Histone modifiers, YY1 and p300, regulate the expression of cartilage-specific gene, chondromodulin-I, in mesenchymal stem cells. J Biol Chem. 2010 Sep 24;285(39]:29842-50.

[56] Baritaki S, Huerta-Yepez S, Sakai T, Spandidos DA, Bonavida B. Chemotherapeutic drugs sensitize cancer cells to TRAIL-mediated apoptosis: up-regulation of DR5 and inhibition of Yin Yang 1. Mol Cancer Ther. 2007 Apr;6(4]:1387-99.

[57] Mijatovic S, Maksimovic-Ivanic D, Mojic M, Timotijevic G, Miljkovic D, Mangano K, et al. Cytotoxic and immune-sensitizing properties of nitric oxide-modified Saquinavir in iNOS-positive human melanoma cells. J Cell Physiol. 2011 Jul;226(7]:1803-12.

[58] Mueller JK, Dietzel A, Lomniczi A, Loche A, Tefs K, Kiess W, et al. Transcriptional regulation of the human KiSS1 gene. Mol Cell Endocrinol. 2011 Aug 6;342(1-2]:8-19.

[59] Wang H, Garzon R, Sun H, Ladner KJ, Singh R, Dahlman J, et al. NF-kappaB-YY1-miR-29 regulatory circuitry in skeletal myogenesis and rhabdomyosarcoma. Cancer Cell. 2008 Nov 4;14(5]:369-81.

[60] Song G, Wang L. Nuclear receptor SHP activates miR-206 expression via a cascade dual inhibitory mechanism. PLoS One. 2009;4(9]:e6880.

[61] Santiago FS, Ishii H, Shafi S, Khurana R, Kanellakis P, Bhindi R, et al. Yin Yang-1 inhibits vascular smooth muscle cell growth and intimal thickening by repressing p21WAF1/Cip1 transcription and p21WAF1/Cip1-Cdk4-cyclin D1 assembly. Circ Res. 2007 Jul 20;101(2]:146-55.

[62] Wang X, Feng Y, Xu L, Chen Y, Zhang Y, Su D, et al. YY1 restrained cell senescence through repressing the transcription of p16. Biochim Biophys Acta. 2008 Oct; 1783(10]:1876-83.

[63] Delehouzee S, Yoshikawa T, Sawa C, Sawada J, Ito T, Omori M, et al. GABP, HCF-1 and YY1 are involved in Rb gene expression during myogenesis. Genes Cells. 2005 Jul;10(7]:717-31.

[64] Reddy SD, Pakala SB, Molli PR, Sahni N, Karanam NK, Mudvari P, et al. Metastasis associated protein1/Histone Deacetylase 4-Nucleosome Remodeling and Deacetylase Complex Regulates PTEN Expression and Function. J Biol Chem. 2012 Aug 10;287(33):27843-50.

[65] Franchina M, Woo AJ, Dods J, Karimi M, Ho D, Watanabe T, et al. The CD30 gene promoter microsatellite binds transcription factor Yin Yang 1 (YY1) and shows genetic instability in anaplastic large cell lymphoma. J Pathol. 2008 Jan;214(1]:65-74.

[66] He CQ, Ding NZ, Fan W. YY1 repressing peroxisome proliferator-activated receptor delta promoter. Mol Cell Biochem. 2008 Jan;308(1-2]:247-52.

[67] Cicatiello L, Addeo R, Sasso A, Altucci L, Petrizzi VB, Borgo R, et al. Estrogens and progesterone promote persistent CCND1 gene activation during G1 by inducing transcriptional derepression via c-Jun/c-Fos/estrogen receptor (progesterone receptor) complex assembly to a distal regulatory element and recruitment of cyclin D1 to its own gene promoter. Mol Cell Biol. 2004 Aug;24(16]:7260-74.

[68] Park SY, Lee JH, Ha M, Nam JW, Kim VN. miR-29 miRNAs activate p53 by targeting p85 alpha and CDC42. Nat Struct Mol Biol. 2009 Jan;16(1]:23-9.

[69] Zhou L, Wang L, Lu L, Jiang P, Sun H, Wang H. A Novel Target of microRNA-29, Ring1 and YY1 Binding Protein (Rybp), Negatively Regulates Skeletal Myogenesis. J Biol Chem. 2012 Jul 20;287(30):25255-65.

[70] Deng Z, Wan M, Cao P, Rao A, Cramer SD, Sui G. Yin Yang 1 regulates the transcriptional activity of androgen receptor. Oncogene. 2009 Oct 22;28(42]:3746-57.

[71] Xu J, De Zhu J, Ni M, Wan F, Gu JR. The ATF/CREB site is the key element for transcription of the human RNA methyltransferase like 1(RNMTL1] gene, a newly discovered 17p13.3 gene. Cell Res. 2002 Sep;12(3-4]:177-97.

[72] Affar el B, Gay F, Shi Y, Liu H, Huarte M, Wu S, et al. Essential dosage-dependent functions of the transcription factor yin yang 1 in late embryonic development and cell cycle progression. Mol Cell Biol. 2006 May;26(9]:3565-81.

[73] Thao S, Escalante-Semerena JC. A positive selection approach identifies residues important for folding of Salmonella enterica Pat, an N(epsilon)-lysine acetyltransferase that regulates central metabolism enzymes. Res Microbiol. 2012 Jul;163(6-7):427-35.

[74] Lee JS, Galvin KM, See RH, Eckner R, Livingston D, Moran E, et al. Relief of YY1 transcriptional repression by adenovirus E1A is mediated by E1A-associated protein p300. Genes Dev. 1995 May 15;9(10]:1188-98.

[75] Kadeppagari RK, Sankar N, Thimmapaya B. Adenovirus transforming protein E1A induces c-Myc in quiescent cells by a novel mechanism. J Virol. 2009 May;83(10]: 4810-22.

[76] Li M, Luo J, Brooks CL, Gu W. Acetylation of p53 inhibits its ubiquitination by Mdm2. J Biol Chem. 2002 Dec 27;277(52]:50607-11.

[77] Luo J, Li M, Tang Y, Laszkowska M, Roeder RG, Gu W. Acetylation of p53 augments its site-specific DNA binding both in vitro and in vivo. Proc Natl Acad Sci U S A. 2004 Feb 24;101(8]:2259-64.

[78] Wang L, Brown JL, Cao R, Zhang Y, Kassis JA, Jones RS. Hierarchical recruitment of polycomb group silencing complexes. Mol Cell. 2004 Jun 4;14(5]:637-46.

[79] Wilkinson FH, Park K, Atchison ML. Polycomb recruitment to DNA in vivo by the YY1 REPO domain. Proc Natl Acad Sci U S A. 2006 Dec 19;103(51]:19296-301.

[80] Palacios D, Mozzetta C, Consalvi S, Caretti G, Saccone V, Proserpio V, et al. TNF/ p38alpha/polycomb signaling to Pax7 locus in satellite cells links inflammation to the epigenetic control of muscle regeneration. Cell Stem Cell. 2010 Oct 8;7(4]:455-69.

[81] Wan M, Huang W, Kute TE, Miller LD, Zhang Q, Hatcher H, et al. Yin Yang 1 plays an essential role in breast cancer and negatively regulates p27. Am J Pathol. 2012 May;180(5]:2120-33.

[82] Kim JD, Yu S, Kim J. YY1 is autoregulated through its own DNA-binding sites. BMC Mol Biol. 2009;10:85.

[83] Baritaki S, Katsman A, Chatterjee D, Yeung KC, Spandidos DA, Bonavida B. Regulation of tumor cell sensitivity to TRAIL-induced apoptosis by the metastatic suppressor Raf kinase inhibitor protein via Yin Yang 1 inhibition and death receptor 5 upregulation. J Immunol. 2007 Oct 15;179(8]:5441-53.

[84] Joshi B, Rastogi S, Morris M, Carastro LM, DeCook C, Seto E, et al. Differential regulation of human YY1 and caspase 7 promoters by prohibitin through E2F1 and p53 binding sites. Biochem J. 2007 Jan 1;401(1]:155-66.

[85] Brooks TA, Kendrick S, Hurley L. Making sense of G-quadruplex and i-motif functions in oncogene promoters. FEBS J. 2010 Sep;277(17]:3459-69.

[86] Huang W, Smaldino PJ, Zhang Q, Miller LD, Cao P, Stadelman K, et al. Yin Yang 1 contains G-quadruplex structures in its promoter and 5'-UTR and its expression is modulated by G4 resolvase 1. Nucleic Acids Res. 2012 Feb;40(3]:1033-49.

[87] Safrany G, Perry RP. Characterization of the mouse gene that encodes the delta/YY1/NF-E1/UCRBP transcription factor. Proc Natl Acad Sci U S A. 1993 Jun 15;90(12]:5559-63.

[88] Eddy J, Maizels N. Gene function correlates with potential for G4 DNA formation in the human genome. Nucleic Acids Res. 2006;34(14]:3887-96.

[89] Deng Z, Wan M, Sui G. PIASy-mediated sumoylation of Yin Yang 1 depends on their interaction but not the RING finger. Mol Cell Biol. 2007 May;27(10]:3780-92.

[90] Rizkallah R, Hurt MM. Regulation of the transcription factor YY1 in mitosis through phosphorylation of its DNA-binding domain. Mol Biol Cell. 2009 Nov;20(22]:4766-76.

[91] Rizkallah R, Alexander KE, Kassardjian A, Luscher B, Hurt MM. The transcription factor YY1 is a substrate for Polo-like kinase 1 at the G2/M transition of the cell cycle. PLoS One. 2011;6(1]:e15928.

[92] Flanagan JR. Autologous stimulation of YY1 transcription factor expression: role of an insulin-like growth factor. Cell Growth Differ. 1995 Feb;6(2]:185-90.

[93] Huang HY, Li X, Liu M, Song TJ, He Q, Ma CG, et al. Transcription factor YY1 promotes adipogenesis via inhibiting CHOP-10 expression. Biochem Biophys Res Commun. 2008 Oct 31;375(4]:496-500.

[94] Yang H, Li TW, Peng J, Mato JM, Lu SC. Insulin-like growth factor 1 activates methionine adenosyltransferase 2A transcription by multiple pathways in human colon cancer cells. Biochem J. 2011 Jun 1;436(2]:507-16.

[95] Santiago FS, Lowe HC, Bobryshev YV, Khachigian LM. Induction of the transcriptional repressor Yin Yang-1 by vascular cell injury. Autocrine/paracrine role of endogenous fibroblast growth factor-2. J Biol Chem. 2001 Nov 2;276(44]:41143-9.

[96] Xie J, Briggs JA, Briggs RC. Human hematopoietic cell specific nuclear protein MNDA interacts with the multifunctional transcription factor YY1 and stimulates YY1 DNA binding. J Cell Biochem. 1998 Sep 15;70(4]:489-506.

[97] Krippner-Heidenreich A, Walsemann G, Beyrouthy MJ, Speckgens S, Kraft R, Thole H, et al. Caspase-dependent regulation and subcellular redistribution of the transcriptional modulator YY1 during apoptosis. Mol Cell Biol. 2005 May;25(9]:3704-14.

[98] Palko L, Bass HW, Beyrouthy MJ, Hurt MM. The Yin Yang-1 (YY1) protein undergoes a DNA-replication-associated switch in localization from the cytoplasm to the nucleus at the onset of S phase. J Cell Sci. 2004 Jan 26;117(Pt 3]:465-76.

[99] Li Y, Wang F, Xu J, Ye F, Shen Y, Zhou J, et al. Progressive miRNA expression profiles in cervical carcinogenesis and identification of HPV-related target genes for miR-29. J Pathol. 2011 Aug;224(4]:484-95.

[100] Chen QR, Yu LR, Tsang P, Wei JS, Song YK, Cheuk A, et al. Systematic proteome analysis identifies transcription factor YY1 as a direct target of miR-34a. J Proteome Res. 2011 Feb 4;10(2]:479-87.

[101] Kaller M, Liffers ST, Oeljeklaus S, Kuhlmann K, Roh S, Hoffmann R, et al. Genome-wide characterization of miR-34a induced changes in protein and mRNA expression by a combined pulsed SILAC and microarray analysis. Mol Cell Proteomics. 2011 Aug;10(8]:M111 010462.

[102] Nguyen N, Zhang X, Olashaw N, Seto E. Molecular cloning and functional characterization of the transcription factor YY2. J Biol Chem. 2004 Jun 11;279(24]:25927-34.

[103] Kim JD, Faulk C, Kim J. Retroposition and evolution of the DNA-binding motifs of YY1, YY2 and REX1. Nucleic Acids Res. 2007;35(10]:3442-52.

[104] Chen L, Shioda T, Coser KR, Lynch MC, Yang C, Schmidt EV. Genome-wide analysis of YY2 versus YY1 target genes. Nucleic Acids Res. 2010 Jul;38(12]:4011-26.

[105] Zhang Q, Stovall DB, Inoue K, Sui G. The oncogenic role of Yin Yang 1. Crit Rev Oncog. 2011;16(3-4]:163-97.

[106] Lee MY, Lu A, Gudas LJ. Transcriptional regulation of Rex1 (zfp42] in normal prostate epithelial cells and prostate cancer cells. J Cell Physiol. 2010 Jul;224(1]:17-27.

[107] Tang S, Mishra M, Frazier DP, Moore ML, Inoue K, Deora R, et al. Positive and negative regulation of prostate stem cell antigen expression by Yin Yang 1 in prostate epithelial cell lines. PLoS One. 2012;7(4]:e35570.

[108] Schroder F, Crawford ED, Axcrona K, Payne H, Keane TE. Androgen deprivation therapy: past, present and future. BJU Int. 2012 Jun;109 Suppl 6:1-12.

[109] Jung C, Kim RS, Lee SJ, Wang C, Jeng MH. HOXB13 homeodomain protein suppresses the growth of prostate cancer cells by the negative regulation of T-cell factor 4. Cancer Res. 2004 May 1;64(9]:3046-51.

[110] Jung C, Kim RS, Zhang HJ, Lee SJ, Jeng MH. HOXB13 induces growth suppression of prostate cancer cells as a repressor of hormone-activated androgen receptor signaling. Cancer Res. 2004 Dec 15;64(24]:9185-92.

[111] Hongo F, Garban H, Huerta-Yepez S, Vega M, Jazirehi AR, Mizutani Y, et al. Inhibition of the transcription factor Yin Yang 1 activity by S-nitrosation. Biochem Biophys Res Commun. 2005 Oct 21;336(2]:692-701.

[112] Ross JS, Gray KE, Webb IJ, Gray GS, Rolfe M, Schenkein DP, et al. Antibody-based therapeutics: focus on prostate cancer. Cancer Metastasis Rev. 2005 Dec;24(4]:521-37.

[113] Lessard L, Mes-Masson AM, Lamarre L, Wall L, Lattouf JB, Saad F. NF-kappa B nuclear localization and its prognostic significance in prostate cancer. BJU Int. 2003 Mar;91(4]:417-20.

[114] Suh J, Payvandi F, Edelstein LC, Amenta PS, Zong WX, Gelinas C, et al. Mechanisms of constitutive NF-kappaB activation in human prostate cancer cells. Prostate. 2002 Aug 1;52(3]:183-200.

[115] Zhang L, Altuwaijri S, Deng F, Chen L, Lal P, Bhanot UK, et al. NF-kappaB regulates androgen receptor expression and prostate cancer growth. Am J Pathol. 2009 Aug; 175(2]:489-99.

[116] Wang H, Hertlein E, Bakkar N, Sun H, Acharyya S, Wang J, et al. NF-kappaB regulation of YY1 inhibits skeletal myogenesis through transcriptional silencing of myofibrillar genes. Mol Cell Biol. 2007 Jun;27(12]:4374-87.

[117] Huerta-Yepez S, Vega M, Garban H, Bonavida B. Involvement of the TNF-alpha autocrine-paracrine loop, via NF-kappaB and YY1, in the regulation of tumor cell resistance to Fas-induced apoptosis. Clin Immunol. 2006 Sep;120(3]:297-309.

[118] Caggia S, Libra M, Malaponte G, Cardile V. Modulation of YY1 and p53 expression by transforming growth factor-beta3 in prostate cell lines. Cytokine. 2011 Nov;56(2]: 403-10.

[119] Maehama T, Dixon JE. The tumor suppressor, PTEN/MMAC1, dephosphorylates the lipid second messenger, phosphatidylinositol 3,4,5-trisphosphate. J Biol Chem. 1998 May 29;273(22]:13375-8.

[120] Stambolic V, Suzuki A, de la Pompa JL, Brothers GM, Mirtsos C, Sasaki T, et al. Negative regulation of PKB/Akt-dependent cell survival by the tumor suppressor PTEN. Cell. 1998 Oct 2;95(1]:29-39.

[121] Sun H, Lesche R, Li DM, Liliental J, Zhang H, Gao J, et al. PTEN modulates cell cycle progression and cell survival by regulating phosphatidylinositol 3,4,5,-trisphosphate and Akt/protein kinase B signaling pathway. Proc Natl Acad Sci U S A. 1999 May 25;96(11]:6199-204.

[122] Bonavida B, Baritaki S. The novel role of Yin Yang 1 in the regulation of epithelial to mesenchymal transition in cancer via the dysregulated NF-kappaB/Snail/YY1/RKIP/ PTEN Circuitry. Crit Rev Oncog. 2011;16(3-4]:211-26.

[123] Seligson D, Horvath S, Huerta-Yepez S, Hanna S, Garban H, Roberts A, et al. Expression of transcription factor Yin Yang 1 in prostate cancer. Int J Oncol. 2005 Jul;27(1]: 131-41.

[124] Brooks JD, Bova GS, Ewing CM, Piantadosi S, Carter BS, Robinson JC, et al. An uncertain role for p53 gene alterations in human prostate cancers. Cancer Res. 1996 Aug 15;56(16]:3814-22.

[125] Osman I, Drobnjak M, Fazzari M, Ferrara J, Scher HI, Cordon-Cardo C. Inactivation of the p53 pathway in prostate cancer: impact on tumor progression. Clin Cancer Res. 1999 Aug;5(8]:2082-8.

[126] Sinik Z, Alkibay T, Ataoglu O, Biri H, Sozen S, Deniz N, et al. Nuclear p53 overexpression in bladder, prostate, and renal carcinomas. Int J Urol. 1997 Nov;4(6]:546-51.

[127] Berezovska OP, Glinskii AB, Yang Z, Li XM, Hoffman RM, Glinsky GV. Essential role for activation of the Polycomb group (PcG) protein chromatin silencing pathway in metastatic prostate cancer. Cell Cycle. 2006 Aug;5(16]:1886-901.

Chapter 24

The Role of PARP Activation in Prostate Cancer

Luis A. Espinoza

Additional information is available at the end of the chapter

http://dx.doi.org/10.5772/53297

1. Introduction

Prostate cancer is the most commonly diagnosed cancer in men and the second leading cause of cancer related mortality. Localized prostate cancer is treated by either radical prostatectomy or radiotherapy. Low levels of testosterone have been associated with prostate cancer progression. These tumor presented advanced tumor stage, high Gleason scores, and had significantly worse overall survival rate [1, 2]. Indeed, intraprostatic dihydrotestosterone (DHT) were consistently reduced in patients with high-grade (Gleason scores of 7 to 10) compared to patients diagnosed with low grade tumors (Gleason scores of 6 or less) [3]. Prostate cancer usually is treated using chemotherapy, radiotherapy, or surgery. For advanced prostate cancer, hormonal therapy is currently used as the standard treatment, however; these tumors develop and aggressive phenotype and become hormone–independent (hormone-refractory) (HRPC) that is resistant to chemotherapy or radiotherapy and metastasizes to lymph nodes and bone [4].

Although prostate cancer is the most common cancer in Caucasians, the risk factors associated with increased prostate cancer incidences include mainly in those individuals with sub-Saharan African ancestry, with African-American men having the highest reported incidence rates of all ethnic groups in the United States (239.8 cases/100,000) [5, 6]. Furthermore, mortality from prostate cancer following surgery is nearly two-fold higher in African-American men (56.3/100,000) succumbing to the disease compared to white men (23.9/100,000) [7-9]. Little is currently know whether the type of factors (biological, diet, racial, or lifestyle) that may play a influence role in the increased prostate cancer incidence in this population. The high mortality in death from prostate cancer is generally due to metastatic disease that results from resistance to the treatments described above. Since rates of prostate cancer in the U.S. are 60 percent higher among African-American men, and their mortality rate are two-and-a-half times that of Caucasian men [10, 11], identifying the mechanisms that support indolent against aggressive disease is an important area of research.

Prostate cancer cells that survive chemotherapy or radiation treatment clearly indicate that may be able to repair most of the radiation-induced DNA breaks. Indeed, different prostate cancer cell lines have shown a very efficient DNA repair system in which DNA damage can be removed [4, 12]. Also, there is the possibility that genetic instability occurring in those cancer cells with unrepaired or misrepaired DNA damage might increase prostate cancer aggressiveness. In this regard, there is an increasing interest in the utilization of PARP inhibitors as a strategy for improving cancer therapy [13]. PARP is a nuclear enzyme that plays active roles in DNA repair, DNA replication, and cell death, in response to diverse forms of stimuli from normal metabolic processes, as well as environmental factors [14, 15]. This enzyme binds nonspecifically to DNA breaks and catalyzes the poly(ADP-ribosyl)ation of various nuclear proteins utilizing NAD^+ as a substrate, leading to chromatin decondensation that allows the repair process for DNA damage.

Overexpression of PAPR1 has been described in a variety of tumor cell lines, which was associated with malignant progression [16]. PARP-1 high levels has also been found in malignant lymphoma cells compared to normal lymph nodes [16], adjacent non-tumor tissues, or hyperplastic polyps [17]. High levels of PARP-1 also showed high correlation with poor prognosis in early breast cancer. In this type of cancer, PARP-1 was indicated to be the major component of tumor cells response to DNA damage and a key player in maintaining their genetic stability. Augmented expression of PARP-1 was also observed in moderate differentiate hepatocellular carcinomas (HCC) [18]. In addition, poly(ADP-ribosyl)ation was consistently increased in HCC [19], colon carcinomas [20], cervical cancer [21], and melanoma and basal cell carcinoma [22]. More recent findings have found that overexpression of PARP-1 appear to be related with prostate cancer progression, and also considered as a potential independent predictor of aggressiveness among the clinicopathological features related to this type of tumor [23].

Prostate tumors that initially respond to standard chemotherapy often recur; with selective outgrowth of tumor cell subpopulations that are resistant not only to the original chemotherapeutic agent, but also to other therapeutics. Therefore, the promising results of PARP inhibitors in treating advanced states of prostate cancer provide new avenues for effective treatment of this deadly disease. This chapter focuses on PARP-1 as a potential target to improve the breadth and effectiveness of prostate cancer treatment.

2. The biological roles of PARP-1

PARP-1 is a nuclear protein that catalyzes the covalent long chain poly(ADP-ribosyl)ation of a variety of nuclear proteins utilizing β-nicotinamide adenine dinucleotide (NAD^+) as a substrate, with PARP-1 itself being the major target of modifications [24, 25]. Moreover, many other nuclear DNA binding proteins are also modified. PARP-1 is only activated when bound to single- or double-stranded DNA ends via its two zinc fingers, which recognize DNA breaks independent of the DNA sequence [14, 15, 25] (Table 1). The active protein catalyzes a sequential transfer reaction of ADP-ribose units from NAD^+ to various nuclear proteins, forming a protein-bound polymer of ADP-ribose units [24].

Agents that activatePARP-1	Events inducing DNA breaks
Alkilating agents	Aging
Apoptosis inducers	Chromosomal alterations
Asbestos	Differentiation
Hydrogen peroxide (H_2O_2)	Gene expression
Ionizing radiation	Genetic instability
Oxidising agents	DNA replication
Nitrosative stress	Inflammation
Topoisomerase inhibitors	Necrosis
	Programming cell death

Table 1. List of events that promote DNA breaks and PARP-1 activation

Since PARP-1 activation is strictly proportional to the number of DNA breaks, its activity is strictly proportional to the number of DNA breaks *in vivo* or *in vitro*, and it is particularly inactive in the absence of DNA breaks [15, 25, 26]. DNA damage can occur during DNA replication or as consequence of exposure of cells to different types of genotoxic agents (Table 1). One of the earliest cellular events that follow this phenomenon is the poly(ADP-ribosyl)ation of PARP-1 and an array of DNA binding proteins that are localized predominantly adjacent to the DNA strand breaks, resulting in polymers adjacent to DNA breaks and in the recruitment of additional proteins that are essential in BER/SSBR [27, 28].The covalent poly(ADP-ribosyl)ation of nuclear DNA-binding proteins in eukaryotes is a phenomena that contributes to various physiologic and pathophysiologic events associated with DNA strand breakage, repair of DNA damage, and apoptosis [15, 29-32]. Detailed studies have demonstrated that in addition to its accessory role in DNA repair, PARP-1 also plays regulatory roles in other nuclear processes, including DNA replication and the regulation of transcription, as a longevity assurance factor associated with genome stability, and in redox signaling [26] (Table 2). In addition, the post-translational modifications reaction in which poly(ADP-ribosyl)ation is involved during post-translational reactions is mainly related to the modulation of chromatin and function in DNA-damaged and apoptotic cells [32, 33]. The nuclear protein substrates of PARP-1 include histones, DNA topoisomerases I and II [34, 35], SV40 large T antigen [36], DNA polymerases α and δ, proliferating cell nuclear antigen (PCNA), and several proteins that are components of the DNA synthesome [35].

The interaction of PARP-1 with components of the base excision repair (BER) complex such as DNA ligase III, DNA pol β, and XRCC1 [37-40], suggested that PARP-1 may have protective function in the BER repair process. PARP-1 has also been shown to interact with a number of transcription factors (Table 3), including AP-2 [41], CXC ligand [41], E2F-1 [32], NF-κB [42], MYB [43], Oct-1 [44], PC3/topoisomerase-I [45], SP-1, TEF-1 [46], and YY1 [47]. Although ADP-ribosylation has been indicated as the main mechanism by which PARP-1 modulates most of these transcription factors, consistent reports in which PARP-1 inhibitors and the downstream effects of NF-κB pathways were analyzed [48] have argued against the requirement of PARP-1 as a critical co-activator of NF-κB [49, 50].

Roles of PARP in cellular and molecular processes
Control of cell cycle
Cell differentiation
Cell death
Chromatin architecture
DNA repair
Redox signaling
Transcription
Transformation

Table 2. List of the roles PARP-1 plays in molecular and cellular processes.

The dual roles of PARP-1 in different nuclear processes are based in on the levels of the substrate NAD^+ and the presence of PARP-activating DNA breaks. Indeed, physical interaction of PARP-1 with DNA polymerase α occurs in the absence of NAD^+ activates polymerase α [51], while addition of NAD^+ to the DNA replication complex inhibits polymerase α catalytic activity [52]. Although in the absence of NAD^+, PARP-1 interacts with different transcription factors to enhance activator-dependent transcription, the presence of NAD^+ and consequent PARP-1 activation represses transcription, presumably by poly(ADP-ribosyl)ation of a series of transcription factors [53]. Thus for example, in the absence of NAD, PARP-1 enhances activator-dependent transcription by interacting with RNA polymerase II-associated factors [53], binds to the transcription enhancer factor 1 (TEF1) and enhances muscle-specific gene transcription [46], and transcription factor AP-2 to co-activate AP-2-mediated transcription [41]. Meanwhile, PARP-1 depletion silences the activation of a number of transcription factors, preventing the formation of active transcription complexes and binding to their respective DNA consensus sequences [54].

In most of the cases, the poly(ADP-ribosyl)ation modification of proteins inhibits their affinity for DNA-binding as a result of the electrostatic repulsion between the negatively charged DNA and long chain of approximately 200 units of poly(ADP-ribose) (PAR) [24, 25]. Although unmodified PARP-1 binds tightly to DNA ends, interfering with the repair machinery, the prolonged poly(ADP-ribosyl)ation automodification of PARP-1 itself is essential to modulate its binding to DNA ends during the repair process [55, 56]. The decrease in DNA-binding affinity caused by electrostatic repulsion between DNA and poly(ADP-ribose) (PAR) as a result of the pos-translational modification may explain the reduction on the catalytic activity of some DNA-binding proteins [57, 58]. Modification of other nuclear proteins such as nucleosomal proteins may also allow the access of various replicative and repair enzymes that bind specifically to those regions of the DNA containing strand breaks [59, 60].

http://dx.doi.org/10.5772/53297

Function	Acceptor proteins
Cell cycle regulation	p53
	PCNA
Chromatin structure	Histone
	HGM
	Lamins
	LMG proteins
DNA metabolism	DNA polymerase α
	DNA polymerase β
	DNAS1L3
	Endonuclease
	PARP-1
	Poly(ADP-ribose) synthetase
	Topoisomerase I
	Topoisomerase II
	XRCC1
Others	Tankyrase-1
	Telomeric repeat binding factor-1

Table 3. List of acceptor proteins for poly(DP-ribose).

The elevated levels of sister chromatid exchanges (SCE) found in PARP-1 knockout mice have been associated with increased genomic instability [61, 62]. Similar events have been reported in splenocytes and fibroblasts isolated from PARP-1$^{-/-}$ animals, which also exhibited signaling abnormalities, apoptosis, proliferation, and defects in DNA repair [62, 63]. Accordingly, animals carrying deletion of the exon 1 [64], exon 2 [61], and exon 4 [62], neither evidenced PARP-1 protein nor exhibited signals of poly(ADP-ribosyl)ation. It was also described that thymocytes derived from PARP-1 knockout mice showed a delayed recovery after exposure to gamma-radiation [61]. Also, PARP-1 inhibition/deletion does not alter key cellular events such as apoptosis, DNA replication, and differentiation in cells derived from these mice; however, some evidence has indicated that PARP-1 has supportive roles in all these processes. Indeed, derived PARP-1 deficient cells showed pronounced effects on some of these events that are not observed in wild type cells [65, 66].

3. Involvement of PARP-1 in prostate cancer progression

Localized prostate tumors are treated by either radical prostatectomy or radiotherapy and usually survive many years [67]. For aggressive prostate cancer, hormonal therapy is the standard treatment however; a significant amount (approximately 30%) of these tumors become hormone–independent (hormone-refractory) [11]. Prostate cancer cells that survive chemotherapy or radiation treatment may be capable to repair most radiation-induced DNA breaks. This is supported by evidence showing both in androgen dependent and independent prostate cancer cell lines in which the EGFR-ERK signaling pathway up-regulates a series of DNA repair proteins, including ERCC1, XPC, and XRCC1, in response to DNA damage [68]. These proteins efficiently repaired the damaged DNA, and enhanced the survival of cells following exposure to genotoxics [68, 69]. The activation of PARP-1 in the presence of DNA breaks consistently promotes the recruitment of XRCC1 and the physical interaction of XRCC1 with PARP-1 has been indicated as an efficient process to repair DNA breaks in a coordinated manner [39]. However, it needs to be taken into account that genetic instability may occur in those cells with unrepaired or misrepaired DNA damage. In this respect, the LNCaP prostate cancer cell line, an androgen-responsive is a good model because undergoes growth arrest, but not apoptosis after androgen deprivation, and it is also highly resistant to radiation-induced cell death [70, 71].

Given that activation of PARP-1 is absolutely dependent on DNA strand breaks [15, 26], the substantial poly(ADP-ribosyl)ation modification of PARP-1 detected during early apoptosis in LNCaP cells was consistent with the DNA damage induced by Phenoxodiol, a synthetic analogue of Genistein [72]. Although the level of PARP-1 activation and its subsequent cleavage in LNCaP cells after Phenoxodiol exposure was exhibited in a time dependent manner, the poly(ADP-ribosyl)ation automodification of PARP-1 activation during the early stages of Phenoxodiol-induced apoptosis may thus be required for progression through the death program [72]. In this respect, subsequent cleavage of PARP-1 may have prevented the depletion of NAD^+ and ATP, which are needed for later steps in apoptosis [73]. However, the possibility that inhibition of the topoisomerase II activity may have caused DNA damage in cells exposed to Phenoxodiol, a well-known topoisomerase II poison, was not excluded [74]. As a matter of fact, activation of PARP-1 has also been detected in apoptotic cells exposed to different antineoplastic agents, such as adriamycin, alkylating agents, cisplatin, mitomycin C, radiation, and topoisomerase inhibitors [75].

A combined treatment of isoflavones and curcumin had a potent inhibitory effect on cellular proliferation of LNCaP cells [76]. The effects associated with this treatment were the enhanced phosphorylation of some nuclear proteins, such as ATM and Chk2 when compared to the effects of cells treated with curcumin alone. Similar effects were observed in the histone H2AX and p53. Interesting, curcumin also inhibited the proliferative effects of the dihydrotestosterone (DHT), a stimulator of prostate growth [3]. The augmented levels of testosterone consistently induced activation of the DNA damage response (DDR) pathways in response to curcumin treatment by promoting the phosphorylation of CHK, H2AX and p53. This approach also induced the proteolytic cleavage of PARP-1, suggesting that activation of the DDR by polyphenols might have a suppress effect on malignant transformation, while a combined therapy of testosterone and curcumin may enhances apoptosis by promoting the release of pro-apoptotic factors, restricting thus prostate cancer progression.

To determine the signaling pathways that are induced by radiation-induced PARP-1 activation, two prostate cancer cell lines LNCaP and DU145, which express different levels of EGFR, were exposed to ionizing radiation and EGF [77]. Although the radiosensitivity was much more evident in LNCaP cells, the radiation treatment consistently reduced the clonogenic survival in both cell lines. The addition of EFG or PD184352, a MEK 1/2 inhibitor, had any significant impact on the killing of the cancer prostate cells. In contrast, PJ34, a potent inhibitor of PARP-1 [78], caused a growth arrest and markedly reduced cell death in both cell lines [77]. In support of these data, poly ADP-ribosylation of PARP-1 was also evident in LNCaP and DU145 cells after irradiation or exposure to EGF. These results are supported by findings linking EGF expression to human prostate cancer development [79, 80], the high levels of EGF secreted by LNCaP and DU145 cell lines [81, 82], as well as the enhanced invasive capacity that EGF exert on another human prostate cancer cell line (PC-3) [83]. Although the reduction of cell death was evident in cells exposed to PJ34 and EGF; however, an opposite effect was observed when PD184352 or the inhibitor of EGF receptor kinase, AG1478, alone was added to the cultures. When the same experimental approaches were applied to PARP-1-depleted cells, expression of poly ADP-ribose production was practically eliminated [78]. This study indicated that PARP-1 activation in both cell lines is linked to the EGF-ERK signaling pathway, which may be critical for the poly ADP-ribosylation and regulation of NAD^+ content following irradiation, and may also be critical for cell survival after treatment for prostate cancer.

Similar apoptotic effects including, annexin-V binding and TUNEL staining, loss of mitochondrial membrane potential the release of cytochrome c, activation of caspase-3, and increase of PARP-1 cleavage were observed in PC-3 cells treated with b-caryophyllene oxide (CPO), wortmannin, and the AKT inhibitor IV [84]. Downregulation of several proteins that are part of the PI3K/AKT/mTOR/S6K1 signaling cascade and ROS-mediate MAPKs activation were also identified, which strongly suggested that multiple cascades are involved in cell survival and proliferation of prostate cancer cells. Accordingly, LNCaP cells exposed to isochaihulactone, a lignin with proved antitumor activity *in vitro* and *in vivo* models [85], evidenced the involvement of the JNK pathway as a potential target for the activation of proteases that are crucial in the induction of caspase-3 activation and PARP-1 cleavage, hallmarks of apoptosis cell death.

4. The relationship between the expression of PARP-1 and p53 in prostate cancer

It is well known that the tumor suppressor gene p53 is a key player in controlling the genetic stability in breast tumor cells [86]. More recently, it was reported that inhibition of PARP-1 by veliparib enhances DNA damage in BRCA-proficient cancer cells, a process that appears to be regulated by p53. Although a diverse response was observed in p53-mutant or –null cells, the veliparib and topotecan combination enhanced DNA damage response and cell death in these type of cells [87]. Similarly, treatment of LNCaP cells to a new ligan isochaihulactone, a proved inhibitor of cell proliferation and effective inducer of apoptosis in a variety of cancer cell lines, enhanced PARP-1 cleavage and increased levels of p53 in those cells that become irreversible committed to cell death [88].

Considering that PARP-1 is thought to be an important modulator of p53 [89], either by covalent modification or by non-covalent binding of poly(ADP-ribose) on specific domains of p53, which alter its DNA binding functions [47], the binding of p53 to DNA damage promotes activation of downstream signal cascades, leading to cell cycle arrest and apoptosis. A recent report have demonstrated the efficacy of a novel CDK1, CDK2 inhibitor, dansylated VMY-1-103, in inhibiting Erb-2/Erb-3/heregulin-induced cell proliferation in LNCaP cells. Apoptosis via decreased mitochondrial membrane polarity, induction of p53 phosphorylation, caspase-3 activation, and PARP-1 cleavage in these prostatic tumor cells, were also among the most relevant findings [90]. The stability of p53 as evidenced by an increase of p53 content is crucial for blocking cell cycle progression or for initiating cell death apoptosis in response to DNA damage [91, 92]. However, it cannot be excluded that other DNA repair proteins can also bind simultaneously to the damaged site and may activate alternative signaling pathways in response to genotoxic insults. The determinant of which of these mechanisms is chosen can be dependent on the magnitude of damage to the DNA.

Although p53 and PARP-1 are both damage sensor proteins and can be functionally activated by DNA damage [92, 93], evidence indicated that PARP-1 is not essential for p53 accumulation induced by DNA damage. However, PARP-1 appear to be required for the appropriate response of p53 to DNA damage [89], including its rapid and enhanced protein expression [91]. In this respect, immunoblotting analysis with antibodies against p53 were able to detect p53 protein in lysates of PARP-1 wild-type cells, but not in PARP-1 deficient cell extracts, which suggested that the reduced protein stability of p53 in cells lacking PARP-1 [94]. The functional interaction between p53 and PARP-1 in response to radiation was also reported in a human glioblastoma cell line A-17 treated with 3-aminobenzamide (3-AB), a well-known PARP-1 inhibitor. The absence of PARP-1 activity by 3-AB dramatically reduced the radiation-induced expression of the p53 downstream, the p21 gene product. In support to this observation, the gel shift analysis evidenced that 3-AB significantly inhibited the irradiation-activated p53-binding activity to its consensus sequences [95]. Similar results were observed in a (1-methyl-4-phenyl-1,2,3,6-tetrahydropyridine) (MPTP)-induced parkinsonism model in which a heavy poly(ADP-ribosyla)tion modification of p53 reduced the DNA-binding activity of p53 to its consensus sequences [96].

Although the specific findings above described clearly proof that PARP-1 expression is implicated in p53 accumulation and stabilization, this effect is different to that observed in PARP-1 knock out cells exposed to N-methyl-N-nitroso urea (MNU), an alkylating agent, in which p53 is accumulated and its activation is consistently enhanced [97]. The findings in this model suggest that PARP-1 regulating p53-mediated response to genotoxic agents is probably dependent on the type of DNA damage. Accordingly the level of MDM-2 transcript, an important negative regulator of the p53, was not increased after gamma-irradiation; however, an increased in the expression of MDM-2 protein was observed in PARP-1 null cells. The increased levels of MDM-2 may provide an alternative explanation for the reduced accumulation and activation of p53 in PARP-1 null cells. Furthermore, the reduced phosphorylation of p53 may also be indicative of a defective activation of the kinases pathways in these cells [97].

Other studies have demonstrated that PARP-1 is dispensable for the repair of DNA double-strand breaks induced by alkylating agents, UV, and gamma-radiation. In this respect, it was proposed the existence of an alternative radiation-induced pathway involving p53 that may function independently of PARP-1 involvement. Although this alternative mechanism may explain the cytotoxic response detected in PARP-1 *null* cells after radiation treatment [61, 98], this does not necessarily support the significant delay in the transient accumulation of p53 in PARP-1-depleted intestinal epithelial stem cells after exposure to irradiation. Similarly, the survival analysis was markedly reduced in crypts of PARP-1 knockout mice, even at radiation doses that have sublethal effects on wild type animals [65]. These observations extended the crucial role of PARP-1 to stem cells survival after DNA damage *in vivo*. Indeed, considering the prolonged regenerative capacity of prostate progenitor stem cells may increase their susceptibility to accumulate genetic or epigenetic alterations during their life cycle, the events may be able to increased proliferative rates, decreased cell death, and overall survival advantages over prostate progenitor stem cells, contributing thus to transformation [6, 99-104]. Along with these studies, PARP-1 inhibition may be a critical component in the treatment of some types of cancer. Additionally, other components of the cell cycle checkpoints such p53 also need to be considered in order to develop an appropriate therapy strategy to avoid relapse.

5. The prostate cancer microenvironment

The morphology of a tumor may also influence in the biological responses of cancer cells to a specific therapy. Although most of the reports in cancer therapy utilize monolayer cultures, multicellular aggregates (spheres) are probably more important because reflects the three-dimensional structure for a real-time *model* representing a tumor, allowing to study the interaction of tumor cells with the microenvironment [105]. The fact that spheroids mimic the tumor microenvironment is also an important tool that may provide more accurate information about the biological and biochemical events occurring in solid tumors [106]. Therefore, the utilization of the spheres assay is an important approach for the in serial in vivo transplantation to verify self-renewal potential.

Although, sphere cells are generated, serially passaged, and maintained in undifferentiated phenotype under appropriate cell culture conditions, they need to be inoculated into animal models to confirm their ability to generate tumor growth [107, 108]. Indeed, substantial differences has been reported in the gene expression signatures on PC3 holoclones compared to parental PC3 cells, which appeared to be consequence of the distinct culture conditions used to growth each cell population [109]. Consistent with these observations, growing conditions also affected the expression of several genes in LNCaP cells [106]. A number of other variables such as the manner in which cells are isolated and the *in vitro* propagation of these cells before transplantation can cause tumor cells to become more aggressive as a result of new acquired mutations, which may affect the outcome of *in vivo* assays. Another critical parameters are to determine the variation on experimental conditions that may influence frequency estimates and to ensure the best animal model available in order to reproduce the tumor biology as it occurs in humans. For example, the limiting dilution data might be dramatically affected by the duration of data analysis [110] or by modification of xenotransplantation assay in non-obese diabetic severe combined immunodeficient (NOD/SCID) mice [111]. Therefore, a main concern for the application of this methodology is that sometimes, the animal models overstate the biology of cancer formation in humans.

Most of human prostate tumor cells have the ability to form spheres; however, the frequency of cells forming spheres is very heterogeneous across all cell lines. In this regard, the adaptation of tumor cells to non-adherent culture conditions may be a determinant in forming spheres [112]. Also, the holoclone-forming cells, which are smaller than paraclone cells, more adherent, highly clonogenic, and whose progeny forms almost exclusively growing colonies, in prostate cancer specimens with the highest clonogenic potential has been associated with stem cell phenotypes [113]. Of great importance is the fact that large holoclones were also consistently present in prostate cancer cell spheres [109, 114], suggesting that these spheres, which are sustained by tumor initiating cells with stem cell-like features, may have a strong self-renewal and pro-angiogenic capability [115]. These spheres were capable of forming new generations of spheres and retained proliferative capacity as well as clonogenic potential after serial passages [116]. These reports were supported by studies in which a minor subpopulation of spheres propagating cells with stem cell-like properties isolated from a series of prostate cancer models were capable of forming spheres, display significant increase in proliferation potential, initiate xenograft tumors with enhanced capacity, and were more drug resistant compared to monolayer cells [109, 117]. Accordingly, the expression of putative cancer stem cell markers such as ALDH1A1, CD44, CD133, showed strong correlation with prostate tumor progression and metastasis [92, 118, 119], while Nanog induction promoted castration-resistant tumor phenotype and tumor regeneration in the LNCaP cells [120].

There is no doubt that the microenvironment definitely affects the expression of multiples genes that may be more evident in spheroids in which the tumor cell interaction with the extracellular matrix may influence responses to prostate cancer treatment. Thus, the three-dimensional system should be included in pre-clinical experimental models to identify in prostate tumors the mechanisms that are related with tumor progression, and those that confer resistant to cancer therapies.

6. Treating prostate cancer

Despite recent therapeutic approaches that have significantly increased survival, most prostate aggressive tumors become resistant to current treatment protocols [8, 121]. Prostate cancers that initially respond to standard chemotherapy often recur with selective outgrowth of tumor cell subpopulations that are resistant not only to the original chemotherapeutic agents, but also to other therapeutics [122]. Several events are thought to be involved in the dysregulation of pathways, which may activate a different pathway(s) for androgen independence probably through a paracrine androgen-independent pathway, which may explain the multifocality and heterogeneity of prostate cancer and for hormone therapy resistance. Indeed, in a xenograft model, most of androgen-responsive genes that were initially downregulated under conditions of androgen deprivation were later re-expressed in recurrence tumors, indicating failure of androgen-derivation therapy as well as irreversible commitment to tumor progression [123].

The array of genes that comprise the proliferation status may differ in different type of tumors. Evidence has demonstrated that the cell cycle regulation is frequently altered in prostate cancers, in part, by the interplay of oncogenic cascades activation with diverse hormones, growth factors, and cytokines. Moreover, the accumulation of mutations in prostate cancer cells may eventually lead to a more poorly differentiated and aggressive tumor behavior, leading to overall higher rates of progression and worse prognosis, irrespective of the size of the lesion [124-127]. Multiple cellular signaling pathways including, protein kinase B (Akt), mitogen-activated protein kinase (MAPK), the nuclear factor kappa B (NF-κB), transforming growth factor beta (TGF-β), the vascular endothelial growth factor (VEGF), and the Wnt have been shown to enhance androgen receptor signaling and promote development of hormone-independent/castration-resistance in preclinical models [128, 129]. Moreover, the increased expression of the androgen receptor transcript was critical for tumor cells resistance to anti-androgen therapy [75]. In this regard, inhibitors of cell cycle regulatory proteins has become an area of increased interest in targeting both cancer cells per se and a subpopulation of stem cell-like that initiates and maintains tumor growth, metastasis, and resistance to therapy [130].

Recently, we have demonstrated that Phenoxodiol induces DNA damage in different types of prostate cancer cell lines (DU145, LNCaP, and PC3), leading to the activation and cleavage of PARP-1 as well as the onset of the cell death program [72]. Interesting, the expression of PARP-1 is highly expressed in LNCaP cells before and after treatment with H_2O_2 [131]. Also accompanying Phenoxodiol-induced cell death we observed a reduction in the availability of NAD^+, which potentially compromises ATP production via glycolysis [132]. A major component of the injury is the alteration of membrane permeability caused by decreased activity of ATP-dependent ionic pumps [133]. Massive NAD^+ depletion is lethal in cells that divide rapidly and have a high-energy requirement. Since the three prostate cancer cell lines, LNCaP, PC3, and DU145 have high metastatic potential and are very resistance to several antitumoral drugs and radiation-induced apoptosis, the fact that this synthetic analogue of Genistein induces death in this tumor type, strongly suggested that this synthetic drug may be a useful treatment for metastatic prostate tumors [72]. A recent study has reported that decreased PSA production and the expression of the androgen receptor in LNCaP cells were observed following a combined treatment with curcumin and isoflavones. Similarly, modulation of PSA levels was observed in a cohort of patients that received prostate biopsies [134]. Finally, cannabidol and the synthetic cannabinoid WIN-55,212 were also determinant in inhibit proliferation and cleavage of PARP-1, caspase-3, as well as activation of phosphatases, and pro-apoptotic phosphatase on LNCaP cells. These compounds also exhibited antitumorigenic activity against different types of tumors and are now being tested in clinical trials for the treatment of brain tumors [135, 136]. The modulation of specific phosphatases in the LNCaP cell line suggested the potential antitumorigenic activity of cannabinoids against the treatment of prostate cancers [137].

7. Treating prostate cancer with PARP-1 inhibitors

Recently, the augmented immunodetection of PARP-1 was associated with prostate cancer progression and prediction of biochemical recurrence [138]. Preclinical data also indicated that PARP inhibitors might sensitize cancer cells and potentiate the effects of radiotherapy and chemotherapy. Interesting, inhibition or depletion of PARP-1 by antisense RNA [139], chemical inhibitors [140-142], or by the expression of dominant negative mutants (4-5), promotes genomic instability [143], as revealed by increased DNA strand breakage, gene amplification, micronuclei formation, and sister chromatide exchanges (SCE) in cells exposed to genotoxic agents. Marked SCE frequency has been observed in PARP-1 deficient cell lines and treated with different inhibitors against PARP-1 activity [144]. Depletion of PARP-1 was indicated as the main contribution to genomic alterations that may promote aberrant expression of cell proliferative genes, which may initiate cancer formation or progression. These observations implicate PARP-1 as a guardian of the genome, facilitating DNA repair and protection against DNA recombination by DNA lesion recognition [144] Accordingly, nuclear PARP-1 protein overexpression was associated with poor overall survival in early breast cancer [145]. PARP inhibitors have also been implicated in the modulation of the mechanisms driving apoptotic cell death [146]. Therefore, evidence correlating increased PARP-1 activity with tumor progression has opened a new avenue for the utilization of PARP inhibitors, which may impair the DNA repair machine. These effects may increase sensitivity of prostate tumor cells to DNA damaging agents by improving the efficiency of cancer therapeutics.

An early innovative therapy to treat prostate cancer cells was to enforce the binding of DNA strand breaks to a dominant-negative mutant of the DNA-binding domain of PARP. The recombinant plasmid inhibited the function of PARP-1 and sensitized prostate tumor cells to the lethal effects of ionizing radiation or etoposide (VP-16), with a markedly reduction of cell survival and induction of apoptosis [12]. The pharmacological inhibition of PARP-1 by benzamide pharmacaphores mimics the nicotinamide moiety of NAD^+, occupying the donor site [147]. For example, the 3-aminobenzamide (3-AB) was shown to inhibit DNA excision repair and radiosensitize cells to ionizing radiation through impaired DNA repair [148, 149]. 3-AB is also know to inhibit the family of mono(ADP-ribose) transferases, which can produce non-specific effects independent of PARP-1 inhibition (Milam, 1984). Therefore, more potent and highly specific PARP inhibitors that promote oxid radiation sensitizer enhancement ratios have been developed. These new specific compounds (Table 4) are dependent of the cell line and inhibitor tested [150]. Thus, for example ABT-888 (veliparib) inhibited recombinant and intracellular PARP-1 activity and was also toxic to both oxic and hypoxic cells. This PARP inhibitor radiosensitize the human prostate carcinoma cell lines DU145 and 22RV1, as evidenced by the reduced clonogenic survival followed by ionizing radiation exposure (Stanley, 2008). Further support for the utilization of ABT-888 in combination therapy comes from studies showing that ABT-888 enhanced the effects of ionizing radiation in DU145 and PC-3 cells [151]. Interestingly, only PC-3 cells undergo enlarged flat morphology and positive staining for SA-β-Gal, and significant overexpression of p21, hallmarks of cell senescence. These findings were confirmed using PC-3 tumor xenografts in which tumor growth was delayed and presented a senescent phenotype. These results appear to indicate that combined ionizing radiation and PARP inhibition may improve therapeutic response in specific types of prostate cancer.

Function	Acceptor proteins
ABT888 (Veliparib)	Enhances cell death and tumor growth delay in irradiated cancer models
5-AIQ hydrochloride	Decreases expression of inflammatory mediators activated by neutrophils
3-Methil-5-AIQ hydrochloride l	Therapeutic benefits on myocardial infarction, ischaemia-reperfusion of the liver and kidney, heart transplantation, and acute lung inflammation
3-Aminobenzamide	Potentiate anticancer therapy
4-Amino-1,8-naphthalimide	Radiation sensitizer
Benzamide	Neuroprotectant
3-(4-Chlorophenyl)quinoxaline-5-carboxamide	Ameliorates methamphetamine-induced dopaminergic neurotoxicity
(3,4-dihydro-5-[4-(1-piperidinyl)butoxyl]-1(2H)-isoquinolinone DPQ	Reduces pre-neoplastic foci, expression of pre-neoplastic markers, and pro-inflammatory genes in hepatocarcinomas
DR2313	Neuroprotectan
EB-47.dihydrochloride.dihydrate	Antioxidant
4-Hydroxyquinazoline	Antioxidant
5-Iodo-6-amino-1,2-benzopyrone	Neuroprotectan
1,5-Isoquinolinediol	Reduces repair of DNA damaged
Minocycline hydrocloride	Anti-inflammatory and neuroprotectan
Nicotinamide	Chemo- and radio-sensitizer
NU1025	Neuroprotectant
6(5*H*)-Phenanthridinone	Immunosuppressant
PJ-34 [*N*-(6-oxo-5,6-dihydrophenanthridin-2-yl)-*N*, *N*-dimethylacetamide.HCl]	Anti-inflammatory
TIQ-A	Neuroprotectant

Table 4. A panel of PARP inhibitors

The clinical experiences with PARP inhibitors are now focus on patients carrying mutations of the BRCA1 or BRCA2 genes, which have been linked to increased sensitivity to PARP-1 inhibitors. For example Olaparib has proved to be very efficient in patients with breast or ovarian cancer with germline mutations in these two genes [152-154]. Although mutations on BCRA2 mutations have a major impact on breast cancer growth, males carrying alteration on this gene also have a high risk of develop prostate cancer [153, 155]. Additional evidence has shown that impaired DNA repair might benefit from treatment with PARP inhibitors. In deed several evidences have proved that PARP inhibitors sensitize human prostate cancer cell lines [148, 149, 156]. It is also know that treatment with high doses of chemotherapy induces massive DNA damage leading to PARP-1 overactivation with the subsequent energy depletion and cell death of tumor cells that are highly resistant [157]. More recently, it was described that PARP-1 mediates the oncogenic EST transcription factor ERG, which is frequently observed in fusion to the androgen-regulated gene TMPRSS2 in a significant amount of prostate tumors [158]. PARP-1 inhibition (treatment with Olaparib) in this group of tumors increases expression of the ETS gene, which promotes accumulation of DNA damage. This study also demonstrated that ERG physically interacts with PARP-1 and DNA-PKCsPARP-1 and that PARP-1 has a critical role on ERG-mediated transition from high-grade prostatic intraepithelial neoplasia to invasive carcinoma [159]. These findings clearly showed that PARP-1 inhibition could potentially increase survival of patients with tumors ETS-positive. Interesting, Olaparib remained ineffective on tumors that did not show the gene fusion. Altogether this evidence support the enormous interest in stimulate the utilization of a new generation of relatively non-toxic, orally administered PARP inhibitors in a series of cancer in clinical trials to induce genomic instability and cell death, blocking the grow and spread of cancer cells. The fact that PARP inhibition is specific against prostate cancer cells is an exciting and promising therapy approach, in part, because they may cause less severe effects than traditional therapies or radiotherapy.

8. Conclusion

This review has highlighted the therapeutic potential of PARP inhibitors in prostate cancer as a monotherapy or in combination with another type therapy. PARP-1 is implicated in stabilizing the genomic content as well as in the selection of cells with unrepaired DNA damaged. A large body of evidence has demonstrated that inhibition of PARP-1 was sufficient to promote the development of tetraploidy in normal cells and effectively enhanced DNA damage in response to genotoxic agents. These results proved that the physical disruption of PARP-1 is essential for the maintenance of genomic instability. The increased expression of PARP-1 in a series of tumors has been related with cell proliferation and determination of the biological behavior of tumors, events that may predict the overall prognosis of the cancer. In this regard, studies on prostate cancer models in vitro and in vivo have shown that PARP inhibitions regulated the growth of tumors or prevented tumor invasion to other organs. Although several studies have provided promising results in treating advanced tumors, few clinical trials are available in prostate cancer, one of the most prevalent cancers affecting men. Indeed, PARP inhibitors are currently tested in breast cancer patients with mutations in the BRCA1 and BRCA2, which are also mutated in a significant number of prostate cancers. Since advanced prostate cancer generally develops resistance to chemotherapeutic and hormone therapies, the identification of mechanisms underlying prostate cancer progression is vital to identify potential targets for prostate cancer therapy. Recent findings have demonstrated that BRCA1 and BRCA2 mutations confer sensitivity to PARP inhibitors, promoting genomic instability and cell death, and that tumors with BRCA1 mutated are potential targets for a new generation of non-toxic PARP inhibitors. Moreover, the mechanism by which PARP-1 inhibition and BRCA mutations allow the accumulation of DNA errors and the promotion of tumor growth in prostate cells may provide the basis to develop more effective strategies for therapeutic intervention. However, the identification of new genetic markers are necessary to define the feasibility of PARP-1 as a therapeutically target for the treatment of patients with prostate cancer.

Author details

Luis A. Espinoza

Department of Biochemistry and Molecular & Cell Biology, Georgetown University, Washington, DC, USA

References

[1] Morgentaler A 2006. Testosterone and prostate cancer: an historical perspective on a modern myth. Eur Urol 2006; 50(5): 935-9.

[2] Morgentaler A, Bruning CO, 3rd, DeWolf WC 1996. Occult prostate cancer in men with low serum testosterone levels. JAMA 1996; 276(23): 1904-6.

[3] Nishiyama T, Ikarashi T, Hashimoto Y, Suzuki K, Takahashi K 2006. Association between the dihydrotestosterone level in the prostate and prostate cancer aggressiveness using the Gleason score. J Urol 2006; 176(4 Pt 1): 1387-91.

[4] Mahler C, Denis L 1992. Management of relapsing disease in prostate cancer. Cancer 1992; 70(1 Suppl): 329-34.

[5] Chu KC, Tarone RE, Freeman HP 2003. Trends in prostate cancer mortality among black men and white men in the United States. Cancer 2003; 97(6): 1507-16.

[6] Odedina FT, Akinremi TO, Chinegwundoh F, Roberts R, Yu D, Reams RR, et al. 2009. Prostate cancer disparities in Black men of African descent: a comparative literature review of prostate cancer burden among Black men in the United States, Caribbean, United Kingdom, and West Africa. Infect Agent Cancer 2009; 4 Suppl 1(S2.

[7] Abbott RR, Taylor DK, Barber K 1998. A comparison of prostate knowledge of African-American and Caucasian men: changes from prescreening baseline to postintervention. Cancer J Sci Am 1998; 4(3): 175-7.

[8] Chornokur G, Dalton K, Borysova ME, Kumar NB 2011. Disparities at presentation, diagnosis, treatment, and survival in African American men, affected by prostate cancer. Prostate 2011; 71(9): 985-97.

[9] Talcott JA, Spain P, Clark JA, Carpenter WR, Do YK, Hamilton RJ, et al. 2007. Hidden barriers between knowledge and behavior: the North Carolina prostate cancer screening and treatment experience. Cancer 2007; 109(8): 1599-606.

[10] McIntosh H 1997. Why do African-American men suffer more prostate cancer? J Natl Cancer Inst 1997; 89(3): 188-9.

[11] Jemal A, Siegel R, Ward E, Hao Y, Xu J, Thun MJ 2009. Cancer statistics, 2009. CA Cancer J Clin 2009; 59(4): 225-49.

[12] Trofimova I, Dimtchev A, Jung M, Rosenthal D, Smulson M, Dritschilo A, et al. 2002. Gene therapy for prostate cancer by targeting poly(ADP-ribose) polymerase. Cancer Res 2002; 62(23): 6879-83.

[13] Kummar S, Chen A, Parchment RE, Kinders RJ, Ji J, Tomaszewski JE, et al. 2012. Advances in using PARP inhibitors to treat cancer. BMC Med 2012; 10(25.

[14] Gradwohl G, Menissier de Murcia JM, Molinete M, Simonin F, Koken M, Hoeijmakers JH, et al. 1990. The second zinc-finger domain of poly(ADP-ribose) polymerase determines specificity for single-stranded breaks in DNA. Proc Natl Acad Sci U S A 1990; 87(8): 2990-4.

[15] Menissier-de Murcia J, Molinete M, Gradwohl G, Simonin F, de Murcia G 1989. Zinc-binding domain of poly(ADP-ribose)polymerase participates in the recognition of single strand breaks on DNA. J Mol Biol 1989; 210(1): 229-33.

[16] Zaremba T, Ketzer P, Cole M, Coulthard S, Plummer ER, Curtin NJ 2009. Poly(ADP-ribose) polymerase-1 polymorphisms, expression and activity in selected human tumour cell lines. Br J Cancer 2009; 101(2): 256-62.

[17] Nosho K, Yamamoto H, Mikami M, Taniguchi H, Takahashi T, Adachi Y, et al. 2006. Overexpression of poly(ADP-ribose) polymerase-1 (PARP-1) in the early stage of colorectal carcinogenesis. Eur J Cancer 2006; 42(14): 2374-81.

[18] Shimizu M, Suzui M, Deguchi A, Lim JT, Xiao D, Hayes JH, et al. 2004. Synergistic effects of acyclic retinoid and OSI-461 on growth inhibition and gene expression in human hepatoma cells. Clin Cancer Res 2004; 10(19): 6710-21.

[19] Nomura F, Yaguchi M, Togawa A, Miyazaki M, Isobe K, Miyake M, et al. 2000. Enhancement of poly-adenosine diphosphate-ribosylation in human hepatocellular carcinoma. J Gastroenterol Hepatol 2000; 15(5): 529-35.

[20] Hirai K, Ueda K, Hayaishi O 1983. Aberration of poly(adenosine diphosphate-ribose) metabolism in human colon adenomatous polyps and cancers. Cancer Res 1983; 43(7): 3441-6.

[21] Fukushima M, Kuzuya K, Ota K, Ikai K 1981. Poly(ADP-ribose) synthesis in human cervical cancer cell-diagnostic cytological usefulness. Cancer Lett 1981; 14(3): 227-36.

[22] Ikai K, Ueda K, Fukushima M, Nakamura T, Hayaishi O 1980. Poly(ADP-ribose) synthesis, a marker of granulocyte differentiation. Proc Natl Acad Sci U S A 1980; 77(6): 3682-5.

[23] Thomas C, Pfirrmann K, Pieles F, Bogumil A, Gillitzer R, Wiesner C, et al. 2012. Predictors for clinically relevant Gleason score upgrade in patients undergoing radical prostatectomy. BJU Int 2012; 109(2): 214-9.

[24] Alkhatib HM, Chen DF, Cherney B, Bhatia K, Notario V, Giri C, et al. 1987. Cloning and expression of cDNA for human poly(ADP-ribose) polymerase. Proc Natl Acad Sci U S A 1987; 84(5): 1224-8.

[25] Cherney BW, McBride OW, Chen DF, Alkhatib H, Bhatia K, Hensley P, et al. 1987. cDNA sequence, protein structure, and chromosomal location of the human gene for poly(ADP-ribose) polymerase. Proc Natl Acad Sci U S A 1987; 84(23): 8370-4.

[26] Schreiber V, Dantzer F, Ame JC, de Murcia G 2006. Poly(ADP-ribose): novel functions for an old molecule. Nat Rev Mol Cell Biol 2006; 7(7): 517-28.

[27] de Murcia G, Schreiber V, Molinete M, Saulier B, Poch O, Masson M, et al. 1994. Structure and function of poly(ADP-ribose) polymerase. Mol Cell Biochem 1994; 138(1-2): 15-24.

[28] El-Khamisy SF, Masutani M, Suzuki H, Caldecott KW 2003. A requirement for PARP-1 for the assembly or stability of XRCC1 nuclear foci at sites of oxidative DNA damage. Nucleic Acids Res 2003; 31(19): 5526-33.

[29] Bhatia K, Kang VH, Stein GS, Bustin M, Cherney BW, Notario V, et al. 1990. Cell cycle regulation of an exogenous human poly(ADP-ribose) polymerase cDNA introduced into murine cells. J Cell Physiol 1990; 144(2): 345-53.

[30] Hassa PO, Hottiger MO 2002. The functional role of poly(ADP-ribose)polymerase 1 as novel coactivator of NF-kappaB in inflammatory disorders. Cell Mol Life Sci 2002; 59(9): 1534-53.

[31] Kidwell WR, Mage MG 1976. Changes in poly(adenosine diphosphate-ribose) and poly(adenosine diphosphate-ribose) polymerase in synchronous HeLa cells. Biochemistry 1976; 15(6): 1213-7.

[32] Simbulan-Rosenthal CM, Rosenthal DS, Luo R, Samara R, Espinoza LA, Hassa PO, et al. 2003. PARP-1 binds E2F-1 independently of its DNA binding and catalytic domains, and acts as a novel coactivator of E2F-1-mediated transcription during re-entry of quiescent cells into S phase. Oncogene 2003; 22(52): 8460-71.

[33] Espinoza LA, Crotti LB 2007. Roles of PARP-1 and p53 in the maintenance of genome integrity. Hauppauge, NY: Nova Science Publishers.

[34] Kasid UN, Halligan B, Liu LF, Dritschilo A, Smulson M 1989. Poly(ADP-ribose)-mediated post-translational modification of chromatin-associated human topoisomerase I. Inhibitory effects on catalytic activity. J Biol Chem 1989; 264(31): 18687-92.

[35] Simbulan-Rosenthal CM, Rosenthal DS, Hilz H, Hickey R, Malkas L, Applegren N, et al. 1996. The expression of poly(ADP-ribose) polymerase during differentiation-linked DNA replication reveals that it is a component of the multiprotein DNA replication complex. Biochemistry 1996; 35(36): 11622-33.

[36] Baksi K, Alkhatib H, Smulson ME 1987. In vivo characterization of the poly(ADP-ribosylation) of SV40 chromatin and large T antigen by immunofractionation. Exp Cell Res 1987; 172(1): 110-23.

[37] Molinete M, Vermeulen W, Burkle A, Menissier-de Murcia J, Kupper JH, Hoeijmakers JH, et al. 1993. Overproduction of the poly(ADP-ribose) polymerase DNA-binding domain blocks alkylation-induced DNA repair synthesis in mammalian cells. Embo J 1993; 12(5): 2109-17.

[38] Dantzer F, de La Rubia G, Menissier-De Murcia J, Hostomsky Z, de Murcia G, Schreiber V 2000. Base excision repair is impaired in mammalian cells lacking Poly(ADP-ribose) polymerase-1. Biochemistry 2000; 39(25): 7559-69.

[39] Masson M, Niedergang C, Schreiber V, Muller S, Menissier-de Murcia J, de Murcia G 1998. XRCC1 is specifically associated with poly(ADP-ribose) polymerase and negatively regulates its activity following DNA damage. Mol Cell Biol 1998; 18(6): 3563-71.

[40] Vodenicharov MD, Sallmann FR, Satoh MS, Poirier GG 2000. Base excision repair is efficient in cells lacking poly(ADP-ribose) polymerase 1. Nucleic Acids Res 2000; 28(20): 3887-96.

[41] Kannan P, Yu Y, Wankhade S, Tainsky MA 1999. PolyADP-ribose polymerase is a co-activator for AP-2-mediated transcriptional activation. Nucleic Acids Res 1999; 27(3): 866-74.

[42] Kameoka M, Ota K, Tetsuka T, Tanaka Y, Itaya A, Okamoto T, et al. 2000. Evidence for regulation of NF-kappaB by poly(ADP-ribose) polymerase. Biochem J 2000; 346 Pt 3(641-9.

[43] Cervellera MN, Sala A 2000. Poly(ADP-ribose) polymerase is a B-MYB coactivator. J Biol Chem 2000; 275(14): 10692-6.

[44] Nie J, Sakamoto S, Song D, Qu Z, Ota K, Taniguchi T 1998. Interaction of Oct-1 and automodification domain of poly(ADP-ribose) synthetase. FEBS Lett 1998; 424(1-2): 27-32.

[45] Ko L, Cardona GR, Chin WW 2000. Thyroid hormone receptor-binding protein, an LXXLL motif-containing protein, functions as a general coactivator. Proc Natl Acad Sci U S A 2000; 97(11): 6212-7.

[46] Butler AJ, Ordahl CP 1999. Poly(ADP-ribose) polymerase binds with transcription enhancer factor 1 to MCAT1 elements to regulate muscle-specific transcription. Mol Cell Biol 1999; 19(1): 296-306.

[47] Oei SL, Griesenbeck J, Schweiger M, Babich V, Kropotov A, Tomilin N 1997. Interaction of the transcription factor YY1 with human poly(ADP-ribosyl) transferase. Biochem Biophys Res Commun 1997; 240(1): 108-11.

[48] Ha HC, Hester LD, Snyder SH 2002. Poly(ADP-ribose) polymerase-1 dependence of stress-induced transcription factors and associated gene expression in glia. Proc Natl Acad Sci U S A 2002; 99(5): 3270-5.

[49] Chang WJ, Alvarez-Gonzalez R 2001. The sequence-specific DNA binding of NF-kappa B is reversibly regulated by the automodification reaction of poly (ADP-ribose) polymerase 1. J Biol Chem 2001; 276(50): 47664-70.

[50] Hassa PO, Covic M, Hasan S, Imhof R, Hottiger MO 2001. The enzymatic and DNA binding activity of PARP-1 are not required for NF-kappa B coactivator function. J Biol Chem 2001; 276(49): 45588-97.

[51] Simbulan CM, Suzuki M, Izuta S, Sakurai T, Savoysky E, Kojima K, et al. 1993. Poly(ADP-ribose) polymerase stimulates DNA polymerase alpha by physical association. J Biol Chem 1993; 268(1): 93-9.

[52] Simbulan-Rosenthal CM, Rosenthal DS, Boulares AH, Hickey RJ, Malkas LH, Coll JM, et al. 1998. Regulation of the expression or recruitment of components of the DNA synthesome by poly(ADP-ribose) polymerase. Biochemistry 1998; 37(26): 9363-70.

[53] Meisterernst M, Stelzer G, Roeder RG 1997. Poly(ADP-ribose) polymerase enhances activator-dependent transcription in vitro. Proc Natl Acad Sci U S A 1997; 94(6): 2261-5.

[54] Oei SL, Griesenbeck J, Schweiger M, Ziegler M 1998. Regulation of RNA polymerase II-dependent transcription by poly(ADP-ribosyl)ation of transcription factors. J Biol Chem 1998; 273(48): 31644-7.

[55] Satoh MS, Lindahl T 1992. Role of poly(ADP-ribose) formation in DNA repair. Nature 1992; 356(6367): 356-8.

[56] Satoh MS, Poirier GG, Lindahl T 1993. NAD(+)-dependent repair of damaged DNA by human cell extracts. J Biol Chem 1993; 268(8): 5480-7.

[57] Yoshihara K, Itaya A, Tanaka Y, Ohashi Y, Ito K, Teraoka H, et al. 1985. Inhibition of DNA polymerase alpha, DNA polymerase beta, terminal deoxynucleotidyl transfer-

ase, and DNA ligase II by poly(ADP-ribosyl)ation reaction in vitro. Biochem Biophys Res Commun 1985; 128(1): 61-7.

[58] Ikeguchi M, Saito H, Kondo A, Tsujitani S, Maeta M, Kaibara N 1999. Mutated p53 protein expression and proliferative activity in advanced gastric cancer. Hepatogastroenterology 1999; 46(28): 2648-53.

[59] Poirier GG, de Murcia G, Jongstra-Bilen J, Niedergang C, Mandel P 1982. Poly(ADP-ribosyl)ation of polynucleosomes causes relaxation of chromatin structure. Proc Natl Acad Sci U S A 1982; 79(11): 3423-7.

[60] Frechette A, Huletsky A, Aubin RJ, de Murcia G, Mandel P, Lord A, et al. 1985. Poly(ADP-ribosyl)ation of chromatin: kinetics of relaxation and its effect on chromatin solubility. Can J Biochem Cell Biol 1985; 63(7): 764-73.

[61] Wang ZQ, Auer B, Stingl L, Berghammer H, Haidacher D, Schweiger M, et al. 1995. Mice lacking ADPRT and poly(ADP-ribosyl)ation develop normally but are susceptible to skin disease. Genes Dev 1995; 9(5): 509-20.

[62] de Murcia JM, Niedergang C, Trucco C, Ricoul M, Dutrillaux B, Mark M, et al. 1997. Requirement of poly(ADP-ribose) polymerase in recovery from DNA damage in mice and in cells. Proc Natl Acad Sci U S A 1997; 94(14): 7303-7.

[63] Trucco C, Oliver FJ, de Murcia G, Menissier-de Murcia J 1998. DNA repair defect in poly(ADP-ribose) polymerase-deficient cell lines. Nucleic Acids Res 1998; 26(11): 2644-9.

[64] Masutani M, Nozaki T, Nishiyama E, Shimokawa T, Tachi Y, Suzuki H, et al. 1999. Function of poly(ADP-ribose) polymerase in response to DNA damage: gene-disruption study in mice. Mol Cell Biochem 1999; 193(1-2): 149-52.

[65] Ishizuka S, Martin K, Booth C, Potten CS, de Murcia G, Burkle A, et al. 2003. Poly(ADP-ribose) polymerase-1 is a survival factor for radiation-exposed intestinal epithelial stem cells in vivo. Nucleic Acids Res 2003; 31(21): 6198-205.

[66] Wesierska-Gadek J, Schloffer D, Gueorguieva M, Uhl M, Skladanowski A 2004. Increased susceptibility of poly(ADP-ribose) polymerase-1 knockout cells to antitumor triazoloacridone C-1305 is associated with permanent G2 cell cycle arrest. Cancer Res 2004; 64(13): 4487-97.

[67] Potosky AL, Davis WW, Hoffman RM, Stanford JL, Stephenson RA, Penson DF, et al. 2004. Five-year outcomes after prostatectomy or radiotherapy for prostate cancer: the prostate cancer outcomes study. J Natl Cancer Inst 2004; 96(18): 1358-67.

[68] Hagan MP, Yacoub A, Dent P 2007. Radiation-induced PARP activation is enhanced through EGFR-ERK signaling. J Cell Biochem 2007; 101(6): 1384-93.

[69] Wollman R, Yahalom J, Maxy R, Pinto J, Fuks Z 1994. Effect of epidermal growth factor on the growth and radiation sensitivity of human breast cancer cells in vitro. Int J Radiat Oncol Biol Phys 1994; 30(1): 91-8.

[70] Kimura K, Bowen C, Spiegel S, Gelmann EP 1999. Tumor necrosis factor-alpha sensitizes prostate cancer cells to gamma-irradiation-induced apoptosis. Cancer Res 1999; 59(7): 1606-14.

[71] Kimura K, Gelmann EP 2000. Tumor necrosis factor-alpha and Fas activate complementary Fas-associated death domain-dependent pathways that enhance apoptosis induced by gamma-irradiation. J Biol Chem 2000; 275(12): 8610-7.

[72] Aguero MF, Venero M, Brown DM, Smulson ME, Espinoza LA 2010. Phenoxodiol inhibits growth of metastatic prostate cancer cells. Prostate 2010; 70(11): 1211-21.

[73] Silasi DA, Alvero AB, Rutherford TJ, Brown D, Mor G 2009. Phenoxodiol: pharmacology and clinical experience in cancer monotherapy and in combination with chemotherapeutic drugs. Expert Opin Pharmacother 2009; 10(6): 1059-67.

[74] Alvero AB, O'Malley D, Brown D, Kelly G, Garg M, Chen W, et al. 2006. Molecular mechanism of phenoxodiol-induced apoptosis in ovarian carcinoma cells. Cancer 2006; 106(3): 599-608.

[75] Chen CD, Welsbie DS, Tran C, Baek SH, Chen R, Vessella R, et al. 2004. Molecular determinants of resistance to antiandrogen therapy. Nat Med 2004; 10(1): 33-9.

[76] Ide H, Yu J, Lu Y, China T, Kumamoto T, Koseki T, et al. 2011. Testosterone augments polyphenol-induced DNA damage response in prostate cancer cell line, LNCaP. Cancer Sci 2011; 102(2): 468-71.

[77] Yacoub A, Hawkins W, Hanna D, Young H, Park MA, Grant M, et al. 2007. Human chorionic gonadotropin modulates prostate cancer cell survival after irradiation or HMG CoA reductase inhibitor treatment. Mol Pharmacol 2007; 71(1): 259-75.

[78] Iwashita A, Tojo N, Matsuura S, Yamazaki S, Kamijo K, Ishida J, et al. 2004. A novel and potent poly(ADP-ribose) polymerase-1 inhibitor, FR247304 (5-chloro-2-[3-(4-phenyl-3,6-dihydro-1(2H)-pyridinyl)propyl]-4(3H)-quinazolinone), attenuates neuronal damage in in vitro and in vivo models of cerebral ischemia. J Pharmacol Exp Ther 2004; 310(2): 425-36.

[79] Fowler JE, Jr., Lau JL, Ghosh L, Mills SE, Mounzer A 1988. Epidermal growth factor and prostatic carcinoma: an immunohistochemical study. J Urol 1988; 139(4): 857-61.

[80] Yang Y, Chisholm GD, Habib FK 1993. Epidermal growth factor and transforming growth factor alpha concentrations in BPH and cancer of the prostate: their relationships with tissue androgen levels. Br J Cancer 1993; 67(1): 152-5.

[81] Connolly JM, Rose DP 1990. Production of epidermal growth factor and transforming growth factor-alpha by the androgen-responsive LNCaP human prostate cancer cell line. Prostate 1990; 16(3): 209-18.

[82] Connolly JM, Rose DP 1989. Secretion of epidermal growth factor and related polypeptides by the DU 145 human prostate cancer cell line. Prostate 1989; 15(2): 177-86.

[83] Jarrard DF, Blitz BF, Smith RC, Patai BL, Rukstalis DB 1994. Effect of epidermal growth factor on prostate cancer cell line PC3 growth and invasion. Prostate 1994; 24(1): 46-53.

[84] Saadat M, Khalili M, Omidvari S, Ansari-Lari M 2011. Parental consanguineous marriages and clinical response to chemotherapy in locally advanced breast cancer patients. Cancer Lett 2011; 302(2): 109-12.

[85] Chen YL, Lin SZ, Chang JY, Cheng YL, Tsai NM, Chen SP, et al. 2006. In vitro and in vivo studies of a novel potential anticancer agent of isochaihulactone on human lung cancer A549 cells. Biochem Pharmacol 2006; 72(3): 308-19.

[86] Bieche I, de Murcia G, Lidereau R 1996. Poly(ADP-ribose) polymerase gene expression status and genomic instability in human breast cancer. Clin Cancer Res 1996; 2(7): 1163-7.

[87] Nguyen D, Zajac-Kaye M, Rubinstein L, Voeller D, Tomaszewski JE, Kummar S, et al. 2011. Poly(ADP-ribose) polymerase inhibition enhances p53-dependent and -independent DNA damage responses induced by DNA damaging agent. Cell Cycle 2011; 10(23): 4074-82.

[88] Chiu SC, Wang MJ, Yang HH, Chen SP, Huang SY, Chen YL, et al. 2011. Activation of NAG-1 via JNK signaling revealed an isochaihulactone-triggered cell death in human LNCaP prostate cancer cells. BMC Cancer 2011; 11(146.

[89] Mendoza-Alvarez H, Alvarez-Gonzalez R 2001. Regulation of p53 sequence-specific DNA-binding by covalent poly(ADP-ribosyl)ation. J Biol Chem 2001; 276(39): 36425-30.

[90] Ringer L, Sirajuddin P, Yenugonda VM, Ghosh A, Divito K, Trabosh V, et al. 2010. VMY-1-103, a dansylated analog of purvalanol B, induces caspase-3-dependent apoptosis in LNCaP prostate cancer cells. Cancer Biol Ther 2010; 10(4): 320-5.

[91] Oren M 1999. Regulation of the p53 tumor suppressor protein. J Biol Chem 1999; 274(51): 36031-4.

[92] Selivanova G, Wiman KG 1995. p53: a cell cycle regulator activated by DNA damage. Adv Cancer Res 1995; 66(143-80.

[93] Tong WM, Cortes U, Wang ZQ 2001. Poly(ADP-ribose) polymerase: a guardian angel protecting the genome and suppressing tumorigenesis. Biochim Biophys Acta 2001; 1552(1): 27-37.

[94] Schmid G, Wang ZQ, Wesierska-Gadek J 1999. Compensatory expression of p73 in PARP-deficient mouse fibroblasts as response to a reduced level of regularly spliced wild-type p53 protein. Biochem Biophys Res Commun 1999; 255(2): 399-405.

[95] Wang X, Ohnishi K, Takahashi A, Ohnishi T 1998. Poly(ADP-ribosyl)ation is required for p53-dependent signal transduction induced by radiation. Oncogene 1998; 17(22): 2819-25.

[96] Mandir AS, Simbulan-Rosenthal CM, Poitras MF, Lumpkin JR, Dawson VL, Smulson ME, et al. 2002. A novel in vivo post-translational modification of p53 by PARP-1 in MPTP-induced parkinsonism. J Neurochem 2002; 83(1): 186-92.

[97] Valenzuela MT, Guerrero R, Nunez MI, Ruiz De Almodovar JM, Sarker M, de Murcia G, et al. 2002. PARP-1 modifies the effectiveness of p53-mediated DNA damage response. Oncogene 2002; 21(7): 1108-16.

[98] Wang ZQ, Stingl L, Morrison C, Jantsch M, Los M, Schulze-Osthoff K, et al. 1997. PARP is important for genomic stability but dispensable in apoptosis. Genes Dev 1997; 11(18): 2347-58.

[99] Al-Hajj M, Clarke MF 2004. Self-renewal and solid tumor stem cells. Oncogene 2004; 23(43): 7274-82.

[100] Mimeault M, Batra SK 2006. Recent advances on multiple tumorigenic cascades involved in prostatic cancer progression and targeting therapies. Carcinogenesis 2006; 27(1): 1-22.

[101] Miller SJ, Lavker RM, Sun TT 2005. Interpreting epithelial cancer biology in the context of stem cells: tumor properties and therapeutic implications. Biochim Biophys Acta 2005; 1756(1): 25-52.

[102] Mimeault M, Batra SK 2007. Functions of tumorigenic and migrating cancer progenitor cells in cancer progression and metastasis and their therapeutic implications. Cancer Metastasis Rev 2007; 26(1): 203-14.

[103] Beachy PA, Karhadkar SS, Berman DM 2004. Tissue repair and stem cell renewal in carcinogenesis. Nature 2004; 432(7015): 324-31.

[104] Bapat SA, Mali AM, Koppikar CB, Kurrey NK 2005. Stem and progenitor-like cells contribute to the aggressive behavior of human epithelial ovarian cancer. Cancer Res 2005; 65(8): 3025-9.

[105] Sutherland RM 1988. Cell and environment interactions in tumor microregions: the multicell spheroid model. Science 1988; 240(4849): 177-84.

[106] Takagi A, Watanabe M, Ishii Y, Morita J, Hirokawa Y, Matsuzaki T, et al. 2007. Three-dimensional cellular spheroid formation provides human prostate tumor cells with tissue-like features. Anticancer Res 2007; 27(1A): 45-53.

[107] Ponti D, Costa A, Zaffaroni N, Pratesi G, Petrangolini G, Coradini D, et al. 2005. Isolation and in vitro propagation of tumorigenic breast cancer cells with stem/progenitor cell properties. Cancer Res 2005; 65(13): 5506-11.

[108] Bao S, Wu Q, Li Z, Sathornsumetee S, Wang H, McLendon RE, et al. 2008. Targeting cancer stem cells through L1CAM suppresses glioma growth. Cancer Res 2008; 68(15): 6043-8.

[109] Zhang K, Waxman DJ 2010. PC3 prostate tumor-initiating cells with molecular profile FAM65Bhigh/MFI2low/LEF1low increase tumor angiogenesis. Mol Cancer 2010; 9(319.

[110] Yamazaki J, Mizukami T, Takizawa K, Kuramitsu M, Momose H, Masumi A, et al. 2009. Identification of cancer stem cells in a Tax-transgenic (Tax-Tg) mouse model of adult T-cell leukemia/lymphoma. Blood 2009; 114(13): 2709-20.

[111] Quintana E, Shackleton M, Sabel MS, Fullen DR, Johnson TM, Morrison SJ 2008. Efficient tumour formation by single human melanoma cells. Nature 2008; 456(7222): 593-8.

[112] Bisson I, Prowse DM 2009. WNT signaling regulates self-renewal and differentiation of prostate cancer cells with stem cell characteristics. Cell Res 2009; 19(6): 683-97.

[113] Patrawala L, Calhoun-Davis T, Schneider-Broussard R, Tang DG 2007. Hierarchical organization of prostate cancer cells in xenograft tumors: the CD44+alpha2beta1+ cell population is enriched in tumor-initiating cells. Cancer Res 2007; 67(14): 6796-805.

[114] Li H, Chen X, Calhoun-Davis T, Claypool K, Tang DG 2008. PC3 human prostate carcinoma cell holoclones contain self-renewing tumor-initiating cells. Cancer Res 2008; 68(6): 1820-5.

[115] Visvader JE, Lindeman GJ 2008. Cancer stem cells in solid tumours: accumulating evidence and unresolved questions. Nat Rev Cancer 2008; 8(10): 755-68.

[116] Guzman-Ramirez N, Voller M, Wetterwald A, Germann M, Cross NA, Rentsch CA, et al. 2009. In vitro propagation and characterization of neoplastic stem/progenitor-like cells from human prostate cancer tissue. Prostate 2009; 69(15): 1683-93.

[117] Rybak AP, He L, Kapoor A, Cutz JC, Tang D 2011. Characterization of sphere-propagating cells with stem-like properties from DU145 prostate cancer cells. Biochim Biophys Acta 2011; 1813(5): 683-94.

[118] Gunia S, May M, Koch S, Dietel M, Erbersdobler A 2009. Expression of CD44s in incidental prostate cancer is more strongly associated with Gleason scores on subsequent radical prostatectomies than conventional prognostic parameters. Pathobiology 2009; 76(6): 286-92.

[119] Hurt EM, Kawasaki BT, Klarmann GJ, Thomas SB, Farrar WL 2008. CD44+ CD24(-) prostate cells are early cancer progenitor/stem cells that provide a model for patients with poor prognosis. Br J Cancer 2008; 98(4): 756-65.

[120] Maitland NJ, Collins AT 2008. Prostate cancer stem cells: a new target for therapy. J Clin Oncol 2008; 26(17): 2862-70.

[121] Gurel B, Iwata T, Koh CM, Yegnasubramanian S, Nelson WG, De Marzo AM 2008. Molecular alterations in prostate cancer as diagnostic, prognostic, and therapeutic targets. Adv Anat Pathol 2008; 15(6): 319-31.

[122] Schalken JA 2005. Validation of molecular targets in prostate cancer. BJU Int 2005; 96 Suppl 2(23-9.

[123] Mousses S, Wagner U, Chen Y, Kim JW, Bubendorf L, Bittner M, et al. 2001. Failure of hormone therapy in prostate cancer involves systematic restoration of androgen responsive genes and activation of rapamycin sensitive signaling. Oncogene 2001; 20(46): 6718-23.

[124] Flavin R, Zadra G, Loda M 2010. Metabolic alterations and targeted therapies in prostate cancer. J Pathol 2010.

[125] Flavin R, Zadra G, Loda M 2011. Metabolic alterations and targeted therapies in prostate cancer. J Pathol 2011; 223(2): 283-94.

[126] Niu Y, Chang TM, Yeh S, Ma WL, Wang YZ, Chang C 2010. Differential androgen receptor signals in different cells explain why androgen-deprivation therapy of prostate cancer fails. Oncogene 2010; 29(25): 3593-604.

[127] Saeki N, Gu J, Yoshida T, Wu X 2010. Prostate stem cell antigen: a Jekyll and Hyde molecule? Clin Cancer Res 2010; 16(14): 3533-8.

[128] Mellado B, Codony J, Ribal MJ, Visa L, Gascon P 2009. Molecular biology of androgen-independent prostate cancer: the role of the androgen receptor pathway. Clin Transl Oncol 2009; 11(1): 5-10.

[129] Wegiel B, Evans S, Hellsten R, Otterbein LE, Bjartell A, Persson JL 2010. Molecular pathways in the progression of hormone-independent and metastatic prostate cancer. Curr Cancer Drug Targets 2010; 10(4): 392-401.

[130] Malumbres M, Barbacid M 2009. Cell cycle, CDKs and cancer: a changing paradigm. Nat Rev Cancer 2009; 9(3): 153-66.

[131] McNealy T, Frey M, Trojan L, Knoll T, Alken P, Michel MS 2003. Intrinsic presence of poly (ADP-ribose) is significantly increased in malignant prostate compared to benign prostate cell lines. Anticancer Res 2003; 23(2B): 1473-8.

[132] Martin DS, Bertino JR, Koutcher JA 2000. ATP depletion + pyrimidine depletion can markedly enhance cancer therapy: fresh insight for a new approach. Cancer Res 2000; 60(24): 6776-83.

[133] Green DR, Reed JC 1998. Mitochondria and apoptosis. Science 1998; 281(5381): 1309-12.

[134] Ide H, Tokiwa S, Sakamaki K, Nishio K, Isotani S, Muto S, et al. 2010. Combined inhibitory effects of soy isoflavones and curcumin on the production of prostate-specific antigen. Prostate 2010; 70(10): 1127-33.

[135] Hall W, Christie M, Currow D 2005. Cannabinoids and cancer: causation, remediation, and palliation. Lancet Oncol 2005; 6(1): 35-42.

[136] Sarfaraz S, Adhami VM, Syed DN, Afaq F, Mukhtar H 2008. Cannabinoids for cancer treatment: progress and promise. Cancer Res 2008; 68(2): 339-42.

[137] Sreevalsan S, Joseph S, Jutooru I, Chadalapaka G, Safe SH 2011. Induction of apoptosis by cannabinoids in prostate and colon cancer cells is phosphatase dependent. Anticancer Res 2011; 31(11): 3799-807.

[138] Thomas E, Gannon PO, Koumakpayi IH, Latour M, Mes-Masson A, Saad F, editors. Implication of PARP-1 expression in prostate cancer progression. ASCO; 2011: J Clin Oncol.

[139] Ding R, Pommier Y, Kang VH, Smulson M 1992. Depletion of poly(ADP-ribose) polymerase by antisense RNA expression results in a delay in DNA strand break rejoining. J Biol Chem 1992; 267(18): 12804-12.

[140] Burkle A, Heilbronn R, zur Hausen H 1990. Potentiation of carcinogen-induced methotrexate resistance and dihydrofolate reductase gene amplification by inhibitors of poly(adenosine diphosphate-ribose) polymerase. Cancer Res 1990; 50(18): 5756-60.

[141] Morgan WF, Cleaver JE 1982. 3-Aminobenzamide synergistically increases sister-chromatid exchanges in cells exposed to methyl methanesulfonate but not to ultraviolet light. Mutat Res 1982; 104(6): 361-6.

[142] Waldman AS, Waldman BC 1991. Stimulation of intrachromosomal homologous recombination in mammalian cells by an inhibitor of poly(ADP-ribosylation). Nucleic Acids Res 1991; 19(21): 5943-7.

[143] Simbulan-Rosenthal CM, Ly DH, Rosenthal DS, Konopka G, Luo R, Wang ZQ, et al. 2000. Misregulation of gene expression in primary fibroblasts lacking poly(ADP-ribose) polymerase. Proc Natl Acad Sci U S A 2000; 97(21): 11274-9.

[144] Chatterjee S, Berger SJ, Berger NA 1999. Poly(ADP-ribose) polymerase: a guardian of the genome that facilitates DNA repair by protecting against DNA recombination. Mol Cell Biochem 1999; 193(1-2): 23-30.

[145] Rojo F, Garcia-Parra J, Zazo S, Tusquets I, Ferrer-Lozano J, Menendez S, et al. 2012. Nuclear PARP-1 protein overexpression is associated with poor overall survival in early breast cancer. Ann Oncol 2012; 23(5): 1156-64.

[146] Horton JK, Stefanick DF, Wilson SH 2005. Involvement of poly(ADP-ribose) polymerase activity in regulating Chk1-dependent apoptotic cell death. DNA Repair (Amst) 2005; 4(10): 1111-20.

[147] Dantzer F, Giraud-Panis MJ, Jaco I, Ame JC, Schultz I, Blasco M, et al. 2004. Functional interaction between poly(ADP-Ribose) polymerase 2 (PARP-2) and TRF2: PARP activity negatively regulates TRF2. Mol Cell Biol 2004; 24(4): 1595-607.

[148] Durkacz BW, Omidiji O, Gray DA, Shall S 1980. (ADP-ribose)n participates in DNA excision repair. Nature 1980; 283(5747): 593-6.

[149] Thraves P, Mossman KL, Brennan T, Dritschilo A 1985. Radiosensitization of human fibroblasts by 3-aminobenzamide: an inhibitor of poly(ADP-ribosylation). Radiat Res 1985; 104(2 Pt 1): 119-27.

[150] Brock WA, Milas L, Bergh S, Lo R, Szabo C, Mason KA 2004. Radiosensitization of human and rodent cell lines by INO-1001, a novel inhibitor of poly(ADP-ribose) polymerase. Cancer Lett 2004; 205(2): 155-60.

[151] Barreto-Andrade JC, Efimova EV, Mauceri HJ, Beckett MA, Sutton HG, Darga TE, et al. 2011. Response of human prostate cancer cells and tumors to combining PARP inhibition with ionizing radiation. Mol Cancer Ther 2011; 10(7): 1185-93.

[152] Audeh MW, Carmichael J, Penson RT, Friedlander M, Powell B, Bell-McGuinn KM, et al. 2010. Oral poly(ADP-ribose) polymerase inhibitor olaparib in patients with BRCA1 or BRCA2 mutations and recurrent ovarian cancer: a proof-of-concept trial. Lancet 2010; 376(9737): 245-51.

[153] Fong PC, Boss DS, Yap TA, Tutt A, Wu P, Mergui-Roelvink M, et al. 2009. Inhibition of poly(ADP-ribose) polymerase in tumors from BRCA mutation carriers. N Engl J Med 2009; 361(2): 123-34.

[154] Tutt A, Robson M, Garber JE, Domchek SM, Audeh MW, Weitzel JN, et al. 2010. Oral poly(ADP-ribose) polymerase inhibitor olaparib in patients with BRCA1 or BRCA2 mutations and advanced breast cancer: a proof-of-concept trial. Lancet 2010; 376(9737): 235-44.

[155] Yap TA, Sandhu SK, Carden CP, de Bono JS 2011. Poly(ADP-ribose) polymerase (PARP) inhibitors: Exploiting a synthetic lethal strategy in the clinic. CA Cancer J Clin 2011; 61(1): 31-49.

[156] Liu SK, Coackley C, Krause M, Jalali F, Chan N, Bristow RG 2008. A novel poly(ADP-ribose) polymerase inhibitor, ABT-888, radiosensitizes malignant human cell lines under hypoxia. Radiother Oncol 2008; 88(2): 258-68.

[157] Mueller T, Voigt W, Simon H, Fruehauf A, Bulankin A, Grothey A, et al. 2003. Failure of activation of caspase-9 induces a higher threshold for apoptosis and cisplatin resistance in testicular cancer. Cancer Res 2003; 63(2): 513-21.

[158] Brenner JC, Chinnaiyan AM 2009. Translocations in epithelial cancers. Biochim Biophys Acta 2009; 1796(2): 201-15.

[159] Brenner JC, Ateeq B, Li Y, Yocum AK, Cao Q, Asangani IA, et al. 2011. Mechanistic rationale for inhibition of poly(ADP-ribose) polymerase in ETS gene fusion-positive prostate cancer. Cancer Cell 2011; 19(5): 664-78.

Section 9

Cell Adhesion Proteins in Prostate Cancer

Chapter 25

Integrins in Prostate Cancer Invasion and Metastasis

Paulynn Chin Suyin, Joanne Louise Dickinson and
Adele Frances Holloway

Additional information is available at the end of the chapter

http://dx.doi.org/10.5772/53482

1. Introduction

Prostate cancer is the most commonly diagnosed cancer in men and is the second leading cause of cancer deaths in men after non-melanoma skin cancer. According to the United States National Cancer Institute, it was estimated that almost 241 740 men would be diagnosed with prostate cancer in the United States alone in 2012 and more than 28 170 would die of prostate cancer. Despite considerable advances in prostate cancer research, this cancer is still associated with significant mortality and morbidity [1]. The risk factors involved in the development of prostate cancer include advancing age, race and family history. If detected in the early stage of disease, prostate cancer is considered curable by surgical excision methods, radiotherapy and androgen deprivation therapy [2]. However, in a percentage of men disease recurs, is frequently refractory to treatment and this is associated with poor prognosis. It is thought there is a population of prostate tumour cells that have the capacity to invade and metastasize, with bone being the most common metastatic site. Autopsy studies have found that more than 80% of men who die of prostate cancer have metastatic boney lesions [3].

The current prostate specific antigen (PSA) screening tool has allowed early detection of prostate cancer, when still locally confined. PSA is a protein produced by the cells in the prostate gland. The PSA screening tool measures the level of PSA in the blood where a high PSA level is indicative of the presence of cancer. However, benign conditions may also show elevated levels of PSA. Therefore, the PSA screening tool has significant limitations resulting in false positives. Further, it is unable to distinguish the aggressive tumours requiring immediate intervention from those that are more appropriately managed by regular surveillance. Thus, there is considerable interest in identifying and discovering new prognostic and diagnostic markers for prostate cancer, particularly markers that can identify those tumours likely to progress to a more aggressive state.

Prostatic intraepithelial neoplasia (PIN), in particular high-grade PIN have been identified as precursors to prostate cancer. High-grade PIN is an abnormal condition of the prostate gland and is considered a pre-malignant condition. Studies have reported that approximately 30% of men with high-grade PIN lesions will develop prostate cancer [4]. Atypical small acinar proliferation (ASAP) is also a precursor to prostate cancer. ASAP lesions mimic cancer and have been found to be strongly predictive of subsequent prostate cancer, with approximately 60% of men with ASAP found to subsequently develop prostate cancer [5]. The progression of prostate cancer may be driven by the accumulation of genetic and epigenetic changes, leading to the activation of oncogenes and inactivation of tumour suppressor genes [6]. These changes lead to the development of PIN and ASAP which may progress into localised invasive cancer and finally metastatic tumours.

Metastasis is a multistep event and it arises when there is a loss of tumour cell adhesion to the primary site leading to cell detachment. These cells then invade through the extracellular matrix (ECM) and subsequently adhere to secondary sites. The transition from a normal prostate gland to the formation of PIN and to invasive and metastatic cancers involves alterations in the cell surface adhesive receptors, integrins. Integrins play important roles in normal prostate development where they are involved in the interaction of the prostate epithelial cells with the ECM and also influence cell signalling, growth, survival and differentiation. During metastasis, changes in integrin expression results in changes in the tumour cell adhesion to adjacent cells and to the ECM leading to increased cell motility. Thus, integrins are key players in metastatic events since they mediate cell to cell (homotypic) and cell to ECM (heterotypic) interactions of prostate cells.

2. Integrins

Integrins belong to a superfamily of transmembrane glycoprotein receptors involved in mediating cell to cell and cell to ECM interactions. They exist as heterodimers composed of α and β subunits bound by non-covalent bonds. To date, 18 α subunits and 8 β subunits have been identified, which can associate to form 24 unique complexes (Table 1) with the different $\alpha\beta$ combinations possessing distinct ligand binding specificities [7, 8]. There are three distinct regions in each integrin subunit with each subunit containing an extracellular domain, a transmembrane domain and a short intracellular domain.

The extracellular regions of the α and β subunits together form the ligand binding site. The most common ligands for integrins are large ECM proteins such as laminin, fibronectin, collagen and vitronectin. These ECM proteins (except for laminin and collagen) have a common arginine-glycine-aspartic acid (RGD) motif, whereas integrins recognise laminin and collagen through cryptic RGD sites. In addition, there are some integrins that interact with other adhesion molecules such as cadherins, intracellular adhesion molecules (ICAMs) and vascular adhesion molecules (VCAMs), expressed on leukocytes and endothelial cells. By grouping the integrins according to integrin ligand specificity, the collagen binding integrins are α1β1, α2β1, α3β1, α10β1, α11β1 and α6β4, the laminin binding integrins are α1β1, α2β1, α3β1, α6β1, α7β1 and α6β4 and the RGD recognising integrins are α5β1,αvβ1, αvβ3, αvβ5, αvβ6, αvβ8 and $\alpha_{IIb}\beta 3$. However, integrins can frequently bind several ligands (as outlined in Table 1), permitting redundancy in signalling as multiple integrins are generally present on any particular cell surface.

Integrin	**Ligand**	
α1β1	Collagen IV and VI, Laminin-1	Collagen binding
α2β1	Collagen I, Laminin-1,-2 and -10	
α10β1	Collagen IV and VI	
α11β1	Collagen I	
α3β1	Laminin-5, Collagen IV, Fibronectin	Laminin binding
α6β1	Laminin-1, Merosis, Kalinin	
α7β1	Laminin-1 and -2	
α6β4	Laminin-1, -2, -5 and -10	
α4β1	Fibronectin, VCAM	RGD motif binding
α5β1	Fibronectin	
α8β1	Fibronectin	
α9β1	Fibronectin, Tenascin, Laminin-1	
αvβ1	Fibronectin, Vitronectin	
αvβ3	Fibronectin, Vitronectin	
αvβ5	Vitronectin	
αvβ6	Fibronectin	
αvβ8	Fibronectin, Collagen IV, Laminin-5	
$\alpha_{IIb}\beta 3$	Fibronectin, Vitronectin	
α4β7	Fibronectin, VCAM	Leukocyte binding
αEβ7	E-cadherin	
αDβ7	ICAM3, VCAM	
αLβ2	ICAM1-5	
αMβ2	ICAM1, VCAM, fibrinogen	
αXβ2	Fibrinogen	

Table 1. List of integrins and their ligands

As an integrin binds to its ligand, it undergoes structural changes which affect the ligand binding affinity [9]. This affinity is also determined by the cytoplasmic signals from within the cell which affects the molecular interactions at the integrin cytoplasmic domain influencing the degree of cell adhesion. This is refered to as inside-out signaling. Integrins also play a role in signal transduction where they transduce extracellular signals to the interior of the cell, refered to as outside-in signaling. Such signalling can affect cell migration, differentiation, survival and proliferation [10-12]. When bound to the ECM proteins, integrins recruit a range of adaptor proteins, and activate various signalling pathways. For example, integrin clustering activates the focal adhesion kinases (FAK), Src family kinases, Rac and Rho GTPases leading to the recruitment of cytoskeleton proteins such as talin, α-actinin, vinculin, paxillin and tensin [13]. Activation of these kinase pathways and cytoskeleton proteins contributes to changes in cell architecture, adhesion and migration on the ECM [14].

3. Roles of integrins in cancer progression

While integrins mediate cell attachment, ligation of integrins by the ECM proteins induces cell migration by generating the traction required for invasion. In cancer, expression of integrins that are involved in cell adhesion are frequently altered, leading to cell proliferation, migration and metastasis. Previous studies in which integrin expression levels were correlated to the different stages of human tumours and the pathological outcomes (metastasis, recurrence, survival), implicated a number of integrins in cancer progression [15-25]. These integrins include $\alpha v\beta 3$, $\alpha 2\beta 1$, $\alpha 3\beta 1$ and $\alpha 6\beta 1$. In contrast integrin $\alpha 4\beta 1$ is associated with tumour suppression [26].

Integrin $\alpha v\beta 3$ has been associated with tumour progression in a range of cancers including lung cancer, gastric cancer, breast cancer and prostate cancer [15-18]. Integrin $\alpha v\beta 3$ remains the most well-studied integrin involved in tumour progression. Interestingly, integrin $\alpha v\beta 3$ is usually only expressed in activated leukocytes, macrophages, platelets and osteoclasts and not normally expressed in epithelial cells. It has been found to mediate adhesion of breast cancer cells to bone matrix and also facilitate migration of breast cancer cells in bone sialoprotein [19, 27]. In colon cancer, blocking integrin $\alpha v\beta 3$ resulted in a decrease in tumour metastasis and improved survival in mice [21]. This integrin was also found to bind to periostin, which is upregulated in epithelial ovarian cancer cells, and promotes cell adhesion and migration [22].

Changes in integrin $\alpha 2\beta 1$ have also been associated with tumour progression with loss of integrin $\alpha 2\beta 1$ resulting in the induction of breast cancer cell metastasis *in vivo*, suggesting that integrin $\alpha 2\beta 1$ is a metastasis suppressor [23]. The re-expression of $\alpha 2\beta 1$ in breast cancer cells reversed some of the tumourigenic properties of the cells [24]. In contrast, in prostate cancer, integrin $\alpha 2\beta 1$ was found to induce prostate cancer cell metastasis to the bone [25]. Thus, this suggests that integrin function is cell type and context dependent. This was evident in a study by Zhang et al., where integrin $\alpha 2$ knockout mice, when challenged with B16F10 melanoma cells showed increased tumour angiogenesis correlating with increased vascular endothelial growth factor receptor 1 (VEGFR-1) [28]. However, the $\alpha 2$ knockout mice bearing Lewis Lung carcinoma (LLC) cells showed no difference in tumour angiogenesis. Further analysis showed that the integrin $\alpha 2\beta 1$-dependent angiogenesis involves the secretion of placental growth factor (PLGF) which was produced by B16F10 cells but not the LLC cells. These data suggest that integrin expression is cell type and context dependent where it is dependent on the interactions of the host factors with the surrounding microenvironment.

4. Roles of integrins in prostate cancer progression

Integrins are expressed in normal prostate basal cells and are required for the interaction of the cells with surrounding stroma which influences their growth, survival and differentiation potential. These integrins include $\alpha2\beta1$, $\alpha3\beta1$, $\alpha5\beta1$ and $\alpha6\beta4$ [29-33]. Altered expression of integrins affects cell adhesion to adjacent cells and to the ECM and such affects have been observed in solid tumours and prostate cancer cell lines. Table 2 highlights the most well characterised integrins involved in prostate cancer progression, migration and invasion, and these integrins are discussed below.

Bonkhoff et al. (1993) investigated the expression of integrin $\alpha2\beta1$ in normal, hyperplastic and neoplastic human prostate tissue as well as lymph node metastases samples. Results showed downregulated $\alpha2\beta1$ in 70% of the hyperplastic samples compared to normal prostate tissues. However, $\alpha2\beta1$ was upregulated in the lymph node metastases compared to primary lesions. In another study, the role of integrin $\alpha2$ in prostate cancer metastasis was investigated [34]. Immunofluorescence staining showed the presence of $\alpha2$ and $\beta1$ subunit clusters in bone metastatic prostate cancer cells (C4-2B) and not in the lymph node metastatic prostate cancer cells (LNCaP), in contrast to the findings of Bonkhoff et al. which reported $\alpha2\beta1$ upregulation in lymph node metastasis. The functional blocking of the integrin $\alpha2$ subunit with antibodies in the C4-2B bone metastatic prostate cancer cell line resulted in reduced adhesion and inhibiton of invasion to collagen I [34]. The role of $\alpha2\beta1$ in bone metastasis is further supported by a study by Hall et al. (2006). A collagen-binding LNCaP cell line was derived (LNCaPcol) and showed increased levels of $\alpha2\beta1$ with associated increased migration towards collagen I [35]. In an *in vivo* analysis of these cells, in which LNCaPcol was injected into the tibia of nude mice, the LNCaPcol injected mice developed bone tumours. A follow-on study was conducted to investigate the signalling pathways involved in $\alpha2\beta1$ stimulated migration [25]. RhoC guanosine triphosphatase activity was increased by five to eight fold in collagen binding cell lines, CB-2B and LNCaPcol compared to non-collagen binding LNCaP. These results support the idea that ligation of collagen I to $\alpha2\beta1$ activates the RhoC signalling pathway, which mediates prostate cancer invasion and metastasis to the bone.

A microarray study was conducted on 111 individuals with localised prostate cancer who had undergone radical prostectomy, including 60 individuals who had tumour recurrence after a follow-up of 123 months [36]. In this study increased integrin $\alpha3$ and $\alpha3\beta1$ expression were found to be related to worse outcome with strong $\alpha3$ and $\alpha3\beta1$ expression associated with higher incidence of recurrence. In another microarray study performed on five prostate cancer cell lines (LNCaP, DU145, PC3, LAPC-4 and 22Rv1) and 13 prostate cancer xenografts, integrin $\alpha4$ showed decreased expression associated with deletion of the integrin $\alpha4$ locus [26]. Since all samples were derived from metastases, it suggests that integrin $\alpha4$ could be a tumour suppressor. Interestingly, integrin $\alpha7$ has also been identified as a tumour suppressor [13]. The prostate cancer cell lines, PC3 and DU145 were transfected with integrin $\alpha7$ expression vector and implanted in SCID mice. After six weeks, the volume of the tumours were measured and compared to mice transfected with control vector. Results showed reduced tumour volume and fewer metastases in the integrin $\alpha7$ vector transfected mice. Further analysis of metastasic potential using a wound-healing assay showed reduced rates of migration in both PC3 and DU145 cells overexpressing integrin $\alpha7$. Thus, these studies support the notion that integrin $\alpha7$ inhibits cell migration and acts as a tumour suppressor.

An early study using DU145 and PC3 cells, which express integrin $\alpha_{IIb}\beta3$, suggested that integrin $\alpha_{IIb}\beta3$ is also involved in prostate cancer metastasis [37]. Although both cell lines express integrin $\alpha_{IIb}\beta3$, immunofluorescence data showed different localisation patterns of the integrin. In DU145 cells the integrin localizes to focal contact sites whereas in PC3 cells, it is mainly intracellular. Interestingly, when both the tumourigenic cell lines were injected intraprostatically into SCID mice, only the DU145 cells metastasized. Further analysis by flow cytometry with an antibody to $\alpha_{IIb}\beta3$ showed higher expression of $\alpha_{IIb}\beta3$ in DU145 cells isolated from the prostate when compared to DU145 cells from the subcutaneous tissue. Therefore, the data suggests that integrin $\alpha_{IIb}\beta3$ is involved in the metastatic progression of prostate tumours. Recently, integrin $\alpha5\beta1$ also has been found to be important in cell adhesion in prostate cancer cells [38]. When integrin $\alpha5\beta1$ was blocked with an antibody, a decrease in the number of adherent PC3 cells to fibronectin was observed. Partial inhibition of the PC3 cell migration and the formation of quasi-spherical cell shape changes were observed, suggesting a reversal to a less mesenchymal phenotype. In addition, the blocking of $\alpha5\beta1$ resulted in weak expression of the cytoskeletal proteins F-actin and α-actinin suggesting a weak cell-fibronectin interaction. Thus, these results support the idea that integrin $\alpha5\beta1$ plays an important role in the adhesion of PC3 cells to fibronectin and the migration of PC3 cells.

Integrin $\alpha v\beta3$ has also been identified to be involved in prostate cancer metastasis. Zheng et al. (1999), found expression of integrin $\alpha v\beta3$ in 16 prostate cancer specimens but not in normal prostate epithelial cells. The highly metastatic and invasive PC3 cell line also expresses integrin $\alpha v\beta3$ but not the non-invasive LNCaP cell line [39]. These $\alpha v\beta3$ expressing PC3 cells and the primary prostate cancer cells were found to adhere and migrate on vitronectin. When LNCaP cells were transfected with a $\alpha v\beta3$ expression plasmid to induce $\alpha v\beta3$ expression, LNCaP cells also adhered to and migrated on vitronectin. Thus, this study suggests that $\alpha v\beta3$ is potentially involved in prostate cancer invasion and metastasis. A following study found integrin $\alpha v\beta3$ to be involved in bone metabolism and angiogenesis [40]. To investigate how inhibition of integrin $\alpha v\beta3$ in cells native to the bone would affect prostate cancer bone metastasis, a prostate cancer cell line that expresses little or no integrin $\alpha v\beta3$ was chosen. Interestingly, in this study, PC3 cells were used as they found undetectable levels of $\alpha v\beta3$ by FACS analysis and by using antibody staining. This is conflicting with the previous study which reported expression of $\alpha v\beta3$ in PC3 cells and it is possible that this is due to the use of different types of antibodies. Regardless, PC3 cells were injected directly into human bone fragments which were previously implanted subcutaneously in SCID mice and the mice were treated with anti-β3 antibody fragment (m7E3 F(ab')$_2$). This antibody only blocks the human bone-derived $\alpha v\beta3$. After two weeks of treatment, inhibition of integrin $\alpha v\beta3$ resulted in a reduced proportion of antigenically-human blood vessels within tumour-bearing bone implants. In addition, a reduction in the rate of tumour cell proliferation within the bone implants, reduced osteoclast number and degradation of calcified bone tissue were observed.

The integrin α6 can pair with either β1 or β4 subunits and it binds to laminin. The integrin α6β4 is a laminin receptor and is known as a hemidesmosome complex, mediating cell attachment to the ECM. It acts as the junctional complex on the basal cell surface and is involved in the attachment of epithelial cells to the adjacent basement membrane. In contrast, integrin α6β1 has been found to be involved in the cell migratory phenotype. The expression and distribution of integrin α6β1 in normal, hyperplastic and neoplastic prostate tissue and lymph node metastases was examined [33]. Approximately 85% of the grade I and grade II tumours and also the lymph node metastases showed upregulation of integrin α6β1, compared to normal and hyperplastic samples. Staining showed clusters of α6β1 receptors in acinar basement membranes which suggests integrin α6β1 is important in mediating cell attachment to the basement membrane. Then, Nagle et al. (1994), found that while most of the prostate carcinoma tissues they tested displayed downregulation of integrins, the majority of these samples expressed α6β1 [41]. This is consistent with the loss of integrin β4 in the carcinoma samples. In a separate study, integrin β4 was found to be absent in prostate carcinoma tissues and only present in normal prostate glands and PIN lesions [42], supporting the previous study. Therefore, these data suggest that integrin β4 is lost during cancer progression and therefore, integrin α6 is preferentially paired with the β1 subunit, forming α6β1. A following study found a variant form of integrin α6, α6p which was expressed in DU145, LNCaP and PC3 prostate cancer cell lines but not expressed in the normal prostate cells, PrEC [32]. This α6p variant also binds to both the β1 and the β4 subunits and has three times longer half-life than α6. Recently, King et al. (2008) investigated the role of integrin α6β1 in prostate cancer migration and bone pain in a novel xenograft mouse model [43]. The human prostate cancer cells (PC3N), were stably transfected to overexpress either the cleavable wild type (PC3N-α6-WT) which forms the α6p variant or the uncleavable (PC3N-α6-RR) form of integrin α6. The α6 subunit can be cleaved via Urokinase-type Plasminogen Activator (uPA) treatment and the cells were directly injected and sealed into the femur of a mouse. After 21 days, tumour cells expressing wild-type integrin α6 (non-cleavable) showed a significant decrease in bone loss, unicortical or bicortical fractures and decreased ability of tumour cells to reach the epiphyseal plate of bone and prevented movement evoked pain, compared to the cleavable a6 integrin. Thus, these results suggest that blocking of integrin α6 cleavage in prostate tumour cells results in decreased tumour cell migration within the bone and reduced bone fractures and pain.

5. Epithelial-mesenchymal transition

Epithelial cell structure is maintained by cell-cell interactions involving tight junctions and desmosomes and these cells are non-motile. In contrast, mesenchymal cells do not have cell-cell contacts but have distinct cell-ECM interactions and cytoskeletal structures and are motile. Epithelial-mesenchymal transition (EMT) is a series of events where the cell-cell and cell-ECM interactions are altered resulting in detachment of epithelial cells from the surrounding tissue followed by rearrangement of the cytoskeleton to confer the ability to move through a three-dimensional ECM and the induction of a series of new transcriptional signaling pathways to maintain the mesenchymal phenotype [42]. This process is important in embryonic development, particularly in gastrulation and segment formation. However, more recently, EMT has been implicated in carcinogenesis. EMT involves a multistep process in which the non-motile epithelial cells are tranformed into motile invasive cells [43]. This process is quite similar to the onset of the invasive metastasis process where there is a transition from a benign to aggressive tumour phenotype, involving the detachment of tumour cells from the primary site followed by invasion through the ECM (Figure 1). The reverse of the EMT process is known as mesenchymal-epithelial transition (MET), which facilitates tumour cell attachment at secondary sites.

Integrin	Integrin expression	Reference
$\alpha2\beta1$	↓ Prostate hyperplastic tissue ↑ Metastatic prostate cancer tissue ↑ Metastatic prostate cancer cell lines	Bonkhoff et al. (1993) Hall et al. (2006), Bostwick DG et al. (2006)
$\alpha3\beta1$	↑ Associated with higher recurrence	Pontes-Junior et al. (2010),
$\alpha_{IIb}\beta3$	↑ Metastatic prostate cell lines	Trikha et al. (1998)
$\alpha4$	↓ Metastatic prostate cencer cell lines and xenograft samples	Saramaki et al. (2006)
$\alpha7$	↓ Metastatic xenograft samples	Ren et al. (2007)
$\alpha v\beta3$	↑ Prostate cancer tissue samples, metastatic prostate cancer cell lines	Zheng et al. (1999), Nameth et al. (2003)
$\alpha5\beta1$	↑ Metastatic prostate cancer cell line	Stachrurska et al. (2012)
$\alpha6\beta1$	↑ Metastatic prostate cancer tissue and metastatic prostate cancer cell lines	Davis et al. (2001), Bonkhoff et al. (1993), Trikha et al. (1998), King et al. (2008)
$\alpha6\beta4$	↓ Metastatic prostate cancer tissue	Davis et al. (2001)

Table 2. Integrin expression in prostate cancer progression

EMT involves a series of signalling processes. Firstly, it involves the break-down of cell-cell interactions leading to loss of E-cadherin expression and the upregulation of mesenchymal markers such as N-cadherin, vimentin and the transcription factors Snail, TWIST and ZEB family members. Then, it is followed by a loss of cell polarisation and cytoskeleton remodelling. Finally, changes in cell adhesion occur leading to cell detachment and the activation of proteolytic enzymes; matrix metalloproteinases (MMPs) [44]. The initiation of EMT is tissue and context dependent and may not involve all EMT markers [45]. There are various stimuli from outside the cell which regulate EMT within the tumour microenvironment. These include the binding of transforming growth factor-β (TGFβ) to the TGFβ receptor (TGFβr), growth factors such as epidermal growth factor (EGF), fibroblast growth factor (FGF) and hepatocyte growth factor (HGF) which bind to the tyrosine-kinase receptor (TKR), the highly conserved Wnt/β-catenin pathway and also integrin signalling which activates the FAK signalling pathway [46, 47]. Since integrins are involved in cell adhesion and signalling, it is possible that integrins can initiate and mediate EMT and invasion in tumour progression (Figure 1).

E-cadherin is a type-I cell-cell adhesion glycoprotein and is a major inducer of EMT as loss of E-cadherin results in decreased cell adhesion and thus, increased cell motility. It is expressed by most epithelial tissues and it forms the tight junction connecting adjacent cells and thus, the formation of stable cell-cell contact. Loss of E-cadherin has been associated with tumour progression and metastasis in breast cancer, prostate cancer, colorectal cancer and gastric cancer [44-48]. Besides genetic and epigenetic factors, transcription factors such as the zinc finger proteins, Snail, Slug, ZEB1, ZEB2 and the basic helix-loop-helix protein, TWIST are involved in the repression of E-cadherin. The zinc finger proteins repress E-cadherin by binding to the E-box motif in the E-cadherin promoter. The role of the Snail transcription factor on E-cadherin has been studied in epithelial tumour cell lines of different origins including bladder cancer, pancreatic cancer and colon cancer. Most of the cell lines showed an inverse correlation between E-cadherin and Snail expression levels and when Snail was transfected into the cell lines that express high E-cadherin levels, it resulted in down-regulation of E-cadherin [49]. It has been proposed that Snail and ZEB2 initiate the silencing of E-cadherin by modifying chromatin organisation of the gene [50]. Subsequently, Slug and ZEB1 have been proposed to be responsible for maintaining the repression of E-cadherin and thus, maintenance of the mesenchymal phenotype [51].

TGFβ signaling is the main inducer of EMT in the development of cancer. Interestingly however, the TGFβ response is context-dependent where it can either act as a growth inhibitor or it can induce tumour progression by promoting angiogenesis, immune suppression and preventing apoptosis [52, 53]. The main role of TGFβ is to induce apoptosis and thus, it generally acts as a tumour suppressor during the early stages of cancer progression. However, frequent loss-of-function mutations in TGFβ have been observed in cancer, which is associated with the progression of cancer by inducing cell metastasis. Multiple signalling pathways are involved in the induction of EMT by TGFβ including the Wnt/β-catenin pathway and integrin signalling pathways. Ligation of the TGFβr results in the activation of Smad2 and Smad3 and constitutive phosphorylation of Smad4 [54]. These Smads then bind to ZEB1 and ZEB2 to repress E-cadherin expression [55-57]. Miyaki et al. (1999) found increased mutations in Smad 4 as the stage of colorectal tumours advanced, suggesting that inactivation of Smad 4 in the TGFβ signalling pathway induces tumour metastasis [58].

Activation of the TKR by growth factors has also been found to induce EMT. Stimulation of the breast cancer cell line, PMC42-LA with EGF resulted in E-cadherin downregulation and upregulation of vimentin expression [59]. This is followed by increased cell adhesion and migratory capacity suggesting the upregulation of integrins upon EGF treatment. Integrins have also been linked to EMT as discussed below.

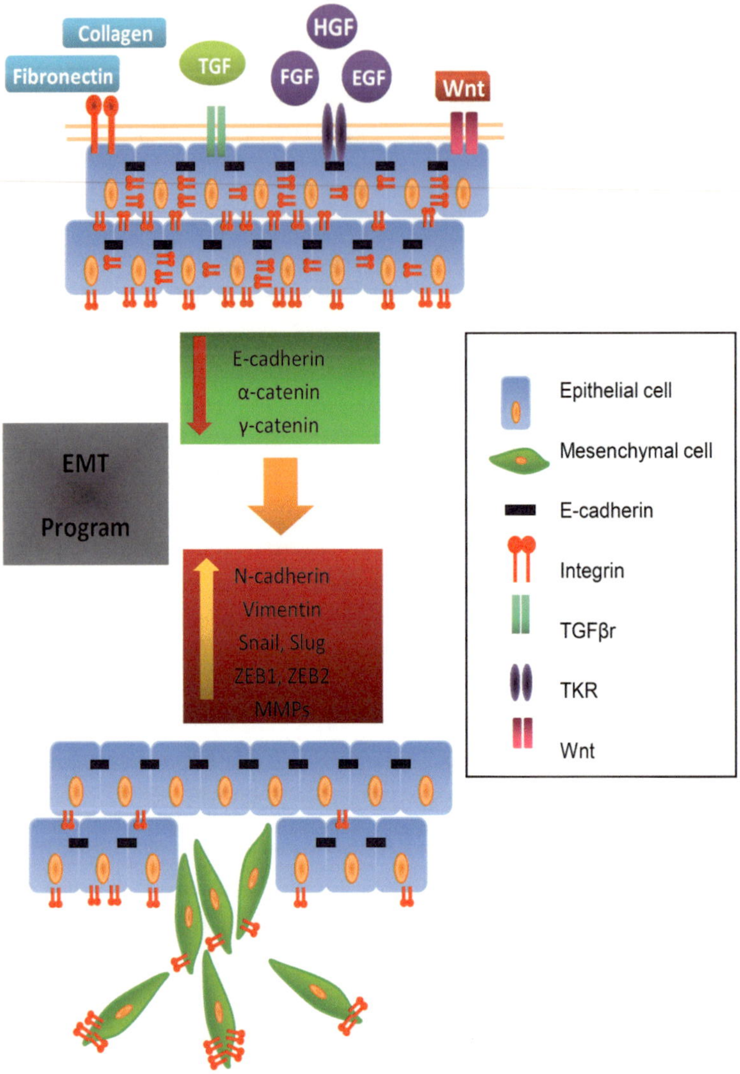

Figure 1. Schematic representation of the EMT process and the roles of integrins in cell adhesion and migration

6. Roles of integrins and EMT in cancer

To date, studies on the involvement of integrins in EMT during cancer progression have been limited, particularly in prostate cancer. Here we highlight the recent studies which correlate integrins (implicated in prostate cancer) and EMT. EMT involving changes in the expression of cadherins has been observed in prostate cancer progression [44]. Loss of E-cadherin (epithelial marker) expression has been correlated with increased tumour grade, with 46 out of 92 prostate tumour samples showing reduced or absence of E-cadherin staining when compared to non-malignant prostate samples [45]. In contrast N-cadherin (mesenchymal marker), was not expressed in normal prostate tissue but expressed in the poorly differentiated areas of prostate cancer specimens, where E-cadherin was absent [44]. These studies suggest that switching of cadherin expression correlates with prostate cancer metastasis.

Collagen type I which is the ligand of integrin α2β1 was found to induce the disruption of E-cadherin adhesion complexes in pancreatic cancer [60]. The study suggested that binding of collagen type I to α2β1 activates FAK phosphorylation which enhances tyrosine phosphorylation of β-catenin and causes the disassembly of the E-cadherin complex. In addition, Shintani et al. (2008) showed that activation of integrin α2β1 by collagen type I together with activation of the discoidin domain receptor 1 (DDR1) induces N-cadherin expression [61]. Furthermore, high E-cadherin was observed in suspended PC3 cells and the expression decreased as cells attached to a fibronectin substrate, whereas N-cadherin expression was 4-fold lower in suspension cells compared with attached cells [62]. Blocking of the integrin β1 by the AIIB2 antibody resulted in no increase of N-cadherin expression in PC3 cells, suggesting that integrin β1-mediated cell adhesion to fibronectin is involved in regulating N-cadherin expression in prostate cancer. The study also investigated the regulation of N-cadherin by Twist1 (a transcription factor that regulates mesenchymal gene expression). Knockdown of Twist1 expression in PC3 cells resulted in decreased N-cadherin expression and inhibition of cell migration. Interestingly, blocking of integrin β1 correlated with inhibition of nuclear accumulation of Twist1 following cell attachment. Therefore, these data suggest that the integrin β1-mediated adhesion is regulated through Twist1 accumulation and activation of N-cadherin.

Integrins have also been shown to activate latent TGFβ. TGFβ is involved in tissue homeostasis and is both a tumour suppressor and tumour inducer, as outlined above. Tumour cells have increased secretion of TGFβ which induces EMT [63]. Studies have found that TGFβ can be activated by integrins. Bates et al. (2005), developed a colon cancer model of EMT, where EMT can be induced in the LIM 1863 colon cancer cell line by exposure to TGFβ. This model showed that EMT resulted in upregulation of integrin αvβ6. This occurs through the Ets-1 transcription factor and integrin αvβ6 was found to promote the activation of autocrine TGFβ in post-EMT to stabilize and sustain EMT and also promote cell migration on fibronectin [64]. In another study, in order to study the role of TGFβ, stable clones of truncated TGFβ were generated in non-transformed mouse mammary ductal epithelial cells (NmuMG) [65]. The truncated TGFβ resulted in blocking of TGFβ-mediated growth inhibition, Smad-mediated transcriptional activation, AKT signaling pathways and EMT. However, this did not block the TGFβ-mediated p38MAPK activation. Further, blocking of integrin β1 with antibody resulted in inhibition of p38MAPK and EMT progression. Therefore, these results suggest that TGFβ-induced EMT is dependent on both p38MAPK activation and integrin β1 which thus suggests the cooperation of TGFβ and integrins in the modulation of EMT progression.

The mesenchymal transcription factor Snail plays a role in EMT by repressing E-cadherin. A study investigated the regulation of integrin αv expression by Snail in epithelial Madin-Darby canine kidney (MDCK) and A431 cells [66]. Upregulation of integrin αv was observed in MDCK Snail transfected cells and A431 Snail transfected cells. Further investigation showed expression of integrin αv was mediated directly through its promoter by the Snail transcription factor. In addition, MDCK Snail transfected cells showed increased cell migration towards osteopontin, the ligand for integrin αvβ3 in bone. Therefore, these data suggest that Snail enhances cell migration, at least in part, by regulating integrin expression in cells. A more recent study which involved stable transfection of Snail into ARCaP and LNCaP prostate cancer cell lines, found a decrease in cell adhesion and increase in cell migration on collagen I and fibronectin [67]. The Snail transfected ARCaP cells were then subjected to flow cytometry and results showed downregulation of integrin α5, α2 and β1, which was reversed by Snail knockdown.

A microarray study undertaken to examine 19 primary prostate tumours showed 65% loss of E-cadherin in metastatic tumour samples compared to primary tumours [18]. The expression levels also correlated with a 71% loss of integrin β4 when comparing metastatic to primary tumours. These results suggest that progression of prostate cancer involves the loss of E-cadherin and a possible involvement of E-cadherin in regulating integrin β4 expression. More recently, a study has found expression of ZEB1 which is a dual zinc finger transcription factor and a known regulator of EMT to repress integrin β4 expression in PC3 cells [68]. Further, transient transfection of ZEB2 in the colon cancer cell line, SW480 was found to upregulate the expression of integrin α5 [69]. Knockdown of ZEB2 resulted in suppression of integrin α5 and the cells displayed reduced cell invasion. In addition, ZEB2 was found to cooperate with the SP1 transcription factor to activate the integrin α5 and vimentin promoters and thus, induction of the mesenchymal gene during EMT in cancer progression.

7. Integrins as therapeutic targets

As previously discussed, integrins have been shown to mediate tumour progression, tumour cell metastasis and EMT in both *in vitro* and *in vivo* models. Thus, these preclinical studies have suggested that integrins could be a novel therapeutic target to prevent cancer progression, including prostate cancer. Currently, studies have been focused on targeting integrin αvβ3 in breast cancer, ovarian cancer and prostate cancer. Integrin αvβ3 is likely to be a good cancer angiogenesis target because it is highly expressed on tumour-associated new blood vessels and the surface of most epithelial tumours cells.

There are currently antibody-type inhibitors (LM609, MEDI-522, CNTO95, c7E3, 17E6) or peptide-type inhibitors (Cilengitide, ATN-161) under investigation. However, here only inhibitors that have been tested specifically on prostate cancer models will be reviewed. MEDI-522 is a humanized monoclonal antibody specific for integrin αvβ3 and a phase I dose escalation trial was conducted in 25 individuals with a variety of metastatic solid tumours which included, breast, colorectal, melanoma, non-small cell lung cancer, ocular melanoma, renal, sarcoma and prostate cancers [70]. Participants in the trial were treated on a daily basis with dosages ranging from 2 to 10 mg/kg/wk, intravenously. Treatment showed a possible effect on tumour perfusion with an increase in mean transit time of blood through target tumour lesions after 8 weeks. There were no significant toxicities observed in the treated individuals, with only mild constitutional and gastrointestinal symptoms observed. Only two individuals with metastatic renal cancer remained on treatment and showed prolonged stable disease for 1 or 2 years, respectively, suggesting MEDI-522 may have clinical activity in metastatic renal cancer. Currently, a phase II, randomized, open-label, two-arm, multicenter study of MEDI-522 in combination with docetaxel (an anti-mitotic, standard chemotherapy drug), prednisone (a glucocorticoid prodrug), and zolendronic acid (a bisphosphonate) in individuals with metastatic androgen-independent prostate cancer has just been completed. However, the results of the trial have not been documented yet.

CNTO95 is a fully human antibody that recognizes the integrin αv. It binds to both integrin $\alpha v\beta 3$ and $\alpha v\beta 5$ [71]. CNTO95 was found to inhibit adhesion and migration of HUVECs (human umbilical vein endothelial) and A375.S2 (human melanoma) cells on vitronectin, fibrinogen, gelatin and fibrin, which are ligands for integrin $\alpha v\beta 3$ and $\alpha v\beta 5$. In an *in vivo* study, CNTO95 inhibited the growth of human melanoma tumours in nude mice by approximately 80% and reduced final tumour weight by 99%, thus suggesting it has antitumour effects. A phase I clinical study was conducted in 24 individuals with a variety of advanced solid tumours. However, there were no individuals with prostate cancer included in this study. CNTO95, administered intravenously, was generally well tolerated with no adverse side effects. Individuals with ovarian cancer showed a prolonged stable disease with CNTO95 treatment and a 9 month partial response was observed in one individual with angiosarcoma. Interestingly, the partial response was observed in an individual with tumour expressing integrin $\alpha v\beta 1$ and not $\alpha v\beta 3$, suggesting a broad specificity for integrin αv. Currently, a phase II study of CNTO95 in combination with docetaxel for the first-line treatment of individuals with metastatic hormone refractory prostate cancer has been completed, although the results have yet to be documented.

Cilengitide is a cyclic peptide that is a potent and selective inhibitor of integrin $\alpha v\beta 3$ and $\alpha v\beta 5$ mediated cell adhesion. In a phase I study, Cilengitide was administrated as a continuous infusion in 4 week cycles at doses of 1, 2, 4, 8, 12, 18, 27, and 40mg/h in 25 individuals with a variety of solid tumours including prostate cancer. This study showed that Cilengitide was generally well tolerated as a continuous infusion and only mild side effects were observed. However, the variable dose did not affect tumour size. This lack of dose-response could be because the lowest dose was as effective as the highest dose. Interestingly, two phase II studies on Cilengitide were conducted by the same research team [72, 73]. In the earlier study, Cilengitide was administrated at 500 mg and 2000 mg, intravenously twice weekly in 44 asymptomatic individuals with metastatic castrate resistant prostate cancer (CRPC) [72]. The treatment was randomized and well tolerated and at the endpoint at 6 months, 9% of participants treated with 500 mg Cilengitide and 23% of participants treated with 2000 mg Cilengitide showed no tumour progression, suggesting better outcomes with the higher dose. The majority of the participants showed stable disease for 9 months. In the second phase II study, Cilengitide was adminitrated at 2000 mg, intravenously twice weekly until toxicity or progression in individuals with non-metastatic CRPC [73]. This treatment was well tolerated although two grade three toxicities (atrial fibrillation) were observed. In addition, Cilengitide showed no detectable clinical activity in this study.

8. Conclusion

The *in vivo, in vitro* and clinical studies reviewed here have shown that integrins are a promising therapeutic target in cancer progression and metastasis including prostate cancer. Since integrins are involved in mediating cell adhesion, deregulation of integrins leads to tumour invasion and metastasis. Studies have also found integrins to be involved in EMT in cancer progression. This occurs by either direct activation of the integrin and its signalling pathway or by activating the TGFβ pathway and also mediating EMT transcription factors. However, studies on the involvement of integrins and the pathways involved in EMT is still very limited. Therefore, further studies are warranted to clarify the processes underlying integrin involvement in EMT in cancer progression. To date, there are still no clinical studies investigating the effect on EMT of integrin inhibitors. These studies will improve our understanding of the integrin mediated EMT pathway and the effects on tumour metastasis. Since bone metastasis is the major cause of prostate cancer related death, targetting integrins using integrin inhibitors could potentially prove valuable in the prevention of the development of prostate cancer boney lesions.

Author details

Paulynn Chin Suyin, Joanne Louise Dickinson and Adele Frances Holloway

Menzies Research Institute Tasmania, University of Tasmania, Hobart, Tasmania, Australia

References

[1] Rider. JR, Sandin F, Andren O, Wiklund P, Hugosson J, Stattin P. Long-term Outcomes Among Noncuratively Treated Men According to Prostate Cancer Risk Category in a Nationwide, Population-based Study. European urology. 2012 Aug 10:aheadofprint.

[2] Fleshner NE, Evans A, Chadwick K, Lawrentschuk N, Zlotta A. Clinical significance of the positive surgical margin based upon location, grade, and stage. Urologic oncology. 2010 Mar-Apr;28(2):197-204.

[3] Bubendorf L, Schopfer A, Wagner U, Sauter G, Moch H, Willi N, et al. Metastatic patterns of prostate cancer: an autopsy study of 1,589 patients. Human pathology. 2000 May;31(5):578-583.

[4] Lefkowitz GK, Taneja SS, Brown J, Melamed J, Lepor H. Followup interval prostate biopsy 3 years after diagnosis of high grade prostatic intraepithelial neoplasia is associated with high likelihood of prostate cancer, independent of change in prostate specific antigen levels. The Journal of urology. 2002 Oct;168(4 Pt 1):1415-1418.

[5] Bostwick DG, Meiers I. Atypical small acinar proliferation in the prostate: clinical significance in 2006. Archives of pathology & laboratory medicine. 2006 Jul;130(7): 952-957.

[6] De Marzo AM, Platz EA, Sutcliffe S, Xu J, Gronberg H, Drake CG, et al. Inflammation in prostate carcinogenesis. Nature reviews Cancer. 2007 Apr;7(4):256-269.

[7] Hynes RO. Integrins: versatility, modulation, and signaling in cell adhesion. Cell. 1992 Apr 3;69(1):11-25.

[8] Rosales C, O'Brien V, Kornberg L, Juliano R. Signal transduction by cell adhesion receptors. Biochimica et biophysica acta. 1995 Jul 28;1242(1):77-98.

[9] Hughes PE, Renshaw MW, Pfaff M, Forsyth J, Keivens VM, Schwartz MA, et al. Suppression of integrin activation: a novel function of a Ras/Raf-initiated MAP kinase pathway. Cell. 1997 Feb 21;88(4):521-530.

[10] Lee JW, Juliano R. Mitogenic signal transduction by integrin- and growth factor receptor-mediated pathways. Molecules and cells. 2004 Apr 30;17(2):188-202.

[11] Hood JD, Cheresh DA. Role of integrins in cell invasion and migration. Nature reviews Cancer. 2002 Feb;2(2):91-100.

[12] Giancotti FG, Ruoslahti E. Integrin signaling. Science (New York, NY). 1999 Aug 13;285(5430):1028-1032.

[13] Ren B, Yu YP, Tseng GC, Wu C, Chen K, Rao UN, et al. Analysis of integrin alpha7 mutations in prostate cancer, liver cancer, glioblastoma multiforme, and leiomyosarcoma. Journal of the National Cancer Institute. 2007 Jun 6;99(11):868-880.

[14] Desgrosellier JS, Cheresh DA. Integrins in cancer: biological implications and therapeutic opportunities. Nature reviews Cancer. 2010 Jan;10(1):9-22.

[15] Mitchell K, Svenson KB, Longmate WM, Gkirtzimanaki K, Sadej R, Wang X, et al. Suppression of integrin alpha3beta1 in breast cancer cells reduces cyclooxygenase-2 gene expression and inhibits tumorigenesis, invasion, and cross-talk to endothelial cells. Cancer Res. 2010 Aug 1;70(15):6359-6367.

[16] Saito Y, Sekine W, Sano R, Komatsu S, Mizuno H, Katabami K, et al. Potentiation of cell invasion and matrix metalloproteinase production by alpha3beta1 integrin-mediated adhesion of gastric carcinoma cells to laminin-5. Clinical & experimental metastasis. 2010 Apr;27(4):197-205.

[17] Tsuji T, Kawada Y, Kai-Murozono M, Komatsu S, Han SA, Takeuchi K, et al. Regulation of melanoma cell migration and invasion by laminin-5 and alpha3beta1 integrin (VLA-3). Clinical & experimental metastasis. 2002;19(2):127-134.

[18] Pontes-Junior J, Reis ST, Dall'Oglio M, Neves de Oliveira LC, Cury J, Carvalho PA, et al. Evaluation of the expression of integrins and cell adhesion molecules through tissue microarray in lymph node metastases of prostate cancer. J Carcinog. 2009;8:3-9.

[19] Sung V, Stubbs JT, 3rd, Fisher L, Aaron AD, Thompson EW. Bone sialoprotein supports breast cancer cell adhesion proliferation and migration through differential usage of the alpha(v)beta3 and alpha(v)beta5 integrins. Journal of cellular physiology. 1998 Sep;176(3):482-494.

[20] Rolli M, Fransvea E, Pilch J, Saven A, Felding-Habermann B. Activated integrin alphavbeta3 cooperates with metalloproteinase MMP-9 in regulating migration of metastatic breast cancer cells. Proceedings of the National Academy of Sciences of the United States of America. 2003 Aug 5;100(16):9482-9487.

[21] Reinmuth N, Liu W, Ahmad SA, Fan F, Stoeltzing O, Parikh AA, et al. Alphavbeta3 integrin antagonist S247 decreases colon cancer metastasis and angiogenesis and improves survival in mice. Cancer Res. 2003 May 1;63(9):2079-2087.

[22] Gillan L, Matei D, Fishman DA, Gerbin CS, Karlan BY, Chang DD. Periostin secreted by epithelial ovarian carcinoma is a ligand for alpha(V)beta(3) and alpha(V)beta(5) integrins and promotes cell motility. Cancer Res. 2002 Sep 15;62(18):5358-5364.

[23] Ramirez NE, Zhang Z, Madamanchi A, Boyd KL, O'Rear LD, Nashabi A, et al. The alpha(2)beta(1) integrin is a metastasis suppressor in mouse models and human cancer. J Clin Invest. 2011 Jan;121(1):226-237.

[24] Zutter MM, Santoro SA, Staatz WD, Tsung YL. Re-expression of the alpha 2 beta 1 integrin abrogates the malignant phenotype of breast carcinoma cells. Proceedings of the National Academy of Sciences of the United States of America. 1995 Aug 1;92(16): 7411-7415.

[25] Hall CL, Dubyk CW, Riesenberger TA, Shein D, Keller ET, van Golen KL. Type I collagen receptor (alpha2beta1) signaling promotes prostate cancer invasion through RhoC GTPase. Neoplasia. 2008 Aug;10(8):797-803.

[26] Saramaki OR, Porkka KP, Vessella RL, Visakorpi T. Genetic aberrations in prostate cancer by microarray analysis. International journal of cancer Journal international du cancer. 2006 Sep 15;119(6):1322-1329.

[27] van der P, Vloedgraven H, Papapoulos S, Lowick C, Grzesik W, Kerr J, et al. Attachment characteristics and involvement of integrins in adhesion of breast cancer cell lines to extracellular bone matrix components. Laboratory investigation; a journal of technical methods and pathology. 1997 Dec;77(6):665-675.

[28] Zhang Z, Ramirez NE, Yankeelov TE, Li Z, Ford LE, Qi Y, et al. alpha2beta1 integrin expression in the tumor microenvironment enhances tumor angiogenesis in a tumor cell-specific manner. Blood. 2008 Feb 15;111(4):1980-1988.

[29] Knox JD, Cress AE, Clark V, Manriquez L, Affinito KS, Dalkin BL, et al. Differential expression of extracellular matrix molecules and the alpha 6-integrins in the normal and neoplastic prostate. Am J Pathol. 1994 Jul;145(1):167-174.

[30] Nagle RB, Hao J, Knox JD, Dalkin BL, Clark V, Cress AE. Expression of hemidesmosomal and extracellular matrix proteins by normal and malignant human prostate tissue. Am J Pathol. 1995 Jun;146(6):1498-507.

[31] Collins AT, Habib FK, Maitland NJ, Neal DE. Identification and isolation of human prostate epithelial stem cells based on alpha(2)beta(1)-integrin expression. Journal of cell science. 2001 Nov;114(Pt 21):3865-3872.

[32] Davis TL, Rabinovitz I, Futscher BW, Schnolzer M, Burger F, Liu Y, et al. Identification of a novel structural variant of the alpha 6 integrin. J Biol Chem. 2001 Jul 13;276(28):26099-26106.

[33] Bonkhoff H, Stein U, Remberger K. Differential expression of alpha 6 and alpha 2 very late antigen integrins in the normal, hyperplastic, and neoplastic prostate: simultaneous demonstration of cell surface receptors and their extracellular ligands. Human pathology. 1993 Mar;24(3):243-248.

[34] Van Slambrouck S, Jenkins AR, Romero AE, Steelant WF. Reorganization of the integrin alpha2 subunit controls cell adhesion and cancer cell invasion in prostate cancer. Int J Oncol. 2009 Jun;34(6):1717-1726.

[35] Hall CL, Dai J, van Golen KL, Keller ET, Long MW. Type I collagen receptor (alpha 2 beta 1) signaling promotes the growth of human prostate cancer cells within the bone. Cancer Res. 2006 Sep 1;66(17):8648-8654.

[36] Pontes-Junior J, Reis ST, de Oliveira LC, Sant'anna AC, Dall'oglio MF, Antunes AA, et al. Association between integrin expression and prognosis in localized prostate cancer. Prostate. 2010 Aug;70(11):1189-1195.

[37] Trikha M, Raso E, Cai Y, Fazakas Z, Paku S, Porter AT, et al. Role of alphaII(b)beta3 integrin in prostate cancer metastasis. Prostate. 1998 May 15;35(3):185-192.

[38] Stachurska A, Elbanowski J, Kowalczynska HM. The role of alpha5ss1 and alphavss3 integrins in relation to adhesion and spreading dynamics of prostate cancer cells interacting with fibronectin under in vitro conditions. Cell biology international. 2012 Jun 11:aheadofprint.

[39] Zheng DQ, Woodard AS, Fornaro M, Tallini G, Languino LR. Prostatic carcinoma cell migration via alpha(v)beta3 integrin is modulated by a focal adhesion kinase pathway. Cancer Res. 1999 Apr 1;59(7):1655-1664.

[40] Nemeth JA, Cher ML, Zhou Z, Mullins C, Bhagat S, Trikha M. Inhibition of alpha(v)beta3 integrin reduces angiogenesis, bone turnover, and tumor cell prolifera-

tion in experimental prostate cancer bone metastases. Clinical & experimental metastasis. 2003;20(5):413-420.

[41] Nagle RB, Knox JD, Wolf C, Bowden GT, Cress AE. Adhesion molecules, extracellular matrix, and proteases in prostate carcinoma. Journal of cellular biochemistry Supplement. 1994;19:232-237.

[42] Davis TL, Cress AE, Dalkin BL, Nagle RB. Unique expression pattern of the alpha6beta4 integrin and laminin-5 in human prostate carcinoma. Prostate. 2001 Feb 15;46(3):240-248.

[43] King TE, Pawar SC, Majuta L, Sroka IC, Wynn D, Demetriou MC, et al. The role of alpha 6 integrin in prostate cancer migration and bone pain in a novel xenograft model. PLoS One. 2008;3(10):3535-3542.

[44] Tomita K, van Bokhoven A, van Leenders GJ, Ruijter ET, Jansen CF, Bussemakers MJ, et al. Cadherin switching in human prostate cancer progression. Cancer Res. 2000 Jul 1;60(13):3650-3654.

[45] Umbas R, Schalken JA, Aalders TW, Carter BS, Karthaus HF, Schaafsma HE, et al. Expression of the cellular adhesion molecule E-cadherin is reduced or absent in high-grade prostate cancer. Cancer Res. 1992 Sep 15;52(18):5104-5109.

[46] Gould Rothberg BE, Bracken MB. E-cadherin immunohistochemical expression as a prognostic factor in infiltrating ductal carcinoma of the breast: a systematic review and meta-analysis. Breast cancer research and treatment. 2006 Nov;100(2):139-148.

[47] Chan AO, Lam SK, Wong BC, Kwong YL, Rashid A. Gene methylation in non-neoplastic mucosa of gastric cancer: age or Helicobacter pylori related? Am J Pathol. 2003 Jul;163(1):371-373.

[48] Dorudi S, Hanby AM, Poulsom R, Northover J, Hart IR. Level of expression of E-cadherin mRNA in colorectal cancer correlates with clinical outcome. British journal of cancer. 1995 Mar;71(3):614-616.

[49] Batlle E, Sancho E, Franci C, Dominguez D, Monfar M, Baulida J, et al. The transcription factor snail is a repressor of E-cadherin gene expression in epithelial tumour cells. Nature cell biology. 2000 Feb;2(2):84-89.

[50] Cano A, Perez-Moreno MA, Rodrigo I, Locascio A, Blanco MJ, del Barrio MG, et al. The transcription factor snail controls epithelial-mesenchymal transitions by repressing E-cadherin expression. Nature cell biology. 2000 Feb;2(2):76-83.

[51] Peinado H, Portillo F, Cano A. Transcriptional regulation of cadherins during development and carcinogenesis. The International journal of developmental biology. 2004;48(5-6):365-375.

[52] Blobe GC, Schiemann WP, Lodish HF. Role of transforming growth factor beta in human disease. The New England journal of medicine. 2000 May 4;342(18):1350-1358.

[53] Derynck R, Akhurst RJ, Balmain A. TGF-beta signaling in tumor suppression and cancer progression. Nature genetics. 2001 Oct;29(2):117-129.

[54] Nakao A, Imamura T, Souchelnytskyi S, Kawabata M, Ishisaki A, Oeda E, et al. TGF-beta receptor-mediated signalling through Smad2, Smad3 and Smad4. The EMBO journal. 1997 Sep 1;16(17):5353-5362.

[55] Comijn J, Berx G, Vermassen P, Verschueren K, van Grunsven L, Bruyneel E, et al. The two-handed E box binding zinc finger protein SIP1 downregulates E-cadherin and induces invasion. Molecular cell. 2001 Jun;7(6):1267-1278.

[56] Postigo AA, Depp JL, Taylor JJ, Kroll KL. Regulation of Smad signaling through a differential recruitment of coactivators and corepressors by ZEB proteins. The EMBO journal. 2003 May 15;22(10):2453-2462.

[57] Verschueren K, Remacle JE, Collart C, Kraft H, Baker BS, Tylzanowski P, et al. SIP1, a novel zinc finger/homeodomain repressor, interacts with Smad proteins and binds to 5'-CACCT sequences in candidate target genes. J Biol Chem. 1999 Jul 16;274(29): 20489-20498.

[58] Miyaki M, Iijima T, Konishi M, Sakai K, Ishii A, Yasuno M, et al. Higher frequency of Smad4 gene mutation in human colorectal cancer with distant metastasis. Oncogene. 1999 May 20;18(20):3098-3103.

[59] Ackland ML, Newgreen DF, Fridman M, Waltham MC, Arvanitis A, Minichiello J, et al. Epidermal growth factor-induced epithelio-mesenchymal transition in human breast carcinoma cells. Laboratory investigation; a journal of technical methods and pathology. 2003 Mar;83(3):435-448.

[60] Koenig A, Mueller C, Hasel C, Adler G, Menke A. Collagen type I induces disruption of E-cadherin-mediated cell-cell contacts and promotes proliferation of pancreatic carcinoma cells. Cancer Res. 2006 May 1;66(9):4662-4671.

[61] Shintani Y, Fukumoto Y, Chaika N, Svoboda R, Wheelock MJ, Johnson KR. Collagen I-mediated up-regulation of N-cadherin requires cooperative signals from integrins and discoidin domain receptor 1. The Journal of cell biology. 2008 Mar 24;180(6): 1277-1289.

[62] Alexander NR, Tran NL, Rekapally H, Summers CE, Glackin C, Heimark RL. N-cadherin gene expression in prostate carcinoma is modulated by integrin-dependent nuclear translocation of Twist1. Cancer Res. 2006 Apr 1;66(7):3365-3369.

[63] Dumont N, Arteaga CL. Transforming growth factor-beta and breast cancer: Tumor promoting effects of transforming growth factor-beta. Breast cancer research : BCR. 2000;2(2):125-132.

[64] Bates RC, Bellovin DI, Brown C, Maynard E, Wu B, Kawakatsu H, et al. Transcriptional activation of integrin beta6 during the epithelial-mesenchymal transition defines a novel prognostic indicator of aggressive colon carcinoma. J Clin Invest. 2005 Feb;115(2):339-347.

[65] Bhowmick NA, Zent R, Ghiassi M, McDonnell M, Moses HL. Integrin beta 1 signaling is necessary for transforming growth factor-beta activation of p38MAPK and epithelial plasticity. J Biol Chem. 2001 Dec 14;276(50):46707-46713.

[66] Haraguchi M, Okubo T, Miyashita Y, Miyamoto Y, Hayashi M, Crotti TN, et al. Snail regulates cell-matrix adhesion by regulation of the expression of integrins and basement membrane proteins. J Biol Chem. 2008 Aug 29;283(35):23514-23523.

[67] Neal CL, McKeithen D, Odero-Marah VA. Snail negatively regulates cell adhesion to extracellular matrix and integrin expression via the MAPK pathway in prostate cancer cells. Cell Adh Migr. 2011 May-Jun;5(3):249-257.

[68] Drake JM, Barnes JM, Madsen JM, Domann FE, Stipp CS, Henry MD. ZEB1 coordinately regulates laminin-332 and {beta}4 integrin expression altering the invasive phenotype of prostate cancer cells. J Biol Chem. 2010 Oct 29;285(44):33940-33948.

[69] Nam EH, Lee Y, Park YK, Lee JW, Kim S. ZEB2 upregulates integrin alpha5 expression through cooperation with Sp1 to induce invasion during epithelial-mesenchymal transition of human cancer cells. Carcinogenesis. 2012 Mar;33(3):563-571.

[70] McNeel DG, Eickhoff J, Lee FT, King DM, Alberti D, Thomas JP, et al. Phase I trial of a monoclonal antibody specific for alphavbeta3 integrin (MEDI-522) in patients with advanced malignancies, including an assessment of effect on tumor perfusion. Clinical cancer research : an official journal of the American Association for Cancer Research. 2005 Nov 1;11(21):7851-7860.

[71] Trikha M, Zhou Z, Nemeth JA, Chen Q, Sharp C, Emmell E, et al. CNTO 95, a fully human monoclonal antibody that inhibits alphav integrins, has antitumor and antiangiogenic activity in vivo. International journal of cancer Journal international du cancer. 2004 Jun 20;110(3):326-335.

[72] Bradley DA, Daignault S, Ryan CJ, Dipaola RS, Cooney KA, Smith DC, et al. Cilengitide (EMD 121974, NSC 707544) in asymptomatic metastatic castration resistant prostate cancer patients: a randomized phase II trial by the prostate cancer clinical trials consortium. Invest New Drugs. 2011 Dec;29(6):1432-1440.

[73] Alva A, Slovin S, Daignault S, Carducci M, Dipaola R, Pienta K, et al. Phase II study of cilengitide (EMD 121974, NSC 707544) in patients with non-metastatic castration resistant prostate cancer, NCI-6735. A study by the DOD/PCF prostate cancer clinical trials consortium. Invest New Drugs. 2012 Apr;30(2):749-757.

Chapter 26

The Role of E-Cadherin-Catenin Complex in Prostate Cancer Progression

Anuradha K. Murali and James S. Norris

Additional information is available at the end of the chapter

http://dx.doi.org/10.5772/52751

1. Introduction

The genetic changes that promote progression of prostate adenocarcinomas are multifactorial and include alterations in several genes. The aberrations include those in genes that affect normal cell adhesion. The long arm of chromosome 16 (16q22.1) is deleted in 30% of primary prostatic tumors and more than 70% of metastatic prostate cancers. The E-cadherin gene is located in this region. E-cadherin is involved in maintaining homotypic cell-cell adhesion between normal prostatic glandular cells. The loss of E-cadherin expression is associated with metastatic progression of prostate cancer (Mason, 2002). Recent data suggests that abnormal expression of E-cadherin, leading to impaired adhesion, correlates with hematogenous spread of primary tumor cells in prostate cancer patients (Loric, 2001). The study further suggests that abnormal E-cadherin expression is a significant independent indicator of prostate cancer recurrence in patients.

Metastatic dissemination of prostate cancer cells occurs via the lymphatic system as well as the vascular system. This complex process of metastasis involves a series of steps starting with neoplastic transformation of prostate cells, tumor angiogenesis/lymphogenesis and cancer growth, loss of cell adhesion molecules and detachment of cancer cells from primary tumor, local invasion of stroma, dissemination of primary tumor cells via the lymphatics or vasculature, avoidance of tumor surveillance by the immune system, homing of primary prostate cancer cells to distant sites, establishment of tumor and growth of tumor at distant metastatic site (Arya et al., 2006). While the majority of metastic lesions are found in the obturator lymph nodes, lesions have also been detected in presacral, presciatic, as well as internal and external iliac nodes. Conversely, hematogenous spread of prostate cancer cells results in the formation of metastatic lesions in the bone, lung, liver and epidural space. Interestingly, in the majority of patients who die from prostate cancer, metastatic lesions have been detected in the bone. One study shows that E-cadherin and β-catenin are downregulated in prostatic bone metastasis, but not in primary prostate tumors (Arya et al., 2006). The spine, femur, pelvis, rib cage, skull and humerus are frequent sites of metastatic prostate cancer lesions. The bone stroma apparently provides a microenvironment suitable for the growth of metastatic prostate cancer cells. While the molecular mechanisms associated with prostate cancer metastasis are not completely elucidated, potential markers of high-risk prostate cancer include the cadherins, catenins, focal adhesin kinase, connexins, integrins and metalloproteinases (Mol et al., 2007).

The E-cadherin-catenin complex and associated proteins have functional roles in cell-adhesion as well as in downstream signaling. It is well known that increased expression of cytoplasmic β-catenin is associated with increased translocation to the nucleus leading to transcriptional activation of β-catenin-TCF responsive genes. β-catenin, γ-catenin and $p120^{ctn}$ proteins are expressed in the nucleus, thereby suggesting that a complex system of checks and balances may exist in normal as well as in tumor cells.

2. Classical cadherins, type I

2.1. E-cadherin

The tight association of individual cells at junctional organelles and the polarized distribution of cytoplasmic and cell surface-components are the primary characteristics of normal epithelial tissues. As a result of this adhesion, normal epithelial cells are less mobile as compared to either cells of mesenchymal origin or to cancer cells of epithelial origin. Normal epithelial cells also have the ability to form selective permeability barriers, and to exhibit vectorial transport in tissues. Four organelles (tight junctions, desmosomes, gap junctions, zonula adherens junctions) are responsible for adhesion between two adjacent cells. In addition, distinct proteins are associated with each of these types of intracellular junctions, suggesting a specific role of each junction in normal cellular processes. First are the tight junctions, which have dual functions: maintenance of cell polarity and inhibition of uncontrolled exchange of small molecules, macromolecules, and water between two adjacent cells. Occludin and ZO-1 protein complexes are typically found in tight junctions in epithelial and endothelial cells (Schnittler et al., 1998). Second, desmosomes typify cells that have undergone epithelial differentiation. Desmosomes function in homophilic adhesion between adjacent cells and link desmosomal proteins to the cytoskeletal proteins called intermediate-sized filaments (Ifs). Desmoglein and desmocollin are pivotal components of desmosomal function (Schafer et al., 1996; Mertens et al., 1999). Third, gap junctions form intracellular channels that allow direct transfer of ions and metabolites. Connexin proteins form these gap junction channels (Dermietzel and Hofstadter, 1998; Windoffer et al., 2000). Zonula adherens junctions, the fourth type of organelles, are specialized structures containing the cell adhesion molecule E-cadherin.

The human E-cadherin gene, CDH1, is located on chromosome 16q22.1 (Rimm et al., 1994). It encodes a 135 kDa precursor form of E-cadherin. In essence, the precursor form cannot function in homophilic adhesion without undergoing N-terminal cleavage. The precursor E-cadherin protein is cleaved in the cytoplasm to form a mature 120 kDa protein containing the newly formed extracellular N-terminal domain. The extracellular domain or N-terminal end of E-cadherin is essential for homophilic calcium-dependent cell-cell adhesion. The mature form of E-cadherin, on the other hand, is transported to the basolateral surface of the epithelial cell where it can function in homophilic adhesion.

The mature E-cadherin contains three distinct domains: the highly conserved carboxy-terminal domain, a single pass transmembrane domain, and an extracellular domain (Figure 1). The extracellular domain consists of five tandem subdomain repeats that bind calcium, referred to as C1-C5 subdomains with the C1 domain being the most distal from the cell membrane. The C1 subdomain contains a histidine-alanine-valine sequence (HAV) that is speculated to be essential for the process of cell-cell adhesion. E-cadherin exists as a *cis* dimer on an individual cell when it is not adhering to an adjacent cell. Subsequent to calcium binding, a conformational change occurs in the HAV structure of the C1 subdomain, allowing the tryptophan-2 residue to move into a hydrophobic cavity. This conformational change allows E-cadherin to form a trans dimer 'zipper' between two adjacent cells. Subsequent linkage to the cytoskeleton stabilizes cell-cell adhesion. The cytoplasmic domain of E-cadherin is required for cadherin-catenin complex formation. The cytoplasmic tail of E-cadherin consists of two regions: the juxtamembrane region and the catenin-binding region. These regions are principally required for clustering of E-cadherin at cell-cell contacts (juxtamembrane) and as a major link to the actin cytoskeleton. These regions are known to stabilize E-cadherin clusters and participate in signal transduction processes via the catenin-binding region. The thirty-two amino acid, hydrophobic transmembrane region separates the extracellular domain from the highly conserved intracellular domain.

E-cadherin forms a complex with four catenin proteins, α-catenin (102 kDa), β-catenin (92 kDa), γ-catenin (83 kDa) and p120 catenin (75-120 kDa). The interaction of E-cadherin with cytoplasmic catenins, α, β, γ and p120 ($p120^{ctn}$) is required for the normal function of E-cadherin. The human genes for all four cadherin-associated catenins have been cloned and characterized; the genes are located on four different chromosomes. While α-Catenin is located on chromosome 5q31, β-catenin is located on chromosome 3p21, γ-catenin on chromosome 17q21, and $p120^{ctn}$ on chromosome 11q11 immediately adjacent to the centromere. All four catenins bind to E-cadherin, but exist as two distinct pools of E-cadherin-catenin complexes in the same cell. E-cadherin binds to either β-catenin or γ-catenin, but does not directly bind to α-catenin. α-catenin, however, binds to either β-catenin or γ-catenin. Therefore, in a single cell, one complex consists of E-cadherin with α− and β-catenin, and the other complex consists of E-cadherin with α and γ-catenin. E-cadherin-catenin complex formation begins shortly after biosynthesis, while still in the endoplasmic reticulum. The sequential order of cadherin-catenin complex formation begins with β-catenin interacting with E-cadherin. If E-cadherin fails to associate with β-catenin, E-cadherin is retained in the endoplasmic reticulum where it is subsequently degraded. A 30 amino-acid region within the cytoplasmic domain of E-cadherin is essential for β-catenin binding. E-cadherin and β-catenin are transported together in a bipartite fashion to the cell surface, where they associate with α-catenin.

The amino-terminal region of α-catenin binds to actin filaments in the cytoplasm, linking the cadherin-catenin complex to the cytoskeleton. Post-translational modification of $p120^{ctn}$ is associated with modulation of cadherin clustering and stablization of adhesion.In summary, a functional cadherin-catenin complex is important for maintaining cellular integrity.

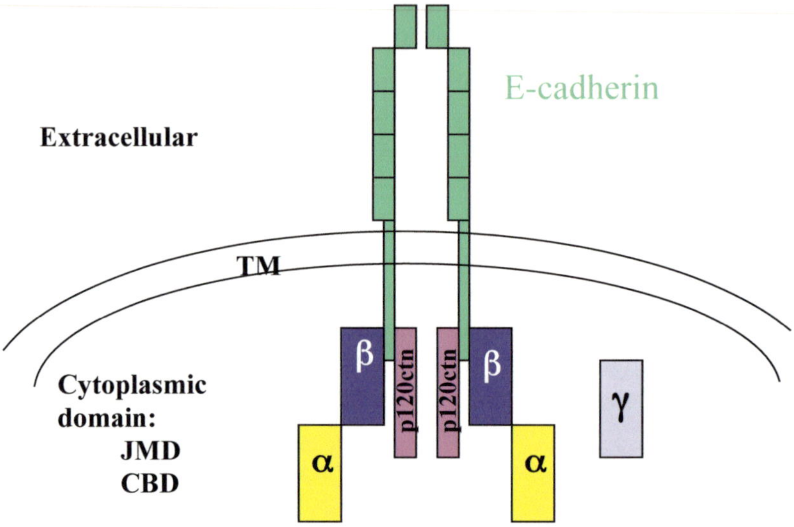

Figure 1. Schematic diagram of E-cadherin-catenin complex. The mature E-cadherin contains three distinct domains: the highly conserved cytoplasmic domain, a single pass transmembrane domain (TM), and an extracellular domain. The cytoplasmic tail of E-cadherin consists of two regions: the juxtamembrane domain (JMD) and the catenin-binding domain (CBD). β- and γ-Catenin bind to the CBD, and $p120^{ctn}$ binds to the JMD regions of E-cadherin. These regions are principally required for clustering of E-cadherin at cell-cell contact and as a major link to the actin cytoskeleton. E-cadherin forms a complex with four catenin proteins, α-catenin (102 kDa), β-catenin (92 kDa), γ-catenin (83 kDa), and p120 catenin (75-120 kDa). α, α-catenin; β, β-catenin; γ, γ-catenin; $p120^{ctn}$, p120 catenin.

2.2. Role of Cadherin in physiological and pathological processes

E-cadherin expression is regulated in both physiological and pathological processes, such as embryonic morphogenesis and tumorigenesis. Tissue and organ formation is regulated in a spatio-temporal manner involving cell proliferation, death, cell-cell adhesion, cell-substrate adhesion, polarization, and migration. One example of this highly regulated process is blastocyst differentiation. E-Cadherin has an essential function in the formation of the blastocyst during mouse embryonic development. Another example of the normal physiological processes associated with E-cadherin regulation is the formation of fluid space in development of murine cochlea. In this embryonic process, E-cadherin is downregulated on the lateral membranes of reticular lamina. This down-regulation allows the process of fluid space opening in the organ of Corti. Wound healing is a third example where a physiological event involves regulation of E-cadherin expression. Injury of the epithelial cell layer in the skin signals the release of cytokines and other factors, such as epidermal growth factor (EGF). These signals reduce cell adhesion and stimulate cell motility, allowing for wound re-

http://dx.doi.org/10.5772/52751

pair. Subsequent to wound repair, cell adhesion is upregulated to restore the epithelial layer to its normal physiological state. Therefore, E-cadherin has to be highly regulated in the above normal physiological processes. Conversely, aberrant growth and differentiation result when E-cadherin is not tightly regulated, such as in cancer.

Association of E-cadherin with neighboring cells acts to inhibit cell mobility and to maintain normal epithelial cell phenotype. Tumorigenesis is an example of a pathological process that involves E-cadherin regulation. The loss or down-regulation of E-cadherin expression has been described in several tumors including stomach (Shino 1995; Tamura, 2000), colon (Van Aken, 1993; Dorudi, 1993), pancreas (Pignatelli, 1994), liver (Joo, 2002), prostate (Morton et al., 1993; Umbas et al., 1994; Ross et al., 1994; Bussemakers et al, 1994; Pan et al., 1998; Noe et al., 1999; Cheng et al., 1996), breast (Lim and Lee, 2002; Hiraguri et al, 1998; Moll et al., 1993; Palacios et al., 1995; Gamallo et al., 1993; Oka et al., 1993; Rasbridge et al., 1993; De Leeuw et al., 1997), uterus (Sakuragi et al., 1994), ovary (Veatch et al., 1994), thyroid (Brabant et al., 1993), and head and neck (Mattijssen et al., 1993). Recent reports suggest that poorly differentiated tumors exhibit reduced E-cadherin expression as a consequence of down-regulation or defects in catenins (Kadowaki et al., 1994; Kawanishi et al., 1995; Navarro et al., 1993; Oyama et al., 1994). Therefore, the results from these studies suggest that the degree of differentiation of tumors is related to the level of E-cadherin expression.

E-cadherin acts as an inhibitor of the invasive and metastatic phenotype of cancer cells. Since tumor invasion and metastasis is a multistep process, E-caderin may play a significant role in regulating invasion and metastasis at the initial steps in the process by promoting homotypic cell-cell adhesion. Numerous mechanisms affecting E-cadheirn-catenin complex formation are associated with a reduction in cell adhesion. While gene mutation is responsible for inactivating E-cadherin-mediated cell adhesion in some breast cancers and gastric adenocarcinomas (Berx et al., 1998a; Berx et al., 1998b), the exact mechanism of E-cadherin down-regulation in other highly invasive tumors is still under investigation. Mechanisms that regulate homophilic cell adhesion include reduction or loss of E-cadherin expression, reduced transcription of genes encoding catenin proteins, redistribution of E-cadherin to different sites within the cell, shedding of E-cadherin, cleavage of E-cadherin, and competition of proteins for binding sites on E-cadherin (Cavallaro and Christofori, 2004).

The proximal E-cadherin promoter contains multiple regulatory elements including three E-boxes, a single CCAAT box, and a GC-rich element. Therefore, the E-cadherin promoter contains more than one site for transcription factors to bind and regulate gene transcription in cancers. These factors include AP-2 (Batsche et al., 1998), SNAIL (Battle et al., 2000), SLUG (Hajra et al., 2002), dEF1/ZEB-1 (Grooteclaes and Frisch, 2000), SIP1/ZEB-2 (Comijn et al., 2001), E12/E47 (Perez-Moreno et al., 2001), and LEF/TCF (Huber et al., 1996). While the retinoblastoma gene and c-myc protooncogene products transactivate the E-cadherin promoter in epithelial cells through interaction with AP-2 transcription factors (Batsche et al., 1998), transcription of E-cadherin is down-regulated by overexpression of ErbB2 (D'Souza and Taylor-Papadimitriou, 1994). SNAIL and SLUG transcription factors have been shown to repress E-cadherin expression in breast cancer cell lines via all three

E-box elements, but particularly, via EboxA and EboxC, located in the proximal E-cadherin promoter (Hajra et al., 2002). Moreover, SLUG is a putative *in vivo* repressor of E-cadherin in breast cancer (Hajra et al., 2002). The E-cadherin promoter also contains binding sites for the lymphoid enhancer factor 1 (LEF1)-β-catenin transcription factor complex; this complex down-regulates E-cadherin expression (Huber et al., 1998). Overexpression of integrin-linked protein kinase ($p59^{ilk}$) stimulates LEF1-β-catenin signaling and causes down-regulation of E-cadherin expression with a concomitant decrease in cell adhesion (Novak et al., 1998). A single nucleotide polymorphism in the E-cadherin promoter has also been associated with a higher risk of prostate cancer in certain ethnic populations with a possible role in transcriptional regulation of E-cadherin gene expression in these individuals (Goto et al., 2007).

Gene transcription can also be regulated by epigenetic inactivation. Many cancer cells have been shown to use this mechanism to inactivate tumor-suppressor genes (Sidransky, 2002). Methylation of genes that encode p16 (cyclin-dependent kinase inhibitor), DAPK (death-associated protein kinase, apoptosis associated protein), and MGMT (a DNA repair protein, methyl O-guanine methyltransferase) has been implicated in lung, and head and neck cancer (Esteller et al., 1999; Sanchez-Cespedes et al., 2000). Aberrant methylation of the hMLH1 promoter has also been associated with microsatellite instability in colon cancer (Grady et al., 2001). Methylation of APC (Usadel et al., 2002), a key component in Wnt-β-catenin signaling, is associated with early-stage lung cancer and esophageal cancer (Kawakami, 2000). E-cadherin expression is downregulated in highly invasive prostate tumors as a result of transcriptional regulation (Morton et al., 1993; Kuczyk et al, 1998). Reduction in E-cadherin expression in prostate cancer cells has been attributed to hypermethylation of CpG islands in the E-cadherin gene promoter (Graff et al., 1995; Graff et al., 1997; Herman et al., 1996; Hirohashi, 1998; Li et al., 2001). This type of silencing of E-cadherin gene expression is also seen in cervical cancer cell lines and tumors (Chen et al., 2003). In summary, epigenetic inactivation of genes is an alternative mechanism used to regulate expression of certain genes in cancer cells. The significance and mechanism of gene inactivations associated with prostate cancer cell invasion remain to be determined.

Post-translational modification is an alternative mechanism to regulate E-cadherin-dependent homophilic cell adhesion (Hirohashi, 1998). Protein tyrosine kinases (PTKs) and phosphatases (PTPs), regulate intracellular phosphotyrosine levels, thereby regulating diverse cellular behaviors such as adhesion, growth and differentiation, and migration. Her2/Neu or ErbB2 tyrosine kinase, as well as transmembrane tyrosine phosphatases such as PTPμ, PTPκ, PTPλ and LAR, have been found to be associated with cadherin-catenin complexes in epithelial cells, suggesting opposing roles for these proteins in regulating cadherin-catenin association (Hellberg et al., 2002). Stimulation of growth factor receptors, i.e. EGF receptor (EGFR), can also regulate E-cadherin expression in tumor cells in a post-translational manner (Hazan and Norton, 1998; Moustafa et al, 1999). A reciprocal and reversible control of intercellular adhesion and cell proliferation occurs with increased expression of EGFR in several epithelial tumors (Jawhari et al, 1999). Restoration of E-cadherin expression in human papilloma virus-transfected keratinocytes reversed the invasive phenotype and, interestingly, down-regulated EGFR expression (Wilding et al., 1996). An inverse relationship between EGFR activation and E-cadherin expression was also observed in lung cancer cells treated with neutralizing monoclonal antibody to EGFR (Moustafa et al., 1999). By blocking EGFR stimulation in lung cancer cells, E-cadherin expression is induced. Activation of Src can also induce tyrosine phosphorylation of E-cadherin and inhibit cell-cell adhesion. As a result of Src activation, the E-cadherin complex is ubiquitinated, leading to its endocytosis and thereby inhibiting homophilic cell adhesion (Fujita et al., 2002). Either transcriptional or post-translational modification of the cadherin-catenin complex can determine the integrity of the adherens junction, as well as regulating downstream signaling.

3. E-cadherin associated catenin proteins

3.1. α-catenin

The α-catenin gene encodes a 102kDa protein that links E-cadherin to the actin cytoskeleton. The amino terminus of α-catenin contains the actin-binding domain essential for linking the cadherin-catenin complex to the cytoskeleton (Beavon, 2000). The cytoplasmic components of the adherens junctions are necessary for linking cadherins to actin (Takeichi, 1991). The association of cadherins with the cytoskeleton is mediated via either α-actinin (Nieset et al., 1997; Knudsen et al., 1995) or vinculin (Hazan et al., 1997a; Weiss et al., 1998; Watabe-Uchida, 1998). α-Catenin is also known to interact with ZO-1 (Itoh et al., 1997). α-catenin associates with either β-catenin or γ-catenin in adherens junctions, but does not form a complex in desmosomes where γ-catenin is bound to desmosomal cadherins and desmoplakin, another desmosomal protein. Therefore, α-catenin links E-cadherin-catenin proteins to the cytoskeleton at adherens junctions, but not at desmosomes. This would suggest that α-cateinin may contribute to the stability of the E-cadherin-catenin complex in normal tissues. Recent studies have suggested that α-catenin is the best prognostic marker for prostate cancer specific survival (van Oort et al., 2007).

3.2. β-catenin

β-catenin is a 92 kDa multifunctional protein that belongs to the armadillo family of proteins, characterized by a central domain of 12 repeats of about 40 amino acids called arm repeats (Figure 2). The arm domain was originally described in armadillo, which is the *Drosophila* homologue of β-catenin (Kodama et al., 1999). β-catenin serves as a link between cadherins and the actin cytoskeleton. β-catenin also binds to numerous other proteins in cadherin-independent complexes (Behrens, 2002) such as APC, lymphoid enhancer factor and T-cell factor (LEF/TCF) transcription factors, RGS domain proteins axin/conductin (Kikuchi, 1999; Kikuchi, 2000; Von Kries et al., 2000; Akiyama, 2000) and prontin 52 (Bauer et al, 1998). β-catenin also associates with fascin, an actin-binding protein, in a cadherin independent manner (Tao et al., 1996).

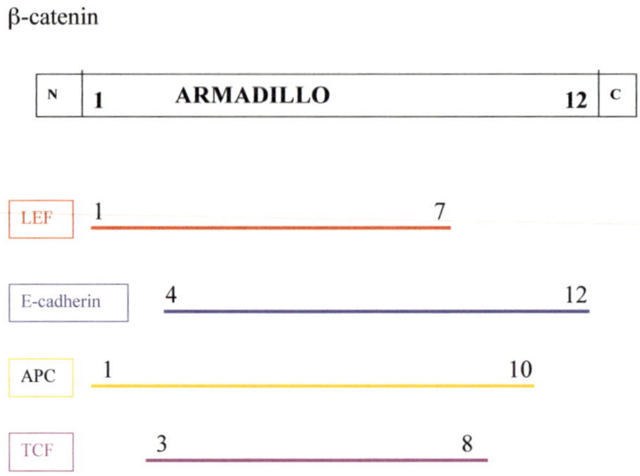

Figure 2. Diagram of the twelve armadillo repeats of β-catenin. The β-catenin protein consists of 12 armadillo repeats designated as 1-12. β-Catenin associates with specific proteins within the indicated region of the 12 repeats, in a mutually exclusive manner. Armadillo repeats 1-7 is designated as the LEF binding region; E-cadherin binds to repeats 4-12; APC binds to repeats 1-10; Tcf binds to repeats 3-8 of the β-catenin protein. Armadillo protein 12 has been shown to be involved in transactivation of Wnt-responsive genes. N, N-terminus; C, Carboxy-terminus; LEF, lymphoid enhancer-binding factor ; APC, adenomatous polyposis coli; TCF, T-cell Transcription factor.

In addition to its role in cell-adhesion, β-catenin is associated with Wnt signal transduction pathway (Figure 3). This pathway is important in regulating embryonic development, and generation of cell polarity. Wnt proteins are differentially expressed in tissues during mammalian development (Cadigan and Nusse, 1997). These proteins are particularly important in regulating tissue differentiation and organogenesis (Behrens, 2002; Parr and McMahon, 1994; Willert and Nusse, 1998; Brown and Moon, 1998; Bullions and Levine, 1998). When Wnt proteins are aberrantly activated, tumor formation ensues (Moon and Kimelman, 1998; Zeng et al., 1997; Wodarz and Nusse, 1998; Peifer and Polakis, 2000; Bienz and Clevers, 2000; Barker and Clevers, 2000). Wnt has also been demonstrated to play a role in cancer development by transmitting a signal via its cytoplasmic component, β-catenin protein (Lejeune et al., 1995; Shimizu et al., 1997; Polakis, 2001; Polakis, 2000; Polakis 1999; Eastman and Grosschedl, 1999; Cadigan and Nusse, 1997). Recent studies have suggested that Wnt proteins may have a role in tumor-induced osteoblastic activity, which is characterized by increased bone production as a result of prostate caner metastasis to the bone (Hall et al., 2006). Wnt proteins bind to cell surface receptors termed Frizzled (Fz). This interaction results in the activation of the cytoplasmic phosphoprotein disheveled (Dvl). Activated Dvl inhibits activation of axin and conductin proteins in the Wnt signaling cascade. Axin and its homolog, conductin (Axin2/Axil) form a multiprotein complex with APC and GSK3β; this activated complex catalyzes the phoshphorylation of β-catenin at specific residues in its N-terminal domain (Behrens, 2002; Ikeda et al., 1998). Axin and conductin act as scaffold proteins that directly bind several components of the Wnt signaling pathway, promoting the phosphorylation of β-catenin by GSK-3β (Jho et al., 2002; Ikeda et al., 1998; Fagotto et al., 1999; Itoh et al., 1998; Hsu et al., 1999; Julius et al., 2000). Four ser/thr residues in the N-terminal region of β-catenin are targets for GSK-3β phosphorylation. In the absence of a Wnt signal, GSK3β phosphorylates β-catenin, which is then targeted for ubiquitination and subsequently degraded by proteasomes. Interestingly, recent studies show that additional proteins are involved in priming β-catenin for phosphorylation by GSK3β. Casein kinase I, Casein kinase II and GSK3β act together in marking β-catenin for phosphorylation (Polakis, 2002; Amit et al., 2002; Liu et al., 2002; Yanagawa e al., 2002; Zhang et al., 2002).

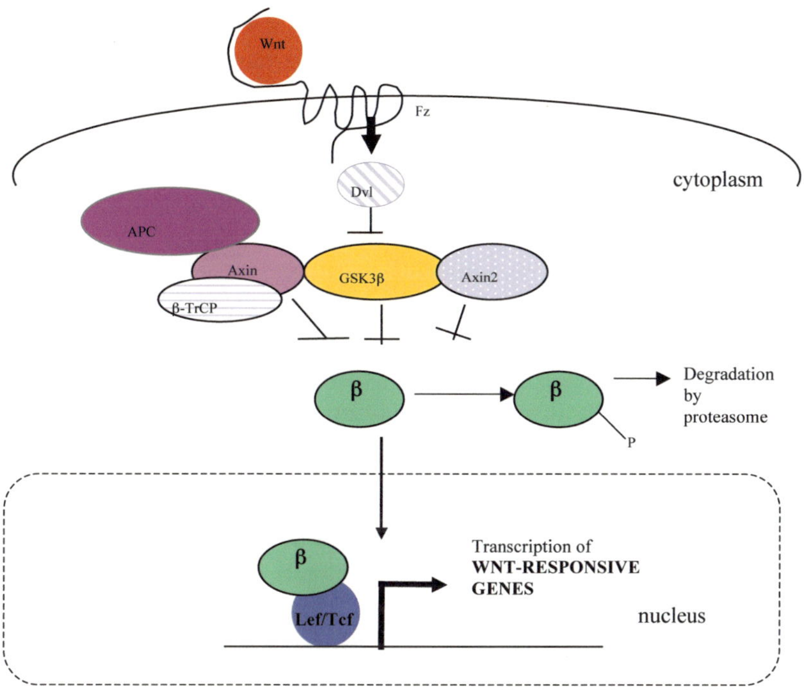

Figure 3. Diagram of Wnt signaling pathway. This schematic represents the Wnt-mediated signaling pathway that functions to stabilize cytoplasmic β-catenin. In the absence of Wnt signaling, β-catenin is degraded by the activity of glycogen synthase kinase 3β (GSK3β) in a complex with APC, axin, axin2 (conductin/Axil), and β-TrCP. The binding of Wnt proteins to its receptor, Frizzled (Fz) at the cell surface leads to the activation of Disheveled (Dvl) in the cytoplasm. Subsequently, GSK3β complex is inactivated and β-catenin accumulates in the cytoplasm, then enters the nucleus to interact with LEF/TCF proteins. β-Catenin-Tcf transcription factor activates the expression of Wnt responsive genes.

Regulation of β-catenin degradation is pivotal in downstream signaling. Several gene mutations have been reported in human cancers that render β-catenin resistant to GSK-3β mediated degradation. First, mutations in APC, a suppressor in human cancers, are associated with aberrant expression of β-catenin in colon cancers (Kawahara et al., 2000; Bienz and Clevers, 2000; Polakis 2000; Bright-Thomas and Hargest, 2002; Kawasaki et al., 2003). Second, oncogenic mutations have been identified in β-catenin at putative GSK-3β phosphorylation sites, which stabilize β-catenin in colorectal cancer and melanoma (Van Noort et al., 2002, Morin et al., 1997 and Korinek et al., 1997). Third, a mutation in human AXIN1 has been found to be associated with hepatocellular carcinoma (Satoh et al., 2000), while a mutation in AXIN2 (also called conductin) is found in colorectal and liver cancers

(Liu et al., 2000; Lustig et al., 2002). Conversely, constitutive Wnt signaling negatively regulates the ubiquitination and degradation of cytosolic β-catenin leading to its stabilization. In summary, stabilization of β-catenin in the cytosol is altered by three independent mechanisms: 1) gene mutation of any one of the degradation complex components: APC, axin, axin2 or GSK-3β, 2) gene mutation of β-catenin, or 3) constitutive Wnt signaling. As a result, the level of cytosolic β-catenin increases, and β-catenin translocates to the nucleus where it interacts with transcription factors of the LEF/TCF family. Several negative feedback loops could limit the duration or intensity of a Wnt-initiated signal. First, the F-box protein β-TrCP is an ubiquitin-ligase complex that has been shown to be involved in the proteasome mediated degradation of phosphorylated β-catenin (Chen et al., 1997; Behrens, 2002; Winston et al., 1999, Hart et al., 1999; Latres et al., 1999; Kitagawa et al., 1999). β-TrCP is post-transcriptionally induced by β-catenin/TCF signaling. As a result of this signal, β-catenin degradation is accelerated. Second, Tcf4/β-catenin signaling regulates transcription of the *Tcf1* gene in epithelial cells. While TCF1 does not bind β-catenin, TCF1 binds to transcriptional repressors such as groucho, which would allow TCF1 to serve as a feedback repressor of β-catenin/Tcf4 target genes (Roose et al., 1999; Polakis 2002). Third, axin2 (conductin) appears to downregulate β-catenin to normal levels after a Wnt signal in a negative feedback loop mechanism (Jho et al., 2002; Leung et al., 2002). This would suggest that, without precise regulation of Wnt-initiated signaling, β-catenin is aberrantly expressed. As a result, downstream target genes that might contribute to tumorigenesis are either up- or downregulated.

Increased concentration of β-catenin in the cytoplasm promotes its binding to LEF/TCF family of DNA-binding proteins. As a result, β-catenin translocates to the nucleus where it transcriptionally activates specific target genes. Although the exact mechanism of nuclear translocation of β-catenin has not been elucidated, association of β-catenin with several nuclear transport proteins, including importin/karyopherin and Ran (Wiechens and Fagotto, 2001; Fagotto et al., 1998), is not responsible. β-catenin lacks a classical nuclear localization sequence, but the armadillo repeats at the C-terminus are essential for nuclear translocation (Figure 2; Giannini et al., 2000; Funayama et al., 1995). Recent studies have suggested that, in prostate cancer cells, β-catenin can translocate into the nucleus as part of a complex with androgen receptor, AR, (Mulholland et al., 2002). This association of β-catenin with the androgen receptor is abrogated in the absence of armadillo repeat 6, further supporting the association of certain armadillo repeats with specific β-catenin functions. Armadillo repeats 4-12 are required for β-catenin to bind to E-cadherin (Hulsken et al., 1994; Orsulic 1996; Piedra et al., 2001). The expression of cadherin proteins could thus sequester β-catenin to the plasma membrane, preventing its nuclear translocation (Heasman et al., 1994; Fagotto et al., 1996; Weng et al., 2002). In the absence of sequestering proteins, β-catenin co-localizes with LEF/TCF in the nucleus to transactivate specific genes that contain LEF/TCF binding sites.

LEF-1 and TCF1-4 were first identified in immune cells (Clevers and van De Wetering, 1997). LEF-1 is a sequence-specific DNA-binding protein that is expressed in pre-B and pre-T lymphocytes of adult mice as well as in the neural crest, mesencephalon, tooth germs and whisker follicles (Van Genderen et al., 1994). In addition to its role in organogenesis and embryogenesis, constitutive LEF/TCF/β-catenin transactivation is associated with oncogenesis in human colon carcinomas and melanomas (Korinek et al., 1997; Morin et al., 1997; Rubinfeld et al., 1997; Aoki et al., 1999). Although LEF/TCFs can bind directly to DNA through their HMG or DNA-binding domain, they are incapable of independently activating gene transcription (Polakis 2000; Polakis 2002, Behrens, 2002; Jiang and Struhl,1998; Kiatagawa et al., 1999; Hecht et al., 1999; Eastman and Grosschedl, 1999; Roose et al., 1999). Specific regions of β-catenin are required to interact with either LEF or TCF proteins. Armadillo repeats 1-7 of β-catenin interact with LEF while armadillo repeats 3-8 interact with TCF (Fig 1-3; Piedra et al., 2001; Sadot 1998; Behrens et al., 1996; Van de Wetering, 1997). β-catenin forms a complex with LEF/TCF proteins, depending on the amount of free β-catenin available. In this complex, LEF/TCF provides the DNA binding domain while β-catenin provides the transactivation domain. β-catenin binds specifically to sequences 1-51 of Tcf-4 (Miravet et al., 2002). Activation of this transcriptional complex between β-catenin and Tcf induces the expression of specific target genes (Mizushima et al., 2002; Behrens, 2002; Polakis 2002). Examples of these genes include ultrabithorax in *Drosophila,* nodal related 3 (McKendry et al., 1997), and siamois in *Xenopus* (Brannon et al., 1997), and c-myc (He 1998; Kolligs et al., 2000) and cyclin D1 (Tetsu and McCormick, 1999; Shtutman et al., 1999) in mammals. The list of target genes also include genes that regulate cellular functions other than stimulating cell growth, such as cyclooxygenase-2 (Howe et al., 2001); multi-drug resistance gene (Yamada et al., 2000); AF17 (Lin et al., 2001); metalloproteinase 7 (MMP-7) (Crawford et al., 1999; Brabletz et al., 1999); peroxisome proliferator-activated receptor δ (He 1999); laminin-5 γ2 (Hlubek 2001); c-jun/fra-1 (Mann et al., 1999) TCF-1 (Roose et al., 1999); axin2 (Jho et al., 2002; Leung et al., 2002); ITF-2 (Kolligs et al., 2002); E-cadherin (Huber et al., 1998; Novak et al., 1998); and mesenchymal genes (Huber et al., 1996; Miller and Moon, 1996; Novak and Dedhar, 1999).

3.3. Post-translational modification of β-catenin

The armadillo repeat domains of β-catenin are essential for binding to its many partners including E-cadherin, α-catenin and TCF-4. This association of β-catenin with various proteins is regulated by post-translational modification at specific sites of the arm repeats (Piedra et al., 2001). Sequences in central arm repeats 4-12 are required for β-catenin to associate with E-cadherin (Hulsken et al., 1994). Moreover, phosphorylation of tyrosine residue 654 (located in arm repeat 12) decreases association of β-catenin with E-cadherin (Roura et al., 1999). Simultaneously, phosphorylation of tyr-654 stimulates binding of β-catenin to the basal transcription factor TATA-binding protein (TBP). Phosphorylation of tyr-654 removes steric hindrance at the C-terminal allowing better access of key components of the transcriptional machinery, such as TBP. Since Tcf-4 binds to armadillo repeats 3-8, its association with β-catenin is not affected by phosphorylation of tyr-654 (arm repeat 12). β-Catenin binding to α-catenin is determined by a short 31 amino-acid sequence in the first armadillo repeat of β-catenin (Aberle et al., 1994). However, this association between β- and α-catenin is not affected by any known post-translational modifications of tyrosine residues.

3.4. γ-catenin

γ-Catenin and β-catenin are closely related and are members of the gene family that includes the Drosophila protein armadillo (Kodama et al., 1999; McCrea et al., 1991). γ-Catenin is identical to plakoglobin (Peifer et al., 1992; Knudsen and Wheelock, 1992). γ-Catenin and β-catenin share 80% sequence identity in the twelve arm repeat domains (Huber and Weis, 2001), but only share 29% and 41% sequence identity in the N- and C-terminal regions, respectively. There are two types of cell-cell junctions: adherens junctions and desmosomes (Takeichi, 1991; Cowin and Burke, 1996). While adherens junctions have one transmembrane component, E-cadherin, desmosomes have two transmembrane components, desmoglein and desmocollin (Buxton et al., 1993). Similar to β-catenin, γ-catenin binds directly to E-cadherin and α-catenin at adherens junctions (Aberle et al., 1994; Hulsken et al., 1994). γ-Catenin is the only component of both desmosome and adherens junctions, suggesting a pivotal role in cell-cell adhesion. In addition to forming a complex with E-cadherin, γ-catenin interacts with the cytoplasmic regions of desmoglein and desmocolin (Kowalczyk et al., 1994; Mathur et al., 1994; Troyanovsky et al., 1994a; Troyanovsky et al., 1994b; Wahl et al., 1996; Witcher et al., 1996). Arm repeats 1-4 of γ-catenin specifically interact with desmoglein. In contrast, γ-catenin arm repeats 11-12 are required for binding desmocolins, but not desmogleins (Witcher et al., 1996). A recent model proposes that the amino- and carboxy-terminal domains of γ-catenin form intramolecular interactions with the armadillo domain, inhibiting its association with desmoglein (Wahl, 2000). Classical cadherins, which include E- and N-cadherin, bind to the same site on γ-catenin as desmocolin (Hulsken et al., 1994; Sacco et al., 1995). Therefore, complexes consisting of E-cadherin, γ- and α-catenins are formed at adherens junctions, while γ-catenin, desmoglein and desmocolin complexes are formed at desmosomes in a mutually exclusive manner. γ-Catenin in adherens junctions and desmosomes may have a potential role in organizing cadherins into an adhesive zipper between two adjacent cells, thereby tightening the association between two cells. γ-Catenin is also found in the cytoplasm, where it forms a homodimer of unknown function (Cowin et al., 1986). The α-catenin binding region maps to the first repeat of γ-catenin, while N-cadherin binding region maps within repeats 7 and 8 (Sacco et al., 1995). γ-Catenin, like β-catenin (Ben Ze'ev and Geiger, 1998), interacts with several proteins, such as classical cadherins (Sacco et al., 1995), α-catenin (Nieset et al., 1997), fascin (Tao et al., 1996), axin (Ikeda et al., 1998; Behrens et al., 1998; Hart et al., 1999; Itoh et al., 1998), APC (Hulsken et al., 1994), and LEF/TCF transcription factors (Simcha et al., 1998; Huber et al., 1996). Tcf-4, however, contains two different sites for binding β- and γ-catenin. Interaction with γ-catenin inhibits transcription of downstream target genes (Miravet et al., 2002). β-Catenin binds to amino acids 1-50 of Tcf-4, whereas γ-catenin binds to residues 51-80. Tcf-4 specifically binds to γ-catenin in the region of arm repeats 1-6. Furthermore, *in vitro* kinase assays have suggested that phosphorylation of Tcf-4 negatively affects its interaction with γ-catenin without altering its association with β-catenin. Therefore, γ-catenin can contribute to homophilic cell-adhesion involving both adherens junctions and zonula adherens junctions.

3.5. p120^{ctn}

p120Catenin (p120^{ctn}) was originally described as a tyrosine-phosphorylated protein in Src-transformed cells (Reynolds et al., 1992; Peifer et al., 1994; Mariner et al., 2000; Noren et al., 2000). Recent evidence suggests pleiotropic functions of p120^{ctn} such as cadherin clustering (Yap, 1998a; Yap et al., 1998b), cell motility (Chen et al., 1997), cadherin turnover at the cell surface (Davis et al., 2004), as well as regulation of neuronal outgrowth and of cadherin-catenin complex stability (Aono et al., 1999; Ohkubo and Ozawa, 1999). While α-, β- and γ-catenins bind to the catenin-binding domain (CBD) of the cadherin cytoplasmic tail, p120^{ctn} binds to the juxtamembrane domain (JMD). Unlike the other catenin proteins, p120^{ctn}does not interact with α-catenin, APC, or transcription factor Lef-1 (Daniel and Reynolds, 1995). Hence, p120^{ctn} does not directly modulate the actin cytoskeleton, implying a distinct role of p120^{ctn} in cadherin-catenin complex and downstream signaling.

p120^{ctn} is thought to indirectly regulate assembly and disassembly of adherens junctions via the Rho family of GTPases (Anastasiadis and Reynolds, 2000; Mariner et al., 2001; Anastasiadis et al, 2000; Grosheva et al., 2001). p120^{ctn} mediates cadherin-dependent activation of RhoA at nascent cell-cell contacts, thereby regulating cadherin clustering and cell junction formation (Anastasiadis et al., 2000). RhoA-GDP forms a complex with p120^{ctn} in the cytoplasm. Dissociation of GDP from RhoA is inhibited because of this trimer formation. In response to post-translational modification, such as tyrosine phosphorylation, p120^{ctn} forms a tighter complex with cadherin-catenin complexes at the cell membrane. The cadherin-bound p120^{ctn} dissociates from RhoA, resulting in the activation of RhoA by guanine nucleotide exchange factors (GEFs) such as Vav2. The exchange of GDP for GTP activates RhoA, which leads to downstream RhoA signaling events that promote cadherin clustering and junction formation. Therefore, cytoplasmic p120^{ctn} regulates specific signaling events at the cell membrane, but this does not preclude the role of nuclear p120^{ctn} in signal transduction.

In response to a putative external signal, p120^{ctn} translocates to the nucleus where it binds Kaiso transcription factor, suggesting that p120^{ctn} regulates transcriptional activity of unidentified target genes (Daniel and Reynolds, 1999; Van Hengel et al., 1999; Mariner et al., 2000). Kaiso interacts with p120, but does not form a complex with E-cadherin, α–catenin or β-catenin, suggesting a mutually exclusive interaction of p120^{ctn} with either Kaiso or E-cadherin. Kaiso is a DNA-binding protein that recognizes a specific consensus sequence and methylated CpG dinucleotides (Daniel et al., 2002; Prokhortchouk et al., 2001). Kaiso is ubiquitously expressed in a panel of cell lines that includes human breast cancer cell lines MCF-7 and MDA-MB-231. However, human prostate cancer cell lines have not yet been characterized with respect to Kaiso protein expression.

3.6. p120^{ctn} isoforms

Most cell types express alternatively spliced isoforms of p120^{ctn} (Anastasiadis and Reynolds, 2000; Thoreson and Reynolds, 2002; Staddon et al., 1995). The following nomenclature is used to distinguish the multiple isoforms of p120^{ctn} (Figure 4). Four different ATG start sites at the N-terminal are used to generate p120 isoforms type 1, 2, 3 and 4. While all four isoforms contain a central armadillo domain with ten arm repeats, only p120 isoform 1 contains a putative coiled-coil domain. The significance of this domain in tumorigenesis is not completely understood. All p120^{ctn} isoforms contain a loop in arm repeat 6, which is thought to act as a nuclear localization signal. C-terminal splicing of p120^{ctn}, where exons A, B, C or none of the C-terminal exons are present adds to the complexity of p120^{ctn} nomenclature. An additional A, B or C designation is included in p120^{ctn} nomenclatrure, based on which C-terminal exon is present. For example, p120^{ctn} 1BC refers to an isoform of p120^{ctn} that is spliced at start site 1 in the N-terminus and contains exons B and C at the C-terminus. These four p120^{ctn} isoforms are differentially expressed based on cell type, suggesting that each isoform may have a specific cellular function. For instance, macrophages and fibroblasts make N-cadherin and express the p120^{ctn} 1A isoform, whereas epithelial cells make E-cadherin and express smaller isoforms such as p120^{ctn} 3A (Anastasiadis and Reynolds, 2000). Based on alternative splicing, possible occurrence of up to 32 isoforms of p120^{ctn} were found in human cells (Anastasiadis and Reynolds, 2000). As discussed above, it is well established that p120^{ctn} interacts with E-cadherin, RhoA and the Kaiso transcription factor. However, the size and specific isoform(s) involved in these interactions remains to be determined. Delineation of the sub-cellular distribution (cytoplasmic vs nuclear) of p120^{ctn} isoforms may provide some insight into the specific function of each.

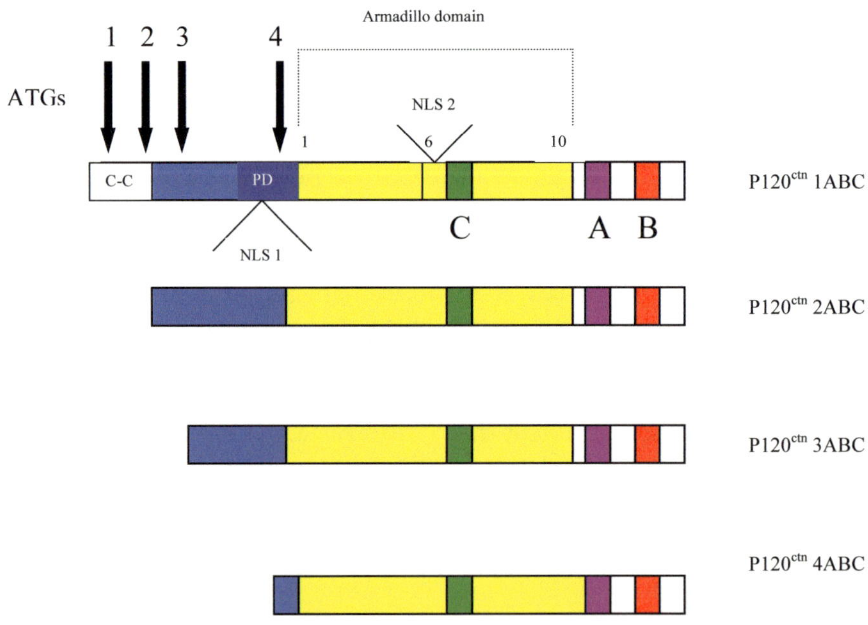

Figure 4. Diagrammatic representations of the multiple isoforms of p120 catenin. Cell-type-specific alternative splicing events result in multiple isoforms of p120 catenin. Four N-terminal ATG start sites generate p120 isoforms 1, 2, 3, and 4. p120 isoform 1 contains a putative coiled-coil domain (C-C), which is absent from isoforms 2-4. Additional alternative splicing generates p120 isoforms using alternative exons in the C-terminal region, exons A, B and C. Isoforms are designated p120^{ctn} 1-4, depending on the N-terminal start site. The A, B, and/or C designations refer to the exons present in the p120 catenin isoform. If none of the C-terminal exons are present, the letter N (for none) is used in the nomenclature (e.g. p120^{ctn}1N). PD, phosphorylation domain; NLS, Nuclear localization sequence.

Similar to the situation with β and γ-catenin, increased levels of $p120^{ctn}$ in the cytoplasm may direct translocation of $p120^{ctn}$ to the nucleus where a downstream signaling cascade is initiated. Although the mechanism of nuclear translocation and the molecular basis for $p120^{ctn}$ isoform specificity has not been described, post-translational modification of $p120^{ctn}$ may be one means of directing $p120^{ctn}$ into either the cytoplasmic or the nuclear compartments. Specific sites of Src-initiated phosphorylation have been identified in murine p120, isoform 1A (Mariner et al., 2001). All of the Src-stimulated phosphorylation sites are present in the amino terminus of $p120^{ctn}$, whereas the tyrosine residues in the armadillo repeat regions are not phosphorylated. Six of these phosphorylated sites cluster in a short-region upstream of the first arm repeat and fourth ATG start site. The significance of Src phosphorylation at these sites remains to be determined. Nonetheless, post-translational modification of $p120^{ctn}$ may be involved in regulating cell-type specific expression patterns, cellular distribution, and/or downstream signaling.

4. N-cadherin

N-cadherin is a member of the classical cadherin family of transmembrane glycoproteins involved in homotypic cell adhesion (Takeichi, 1995). The extracellular domain of N-cadherin consists of five cadherin domains with residues that allow homophilic binding in the first extracellular domain (ECD) (Shan et al., 1999; Koch et al., 1999).In neuronal cells, N-cadherin is involved in the control of axonal growth, synapse formation and synaptic plasticity (Matsunaga et al., 1988; Riehl et al., 1996; Fannon and Colman, 1996; Inoue and Sanes, 1997; Tang et al., 1998; Bozdagi et al., 2000). While it is known that N-cadherin is important in homotypic cell adhesion, there is some evidence that N-cadherin may also be involved in signaling cascades that promote axonal growth (Utton et al., 2001). N-cadherin has been shown to have a role in bone formation (Marie, 2002). In contrast to E-cadherin, which is primarily expressed on cells of epithelial origin, N-cadherin is expressed on mesenchymal cells, such as neuronal tissues, stromal fibroblasts, muscle endothelium and in pleural mesothelial cells (Hazan et al., 1997b).

N-cadherin expression is also altered in pathological processes, such as metastasis of highly invasive cancer cells to regional lymph nodes and bone.The metastatic process is multifactorial, with possible transition of cells from an epithelial to a mesenchymal phenotype promoting migration of cells to distant sites. For example, breast cancer cell lines that have de-differentiated (more primitive) to a mesenchymal phenotype have reduced expression of E-cadherin with concomitant up-regulation of N-cadherin (Hazan et al., 1997b). The de-differentiated breast cancer cells are capable of interacting with surrounding stromal tissues, supporting the invasive phenotype of the breast cancer cells. The epithelial to mesenchymal transition (EMT) is also seen in prostate cancer cell lines, and is correlated with the increased invasive capacity of these cells (Tran et al., 1999). The more invasive prostate cancer cell lines (i.e., JCA-1[1]) and prostate stromal fibroblasts express N-cadherin, with a loss of E-cadherin expression. This would

1 JCA-1 and TsuPr1 have now been identified as derivatives of T24 Bladder Carcinoma cells and are not of prostatic origin (Van Bokhoven et al., 2001). However, JCA-1 and TsuPr1 remain relevant to our theoretical model of cancer cell invasion due to their urogenital origin and therefore, are included in this thesis. JCA-1 and TsuPr1 are indicated with * to emphasize the known origin of these cell lines.

suggest that mutually exclusive expression of either E-cadherin or N-cadherin would establish an epithelial or mesenchymal phenotype, respectively. Homotypic adhesion between prostate cancer cells and stromal fibroblasts (encapsulating the prostate gland) could promote prostate cancer cell invasion and extracapsular metastasis. The loss of E-cadherin and concomitant expression of N-cadherin would allow prostate cancer cells to undergo an epithelial to mesenchymal transition allowing the cells to now become highly invasive.

5. Classical cadherins, Type II

5.1. Cadherin 11

Type II cadherins, cadherins 5, 6, 7, 8, 9, 10, 11, and 12, have structural features similar to Type I cadherins, but differ in amino acid sequence. Type II mesenchymal cadherins are normally expressed on stromal cells and osteoblasts. A mesenchymal cadherin, cadherin 11, and its truncated variant are expressed on highly invasive breast cancer cell lines (Pishvaian et al., 1999), but not on non-invasive cell lines. Previous studies have shown that cadherin 11 is expressed in embryonic mesenchymal tissues, and restricted to certain regions of neural tube (Kimura et al., 1995; Hoffman and Balling, 1995). As tumor cells become more invasive and less differentiated, with concomitant loss of E-cadherin expression, there is an increase in mesenchymal cadherin expression. This pattern would suggest an epithelial to mesenchymal transition of highly invasive, poorly differentiated tumor cells. Although little is known about the expression pattern and function of Type II cadherins in prostate cancer cell lines, expression of cadherin 11 may facilitate metastasis of cancer cells and form distant lesions, particularly in the bone (Bussemakers et al., 2000; Tomita et al., 2000). It is important to note that patients with advanced lung, breast or prostate cancers develop bone metastasis (Mundy, 2002; Soos et al., 1997). In humans, prostate cancer cells invade Batson's vertebral veins, allowing metastatic cancer cells to reach and colonize distant sites within the bone (Geldof, 1997; Oesterling et al, 1997; Lehr and Pienta, 1998). Therefore, successive E-cadherin down-regulation, expression of metalloproteinases, and expression of mesenchymal cadherins allow prostate cancer cells to follow a defined metastatic pathway. The prostate cancer cells may disassociate, invade the basement membrane, metastasize, and colonize distant sites in the bone with concomitant expression of mesenchymal cadherin 11. This type of cancer cell-stromal cell interaction mediated by cadherin 11 is seen in invasive gastric cancers (Shibata et al., 1996). It is possible that E-cadherin acts as a tumor suppressor in cancer progression, while cadherin 11 regulates invasion and formation of metastatic lesions in the bone. This would warrant further investigation of the expression pattern and function of cadherin 11, as well as its role in signalling metastatic progression of prostate cancer cell lines.

6. Matrix metalloproteinases

6.1. Structural motifs

The matrix metalloproteinases (MMPs) are a family of zinc-dependent endopeptidases that consist of more than 21 human MMPs. MMPs are divided into eight distinct structural groups, five of which are secreted and three of which are membrane-localized MMPs, MT-MMPs (Table 1). The existence of multiple MMPs suggests that each MMP subfamily has a specific function that is cell-type specific. Understanding the structural composition of each of the MMP subfamilies may provide some insight into their differential expression and function (Figure 5). MMPs contain an amino-terminal signal sequence (pre) that directs them to the endoplasmic reticulum, a propeptide (pro) sequence with a zinc-interacting thiol group that is cleaved upon activation, and a catalytic domain with a zinc-binding site. Classification of MMPs into the eight subclasses is based on their structural motifs. For example, Group 1 MMPs containing only the pre-, pro- and catalytic domains only, are called the minimal-domain MMP (Sternlicht and Werb, 2001; Egelblad and Werb, 2002). Group 2 MMPs are simple hemopexin-domain containing MMPs with a hemopexin-like domain in addition to the pre-, pro- and catalytic domains found in the minimal-domain MMPs. This additional domain is involved in interactions with tissue inhibitors of metalloproteinases (TIMPS), as well as with their proteolytic substrates. A hinge region connects the catalytic and hemopexin domains. The function of the hinge region is not known, but molecular modeling studies suggest that this region interacts with triple helical collagen (Nagase and Woessner, 1999). Six of the eight structural groups contain the hemopexin domain with the exception of Group 1, minimal- domain MMPs and Group 8, the Type II transmembrane MMPs. While the specific mechanism of proteolytic cleavage is not known, the hemopexin domain is essential for collagenases to cleave triple helical interstitial collagens (Bode, 1995). Note, however, that MMPs have substrate specificity distinct from that of hemopexin domain (Clark and Cawston, 1989). Cell-surface activation of pro-MMP2 requires the presence of hemopexin-domain of MMP-2 (Murphy et al., 1992; Strongin et al., 1995). In addition, recent *in vitro* studies have suggested that the hemopexin domain may assist tumor cells in evasion of immune surveilance. The hemopexin C-terminal domain of MT1-MMP has been suggested to modulate the levels of complement component (gC1qR) in the tumor cell microenvironment (Rozanov et al., 2002). C1q is a subcomponent of the C1 complex of the classical pathway of complement activation. Active MT1-MMP can reduce the levels of soluble gC1qR in the tumor vicinity via proteolytic cleavage. Interestingly, the hemopexin-like C-terminal domain is involved in proteolytic cleavage of gC1qR. These *in vitro* studies imply that tumor cells can evade immune surrveilance by hemopexin domain mediated cleavage of complement components. Group 3 encompasses gelatin-binding MMPs containing fibronectin-like repeats that are associated with binding collagen (FI) and gelatin (Egeblad and Werb, 2002; Allan et al., 1995; Steffensen et al., 1995). Groups 4-8 contain a motif between the propeptide and catalytic domains that is recognized by intracellular furin-like serine proteinases (FU). These MMPs are intracellularly activated by furin-initiated proteolytic cleavage at this site. Groups 5 MMPs contain a vitronectin-like insert in addition to the FU recognition motif. MMPs that are associated with the membrane include the membrane-type MMPs (Group 6) and the glycosylphosphatidylinositol (GPI)-anchored MMPs (Group 7). Membrane-type MMPs (MT-MMPs) have a carboxy-terminal, single-span transmembrane domain (TM) and a very short cytoplasmic domain (Cy). In contrast to the MT-MMPs, the GPI-anchored MMPs are tethered to the membrane by a GPI component at the C-terminal. Group 8 represents the type II transmembrane MMPs with an N-terminal signal anchor (SA) that targets the MMP to the cell membrane. MMP-23 is identified as a type II transmembrane MMPs with unique cysteine array (CA) and immunoglobulin (Ig)-like domains at the C-terminus. The functional significance of these domains has not yet been established.

MMP subfamily	Structural Group	MMP number	MMP name	Substrates
Collagenases	2	1	Interstitial collagenase	Collagens I, II, III and VI, gelatins, aggrecan, entactin
	2	8	Neutrophil collagenase	Collagens I, II, III, aggrecan
	2	13	Collagenase-3	Collagens I, II, III
Gelatinases	3	2	72 kDa Type IV gelatinase	Gelatin, collagens I, IV, V, VII, X, XI, fibronectin, laminin, vitronectin
	3	9	92 kDa Type IV gelatinase	Gelatins, collagens IV, V, XIV, aggrecan, elastin, entactin, vitronectin
Stromelysins	2	3	Stromelysin-1	Aggrecan, gelatins, fibronectin, laminin, collagen III, IV, IX, X, vitronectin
	2	10	Stromelysin-2	Aggrecan, fibronectin, laminin, collagen IV
	4	11	Stromelysin-3	Fibronectin, laminin, collagen IV, aggrecan, gelatins
	2	18	Putative MMP	Collagen I
Membrane-type MMPs	6	14	MT1-MMP	Pro-MMP2, avb3 integrin, CD44, proMMP13, fibronectin, laminin, vitronectin, collagens I, II, III
	6	15	MT2-MMP	Not identified
	6	16	MT3-MMP	ProMMP-2
	7	17	MT4-MMP	Not identified
	6	24	MT5-MMP	Not identified
	7	25	MT6-MMP	Not identified
Other MMPs	1	7	Matrilysin (PUMP-1)	Aggrecan, fibronectin, laminin, collagen IV, elastin, entactin, vitronectin
	2	12	Macrophage elastase	Elastin
	2	19	Rheumatoid arthritis-associated MMP	Not identified
	2	20	Enamelysin	Amelogenin
	5	21	Homologue of *Xenopus* XMMP	
	2	22	CMMP	
	8	23	Cysteine array MMP	
	1	26	Endometase, matrilysin-2	Fibronectin, vitronectin, fibrinogen, type IV collagen, MMP9, gelatin
	2	27	Unkown	
	4	28	Epilysin	

Table 1. Classification and Nomenclature of Human MMPs. MMP superfamily is classified into eight structural groups. While five of these groups are secreted, three groups are membrane-bound. The MMP subfamily, structural group number, corresponding MMP number and the common name are shown in the table. Substrates for each enzyme are also listed in the table (Vincenti, 2000; Nagase and Woessner, 1999; Egelblad and Werb, 2002). MMP Structural Groups: Group 1, Minimal-domain; Group 2, Simple hemopexin-domain-containing; Group 3, Gelatin-binding; Group 4, Furin-activated secreted; Group 5, Vitronectin-like insert; Group 6, Transmembrane; Group 7, GPI-anchored; Group 8, Type II Transmembrane.

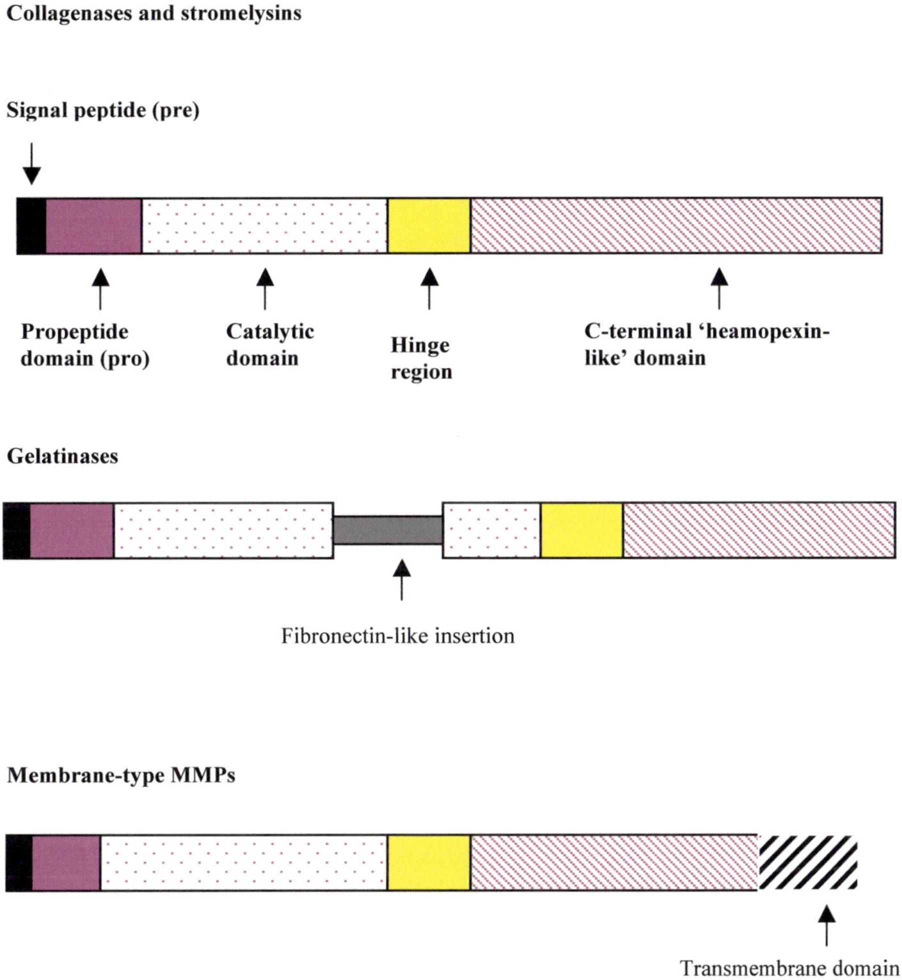

Figure 5. Structure of the matrix metalloproteinase. MMPs contain the following domains: signal peptide (pre-peptide), propeptide, catalytic domain, hinge region, and hemopexin-like domain. The cleavage of N-terminal propeptide domain of the latent MMP yields the active form of the enzyme. The gelatinases contain a fibronectin-like region within their catalytic domain. The membrane-type MMPs are characterised by a C-terminal transmembrane domain. The hemopexin-like repeat is absent in matrilysin (MMP-7).

Common names are also used to distinguish substrate specificity for each of the MMP groups described above. For example, interstitial collagenases, such as MMP-1 (structural group 2), have high specificity for fibrillar collagen types I, II, and III. In contrast, gelatinases, MMP-2 and MMP-9 (structural group 3), have a greater propensity to cleave denatured collagen products, as well as basement membrane components such as collagen type IV. Stromelysins, such as MMP-3 (structural group 2), cleave extracellular components and have the ability to activate other MMPs. Recently, a new subfamily of membrane-tethered or membrane-type MMPs, MT-MMPs (Group 6) has been included in the MMP family. Five enzymes: MT1-, MT2-, MT3-, MT4- and MT5- (Sato et al., 1996; Takino et al., 1995; Will and Hinzmann, 1995; Puente et al., 1996; Pei, 1999) have been identified as members of this group.

MMPs are synthesized as inactive zymogen requiring proteolytic cleavage of the N-terminus in order to be activated. A cysteine-sulphydryl group in the propeptide domain interacts with a zinc ion bound to the catalytic domain. Proteolytic cleavage removes the propeptide domain, leading to the activation of latent MMP (Cao et al., 1998). Generally, MMPs are activated by either serine proteinases or other activated MMPs outside of the cell. In contrast, MMP-11, MMP-28 and MT-MMPs are activated by intracellular furin-like serine proteinases before they are associated with the cell membrane. MMP activity is regulated at three levels: transcription, activation, and inhibition/deactivation.

6.2. Transcriptional regulation of MMPs

Increased MMP expression in tumors is primarily associated with transcriptional changes rather than genetic alterations, although translocation of MMP23 genes in neuroblastoma and amplification of MMP24 gene have been reported (Llano, 1999). Transcriptional regulation of MMP mRNA expression is subject to influences by several chemical reagents, neurohormones, and cytokines (Liotta et al., 1983; Unemori and Werb, 1988; Galis et al., 1994; Werb et al., 1989; Matrisian and Hogan, 1990). For example, tumor necrosis factor alpha (TNF-α) and interleukin-1 can stimulate the production of MMP-1, MMP-3, and MMP-9 (MacNaul et al., 1990). While the pathways by which these factors regulate MMP transcription remain to be determined, it is known that the MMP promoter regions contain response elements that transcriptionally regulate expression. Tumor response element (TRE) and activation protein-1 (AP-1) binding sites are present in MMP-1, MMP-3, MMP-7, MMP-9, MMP-10, MMP-12 and MMP-13 (Benbow and Brinkerhoff, 1997). Transcriptional regulation can be further influenced either by genetic polymorphisms or by growth factor-activated transcription factors. MMP-1 protein expression is influenced by polymorphisms in MMP-1 gene promoter. Promoters of inducible MMPs and TIMPs have specific sites that bind AP-1 and Polyoma Enhancer A-binding Protein-3 (PEA-3), which is pivotal in transcriptional activation. While Fos and Jun families of transcription factors bind to AP-1 sites, PEA-3 binds to the Ets binding sites (EBS). The presence of two guanine nucleotides in the MMP-1 promoter creates a functional Ets-binding site adjacent to an AP-1 site, up-regulating the transcription of MMP-1 gene in multiple cancers, including ovarian cancers (Kanamori, 1999). MMP transcription can also be downregulated in response to certain signals. For example, MMP-1 transcription can be repressed in the presence of the tumor suppressor p53 (Sun et al., 1999). Interestingly, p53 is also known to differentially regulate MMP-13 expression (Sun et al., 2000). Another example of transcriptional regulation of MMPs is the up-regulation of MMP-7 expression in colon tumors (Crawford, 2001). The PEA-3 subfamily of Ets transcription factors and the β-catenin-LEF-1 complex activate MMP-7 expression in colon tumors. These findings suggest that multiple regulatory elements in MMP promoter regions coordinately regulate tissue-specific and temporal expression of MMP.

6.3. Activation of MMPs

While transcriptional regulation is important in determining MMP synthesis, activation of MMPs is a key factor in regulating proteolysis of specific substrates. Newly synthesized MMPs are secreted into the extracellular space in zymogen form. Outside the cell, other MMPs, serine proteinases, growth factors, and chemical/physical reagents can activate the latent MMP. Proteolytic enzymes such as urokinase, plasmin, and cathepsins are known to activate MMPs. In addition, organomercurials (APMA) are used routinely to activate MMPs under experimental conditions. MMP activity *in vivo* has been associated with the interstitial form urokinase plasminogen activator (uPA). Recent evidence has shown that latent MMP-2 is activated at the cell surface in a highly regulated pathway involving tissue inhibitors of metalloproteinases-2 (TIMP-2) and MT1-MMP (Hernandez-Barrantes et al., 2000). TIMP-2 binds MT1-MMP at its N-terminus and proMMP-2 at its C-terminus. Another free MT1-MMP molecule cleaves the bound proMMP-2, leading to partial activation of MMP-2. Another fully activated MMP-2 is required to remove a residual portion of the MMP-2 propeptide (Deryugina, 2001). At low concentrations, TIMP-2 stimulates proMMP-2 activation; at high concentrations, it inhibits MMP-2 activation.

6.4. Inhibition of MMP activity

Inhibition/deactivation of MMPs can be accomplished by several factors including α-2-macroglobulin, tissue inhibitors of metalloproteinases (TIMPs), small molecules with TIMP-like domains, and the membrane-bound inhibitor RECK (reversion-inducing cysteine-rich protein with kazal motifs) (Sasahara et al., 2002). In tissue fluids, α2-macroglobulin forms a complex with MMPs that can bind to a scavenger receptor. Endocytosis removes the trimeric complex, α2-macroglobulin-MMP-scavenger receptor, in an irreversible manner. The activity of MMPs is regulated by the presence of endogenous protein inhibitors, Tissue Inhibitors of Metalloproteinases (TIMP). Four TIMPs (TIMPs1-4) have been identified, each with a specific function (Gomez et al., 1997). TIMPs inhibit tumorigenesis, cell invasion, metastasis and angiogenesis. A fine balance between MMPs and TIMPs regulates tumor progression. TIMP binds to the active site of MMP, leading to a conformational change in the enzyme. The ratio of MMP to its specific TIMP determines the metastatic potential of a tumor cell. Recent evidence suggests that an increase in MMP2 to TIMP2 ratio is associated with high-grade and high-stage prostate tumors (Still et al., 2000).

6.5. Normal and pathological processes involving MMP expression

MMPs are involved in normal embryonic development (Alexander et al., 1996b; Lelongt et al., 1997), renal organogenesis (Lelongt et al., 1997), and invasion and metastasis of cancer (Stetler-Stevenson et al., 1993). There are several examples of normal embryonic development that require MMP expression, including trophoblast implantation, embryonic growth, and tissue morphogenesis. In addition, MMPs are required for normal wound repair. As part of the wound repair process, development of new tissue at the site of injury involves a series of highly regulated events. MMPs degrade several components of the extracellular matrix (ECM), followed by migration of new cells to the site leading to formation of new

ECM at the injured site. The level as well as the tissue-specificity of MMPs can determine the degree of wound repair. For example, MMP-7 is the only MMP expressed by lung epithelial cells under conditions of tracheal damage (Dunsmore et al., 1998). In contrast, more than one MMP is required for epithelial cell migration during normal wound repair (Sudbeck et al., 1997). While different levels of MMP-1, -2, and –9 have been detected at the wound site, neutrophil-derived MMP-8 is the primary collagenase present in normal healing wounds. However, unregulated expression of MMP-8 is associated with chronic leg ulcers (Armstrong and Jude, 2002; Nwomeh et al., 1999). Mammary gland development and involution is another example of a physiological process that requires tightly regulated expression of MMPs (Lund et al., 1996). In summary, regulation of MMP expression and MMP activity is essential for normal cellular processes.

Pathological processes that are associated with aberrant MMP expression include cardiovascular disease (Libby, 1995; Thompson et al., 1995), interstitial fibrosis (Norman et al., 1995), glomerulosclerosis (Schaefer et al., 1997; Jacot et al., 1996), pulmonary emphysema (D'Armiento et al., 1992), and bullous pemphigoid (Liu et al., 1998), an autoimmune subepidermal blistering disease. MMPs are also associated with tumor progression and contribute to tumor invasion and metastasis. MMPs are associated with five principal processes promoting tumor progression (Egeblad and Werb, 2002). First, MMPs can promote cancer cell proliferation by three known mechanisms. These include release of cell-membrane-bound precursors of some growth factors, such as TGF-α, degradation of ECM proteins resulting in the release of peptide growth factors, or indirect proliferative signals through integrins. Second, MMPs regulate apoptosis as well as anti-apoptosis. MMP-3, -7, -9 and –11 are known to regulate apoptosis involving different signaling processes. Overexpression of MMP-3 is known to induce apoptosis in mammary epithelial cells by degrading laminin (Alexander et al., 1996a; Witty et al., 1995) and MMP-7 cleaves FAS ligand, a ligand for the death receptor FAS, from its membrane-bound precursor. As a result of this cleavage, a pro-apoptotic molecule is released into the surrounding microenvironment (Powell et al., 1999; Mitsiades et al., 2001). MMPs can also induce apoptosis of endothelial cells or epithelial cells by shedding the adhesion molecules VE-cadherin (Herren et al., 1998), PECAM-1 (Ilan et al., 2001) and E-cadherin (Steinhusen et al., 2001). Third, MMPs are positive regulators of angiogenesis, which is required for tumor growth. MMP-2, -9 and –14 and –19 have been shown to regulate angiogenesis by promoting the availability of factors involved in angiogenesis, such as vascular endothelial growth factor (VEGF), fibroblast growth factor 2 (FGF-2) and TGF-β. These factors are required for endothelial cell proliferation and migration. Moreover, MMP-2 is required for transition to an angiogenic phenotype in a tumor model (Fang et al., 2000), suggesting that MMPs are important for maintenance of tumor growth and proliferation. Fourth, MMPs allow cancer cells to evade immune surveillance. For example, MMP-9 can cleave interleukin-2 receptor-a (IL-2Ra) from the surface of activated T lymphocytes, thereby suppressing their proliferation (Sheu et al., 2001). As a result of this suppression, tumor-specific T lymphocytes cannot infiltrate tumor cells. MMP-11 also generates a cleavage product that allows tumor cells to evade the tumor-targeted activity of natural killer cells. MMP-11 cleaves α1-proteinase-inhibitor, which decreases natural killer cell cytotoxicity (Kataoka et al., 1999). Active membrane-type 1 MMP (MT1-MMP) has also been suggested to assist tumor cells in evasion of immune surveillance (Rozanov et al., 2002). Therefore, tumor cells escape immune surveillance leading to uncontrolled tumor growth. Fifth, MMPs degrade extracellular matrix components and allow tumor cells to migrate across epithelial basement membranes and metastasize to a new site. While the exact mechanism triggering MMP release by tumor cells is not yet completely understood, MMPs are the only enzymes known to degrade fibrillar collagen types I, II, III and IV. MMP-2, -3, -13 and –14 promote invasion of cell lines in *in vitro* models of invasion (Lochter et al., 1997; Belien et al., 1999; Deryugina et al., 1997; Polette and Birembaut, 1998). Furthermore, MMP-2 and MMP-14 cleave laminin-5 leading to cell motility (Koshikawa et al., 2000). Proteolytic cleavage of CD44 as well as integrin αv subunit by MMP-14 promotes cell migration (Kajita et al., 2001; Deryugina, 2001). Recently, MT-MMP1 has been identified as a downstream target of the β-catenin/Tcf4 complex in colorectal cancers, suggesting that E-cadherin-catenin signaling is important in regulating MT-MMP1 expression (Takahashi et al., 2002). Interestingly, MMP-14 has recently been shown to function as an integrin convertase promoting cell adhesion, migration and focal adhesion kinase phosphorylation of breast cancer cells (Ratnikov et al., 2002). These findings suggest that MMP-14 may be important in regulating cross-talk between integrin and cell-adhesion molecules. MMP-3 as well as MMP-7 cleaves E-cadherin leading to tumor progression (Noe et al., 2001). The newly released E-cadherin cleavage product could interfere with another unprocessed E-cadherin molecule such that E-cadherin function is impaired and, as a result, tumor-cell invasion ensues. Taken together, MMPs are important in many aspects of tumor progression in addition to tumor cell migration and invasion.

6.6. Role of MMP in prostate cancer

Growth factors and receptor kinases can also influence transcriptional regulation of MMPs. MMPs have been shown to play a significant role in prostate cancer metastasis (Wood et al., 1997; Sehgal et al, 1998; Pajouh et al, 1991; Powell et al, 1993). Moreover, recent evidence suggests an increase in MMP-2 and TIMP-2 ratio is associated with high-grade and high-stage prostate tumors (Still et al., 2000). MMP expression could be induced by two possible mechanisms. First, prostate stromal cells could secrete growth factors such as epidermal growth factor (EGF) and induce expression of downstream effectors such as metalloproteinases. Growth factors and their receptors have been shown to be key components of tumor development and progression (Sundareshan et al., 1999). Epidermal growth factor receptor (EGFR) expression in bladder cancer cells, for example, is associated with high tumor stage and grade (Nutt et al., 1998). EGF has been shown to induce the AP-1 transcriptional regulatory complex, which transcriptionally activates MMP-1 expression and MMP-3 expression in fibroblasts. EGFR stimulation promotes both breast cancer cell migration (Price et al., 1999) and induces MMP-1 expresssion (Nutt and Lunec, 1996). Second, MMP expression is also regulated by E-cadherin expression (Nawrocki-Raby et al., 2003). Restoration of E-cadherin expression in E-cadherin negative Dunning rat prostate tumor cells inhibits *in vitro* invasion and MMP-2 activity in these cells (Luo et al., 1999).

7. Concluding remarks

The cellular localization of E-cadherin and the catenin proteins has a significant role in regulating cancer progression. β-, γ- and $p120^{ctn}$ proteins are important components of the E-cadherin-catenin signal transduction pathway. Elucidating the mechanisms of nuclear localization or nuclear retention of β-, γ- and $p120^{ctn}$ proteins, may help us to understand the role of these catenins in regulating E-cadherin downstream signaling events associated with prostate cancer invasion.

Acknowledgements

This project was supported by a grant from NIH (CA97132) to JSN. The authors wish to thank Dr. Christina Voelkel-Johnson and Lucille London for carefully reading the manuscript.

Author details

Anuradha K. Murali and James S. Norris

*Address all correspondence to: muraliak@musc.edu

Microbiology and Immunology, Medical University of South Carolina, Charleston, USA

References

[1] Aberle, H., Butz, S., Stappert, J., Weissig, H., Kemler, R., & , H. Hoschuetzky ((1994). Assembly of the cadherin-catenin complex in vitro with recombinant proteins. Journal of Cell Science, 107, 3655-3663.

[2] Aberle, H., Bauer, A., Stappert, J., Kispert, A., & Kemler, R. (1997). catenin is a target for the ubiquitin-proteasome pathway." EMBO Journal, 16(13), 3797-3804.

[3] Akiyama, T. (2000). Wnt/b-catenin signaling. *Cytokine and Growth Factor Reviews*, 11, 273-282.

[4] Alexander, C. M., Howard, E. W., Bissell, M. J., & Werb, Z. (1996a). Rescue of mammary epithelial cell apoptosis and entactin degradation by a tissue inhibitor of metalloproteinase-1 transgene. Journal of Cell Biology, 135, 1669-1677.

[5] Alexander, C. M., Hansell, E. J., Behrendtsen, O., Flannery, M. L., Kishnani, N. S., Hawkes, S. P., & , Z. Werb ((1996b). Expression and function of matrix metalloprotei-

nases and their inhibitors at the maternal-embryonic boundary during mouse embryo implantation. Development , 122, 1723-1736.

[6] Allan, J. A., Docherty, A. J. P., Barer, P. J., Huskisson, N. S., Reynolds, J. J., & , G. Murphy ((1995). Binding of gelatinases A and B to type-1 collagen and other matrix components."Biochemistry Journal , 309, 299-306.

[7] Amit, S., Hatzubai, A., Birman, Y., Andersen, J. S., Ben-Shushan, E., Mann, M., Ben-Neriah, Y., & Alkalay, I. (2002). Axin-mediatedCKI phosphorylation of beta-catenin at Ser 45: a molecular switch for the Wnt pathway." Genes and Development , 16, 1066-1076.

[8] Anastasiadis, P.Z. and A.B. Reynolds (2000). "The p120 catenin family: complex roles in adhesion, signaling and cancer." Journal of Cell Science 113: 1319-1334.

[9] Anastasiadis, P.Z., S.Y. Moon, M.A. Thoreson, D.J. Mariner, H.C. Crawford, Y. Zheng and A.B. Reynolds (2000)."Inhibition of RhoA by p120 catenin."Nature Cell Biology 2(9): 637.

[10] Aoki, M., Hecht, A., Kruse, U., Kemler, R., & , P. K. Vogt ((1999). Nuclear endpoint of Wnt signaling: Neolastic transformation induced by transactivating lymphoid-enhancing factor 1." Proceedings of the National Academy of Sciences , 96(1), 139-144.

[11] Aono, S., S. Nakagawa, A.B. Reynolds and M. Takeichi (1999). "P120^{ctn} acts as an inhibitory regulator of cadherin function in colon carcinoma cells." Journal of Cell Biology 145: 551-562.

[12] Armstrong, D.G. and E.B. Jude(2002). The role of matrix metalloproteinases in wound healing. American Podiatric Medical Association , 92(1), 12-8.

[13] Arya, M., Bott, S. R., Shergill, I. S., Ahmed, H. U., Williamson, M., & , H. R. Patel ((2006). The metastatic cascade in prostate cancer. Surgical Oncology, 15, 117-128.

[14] Barker, N., & , H. Clevers ((2000). Catenins.Wnt signaling and cancer."Bioessays, 22, 961-965.

[15] Batsche, E., Muchardt, C., ehrens, J., & , H. C. Hurst and C.Cremisi ((1998). RB and c-Myc activate expression of the E-cadherin gene in epithelial cells through interaction with transcription factor AP-2. Molecular and Cellular Biology, 18(7), 3647-3658.

[16] Battle, E., Sancho, E., Franci, C., Dominguez, D., Monfar, M., Baulida, J., & , A. Garcia de Herreros ((2000). The transcription factor Snail is a repressor of E-cadherin gene expression in epithelial tumour cells." Nature Cell Biology , 2, 84-89.

[17] Bauer, A., Otmar, H., & Kemler, R. (1998). Pontin52, an interaction partner of β-catenin, binds to the TATA box binding protein." Proceedings of the National Academy of Sciences , 95, 14787-14792.

[18] Beavon, I.R.G(2000). The E-cadherin-catenin complex in tumour metastasis: structure, function and regulation. European Journal of Cancer , 36, 1607-1620.

[19] Behrens, J., Von, J. P., Kries, M., Kuhl, L., Bruhn, D., Wedlich, R., Grosschedl, , & , W. Bichmeier ((1996). Functional interaction of β-catenin with the trnscription factor Lef1."Nature , 382, 638-642.

[20] Behrens, J., Jerchow, B. A., Wurtele, M., Grimm, J., Asbrand, C., Wirtz, R., Kuhl, M., Wedlich, D., & Birchmeier, W. (1998). Functional interaction of an Axin homolog, conductin, with β-catenin, APC, and GSK3β." Science , 280, 596-599.

[21] Behrens, J. (2002). Control of beta-catenin signaling in tumor development. Annals ofNew York Academy of Sciences , 910, 21-35.

[22] Belien, A. T., Paganetti, P. A., & Schwab, M. E. (1999). Membrane-type 1 matrix metalloprotease (MT1-MMP) enables invasive migration of glioma cells in central nervous system white matter. Journal of Cell Biology , 144(2), 373-384.

[23] Benbow, U., & Brinkerhoff, C. (1997). The AP-1 site and MMP gene regulation: what is all the fuss about? Matrix Biology , 15, 519-526.

[24] Ben, Ze'ev. A., & , B. Geiger ((1998). Differential molecular interactions of beta-catenin and plakoglobin in adhesion, signaling and cancer. Current Opinion in Cell Biology, 10(5), 629-639.

[25] Berx, G., Staes, K., Hengel, J. V., Molemans, F., Bussemakers, M. J. G., Bokhoven, A. V., & , F. and Roy ((1995). Cloning and Characterization of the Human invasion Suppressor Gene E-cadherin (CDH1). Genomics, 26, 281-289.

[26] Berx, G., Becker, K. F., Hofler, H., & van Roy, F. (1998a). Mutations of the human E-cadherin (CDH1) gene. *Human Mutation,* 12(4), 226-237.

[27] Berx, G., Nollet, F., & van Roy, F. (1998b). Dysregulation of the E-cadheirn/catenin complex by irreversible mutations in human carcinomas."Cell Adhesion and Communication 6(2-3): 171-184.

[28] Bienz, M., & , H. Clevers ((2000). Linking colorectal cancer to Wnt signaling. Cell, 103(2), 311-320.

[29] Bode, W. (1995). A helping hand for collagenases: the haemopexin-like domain. Structure , 3, 527-530.

[30] Bozdagi, O., Shan, W., Tanaka, H., Benson, D. L., & Huntley, G. W. (2000). Increasing numbers of synaptic puncta during late-phase LTP: N-cadherin is synthesized, recruited to synaptic sites, and required for potentiation. *Neuron,* 28(1), 245-259.

[31] Brabant, G., Hoang-Vu, C., Cetin, Y., Dralle, H., Scheumann, G., Molne, J., Hansson, G., Jansson, S., Ericson, L. E., & Nilsson, M. (1993). E-cadherin: a differentiation marker in thyroid malignancies. *Cancer Research,* 53(20), 4987-4993.

[32] Brabletz, T., Jung, A., Dag, S., Hlubek, F., & Kirchner, T. (1999). Beta-catenin regulates the expression of the matrix metalloproteinase-7 in human colorectal cancer. American Journal of Pathology, 155(4), 1033-1038.

[33] Bracke, M. E., & , F. M. Van Roy and M. Mareel ((1996). The E-cadherin/catenin complex in invasion and metastasis. Current Topics in Microbiology and ImmunologyPt 1):, 123 EOF-61 EOF.

[34] Brannon, M., Gomperts, M., Sumoy, L., Moon, R. T., & Kimelman, D. (1997). A beta-catenin/XTcf-3 complex binds to the siamois promoter to regulate dorsal axis specification in Xenopus. Genes and Development , 11, 2359-2370.

[35] Bright-Thomas, R. M., Hargest, R., & (2002).", A. P. (2002). APC, β-catenin and hTCF-4; an unholy trinity in the genesis of colorectal cancer."European Journal of Surgical Oncology , 29, 107-117.

[36] Brown, J.D. and R.T. Moon. (1998). Wnt signaling: why is everything so negative? *Current Opinion in Cell Biology*, 10, 182-187.

[37] Bryden, A.A.G., J. A. Hoyland, A.J. Freemont, N.W. Clarke, D.S. Wismayer and N.J.R. George (2002). "E-cadherin and β-catenin are downregulated in prostatic bone metastases." British Journal of Urology International 89(4): 400.

[38] Bukholm, I. K., Nesland, J. M., Karesen, R., & , U. Jacobsen and A.-L.Borresen-Dale ((1998). E-cadherin and α-, β-, and γ-catenin protein expression in relation to metastasis in human breast carcinoma."Journal of Pathology , 185, 262-266.

[39] Bullions, L. C., & , A. Levine ((1998). The role of beta-catenin in cell adhesion, signal transduction, and cancer. Current Opinion in Oncology, 10, 81-87.

[40] Bussemakers, M. J. G., Giroldi, L. A., & , A. van Bokhoven and J.A. Schalken ((1994). Transcriptional regulation of the human E-cadherin gene in human prostate cancer cell lines: characterization of the human E-cadherin gene promoter. Bio.Biophy. Res. Com. , 203(2), 1284-1290.

[41] Bussemakers, M. J. G., Van Bokhoven, A., Tomita, K., Jansen, C. F. J., & , J. A. Schalken ((2000). Complex cadherin expression in human prostate cancer cells. InternationalJournal of Cancer85: , 446 EOF-50 EOF.

[42] Butz, S., & , R. Kemler ((1994). Distinct cadherin-catenin complexes in Ca^{2+} dependent cell-cell adhesion."*FEBS Letters* . , 355, 195-200.

[43] Buxton, R. S., Cowin, P., Franke, W. W., Garrod, D. R., Green, K. J., King, I. A., Koch, P. J., Magee, A. I., Rees, D. A., Stanley, J. R., & Steinberg, M. S. (1993). Nomenclature of the desmosomal cadherins. Journal of Cell Biology , 121, 481-483.

[44] Cadigan, K. M., & Nusse, R. (1997). Wnt singnaling: a common theme in animal development." Genes and Development , 11, 3286-3305.

[45] Cao, J., Drews, M., Lee, H. M., Conner, C., Bahou, W. F., & Zucker, S. (1998). The propeptide domain of membrane type 1 matrix metalloproteinase is required for binding of tissue inhibitor of metalloproteinases and for activation of pro-gelatinase A. Journal of Biological Chemistry , 273(52), 34745-34752.

[46] Cavallaro, U., & , G. Christofori ((2004). Cell adhesion and signaling by cadherins and Ig-CAMs in cancer."*Nature Reviews Cancer*. Cancer , 4, 118-132.

[47] Chen, H., Paradies, N. E., Fedor-Chaiken, M., & Brackenbury, R. (1997). E-cadherin mediates adhesion and suppresses cell motility via distinct mechanisms. *Journal of Cell Science*, 110, 345-356.

[48] Chen, C., , L., Liu, S. S., , S., Ip, M., Wong, L. C., Ng, T. Y., & Ngan, H. Y. S. (2003). E-cadherin expression is silenced by DNA methylation in cervical cancer cell lines and tumours. European Journal of Cancer, 39, 517-523.

[49] Cheng, L., Nagabhushan, M., & Pretlow, T. P. (1996). Expression of E-cadherin in primary and metastatic prostate cancer. American Journal of Pathology 148: , 1375 EOF-80 EOF.

[50] Clark, I. M., & , T. E. Cawston ((1989). Fragments of human fibroblast collagenase. Purification and characterization. Biochemistry Journal , 263, 201-206.

[51] Clevers, H., & , M. van De Wetering ((1997). TCF/LEF factors earn their wings. Trends in Genetics, 13, 485-489.

[52] Comijn, J., Berx, G., Vermassen, P., Verschueren, K., Van Grunsve, L., Bruyneel, E., Mareel, M., Huylebroeck, D., & van Roy, F. (2001). The two-handed E box binding zinc finger protein SIP1 downregulates E-cadherin and induces invasion. *Molecular Cell*, 7, 1267-1278.

[53] Cowin, P., , H., Kapprell, P., Franke, W. W., Tamkum, J., & Hynes, R. O. (1986). Plakoglobin: a protein common to different kinds of intercellular adhering junctions. *Cell*, 46, 1063-1073.

[54] Cowin, P., & , B. Burke ((1996). Cytoskeleton-membrane interactions. Current Opinion in Cell Biology, 8, 56-65.

[55] Crawford, H. C., Fingleton, B. M., Rudolph-Owen, L. A., Goss, K. J., Rubinfeld, B., Polakis, P., & Matrisian, L. M. (1999). The metalloproteinase matrilysin is a target of beta-catenin transactivation in intestinal tumors. *Oncogene*, 18(18), 2883-2891.

[56] Crawford, H. C., Fingleton, B., Gustavson, M. D., Kurpios, N., Wagenaar, R. A., Hassell, J. A., & Matrisian, L. M. (2001). The PEA3 subfamily of Ets transcription factors synergizes with β-catenin-LEF-1 to activate matrilysin transcription in intestinal tumors." Mol. Cell Biol., 21, 1370-1383.

[57] D'Armiento, J., Dalal, S. S., Okada, Y., Berg, R. A., & Chada, K. (1992). Collagenase expression in the lungs of transgenic mice causes pulmonary emphysema. *Cell*, 71, 955-961.

[58] D'Souza, B., & Taylor-Papadimitriou, J. (1994). Overexpression of ERBB2 in human mammary epithelial cells signals inhibition of transcription of the E-cadherin gene. Proceedings of the National Academy of Sciences, 91, 7202-7206.

[59] De Leeuw, W. J. G., Berx, C. B., Vos, J. L., Peterse, M. J., Van de Vijver, S., Litvinov, F., Van Roy, C. J., Corneliss, A. M., & Cleton-Jansen, . (1997). Simultaneous loss of E-cadherin and catenins in invasive lobular breast cancer and lobular carcinoma in situ. Journal of Pathology , 183, 404-411.

[60] Daniel, J.M. and A.B. Reynolds (1995). "The tyrosine kinase substrate p120cas binds directly to E-cadherin but not to the adenomatous polyposis coli protein or alpha-catenin." Molecular Cellular Biology 15: 4819-4824.

[61] Daniel, J.M. and A.B. Reynolds (1999). "The Catenin p120^{ctn} interacts with Kaiso, a novel BTB/POZ domain zinc finger transcription factor." Molecular Cellular Biology 19(5): 3614-3623.

[62] Daniel J.M., C.M. Spring, H.C. Crawford, A.B. Reynolds and A. Baig (2002). "The p120ctn-binding partner Kaiso is a bi-modal DNA-binding protein that recognizes both a sequence-specific consensus and methylated CpG dinucleotides." Nucleic Acids Research 30(13): 2911-2919.

[63] Davis, M.A., Ireton, R.C. and A.B. Reynolds (2003). "A core function of p120-catenin in cadherin turnover." Journal of Cell Biology 163(3): 525-534.

[64] Dermietzel, R., & , F. Hofstadter ((1998). Gap junctions in health and disease. Virchows Arch , 432, 177-186.

[65] Deryugina, E. I., Luo, G. X., Reisfeld, R. A., Bourdon, M. A., & Strongin, A. (1997). Tumor cell invasion through matrigel is regulated by activated matrix metalloproteinase-2. *Anticancer Research*, 17, 3201-3210.

[66] Deryugina, E.I(2001). MT1-MMP initiates activation of proMMP-2 and integrin avb3 promotes maturation of MMP-2 in breast carcinoma cells." Experimental Cell Research , 263, 209-223.

[67] Dorudi, S., Sheffield, J. P., Poulsom, R., Northover, J. M., & , I. R. Hart ((1993). E-cadherin expression in colorectal cancer. An immunocytochemical and in situ hybridization study. American Journal of Pathology , 142(4), 981-986.

[68] Dunsmore, S. E., Saarialh-Kere, U. K., Roby, J. D., Wilson, C. L., Matrisian, L. M., Welgus, H. G., & Parks, W. C. (1998). Matrilysin expression and function in airway epithelium. Journal of Clinical Investigations , 102, 1321-1331.

[69] Eastman, Q., & Grosschedl, R. (1999). Regulation of LEF-1/TCF transcription factors by Wnt and other signals. *Current Opinion in Cell Biology*, 11, 233-240.

[70] Egelblad, M., & , Z. Werb ((2002). New functions for the matrix metalloproteinases in cancer progression."Nature Reviews Cancer , 2(3), 161-174.

[71] Esteller, M. M., Sanchez-Cespedes, R., Rosell, D., Sidransky, S. B., Baylin, , & , J. G. Herman ((1999). Detection of aberrant promoter hyermethylation of tumor suppressor genes in serum DNA from non-small cell lung cancer patients."Cancer Research , 59, 7-70.

[72] Fagotto, F., Funayama, N., Gluck, U., & Gumbiner, B. M. (1996). Binding to cadherins antagonizes the signaling activity of beta-catenin during axis formation in Xenopus. Journal of Cell Biology , 132(6), 1105-1114.

[73] Fagotto, F., Gluck, U., & , B. M. Gumbiner ((1998). Nuclear localization signal-independent and importin/karyopherin-independent nuclear import of β-catenin."Current Biology , 8, 181-190.

[74] Fagotto, F., E-h, Jho. L., Zeng, T., Kurth, T., Joos, C., Kaufmann, , & Costantini, F. (1999). Domains of Axin involved in protein-protein interactions, Wnt pathway inhibition, and intracellular localization. Journal of Cell Biology , 145(4), 741-756.

[75] Fang, J., Shing, Y., Wiederschain, D., Yan, L., Butterfield, C., Jackson, G., Harper, J., Tamvakopoulos, G., & Moses, M. A. (2000). Matrix metalloproteinase-2 is required for the switch to the angiogenic phenotype in a tumor model. Proc. Natl. Acad. Sci. USA , 97, 3884-3889.

[76] Fannon, A. M., & Colman, D. R. (1996). A model for central synaptic junctional complex formation based on the differential adhesive specificities of the cadherins. *Neuron*, 17(3), 423-434.

[77] Fujita, Y., Krause, G., Scheffner, M., Zechner, D., Leddy, H. E. M., Behrens, J., Sommer, T., & Birchmeier, W. (2002). Hakai, a c-Cbl-like protein, ubiquitinates and induces endocytosis of the E-cadherin complex." Nature Cell Biology , 4, 222-231.

[78] Funayama, N. F., Fagotto, P., Mc Crea, , & Gumbiner, B. M. (1995). Embryonic axis induction by the armadillo repeat domain of β-catenin: evidence for intracellular signaling." Journal of Cell Biology , 128(5), 959-968.

[79] Galis, Z. S., Sukhova, G. K., Lark, M. W., & Libby, P. (1994). Increased expression of matrix metalloproteinases and matrix degrading activity in vulnerable regions of human atherosclerotic plaques. Journal of Clinical Investigations , 94(6), 2493-503.

[80] Gamallo, C., Palacios, J., Suarez, A., , A., Pizarro, M., Quintanilla, , & Cano, A. (1993). Correlation of E-cadherin expression with differentiation grade and histological type in breast carcinoma. American Journal of Pathology , 142, 987-993.

[81] Geldof, A. A. (1997). Models for cancer skeletal metastasis: A reappraisal of Batson's Plexus. *Anticancer Research*, 17, 1535-1540.

[82] Giannini, A. L., M.d, M., Vivanco, , & Kypta, R. M. (2000). Analysis of β-catenin aggregation and localization using GFP fusion proteins: nuclear import of α-catenin by the β-catenin/Tcf complex." Experimental Cell Research , 255(2), 207-220.

[83] Gomez, D. E., Alonso, D. F., Yoshiji, H., & Thorgeirsson, U. P. (1997). Tissue inhibitors of metalloproteinases: structure, regulation and biological functions. *European Journal of Cell Biology*, 74, 111-122.

[84] Goto, T., Nakano, M., Ito, S., Ehara, H., Yamamoto, N., & , T. Deguchi ((2007). Significance of an E-cadherin gene promoter polymorphism for risk and disease severity of prostate cancer in a Japanese population. Urology, 70(1), 127-30.

[85] Grady, W. M., Rajput, A., Lutterbaugh, J. D., & , S. D. Markowitz ((2001). Detection of aberrantly methylated hMLH1 promoter DNA in the serum of patients with microsatellite unstable colon cancer. Cancer Research, 61, 900-902.

[86] Graff, J. R., Herman, J. G., & Lapidus, R. G. (1995). E-cadherin expression is silenced by DNA hypermethylation in human breast and prostate carcinomas. *Cancer Research*, 5195 EOF-9 EOF.

[87] Graff, J. R., Herman, J. G., Myohanen, S., Baylin, S. B., & Vertino, P. M. (1997). Mapping Patterns of CpG Island Methylation in Normal and Neoplastic Cells Implicates Both Upstream and Downstream Regions in de Novo Methylation. Journal of Biological Chemistry , 272(35), 22322-22329.

[88] Grooteclaes, M. L., & , S. M. Frisch ((2000). Evidence for a function of CtBP in epithelial gene regulation and anoikis. Oncogene, 19, 3823-3828.

[89] Grosheva, I., M. Shtutman, M. Elbaum and A.D. Bershadsky (2001). "p120 catenin affects cell motility via modulation of activity of Rho-family GTPases: a link between cell-cell contact formation and regulation of cell locomotion." Journal of Cell Science 114: 695-707.

[90] Hajra, K. M., -S, D. Y., Chen, , & Fearon, E. R. (2002). The SLUG Zinc-finger protein represses E-cadherin in Breast Cancer. *Cancer Research*, 62, 1613-1618.

[91] Hall, C. L., Kang, S., Mac, O. A., & Dougald, E. T. Keller ((2006). Role of Wnts in Prostate Cancer Bone Metastases. Journal of Cellular Biochemistry , 97, 661-672.

[92] Hart, M., -P, J., Concordet, I., Lassot, I., Albert, R., del los, Santos. H., Durand, C., Perret, B., Rubinfeld, F., Margottin, R., Benarous, , & Polakis, P. (1999). The F-box protein β-TrCP associates with phosphorylated β-catenin and regulates its activity in the cell." Current Biology , 9, 207-210.

[93] Hazan, R. B., Kang, L., Roe, S., Borgen, P. I., & Rimm, D. L. (1997a). Vinculin is associated with the E-cadherin adhesion complex. Journal of Biological Chemistry , 272(51), 32448-32453.

[94] Hazan, R. B., Kang, L., Wooley, B. P., & Borgen, P. I. (1997b). N-cadherin promotes adhesion between invasive breast cancer cells and the stroma. *Cell Adhesion and Communication*, 4(6), 399-411.

[95] Hazan, R. B., & Norton, L. (1998). The Epidermal Growth Factor Receptor Modulates the interaction of E-cadherin with the Actin Cytoskeleton. Journal of Biological Chemistry, 273(15), 9078-9084.

[96] He, T. C., Sparks, A. B., Rago, C., Hermeking, H., Zawel, L., Da, L. T., Costa, P. J., Morin, B., Vogelstein, , & Kinzler, K. W. (1998). Identification of c-MYC as a target of the APC pathway. Science , 281, 1509-1512.

[97] He, T. C., Chan, T. A., Vogelstein, B., & Kinzler, K. W. (1999). PPARdelta is an APC-regulated target of nonsteroidal anti-inflamatory drugs." Cell , 99(3), 335-345.

[98] Heasman, J., Crawford, A., Goldstone, K., Garner-Hamrick, P., Gumbiner, B., Mc Crea, P., Kintner, C., Noro, C. Y., & Wylie, C. (1994). Overexpression of cadherins and underexpression of beta-catenin inhibit dorsal mesoderm induction in early Xenopus embryos. *Cell*, 79(5), 791-803.

[99] Hecht, A., Litterst, C. M., Huber, O., & Kemler, R. ((1999). Functional characterization of multiple transactivating elements in β-catenin, some of which interact with the TATA-binding protein in vitro."Journal of Biological Chemistry , 274, 18017-18025.

[100] Hellberg, C. B., Burden-Gulley, S. M., Pietz, G. E., & Brady-Kalnay, S. M. (2002). Expression of the receptor protein-tyrosine phosphatase, PTPm, restores E-cadherin-dependent adhesion in human prostate carcinoma cells.". Journal of Biological Chemistry , 277(13), 11165-11173.

[101] Herman, J. G., Graff, J. R., Myohanen, S., Nelkin, B. D., & Baylin, S. B. (1996). Methylation-specific PCR: A novel PCR assay for methylation status of CpG islands. Proceedings of the National Academy of Sciences , 93, 9821-9826.

[102] Hernandez-Barrantes, S., Toth, M., Bernardo, M. M., Yurkova, M., Gervasi, D. C., Raz, Y., Sang, Q. A., & Fridman, R. (2000). Binding of Active 57kDa Membrane Type 1-Matrix metalloproteinase (MT1-MMP) to tissue inhibitor of metalloproteinase (TIMP-2) regulates MT1-MMP processing and proMMP-2 activation." Journal of Biological Chemistry , 275(16), 12080-12089.

[103] Herren, B., Levkau, B., Raines, E. W., & Ross, R. (1998). Cleavage of beta-catenin and plakoglobin and shedding of VE-cadherin during endothelial apoptosis: evidence for a role for caspases and metalloproteinases. Molecular Biology Cell , 9(6), 1589-1601.

[104] Herrenknecht, K., Ozawa, M., Eckerskorn, C., Lottspeich, F., Lenter, M., & Kemler, R. (1991). The uvomorulin-anchorage protein α catenin is α vinculin homologue." Proceedings of the National Academy of Sciences , 88, 9156-9160.

[105] Hinck, L., Nathke, I. S., Papkoff, J., & Nelson, W. J. (1994). Dynamics of cadherin/catenin complex formation: novel protein interactions and pathways of complex assembly. Journal of Cell Biology , 125, 1327-1340.

[106] Hiraguri, S., Godfrey, T., Nakamura, H., Graff, J., Collins, C., Shayesteh, L., Doggett, N., Johnson, K., Wheelock, M., Herman, J., Baylin, S., Pinkel, D., & Gray, J. (1998). Mechanisms of inactivation of E-cadherin in breast cancer cell lines. *Cancer Research*, 58, 1972-1977.

[107] Hirohashi, S., & (1998).", . (1998). Inactivation of the E-cadherin-mediated cell adhesion system in human cancers. American Journal of Pathology, 153(2), 333-339.

[108] Hlubek, F., Jung, A., Kotzor, N., Kirchner, T., & Brabletz, T. (2001). Expression of the invasion factor laminin γ2 in colorectal carcinomas is regulated by β-catenin." Cancer Research , 61, 8089-8093.

[109] Hoffmann, I., & Balling, R. (1995). Cloning and expression analysis of a novel mesodermally expressed cadherin. *Developmental Biology*, 169, 337-346.

[110] Howe, L., Crawford, H. C., Subbaramaiah, K., Hassell, J. A., Dannenberg, A. J., & Brown, A. M. C. (2001). PEA3 is up-regulated in response to Wnt1 and activates the expression of cyclooxygenase-2. Journal of Biological Chemistry , 276(23), 20108-20115.

[111] Hsu, W., Zeng, L., & , F. Costantini((1999). Identification of a domain of axin that binds to the serine/threonine protein phosphatase 2A and a self-binding domain. Journal of Biological Chemistry , 274, 3439-3445.

[112] Huber, O., Korn, R., & Mc Laughlin, R. (1996). Nuclear localization of beta-catenin by interaction with transcription factor LEF-1. *Mechanisms of Development*, 3 EOF-10 EOF.

[113] Huber, O., Bierkamp, C., & , R. Kemler ((1998). Cadherins and Catenins in development. Current Opinion in Cell Biology, 8, 685-691.

[114] Huber, A.H. and W.I. Weis(2001). The structure of the β-catenin/E-cadherin complex and the molecular basis of diverse ligand recognition by β-catenin."Cell , 105, 391-402.

[115] Hulsken, J., Birchmeier, W., & Behrens, J. (1994). E-cadherin and APC compete for the interaction with β-catenin and the cytoskeleton." Journal of Cell Biology , 127, 2061-2069.

[116] Ikeda, S., Kishida, S., Yamamoto, H., , H., Murai, S., Koyama, , & Kikuchi, A. (1998). Axin, a negative regulator of the Wnt signaling pathway, forms a complex with GSK3β and β-catenin and promotes GSK3β-dependent phosphorylation of β-catenin." EMBO Journal , 17(5), 1371-1384.

[117] Ilan, N., Mohsenin, A., Cheung, L., & Madri, J. A. (2001). PECAM-1 shedding during apoptosis generates a membrane-anchored truncated molecule with unique signaling characteristics. FASEB Journal, 15, 362-372.

[118] Inoue, A., & Sanes, J. R. (1997). Lamina-specific connectivity in the brain: regulation by N-cadherin, neurotrophins, and glycoconjugates. Science , 276, 1428-1431.

[119] Itoh, M., Nagafuchi, A., Moroi, S., & , S. Tsukita ((1997). Involvement of ZO-1 in cadherin-based cell adhesion through its direct binding to alpha-catenin and actin filaments. Journal of Cell Biology , 138, 181-192.

[120] Itoh, K., Krupnik, V. E., & Sokol, S. Y. (1998). Axis determination in Xenopus involves biochemical interactions of axin, glycogen synthase kinase 3 and β-catenin." Current Biology , 8, 591-594.

[121] Jacot, T. A., Striker, G. E., Stetler-Stevenson, M., & Striker, L. J. (1996). Mesangial cells from transgenic mice with progressive glomerlosclerosis exhibit stable, phenotypic changes including undetectable MMP-9 and increased type IV collagen." Laboratory Investigations , 75, 79-799.

[122] Jawhari, A. U., Farthing, M. J. G., & Pignatelli, M. (1999). The E-cadherin/Epidermal Growth Factor Receptor Interaction: A Hypothesis of Reciprocal and Reversible Control of Intercellular Adhesion and Cell Proliferation. Journal of Pathology , 187, 155-157.

[123] Jho-H, E., Zhang, T., Domon, C., -K, C., Joo-N, J., Freund, , & Costantini, F. (2002). Wnt-β-catenin/Tcf signaling induces the transcription of Axin2, a negative regulator of the signaling pathway." Molecular and Cellular Biology , 22(4), 1172-1183.

[124] Jiang, J., & , G. Struhl ((1998). Regulation of the hedgehog and wingless signaling pathways by the F-box/WD40-repeat protein slimb."*Nature.* , 391, 493-496.

[125] Joo, Y. E., Rew, J. S., Park, C. S., & Kim, S. J. ((2002). Expression of E-cadherin, alpha- and beta-catenins in patients with pancreatic adenocarcinomas."Pancreatology , 2(2), 129-137.

[126] Joseph-Silverstein, J., & Silverstein, R. L. (1998). Cell Adhesion Molecules: An Overview. *Cancer Investigation,* 16(3), 176-182.

[127] Jou, T. S., Stewart, D. B., & , J. Stappert ((1995). Genetic and biochemical dissection of protein linkages in the cadherin-catenin complex. Procedings of the National Academy of Sciences , 92, 5067-5071.

[128] Julius, M. A., Schelbert, B., Hsu, W., Fitzpatrick, E., Jho, E., Fagotto, F., Costantini, F., & Kitajewski, J. (2000). Domains of axin and disheveled required for interaction and function in Wnt signalins." Biochemical and Biophysical Research Communications , 276, 1162-1169.

[129] Kadowaki, T., Shiozaki, H., Inoue, M., Tamura, S., Oka, H., Doki, Y., Iihara, K., Matsui, S., Iwazawa, T., & Nagafuchi, A. (1994). E-cadherin and alpha-catenin expression in human esophageal cancer. *Cancer Research,* 54, 291-296.

[130] Kajita, M., Itoh, Y., Chiba, T., Mori, H., Okada, A., Kinoh, H., & Seiki, M. (2001). Membrane-tye 1 matrix metalloproteinase cleaves CD44 and promotes cell migration." Journal of Cell Biology , 153(5), 893-904.

[131] Kanamori, Y. (1999). Correlation between expression of the matrix metalloproteinase-1 gene in ovarian cancers and an insertion/deletion polmorphism in its promoter region." Cancer Research , 59, 4225-4227.

[132] Kataoka, H., Uchino, H., Iwamura, T., Seiki, M., Nabeshima, K., & , M. Koono ((1999). Enhanced tumor growth and invasiveness in vivo by a carboxyl-terminal fragment of a1-proteinase inhibitor generated by matrix metalloproteinases: a possible modulatory role in natural killer cytotoxicity." American Journal of Pathology , 154(2), 457-468.

[133] Kawahara, K., Morishita, T., Nakamura, T., Hamada, F., Toyoshima, K., & Akiyama, T. (2000). Down-regulation of β-catenin by the colorectal tumor suppressor APC requires association with axin and β-catenin." Journal of Biological Chemistry , 275(12), 8369-8374.

[134] Kawakami, K. (2000). Hypermethylated APC DNA in plasma and prognosis of patients with esophageal adenocarcinoma. Journal of National Cancer Institute , 92, 1805-1811.

[135] Kawasaki, Y., Sato, R., & Akiyama, T. (2003). Mutated APC and Asef are involved in the migration of colorectal tumour cells. *Nature Cell Biology*, 5, 211-215.

[136] Kawanishi, J., Kato, J., Sasaki, K., Fujii, S., Watanabe, N., & , Y. Niitsu ((1995). Loss of E-cadherin-dependent cell-cell adhesion due to mutation of the β-catenin gene in a human cancer cell line, HSC-39." Molecular and Cellular Biology , 15(3), 1175-1181.

[137] Kikuchi, A. (1999). Roles of axin in the Wnt signaling pathway.". Cell Signaling , 11(11), 777-788.

[138] Kikuchi, A. (2000). Regulation of beta-catenin signaling in the Wnt pathway. *Biochemical and Biophysical Research Communications*, 268(2), 243-248.

[139] Kimura, Y., Matsunami, H., Inoue, T., Shimamura, K., Uchida, N., Ueno, T., & , T. Miyazaki and M.Takeichi ((1995). Cadherin 11 Expressed in association with mesenchymal morphogenesis in the head, somite, and limb bud of early mouse embryos." Developmental Biology, 169, 347-358.

[140] Kitagawa, M., Hatekeyama, S., Shirane, M., Matsumoto, M., Ishida, N., Hatori, K., Nakamichi, I., Kikuchi, K., & Nakayama, K. (1999). An F-box protein, FWD1, mediates ubiquitin-dependent proteolysis of beta-catenin." EMBO Journal , 18, 2401-2410.

[141] Knudsen, K., & Wheelock, M. (1992). Plakoglobin, or an 83-kDa homologue distinct from β-catenin, interacts with E-cadherin and N-cadherin." Journal of Cell Biology , 118, 671-679.

[142] Knudsen, K. A., Solar, A. P., Johnson, K. R., & , M. J. Wheelock ((1995). Interaction of alpha-actinin with the cadherin/catenin cell-cell adhesion complex via alpha-catenin. Journal of Cell Biology , 130, 67-77.

[143] Koch, A. W., Bozic, D., Pertz, O., & , J. Engel ((1999). Homophilic adhesion by cadherins. Current Opinion in Structural Biology, 9(2), 275-281.

[144] Kodama, S., Ikeda, S., Asahara, T., Kishida, M., & Kikuchi, A. (1999). Axin directly interacts with plakoglobin and regulates its stability. Journal of Biological Chemistry , 274(39), 27682-27688.

[145] Kolligs, F. T., Kolligs, B., Hajra, K. M., Hu, G., Tani, M., Cho, K. R., & Fearon, F. R. (2000). Gamma-catenin is regulated by the APC tumor suppressor and its oncogenic activity is distinct from that of β-catenin." Genes and Development , 14(11), 1319-1331.

[146] Kolligs, F. T., Nieman, M. T., Winer, I., Hu, G., Van Mater, D., Feng, Y., Smith, I. M., Wu, R., Zhai, Y., Cho, K. R., & Fearon, E. R. (2002). ITF-2, a downstream target of the Wnt/TCF pathway, is activated in hum. an cancers with beta-catenin defects and promotes neoplastic transformation." Cancer Cell , 1(2), 145-155.

[147] Korinek, V., Barker, N., Morin, P. J., Van Wichen, D., de Weger, R., Kinzler, K. W., Vogelstein, B., & Clevers, H. (1997). Constitutive transcriptional activation by a beta-catenin-Tcf complex in APC-/- colon carcinoma. Science , 275, 1784-1787.

[148] Koshikawa, N. G., Giannelli, V., Cirulli, K., Miyazaki, , & , V. Quaranta ((2000). Role of cell surface metalloprotease MT-MMP in epithelial cell migration over laminin-5." Journal of Cell Biology , 148(3), 615-624.

[149] Kowalczyk, A. P., Palka, H. L., Luu, H. H., Nilles, L. A., Anderson, J. E., Wheelock, M. J., & , K. J. Green ((1994). Posttranslational regulation of plakoglobin expression. Influence of the desmosomal cadherins on plakoglobin metabolic stability. Journal of Biological Chemistry , 269, 31214-31223.

[150] Kraus, C., T. Liehr, J. Hulsken, J. Behrens, W. Birchmeier, K.-H.Grzeschik and W.G. Ballhausen (1994). "Localization of the human ▪ -catenin gene (CTNNB1) to 3p21: A region implicated in tumor development." Genomics 23: 272-274.

[151] Kuczyk, M., Serth, J., Machtens, S., Bokemeyer, C., Bathke, W., Stief, C., & Jonas, U. (1998). Expression of E-cadherin in primary prostate cancer: correlation with clinical features." British Journal of Urology , 81, 406-412.

[152] Larue, L., Ohsugi, M., Hirchenhain, J., & Kemler, R. (1994). E-cadherin null mutant embryos fail to form a trophectoderm epithelium." Procedings of the National Academy of Sciences , 91, 8263-8267.

[153] Latres, E., Chiaur, D. S., & Pagano, M. (1999). The human F box protein β-Trcp associates with the Cul1/Skp1 complex and regulates the stability of β-catenin." Oncogene , 18(4), 849-854.

[154] Lehr, J.E. and K.J. Pienta(1998). Preferential adhesion of prostate cancer cells to a human bone marrow endothelial cell line." Journal of National Cancer Institute, 90, 118-23.

[155] Lejeune, S., Huguet, E. L., Hamby, A., Poulson, R., Haris, A. L., & (1995).", . (1995). Wnt5a cloning, expression, and up-regulation in human primary breast cancers." Clinical Cancer Research , 1(2), 215-222.

[156] Lelongt, B., Trugnan, G., Murphy, G., & Ronco, P. M. (1997). Matrix metalloproteinases MMP2 and MMP9 are produced in earl stages of kidney morphogenesis but only MMP9 is required for renal organogenesis in vitro." Journal of Cell Biology , 136, 1363-1373.

[157] Leung, J. Y., Kolligs, F. T., Wu, R., Zhai, Y., Kuick, R., Hanash, S., Cho, K. R., & , E. R. Fearon ((2002). Activation of AXIN2 expression by beta-catenin-T cell factor.A feed-

back repressor pathway regulating Wnt signaling." Journal of Biological Chemistry , 277(24), 21657-21665.

[158] Li-C, L., Zhao, H., Nakajima, K., Oh, B. R., Filho, L. A. R., Carroll, P., & Dahiya, R. (2001). Methylation of the E-cadherin gene promoter correlates with progression of prostate cancer." Journal of Urology , 166, 705-709.

[159] Libby, P. (1995). Molecular bases of the acute coronary syndromes." Circulation , 91, 2844-2850.

[160] Lickert, H., Bauer, A., Kemler, R., & Stappert, J. (2000). Casein Kinase II Phosphorylation of E-cadheirn increases E-cadherin/β-catenin interaction and strengthens cell-cell adhesion." Journal of Biological Chemistry , 275(7), 5090-5095.

[161] Lim, S. C., & , M. S. Lee ((2002). Significance of E-cadherin/beta-catenin and cyclin D1 in breast cancer." Oncology Reports , 9(5), 915-28.

[162] Lin-M, Y., Ono, K., Satoh, S., Ishiguro, H., Fujita, M., Miwa, N., Tanaka, T., Tsunoda, T., , K., Yang, C., Nakamura, Y., & , Y. Furukawa ((2001). Identification of AF17 as a downstream gene of the β-catenin/T-Cell Factor pathway and its involvement in colorectal carcinogenesis." Cancer Research , 61, 6345-6349.

[163] Liotta, L. A., Rao, C. N., & , S. H. Barskey ((1983). Tumor invasion by the extracellular matrix." Lab Investigation , 49, 636-649.

[164] Liu, Z., Shipley, J. M., Vu, T. H., Zhou, X., Diaz, L. A., Werb, Z., & Senior, R. M. (1998). Gelatinase B-deficient mice are resistant t experimental bullous pemphigoid." Journal of Experimental Medicine , 188, 475-482.

[165] Liu, W., Dong, X., Mai, M., Seelan, R. S., Taniguchi, K., Krishnadath, K. K., Halling, K. C., Cunningham, J. M., Boardman, L. A., Qian, C., Christensen, E., Schmidt, S. S., Roche, P. C., Smith, D. I., & Thibodeau, S. N. (2000). Mutations in AXIN2 cause colorectal cancer with defective mismatch repair by activating beta-catenin/TCF signaling." Nature Genetics , 26(2), 146-147.

[166] Liu, C., Li, Y., Semenov, M., Han, C., Baeg, G. H., Tan, Y., Zhang, Z., Lin, X., & , X. He ((2002). Control of beta-catenin phosphorylation/degradation by a dual-kinase mechanism."Cell , 108, 837-847.

[167] Llano, E. (1999). Identification and characterization of human MT5-MMP, a new membrane-bound actiator of progelatinase A overexpressed in brain tumors." Cancer Research , 59, 2570-2576.

[168] Lochter, A., Galosy, S., Muschler, J., Freedman, N., Werb, Z., & Bissell, M. J. (1997). Matrix metalloproteinase stromelysin-1 triggers a cascade of molecular alterations that leads to stable epithelial-to-mesenchymal conversion and a remalignant phenotype of mammary epithelial cells." Journal of Cell Biology , 139(7), 1861-1872.

[169] Loric, S., Paradis, V., , J., Gala, L., Berteau, P., Bedossa, P., Benoit, G., & Eschwege, P. (2001). Abnormal E-cadherin expression and prostate cell blood dissemination as

markers of biological recurrence in cancer." European Journal of Cancer , 37, 1475-1481.

[170] Lund, L. R., Romer, J., Thomasset, N., Solberg, H., Pyke, C., Bissell, M. J., Dano, K., & Werb, Z. (1996). Two distinct phases of apoptosis in mammary gland involution: Proteinase-independent and dependent pathways." Development , 122, 181-193.

[171] Luo, J., Lubaroff, D. M., & , M. J. C. Hendrix ((1999). Suppression of Prostate Cancer Invasive Potential and Matrix Metalloproteinase Activity by E-cadherin Transfection."Cancer Research , 59, 3552-3556.

[172] Lustig, B., Jerchow, B., Sachs, M., Weiler, S., Pietsch, T., Karsten, U., van de Wetering, M., Clevers, H., Schlag, P. M., Birchmeier, W., & Behrens, J. (2002). Negative feedback loop of Wnt signaling through upregulation of conductin/axin2 in colorectal and liver tumors." Molecular and Cellular Biology , 22(4), 1184-1193.

[173] Mac, Naul. K. L., Chartrain, N., Lark, M., Tocci, M. J., & Hutchinson, N. I. (1990). Discordinate expression of stromelysin, collagenase, and tissue inhibitor of metalloproteinases-1 in rheumatoid human synovial fibroblasts: synergistic effects of interlekin-1 and tumor necrosis factor-a on stromelysin expression." Journal of Biological Chemistry , 265, 17238-17245.

[174] Mann, B., Gelos, M., Siedow, A., Hanski, M. L., Gratchev, A., Ilyas, M., Bodmer, W. F., Moyer, M. P., Riecken, E. O., Buhr, H. J., & Hanski, C. (1999). Target genes of β-catenin-T cell-factor/lymphoid-enhancer factor signaling in human colorectal carcinomas." Procedings of the National Academy of Sciences, 96, 1603-1608.

[175] Marie, P.J(2002). Role of N-cadherin in Bone Formation." Journal of Cellular Physiology , 190, 297-305.

[176] Mariner, D.J., J. Wang and A.B. Reynolds (2000). "ARVCF localizes to the nucleus and adherens junction and is mutually exclusive with p120(ctn) in E-cadherin complexes." Journal of Cell Science 113(Pt 8): 1481-90.

[177] Mariner, D.J., P. Anastasiadis, H. Keilhack, F-D., Bohmer, J. Wang, and A.B. Reynolds (2001). "Identification of Src Phosphorylation sites in the catenin p120." Journal of Biological Chemistry 276(30): 28006-28013.

[178] Mason, M. D., Davies, G., & , W. G. Jiang ((2002). Cell adhesion molecules and adhesion abnormalities in prostate cancer."Critical Reviews in Oncology/Hematology , 41, 11-28.

[179] Mathur, M., Goodwin, L., & Cowin, P. (1994). Interactions of the cytoplasmic domain of the desmosomal cadherin Dsg1 with plakoglobin."Journal of Biological Chemistry , 269, 14075-14080.

[180] Matrisian, L.M. and B.L.M. Hogan(1990). Growth factor regulated proteases and extracellular matrix remodeling during mammalian development." Current Topics in Developmental Biology , 24, 219-259.

[181] Matsunaga, M., Hatta, K., Nagafuchi, A., & , M. Takeichi ((1988). Guidance of optic nerve fibres by N-cadherin adhesion molecules."Nature , 334, 62-64.

[182] Mattijssen, V., Peters, H. M., Schalkwijk, L., Manni, J. J., van Hof-Grootenboer, B., & , P. H. de Mulder and D.J. Ruiter ((1993). E-cadherin expression in head and neck squamous-cell carcinoma is associated with clinical outcome." International Journal of Cancer , 55(4), 580-585.

[183] Mc Crea, P. D., Turck, C. W., & Gumbiner, B. (1991). A homolog of the armadillo protein in Drosohila (plakoglobin) associated with E-cadherin." Science , 254, 1359-1361.

[184] Mc Kendry, R., Hsu, S. C., Harland, R. M., & Grosschedl, R. (1997). LEF-1/TCF proteins mediate wnt-inducible transcription from the Xenopus nodal-related 3 promoter." Developmental Biology , 192, 420-431.

[185] Mertens, C., Kuhn, C., Moll, R., Schwetlick, I., & , W. W. Franke ((1999). Desmosomal plakophilin 2 as a differentiation marker in normal and malignant tissues."Differentiation , 64, 277-290.

[186] Miller, J.R. and R.T. Moon(1996). Signal transduction through beta-catenin and specification of cell fate during embrogenesis." Genes and Development , 10, 2527-2539.

[187] Miravet, S., Piedra, J., Miro, F., Itarte, E., & , A. G. de Herreros and M. Dunach ((2002). The transcriptional factor Tcf-4 contains different binding sites for β-catenin and plakoglobin." Journal of Biological Chemistry , 277(3), 1884-1891.

[188] Mitsiades, N., , W., Yu, H., Poulaki, V., Tsokos, M., & Stamenkovic, I. (2001). Matrix metalloproteinase-7-mediated cleavage of fas ligand protects tumor cells from chemotherapeutic drug cytotoxicity." Cancer Research , 61, 577-581.

[189] Mizushima, T., Nakagawa, H., Kamberov, Y. G., Wilder, E. L., Klein, P. S., & Rustgi, A. K. (2002). Wnt-1 but not Epidermal Growth factor induces β-catenin/T-Cell factor-dependent transcription in Esophageal Cancer Cells." Cancer Research , 62, 277-282.

[190] Mol, , , A. J. M., Gelfof, A. A., Meijer, G. A., & , H. G. van der Poel and R.J.A. van Moorselaar ((2007). New experimental markers for early detection of high-risk prostate cancer: role of cell-cell adhesion and cell-migration." Journal of Cancer Research and Clinical Oncology , 133(10), 687-695.

[191] Moll, R., Mitze, M., Frixen, U. H., & , W. Birchmeier ((1993). Differential loss of E-cadherin expression in infiltrating ductal and lobular breast carcinomas." American Journal of Pathology , 143, 1731-1742.

[192] Moon, R. T., & , D. Kimelman ((1998). From cortical rotation to organizer gene expression, toward a molecular explanation of axis specification in Xenopus."Bioessays , 20, 536-545.

[193] Morin, P., Sparks, A., Korinek, V., Barker, N., Clevers, H., Vogelstein, B., & Kinzler, K. (1997). Activation of β-catenin-Tcf signaling in colon cancer by mutations in β-catenin or APC."Science , 275, 1787-1790.

[194] Morton, R. A., Ewing, C. M., Nagafuchi, A., Tsukita, S., & , W. B. Isaacs ((1993). Reduction of E-cadherin levels and deletion of the α-catenin gene in human prostate cancer cells."Cancer Research , 53, 3585-3590.

[195] Moustafa-E, A., Yansouni, D., Alaoui-Jamali, M. A., & O'Connor Mc, M. O'Connor-McCourt ((1999). Up-Regulation of E-Cadherin by an Anti-Epidermal Growth Factor Receptor Monoclonal Antibody in Lung Cancer Cell Lines."Clinical Cancer Research , 5, 681-686.

[196] Mulholland, D. J., Cheng, H., Reid, K., Rennie, P. S., & Nelson, C. C. (2002). The Androgen Receptor can promote β-catenin nuclear translocation." Journal of Biological Chemistry , 277(20), 17933-17943.

[197] Mundy, G. R. (2002). Metastasis to bone: causes, consequences and therapeutic opportunities." Nature Reviews Cancer , 2, 584-593.

[198] Murphy, G., , F., Willenbrock, R. V., Ward, M. I., Cockett, D., Eaton, D., & Docherty, A. J. P. (1992). The C-terminal domain of 72 kDa gelatinase A is not required for catalysis, but is essential for membrane activation and modulates interactions with tissue inhibitors of metalloproteinases." Biochemistry Journal , 283, 637-641.

[199] Nagase, H., Woessner, J. F., & Jr , . (1999). Matrix Metalloproteinases."Journal of Biological Chemistry , 274(31), 21491-21494.

[200] Nathke, I. S., Hinck, L., Swedlow, J. R., Papkoff, J. R., & , W. J. Nelson ((1994). Defining interactions and distributions of cadherin and catenin complexes in polarized epithelial cells." Journal of Cell Biology , 125, 1341-1352.

[201] Navarro, P., Lozano, E., & Cano, A. (1993). Expression of E- or P-cadherin is not sufficient to modify the morphology and the tumorigenic behavior of murine spindle carcinoma cells." Journal of Cell Science , 105, 923-934.

[202] Nieset, J., Redfield, A., Jin, F., Knudsen, K., , K., Johnson, M., & Wheelock, . (1997). Characterization of the interactions of alpha-catenin with alpha-catenin and beta-catenin/plakoglobin."Journal of Cell Science , 110, 1013-1022.

[203] Noe, V., Chastre, E., Bruyneel, E., Gespach, C., & Mareel, M. (1999). Extracellular regulation of cancer invasion: the E-cadherin-catenin and other pathways." Biochemical Society Symposium , 65, 43-62.

[204] Noe, V., Fingleton, B., Jacobs, K., Crawford, H. C., Vermeulen, S., Steelant, W., Bruyneel, E., Matrisian, L. M., & Mareel, M. (2001). Release of an invasion promoter E-cadherin fragment by matrilysin and stromelysin-1." Journal of Cell Science, 114, 111-118.

[205] Noren, N.K., B.P. Liu, K. Burridge and B. Kreft (2000). "P120 Catenin regulates the actin cytoskeleton via Rho family GTPases." Journal of Cell Biology 150:567-580.

[206] Norman, J. T., Gatti, L., Wilson, P. D., & , M. Lewis ((1995). Matrix metalloproteinases and tissue inhigitor of matrix metalloproteinases expression by tubular epithelia and

interstitial fibroblasts in the normal kidney and in fibrosis."Experimental Nephrology , 3, 88-89.

[207] Novak, A., Hsu, S. C., Leung-Hagesteijn, C., Radeva, G., Papkoff, J., Montesano, R., Roskelley, C., Grosschedl, R., & Dedhar, S. (1998). Cell adhesion and the integrin-linked kinase regulate the LEF-1 and beta-catenin signaling pathways." Proceedings of the National Academy of Sciences , 95(8), 4374-4379.

[208] Novak, A. and S. Dedhar (1999)."Signaling through beta-catenin and Lef/Tcf."Cellular and Molecular Life Sciences 56(5-6): 523-537.

[209] Nawrocki-Raby, B., Gilles, C., Polette, M., Martinella-Catusse, C., Bonnet, N., Puchelle, E., , J., Foidart, M., & , F. van Roy and P. Birembaut ((2003). E-cadherin mediates MMP down-regulation in highly invasive bronchial tumor cells. "American Journal of Pathology , 163(2), 653-661.

[210] Nutt, J. E., & , J. Lunec ((1996). Induction of metalloproteinase (MMP-1) expression by epidermal growth factor (EGF) receptor stimulation and serum deprivation in human breast tumour cells."European Journal of Cancer 32A: , 2127-2135.

[211] Nutt, J. E., Mellon, J. K., Qureshi, K., & Lunec, J. (1998). Matrix Metalloproteinase-1 is induced by epidermal growth factor in human bladder tumour cell lines and is detectable in urine of patients with bladder tumours." British Journal of Cancer , 78(2), 215-220.

[212] Nwomeh, B. C., , H., Liang, X., Cohen, I. K., & Yager, D. R. (1999). MMP-8 is the predominant collagenase in healing wounds and nonhealing ulcers." Journal of Surgical Research , 81, 189-195.

[213] Oesterling, J., Fuks, Z., Lee, C. T., & , H. L. Scher ((1997). Cancer of the prostate. In: Devita, Hellman, Rosenberg eds. Cancer Principles and Practice of Oncology Philadelphia: lippincott-Raven , 2, 1322-1386.

[214] Ohkubo, T and M. Ozawa (1999). "P120^{ctn} binds to the membrane-proximal region of the E-cadherin cytoplasmic domain and is involved in modulation of Adhesion activity." Journal of Biological Chemistry 274(30): 21409-21415.

[215] Ohsugi, M. L., Larue, H., Schwarz, , & , R. Kemler ((1997). Cell-junctional and cytoskeletal organization in mouse blastocysts lacking E-cadherin." Developmental Biology , 185, 261-271.

[216] Oka, H., Shiozaki, H., Kobayashi, K., Inoue, M., Tahara, H., Kobayashi, T., Takatsuka, Y., Matsuyoshi, N., & , S. Hirano and M.Takeichi ((1993). Expression of E-cadherin cell adhesion molecules in human breast cancer tissues and its relationship to metastasis." Cancer Research , 53, 1696-1701.

[217] Orsulic, S., Huber, O., Aberle, H., Arnold, S., & Kemler, R. (1999). E-cadherin binding prevents beta-catenin nuclear localization and beta-catenin/LEF-1-mediated transactivation." Journal of Cell Science , 112(8), 1237-1245.

[218] Oyama, T., Kanai, Y., Ochiai, A., Akimoto, S., Oda, T., Yanagihara, K., Nagafuchi, A., Tsukita, S., Shibamoto, S., & Ito, F. (1994). A truncated beta-catenin disrupts the interaction between E-cadherin and alpha-catenin: a cause of loss of intercellular adhesiveness in human cancer cell lines." Cancer Research , 54, 6282-6287.

[219] Ozawa, M., Baribault, H., & Kemler, R. (1989). The cytoplasmic domain of the cell adhesion molecule uvomorulin associates with three independent proteins structurally related in different species." EMBO Journal , 8, 1711-1717.

[220] Ozawa, M., & , R. Kemler ((1998). Altered Cell Adhesion Activity by Pervanadate Due to the Dissociation of α-Catenin from the E-cadherin-Catenin Complex."Journal of Biological Chemistry , 273(11), 6166-6170.

[221] Ozawa, M. (2002). Lateral Dimerization of the E-cadherin extracellular domain is necessary but not sufficient for adhesive activity." Journal of Biological Chemistry , 277(22), 19600-19608.

[222] Pajouh, M. S., Nagle, R. B., Breathnach, R., Finch, J. S., Brawer, M. K., & , G. T. Bowden ((1991). Expression of metalloproteinase genes in human prostate cancer."Journal of Cancer Research and Clinical Oncology , 117(2), 144-150.

[223] Palacios, J., Benito, N., Pizarro, A., , A., Suarez, J., Espada, A., Cano, , & Gamallo, C. (1995). Anamalous expression of P-cadherin in breast carcinoma. Correlation with E-cadherin expression and pathological features."American Journal of Pathology , 146, 605-612.

[224] Pan, Y., Matsuyama, H., Wang, N., Yoshihiro, S., Haggarth, L., Li, C., Tribukait, B., Ekman, P., & Bergerheim, U. S. R. (1998). Chromosome 16q24 Deletion and decreased E-cadherin expression: possible association with metastatic potential in prostate cancer." Prostate , 36, 31-38.

[225] Parr, B. A., & Mc , A. P. McMahon ((1994). Wnt genes and vertebrate development."Current Opinion in Genetics and Development , 4(4), 523-528.

[226] Pei, D. (1999). Identification and characterization of the fifth membrane-type matrix metalloproteinase MT5-MMP."Journal of Biological Chemistry , 274(13), 8925-8932.

[227] Peifer, M., Mc Crea, P. D., Green, K. J., Wieschaus, E., & Gumbiner, B. M. (1992). The vertebrate adhesive junction proteins β-catenin and plakoglobin and the Drosophila segment polarity gene armadillo form a multigene family with similar properties." Journal of Cell Biology , 118, 681-691.

[228] Peifer, M., Berg, S., & Reynolds, A. B. (1994). A repeating amino acid motif shared by proteins with diverse cellular roles." Cell , 76, 789-791.

[229] Peifer, M., & , P. Polakis ((2000). Wnt signaling in oncogenesis and embryogenesis-a look outside the nucleus."Science , 287, 1606-1609.

[230] Perez-Moreno, M. A., Locasciao, A., Rodrigo, I., Dhondt, G., Portillo, F., Nieto, M. A., Cano, A., & (2001).", . (2001). A new role for E12/E47 in the repression of E-cadherin

expression and epithelial-mesenchymal transitions."Journal of Biological Chemistry , 276, 27424-27431.

[231] Pertz, O., Bozic, D., Koch, A. W., Fauser, C., Brancaccio, A., & Engel, J. (1999). A new crystal structure, Ca2+ dependence and mutational analsis reveal molecular details of E-cadherin homoassociation." EMBO Journal , 18(7), 1738-47.

[232] Piedra, J., Martinez, D., Castano, J., Miravet, S., Dunach, M., & , G. Garcia de Herreros ((2001). Regulation of β-catenin structure and activity by tyrosine phosphorylation."Journal of Biological Chemistry , 276(23), 20436-20443.

[233] Pignatelli, M., Ansari, T. W., Gunter, P., Liu, D., Hirano, S., Takeichi, M., Kloppel, G., & Lemoine, N. R. (1994). Loss of membranous E-cadherin expression in pancreatic cancer: correlation with lymph node metastasis, high grade, and advanced stage." Journal of Pathology , 174(4), 243-248.

[234] Pishvaian, M. J., Feltes, C. M., Thompson, P., Bussemakers, M. J., Schalken, J. A., & Byers, S. W. (1999). Cadherin 11 is expressed in invasive breast cancer cell lines." Cancer Research , 59, 947-952.

[235] Pokutta, S., Drees, F., Takai, Y., Nelson, W. J., & , W. I. Weis ((2002). Biochemical and structural definition of the 1-afadin- and actin-binding sites of α-catenin."Journal of Biological Chemistry , 277(21), 18868-18874.

[236] Polakis, P. (1999). The oncogenic activation of beta-catenin."Current Opinion in Genetics , 9, 15-21.

[237] Polakis, P. (2000). Wnt signaling and cancer." Genes and Development , 14, 1837-1851.

[238] Polakis, P. (2001). More than one way to skin a catenin."Cell , 105(5), 563-566.

[239] Polakis, P. (2002). Casein Kinase 1: a Wnt'er of disconnect." Current Biology 12: RR501., 499.

[240] Polette, M., & , P. Birembaut ((1998). Membrane-type metalloproteinases in tumor invasion."International Journal of Biochemistry and Cell Biology , 30(11), 1195-1202.

[241] Powell, W. C., Knox, J. D., Navre, M., Grogan, T. M., Kittelson, J., Nagle, R. B., & Bowden, G. T. (1993). Expression of the metalloproteinase matrilysin in DU145 cells increases their invasive potential in severe combined immunodeficient mice." Cancer Research , 53, 417-422.

[242] Powell, W. C., Fingleton, B., Wilson, C. L., Boothby, M., & Matrisian, L. M. (1999). The metalloproteinase matrilysin proteolytically generates active soluble fas ligand and potentiates epithelial cell apoptosis." Current Biology , 9, 1441-1447.

[243] Price, J. T., Tiganis, T., Agarwal, A., Djakiew, D., & Thompson, E. W. (1999). Epidermal Growth Factor Promotes MDA-MB-231 Breast Cancer Cell Migration through a Phosphatidylinositol 3'-Kinase and Phospholipase C-dependent Mechanism." Cancer Research , 59, 5475-5478.

[244] Prokhortchouk, A., B. Hendrich, H. Jorgensen, A. Ruzov, M. Wilm, G. Georgiev, A. Bird and E. Prokhortchouk (2001). "The p120 catenin partner kaiso is a DNA methylation-dependent transcriptional repressor." Genes and Development 15: 1613-1618.

[245] Puente, X. S., Pendas, A. M., Llano, E., Velasco, G., & Lopez, C. Lopez-Otin ((1996). Molecular cloning of a novel membrane-type matrix metalloproteinase from a human breast carcinoma." Cancer Research, 56, 944-949.

[246] Rasbridge, S. A. C. E., Gillett, S. A., Sampson, F. S., Walsh, R. R., & Millis, . (1993). Epithelial (E-) and placental (P-) cadherin cell adhesion molecule expression in breast carcinoma." Journal of Pathology , 169(2), 245-250.

[247] Ratnikov, B. I., Rozanov, D. V., Postnova, T. I., Baciu, P. G., Zhang, H., Di Scipio, R. G., Chestukhina, G. G., Smith, J. W., Deryugina, E. I., & Strongin, A. Y. (2002). An alternative processing of integrin av subuit in tumor cells by membrane type-1 matrix metalloproteinase." Journal of Biological Chemistry , 277(9), 7377-7385.

[248] Reima, I. E., Lehtonen, I., & Virtanen, J. E. Flechon ((1993). The cytoskeleton and associated proteins during cleavage, compaction and blastocyst differentiation in the pig." Differentiation , 54(1), 34-45.

[249] Reynolds, A.B., L. Herbert, J.L. Cleveland, S.T. Berg and J.R. Gaut (1992). "P120, a novel substrate of protein tyrosine kinase receptors and of p60v-src, is related to cadherin-binding factors beta-catenin, plakoglobin and armadillo." Oncogene 7: 2439-2445.

[250] Reynolds, A.B., N.A. Jenkins, D.J. Gilbert, N.G. Copeland, D.N. Shapiro, J.Wu and J.M. Daniel (1996). "The gene encoding p120cas, a novel catenin, localizes on human chromosome 11q11 (CTNND) and mouse chromosome 2 (Catns)." Genomics 31(1): 127-9.

[251] Reynolds, A.B., and J.M. Daniel (1997). "P120^{ctn}, a Src-substrate turned catenin." In P. Cowin and M. Klymkowsky (ed.), Cytoskeletal-membrane interactions and signal transduction,vol. 3. Georgetown: Landes Bioscience, p31.

[252] Riehl, R., Johnson, K., Bradley, R., Grunwald, G. B., Cornel, E., Lilienbaum, A., & Holt, C. E. (1996). Cadherin function is required for axon outgrowth in retinal ganglion cells in vivo." Neuron , 17, 837-848.

[253] Rimm, D.L. and J.S. Morrow(1994). Molecular Cloning of Human E-cadherin Suggests a Novel Subdivision of the Cadherin Superfamily." Biochemical and Biophysical Research Communications , 200(3), 1754-1761.

[254] Roczniak-Ferguson, A. and A.B. Reynolds (2003)."Regulation of p120-catenin nucleocytoplasmic shuttling activity."Journal of Cell Science 116: 4201-4212.

[255] Roose, J., Huls, G., Van Beest, M., Moerer, P., Van der Horn, K., Goldschmeding, R., Logtenberg, T., & Clever, H. (1999). Synergy between tumor suppressor APC and the beta-catenin-Tcf target Tcf1." Science , 285, 1923-1926.

[256] Ross, J. S., Figge, H. L., & Bui, H. X. (1994). E-cadherin expression in prostatic carcinoma biopsies: correlation with tumor grade, DNA content, pathologic stage, and clinical outcome." Modern Pathology 7: 835.

[257] Roura, S., Miravet, S., Piedra, J., & , A. Garcia de Herreros and M. Dunach ((1999). Regulation of E-cadherin/catenin association by tyrosine phosphorylation."Journal of Biological Chemistry , 274, 36734-36740.

[258] Rozanov, D. V., Ghebrehiwet, B., Postnova, T. I., Eichinger, A., Deryugina, E. I., & Strongin, A. Y. (2002). The hemopexin-like C-terminal domain of membrane type 1 matrix metalloproteinase regulates proteolysis of a multifunctional protein, gC1qR." Journal of Biological Chemistry , 277(11), 9318-9325.

[259] Rubinfeld, B., Robbins, P., El -Gamil, M., Albert, I., Porfiri, E., & , P. Polakis ((1997). Stabilization of β-catenin by genetic defects in melanoma cell lines."Science , 275, 1790-1792.

[260] Sacco, P. A., Mc Granahan, T. M., Wheelock, M. J., & Johnson, K. R. (1995). Identification of plakoglobin domains required for association with N-cadherin and alpha-catenin." Journal of Biological Chemistry , 270, 20201-20206.

[261] Sadot, E., Simcha, I., Shtutman, M., Ben-Ze'ev, A., & , B. Geiger ((1998). Inhibition of β-catenin-mediated transactivation by cadherin derivatives."Proceedings of the National Academy of Sciences , 95, 15339-15344.

[262] Sakuragi, N., Nishiya, M., Ikeda, K., Ohkouch, T., Furth, E. E., Hareyama, H., Satoh, C., & Fujimoto, S. (1994). Decreased E-cadherin expression in endometrial carcinoma is associated with tumor dedifferentiation and deep myometrial invasion." Gynecologic Oncology, 53, 183-189.

[263] Sanchez-Cespedes, M., Esteller, M., Wu, L., Nawroz-Danish, H., Yoo, G. H., Koch, W. M., Jen, J., Herman, J. G., & Sidransky, D. (2000). Gene promoter hypermethlation in tumors and serum of head and neck cancer patients."Cancer Research , 60, 892-895.

[264] Sasahara, R. M., Brochado, S. M., Takahashi, C., Oh, J., Maria-Engler, S. S., Granjeiro, J. M., Noda, M., & Sogayar, M. C. (2002). Transcriptional control of the RECK metastasis/angiogenesis suppressor gene." Cancer Detection and Prevention , 26(6), 435-443.

[265] Sato, H., Kinoshita, T., Takino, T., Nakayama, K., & Seiki, M. (1996). Activation of a recombinant membrane type-1 matrix metalloproteinase (MT1-MMP) by furin and its interaction with tissue inhibitor of metalloproteinases (TIMP-2)" FEBS Letter , 393, 101-104.

[266] Satoh, S., Daigo, Y., Furukawa, Y., Kato, T., Miwa, N., Nishiwaki, T., Kawasoe, T., Ishiguro, H., Fuita, M., Tokino, T., & (2000).", A. X. I. (2000). AXIN1 mutations in hepatocellular carcinomas, and growth suppression in cancer cells by virus-mediated transfer of AXIN1." Nature Genetics , 24, 245-250.

[267] Schafer, S., Stumpp, S., & , W. W. Franke ((1996). Immunological identification and characterization of the desmosomal cadherin Dsg2 in coupled and uncoupled epithelial cells and in human tissues."Differentiation , 60, 99-108.

[268] Schaefer, L., X. Han, C. August, F. Matzkies, T. Lorenz and R.M. Schaefer (1997)."Differential regulation of glomerular gelatinase B (MMP-9) and tissue inhibitor of metalloproteinase-1 (TIMP-1) in obese Zucker rats."Diabetologia 40: 1035-1043.

[269] Schnittler, H., & , J. (1998). Structural and functional aspects of intercellular junctions in vascular endothelium."Basic Research Cardiology , 93, 30-39.

[270] Sehgal, G., Hua, J., Bernhard, E. J., Sehgal, I., Thompson, T. C., & , R. J. Muschel ((1998). Requirement for matrix metalloproteinase-9 (Gelatinase B) expression in metastasis by murine prostate carcinoma."American Journal of Pathology , 152(2), 591-596.

[271] Shan, W.S., A. Koch, J. Murray, D.R. Colman and L. Shapiro (1999)."The adhesive binding site of cadherins revisted."Biophysical Chemistry 82(2-3): 157-163.

[272] Sheu, B.-C., S-M.Hsu, H-N. Ho, H-C. Lien, S-C Huang, and R-H.Lin (2001)."A novel role of metalloproteinase in cancer-mediated immunosuppression." Cancer Research 61: 237-242.

[273] Shibata, T., Ochiai, A., Gotoh, M., Machinami, R., & Hirohashi, S. (1996). Simultaneous expression of Cadherin 11 in signet-ring cell carcinoma and stromal cells of diffuse-type gastric cancer."Cancer Letter , 99, 147-153.

[274] Shimizu, H., Julius, M. A., Giarre, M., Zheng, Z., Brown, A. M., & Kitajewski, J. (1997). Transformation by Wnt family proteins correlates with regulation of beta-catenin." Cell Growth and Differentiation , 8, 1349-1358.

[275] Shino, Y., Watanabe, A., Yamada, Y., Tanase, M., Yamada, T., Matsuda, M., Yamashita, J., Tatsumi, M., Miwa, T., & , H. Nakano ((1995). Clinicopathologic evaluation of immunohistochemical E-cadherin expression in human gastric carcinomas."Cancer , 76(11), 2193-2201.

[276] Shtutman, M., Zhurinsky, J., Simcha, I., Albanese, C., D'Amico, M., Pestell, R., & Ben, A. Ben-Ze'ev ((1999). The cyclin D1 gene is a target of the beta-catenin/Lef1 pathway." Proceedings of the National Academy of Sciences , 96, 5522-5527.

[277] Sidransky, D. (2002). Emerging Molecular Markers of Cancer."Nature Reviews Cancer , 2(3), 210-219.

[278] Simcha, I., Shtutman, M., Salomon, D., Zhurinsky, J., Sadot, E., Geiger, B., & Ben-Ze'ev, A. (1998). Differential nuclear translocation and transactivation potential of beta-catenin and plakoglobin." Journal of Cell Biology , 141, 1433-1448.

[279] Slagle, B. L., Zhou, Y. Z., Birchmeier, W., & , K. A. Scorsone ((1993). Deletion of the E-cadherin gene in hepatitis B virus-positive Chinese hepatocellular carcinomas." Hepatology , 18(4), 757-762.

[280] Soos, G., Jones, R. F., Haas, G. P., & Wang, C. Y. (1997). Comparative intraosseal growth of human prostate cancer cell lines LNCaP and PC-3 in the nude mouse." Anticancer Research, 17, 4253-4258.

[281] Staddon, J.M., C. Smales, C. Schulze, F.S. Esch and L.L. Rubin (1995)."p120, a p120-related protein (p100), and the cadherin/catenin complex."Journal of Cell Biology 130(2): 369-381.

[282] Stappert, J., & Kemler, R. (1994). A short core region of E-cadherin is essential for catenin binding and is highly phosphorylated." Cell Adhesion and Communication , 2(4), 319-327.

[283] Steffensen, B., Wallon, U. M., & Overall, C. M. (1995). Extracellular matrix binding properties of recombinant fibronectin type II-like modules of humna 72-kDa gelatinase/type IV collagenase." Journal of Biological Chemistry , 270, 11555-11566.

[284] Steinhusen, U., Weiske, J., Badock, V., Tauber, R., Bommert, K., & , O. Huber ((2001). Cleavage and Shedding of E-cadherin after Induction of Apoptosis."Journal of Biological Chemistry , 276(7), 4972-4980.

[285] Sternlicht, M. D., & Werb, Z. (2001). How matrix metalloproteinases regulate cell behavior." Annual Review of Cell Developmental Biology , 17, 463-56.

[286] Stetler-Stevenson, W.G., L.A. Liotta and D.E. Kleiner Jr(1993). Extracellular matrix 6: role of matrix metaloproteinases in tumor invasion and metastasis." FASEB Journal , 7, 1434-1441.

[287] Still, K., Robson, C. N., , P., & , M. C. Autzen ((2000). Robinson and F.C. Hamdy."Localization and quantification of mRNA for matrix metalloproteinase-2 (MMP-2) and tissue inhibitor of matrix metalloproteinase-2 (TIMP-2) in human benign and malignant prostatic tissue."Prostate , 42, 18-25.

[288] Strongin, A. Y., Collier, I., Bannikov, G., Marmer, B. L., Grant, G. A., & , G. I. Goldberg ((1995). Mechanism of cell surface activation of 72-kDa type IV collagenase."Journal of Biological Chemistry , 270(10), 5331-5338.

[289] Sudbeck, B. D., Pilcher, B. K., Welgus, H. G., & Parks, W. C. (1997). Induction and repression of collagenase-1 by keratinocytes is controlled by distinct components of different extracellular matrix components." Journal of Biological Chemistry , 272, 22103-22110.

[290] Sun, Y., Y. Sun, L. Wenger, J.L. Ruter, C.E. Brinckerhoff and H.C. Cheung (1999). "p53 Down-regulates human matrix metalloproteinase-1 (collagenase-1) gene expression." Journal of Biological Chemistry 274(17): 11535-11540.

[291] Sun, Y., J.M. Cheung, J. Martel-Pelletier, J.P. Pelletier, L. Wenger, R.D. Altman, D.S. Howell, and H.S. Cheung (2000). "Wild type and mutant p53 differentially regulate the gene expression of human collagenase-3 (hMMP-13). Journal of Biological Chemistry 275(15): 11327-11332.

[292] Sundareshan, P., Nagle, R. B., & Bowden, G. T. (1999). EGF Induces the expression of matrilysin in the human prostate adenocarcinoma line, LNCaP." The Prostate , 40, 159-166.

[293] Syrigos, K. N., Karayiannakis, A., Syrigou, E. I., Harrington, K., & Pignatelli, M. (1998). Abnormal expression of correlates with poor survival in patients with bladder cancer." European Journal of Cancer 34(13): 2037-2040., 120.

[294] Takahashi, M., Tsunoda, T., Seiki, M., Nakamura, Y., & Furukawa, Y. ((2002). Identification of membrane-type metalloproteinase-1 as a target of the β-catenin/Tcf4 complex in human colorectal cancers."Oncogene , 21, 5861-5867.

[295] Takeichi, M. (1991). Cadherin cell adhesion receptors as a morphogenetic regulator." Science , 251, 1451-1455.

[296] Takeichi, M. (1995). Morphogenetic roles of classic cadherins."Current Opinion in Cell Biology , 7(5), 619-627.

[297] Takino, T., Sato, H., Shinagawa, A., & , M. Seiki ((1995). Identification of the second membrane-type metalloproteinase (MT-MMP2) gene from a human placenta cDNA library. MT-MMPs form a unique membrane-type subclass in the MMP family." Journal of Biological Chemistry , 270(39), 23013-23030.

[298] Tamura, G., Yin, J., Wang, S., Fleisher, A. S., Zou, T., Abraham, J. M., Kong, D., Smolinski, K. N., Wilson, K. T., James, S. P., Silverberg, S. G., Nishizuka, S., Terashima, M., Motoyama, T., & Meltzer, S. J. (2000). E-cadherin gene promoter hypermethylation in primary human gastric carcinomas."Journal of National Cancer Institute , 92(7), 569-73.

[299] Tang, L., Hung, C. P., Schuman, E. M., & (1998).", . (1998). A role for the cadherin family of cell adhesion molecules in hippocampal long-term potentiation."Neuron , 20(6), 1165-1175.

[300] Tao, Y. S., Edwards, R. A., Tubb, B., Wang, S., Bryan, J., & Mc Crea, P. D. (1996). Beta-catenin associates with the actin-bundling protein fascin in a noncadherin complex." Journal of Cell Biology , 134, 1271-1281.

[301] Tetsu, O., & Mc Cormick, F. (1999). Beta-catenin regulates expression of cyclin D1 in colon carcinoma cells." Nature , 398, 422-426.

[302] Thompson, R. W., Mertens, R. A., Liao, S., Holmes, D. R., Mecham, R. P., Welgus, H. G., & Parks, W. C. (1995). Production and localization of 92 kDa gelatinase in abdominal aortic aneurysms: an elastolytic metalloproteinase expressed by aneurysm-infiltrating macrophages." Journal of Clinical Investigations , 96, 318-326.

[303] Thoreson, M.A. and A.B. Reynolds (2002)."Altered expression of the catenin p120 in human cancer: implications for tumor progression."Differentiation 70: 583-589.

[304] Tomita, K., Van Bokhaven, A., Van Leenders, G., Ruijter, E. T. G., Jansen, C. F. J., Bussemakers, M. J. G., & Schalken, J. A. (2000). Cadherin switching in human prostate cancer progression."Cancer Research 60: 3650.

[305] Tran, N. L., Nagle, R. B., Cress, A. E., & , R. L. Heimark ((1999). N-cadherin expression in human prostate carcinoma cell lines."American Journal of Pathology , 155, 787-798.

[306] Troyanovsky, S. M., Troyanovsky, L. G., Eshkind, L. G., Leube, R. E., & Franke, W. W. (1994a). Identification of amino acid sequence motifs in desmocollin, a desmosomal glycoprotein, that are required for plakoglobin binding and plaque formation." Proceedings of the National Academy of Sciences, 91, 10790-10794.

[307] Troyanovsky, S. M., Troyanovsky, R. B., Eshkind, L. G., Krutovskikh, V. A., Leube, R. E., & , W. W. Franke ((1994b). Identification of the plakoglobin-binding domain in desmoglein and its role in plaque assembly and intermediate filament anchorage."Journal of Cell Biology , 127, 151-160.

[308] Umbas, R., Isaacs, W. B., Breinguier, P. P., Schaafsma, H. E., Karthaus, H. F. M., Oosterhof, G. O. N., Debruyne, F. M. J., & Schalken, J. A. (1994). Decreased E-cadherin expression is associated with poor prognosis in patients with prostate cancer." Cancer Research , 54, 3929-3933.

[309] Unemori, E. N., & , Z. Werb ((1988). Collagenase expression and endogenous activation in rabbit synovial fibroblasts stimulated by the calcium ionophore A23187."Journal of Biological Chemistry , 263(31), 16252-16259.

[310] Usadel, H., Brabender, J., Danenberg, K. D., Jeronimo, C., Harden, S., Engles, J., Danenberg, P. V., Yang, S., & Sidransky, D. (2002). Quantitative adenomatous polyposis coli promoter methylation analysis in tumor tissue, serum and plasma DNA of patients with lung cancer."Cancer Research , 62, 371-375.

[311] Utton, M. A., Eickholt, B., Howell, F. V., Wallis, J., & Doherty, P. (2001). Soluble N-cadherin stimulates fibroblast growth factor receptor dependent neurite outgrowth and N-cadherin and the fibroblast growth factor receptor co-cluster in cells." Journal of Neurochemistry , 76, 1421-1430.

[312] Van Aken, J., Cuvelier, C. A., De Wever, N., Roels, J., Gao, Y., & Mareel, M. M. (1993). Immunohistochemical analysis of E-cadherin expression in human colorectal tumours."Pathology Research and Practice , 189, 975-978.

[313] Van Genderen, C., Okamura, R. M., Farinas, I., Quo, R. G., Parslow, T. G., Bruhn, L., & Grosschedl, R. (1994). Development of several organs that require inductive epithelial-mesenchymal interactions is impaired in LEF-1-deficient mice." Genes and Development , 8, 2691-2703.

[314] Van Hengel, J., Vanhoenacker, P., Staes, K., & Van Roy, F. (1999). Nuclear localization of the Armadillo-like catenin is counteracted by a nuclear export signal and by

E-cadherin expression." Proceedings of the National Academy of Sciences 96: 7980-7985., 120ctn.

[315] Van Noort, M., Meeldijk, J., Van der Zee, R., Deshee, O., & Clevers, H. (2002). Wnt Signaling controls the phosphorylation status of β-catenin." Journal of Biological Chemistry , 277(20), 17901-17905.

[316] Van Oort, I. M., Tomita, K., van Bokhoven, A., Bussemakers, M. J. G., Kiemeney, L. A., Karthaus, H. F. M., Witjes, J. A., & Schalken, J. A. (2007). The prognostic value of E-cadherin and the cadherin-associated molecules α-, β-, γ-catenin and in prostate cancer specific survival: a long-term follow-up study." Prostate 67: 1432-1438., 120ctn.

[317] Van de Wetering, M., Cavallo, R., Dooijes, D., van Beest, M., van Es, J., Loureiro, J., Ypma, A., Hursh, D., jones, T., Bejsovec, A., Peifer, M., Mortin, M., & Clevers, H. (1997). Armadillo coactivates transcription driven by the product of the Drosophila segment polarity gene dTCF." Cell , 88, 789-799.

[318] Veatch, A. L., Carson, L. F., & , S. Ramakrishnan ((1994). Differential expression of the cell-cell adhesion molecule E-cadherin in ascites and solid human ovarian tumor cells."International Journal of Cancer , 58(3), 393-399.

[319] Vincenti, M.P(2000). The Matrix Metalloprotienase (MMP) and Tissue inhibitor of metalloproteinase (TIMP) Genes." In: Matrix Metalloproteinase Protocols Totowa: Humana Press, , 122-123.

[320] Von, Kries. J. P., Winbeck, G., Asbrand, C., Schwarz-Romond, T., Sochnikova, N., Dell'Oro, A., Behrens, J., & Birchmeier, W. (2000). Hot spots in beta-catenin for interactions with LEF-1, conductin and APC."Nature Sructural Biology , 7(9), 800-7.

[321] Wahl, J., Sacco, P., Mc Granahan-Sadler, T., Sauppe, L., Wheelock, M., & , K. Johnson ((1996). Plakoglobin domains that define its association with the desmosomal cadherins and the classical cadherins: identification of unique and shared domains." Journal of Cell Science , 109, 1143-1154.

[322] Wahl, J. K., Nieset, J. E., Sacco-Bubulya, P. A., Sadler, T. M., Johnson, K. R., & Wheelock, M. J. (2000). The amino- and carboxyl-terminal tails of β-catenin reduce its affinity for desmoglein 2." Journal of Cell Science , 113, 1737-1745.

[323] Watabe-Uchida, M., Uchida, N., Imamura, Y., nagafuchi, A., Fujimoto, K., Uemura, T., Vermeulen, S., F.van, Roy. E. D., Adamson, , & Takeichi, M. (1998). A-catenin-vinculin interaction functions to organize the apical junctional complex in epithelial cells." Journal of Cell Biology , 142(3), 847-857.

[324] Weiss, E. E., Kroemker, M., , A., Rudiger, H., Jockusch, B. M., & Rudiger, M. (1998). Vinculin is part of the cadherin-catenin junctional complex: complex formation beteen alpha-catenin and vinculin." Journal of Cell Biology , 141, 755-784.

[325] Weng, Z., Xin, M., Pablo, L., Grueneberg, D., Hagel, M., Bain, G., Muller, T., & , J. Papkoff ((2002). Protection againsto anoikis and down-regulation of cadherin expres-

sion by a regulatable beta-catenin protein."Journal of Biological Chemistry , 277, 18677-18686.

[326] Werb, Z., Tremble, P. M., Behrendtsen, O., Crowley, E., & Camsk, C. H. (1989). Signal transduction through the fibronectin receptor induces collagenase and stromelysin gene expression." Journal of Cell Biology , 109, 877-889.

[327] Whitlon, D.S(1993). E-cadherin in the mature and developing organ of Corti of the mouse."Journal of Neurocytochemistry , 22, 1030-1038.

[328] Wiechens, N., Fagotto, F., & (2001).", C. R. (2001). CRM1- and Ran-independent nuclear export of β-catenin."Current Biology , 11, 18-27.

[329] Wilding, J., Vousden, K. H., Soutter, W. P., Mc Crea, P. D., & , R. Del Buono and M. Pignatelli ((1996). E-cadherin Transfection Down-regulates the Epidermal Growth Factor Receptor and Reverses the Invasive Phenotype of Human Papilloma Virus-transfected Keratinocytes." Cancer Research, 56, 5285-5292.

[330] Will, H., & Hinzmann, B. (1995). cDNA sequence and mRNA tissue distribution of a novel human matrix metalloproteinase with a potential transmembrane segment." European Journal of Biochemistry , 231, 602-608.

[331] Willert, K., & Nusse, R. (1998). Beta-catenin: a key mediator of Wnt signaling." Current Opinion in Genetics and Development , 8, 95-102.

[332] Windoffer, R., Beile, B., Leibold, A., Thomas, S., Wilhelm, U., & , R. E. Leube ((2000). Visualization of gap junction mobility in living cells."Cell Tissue Research , 299, 347-362.

[333] Winston, J. T., Strack, P., Beer-Romero, P., Chu, C. Y., Elledge, S. J., & Harper, J. W. (1999). The SCFb-TRCP-ubiquitin ligase complex associates specifically with phosphorylated destruction motifs in IκBα and β-catenin and stimulates IκBα ubiquitination in vitro." Genes and Development , 13, 270-283.

[334] Witcher, L. L., Collins, R., Puttogunta, S., Mechanic, S. E., Munson, M., Gumbiner, B., & Cowin, P. (1996). Desmosomal cadherin binding domains of plakoglobin."Journal of Biological Chemistry , 271(18), 10904-10909.

[335] Witty, J.P., T. Lempka, R.J. Coffey, Jr and L.M. Matrisian (1995). "Decreased tumor formation in 7, 12-dimethylbenzanthracene-treated stromelysin-1 transgenic mice is associated with alterations in mammary epithelial cell apoptosis." Cancer Research 55: 1401-1406.

[336] Wodarz, A., & , R. Nusse ((1998). Mechanisms of Wnt signaling in development."Annual Review of Cell and Developmental Biology , 14, 59-88.

[337] Wood, M., Fudge, K., Mohler, J. L., Frost, A. R., Garcia, F., Wang, M., & Stearns, M. E. (1997). In situ hybridization studies of metalloproteinases 2 and 9 and TIMP1 and TIMP2 expression in human prostate cancer." Clinical Experimental Metastasis , 15, 246-258.

[338] Yamada, T., Takaoka, A. S., Naishiro, Y., Hayashi, R., Maruyama, K., & , C. Maesawa ((2000). Transactivation of the Multidrug Resistance 1 gene by T-Cell Factor 4/β-catenin complex in early colorectal carcinogenesis."Cancer Research , 60, 4761-4766.

[339] Yanagawa, S., , Y., Matsuda, J., lee, H., Matsubayashi, S., Sese, T., Kadowaki, , & Ishimoto, A. (2002). Casein kinase 1 phosphorylates the Armadillo protein and induces its degradation in Drosophila." EMBO Journal , 21, 1733-1742.

[340] Yap, A.S(1998a). The morphogenetic role of cadherin cell adhesion molecules in human cancer: a thematic review." Cancer Investigation , 16(4), 252-261.

[341] Yap, A.S., C.M. Niessen, and B.M. Gumbiner (1998b)."The Juxtamembrane Region of the Cadherin Cytoplasmic Tail Supports Lateral Clustering, Adhesive Strengthening, and Interaction with $p120^{ctn}$."Journal of Cell Biology141(3): 779-789.

[342] Zhang, Y., Qiu, W. J., Chan, S. C., Han, J., He, X., & Lin, S. C. (2002). Casein kinase I and casein kinase II differentially regulate Axin function inWnt and JNK pathways." Journal of Biological Chemistry , 277, 17706-17712.

[343] Zeng, L., Fagotto, F., Zhang, T., Hsu, W., Vasicek, T. J., Perry, W. L., Lee, J. J., Tilghman, S. M., Gumbiner, B. M., & Costantini, F. (1997). The mouse fused locus encodes Axin, an inhibitor of the Wnt signaling pathway that regulates embryonic axis formation." Cell ., 90, 181-192.